The Key to Self-Liberation

Christiane Beerlandt

The Key
to
Self-Liberation

1000 Diseases and their Psychological Origins

Beerlandt Publications
Ostend

The Key to Self-Liberation
Written by Christiane Beerlandt
Original title: De Sleutel tot Zelf-Bevrijding
First edition 1993 – Eighth, revised and enlarged edition 2001
Copyright © by Christiane Beerlandt and Beerlandt Publications

English translation copyright © 2003 by Christiane Beerlandt and Beerlandt Publications

Cover illustration and design by Christiane Beerlandt
copyright © 1993 and © 2003 by Christiane Beerlandt and Beerlandt Publications

Printed in Belgium
by Drukkerij Schaubroeck, Nazareth
ISBN: 9075849354
Legal deposit (Wettelijk depot): Royal Library Albert I, Brussels
(Koninklijke Bibliotheek Albert I) D/2003/8022/10

About "The Key to Self-Liberation"

The Key to Self-Liberation is the first work that I was allowed to write down (in 1992). The information was obtained by tuning myself to the frequency of truth and listening deep inside me, via my heart and consciousness, to the deep language of life itself. Observation and common sense are useful, but the Source of Life — via *"deeper knowing"* — reveals so much more to us: the essence, the "why" of things. No one can possess truth, not I, not you. But we can tune in to the frequency of truth, living and listening "according to truth"/in honesty. In this manner, the chapters of this book have been written. The content has nothing to do with scientific observation, but neither with channeling or guides. Don't try to pigeon-hole this book. You won't succeed. Searching people, with a "heart" and an "open mind," whether they call themselves "conservative" or "alternative," will feel at home in these chapters, which are meant to be their friends.

Even if it's not possible yet, I am convinced that "science" will come to the same conclusions as the information in this book, be it via other routes. But the "equipment" to measure psyche, emotions, and energetic happenings/evolution — the relationship between the inner self and the physical body (illness-health) — does not yet exist or is still inadequate.

For the countless "regular" and "alternative" doctors, care-givers, and laymen who already have worked with the information of this book for years and made contact with me, there doesn't need to be any further "proof." . . . "It simply works like that in daily life." It makes me extremely happy: how the human being can liberate and heal himself, as long as he gains "insight" and suits the action to the word — with or without remedies from the outside. **How the seeds of illness are sown**, and how we can bring about fundamental healing via Insight and Application.

Our "spiritual-energy" influences the body/"matter" and not the reverse. Everything is being directed and driven from within. When we better understand these processes, we can, as conscious people, bring about change in ourselves. I have often seen how, in certain people, acquiring "insight," or something being "triggered off" in one's mind regarding the true cause of one's illness — was enough to bring about sudden recovery. Mostly, however, we are involved with a growth process whereby the (sick) body reacts in a growing way to the changes one brings about in oneself: changes on the psychological and emotional levels, changes in one's convictions. The body reacts to those changes . . . and heals.

I am not at all against medicine or other remedies from the outside. On the contrary, it can be good for many people to use them in a certain phase (even though many heal themselves without them). *Therefore, don't worry about using medicine or healing methods if you feel this is best for you. Here lies the free choice of every human being.* One must realize, however, that one has to work, in the meantime, on **the *"true"* healing** of an ailment — that the FUNDAMENTAL HEALING of an illness will only take place when one **realizes** and **solves** its FUNDAMENTAL CAUSE: and that happens on a deeper level than the purely physiological or chemical. That actually happens on the emotional and psychological levels, in the realm of emotions and convictions, of expectations, and of the image one has of oneself.

I am not interested in "convincing" someone; I only offer deep, called-up Information, and everyone has a free choice either to use it or not. I consider it my task to write down this received Information and place it at the disposal of all good people.

Finally, let this book function as a "Key," but don't cling to it. Go onward, live yourself, and be your own master. Never cling to a signpost. You can only make grateful use of it in order to more quickly get upon *your* track of life.

In the *First Part* of this book, I describe the liberating philosophy according to which I experience life. From out of the depths of my heart, I wish you, too, a wonderful, truthful existence filled with love!

Christiane
Ostend, 6 June 2001

A Message to the Reader

When we feel our especially beautiful planet Earth groan under the suffering, the violence of war, the pains, the power-game, then don't we — don't all human beings — need to take responsibility for ourselves? It is of no use to heal wounds or donate food if the underlying causes of misery are not being resolved. The world changes from within, from the inner consciousness of every human being. Illness, as well as events, are only a consequence of what happens IN the human being. If we can no longer "change" this world, then let us, each for himself, lay building blocks for a new world, where Life in its value will be understood, in Joy. There's no use screaming against, fighting against, going into the streets against. . . . True transformation begins by the human being cleansing himself of negative convictions regarding himself. Reality is only a reflection of, a result of, our unconscious and conscious expectations in life. The future is not pre-determined, nor is life a melancholy, accidental happening about which we don't have any say. Individually and en masse, we constantly create our living world. We are in a dialogue with our planet. We don't have to wait for an Angel, a *Deus ex machina,* or a UFO to come and "save" the world. With the power of our Living Self, we are able to build a new house on an earth which will never be destroyed — because we wish her to be Alive.

This is possible if each of us, convinced of our loving "I AM," accepts our responsibility and no longer looks to others for the causes of illness and misery. When every human being, by himself, creates harmony in his existence, then this positive influence is a reality for all of humanity. After all, we are not separate from each other. There is more than just matter alone; energies are working more and more powerfully, including the energies which we call "emotions, awareness powers, thoughts. . . ." Let's use these energies in a Self-aware way, in growth toward health, toward healing, but also in creating a new Earth, where finally there will no longer be any suffering, pain, hunger, or death. With our feet on the ground, without floating with our heads in the clouds, let's take the helm, and become aware of the possibilities every Human Being carries inside — the possibilities of directing his existence toward something beautiful, and in so doing help lay out a feast in the nature of Mother Earth.

We need to end false determinations such as inflicting on ourselves the punishments of karma and original sin. Self-liberation leads to the liberation of Earth and humanity. The Key that opens the gates to Joyfulness — that Key is to be found in your Self. May this book, called up from the heart "according to truth," declare its servitude as an Information-source to all good people.

Christiane
Ostend, 17 July 2003

Remarks concerning this English translation

- About the meaning of the word "man" in general: Each woman, each man, could call herself or himself "man." It doesn't signify "male"; in the author's language it means "human being," or both elements — male and female — in equality within one person. No question of discrimination.

- About the use of the word "desire": When this word is being used in the text, it always has a negative meaning: absolutely wanting to have or possess something, greediness, wanting to grab things, covetousness, etc.

CONTENTS

PART II

THE KEY TO HEALTH AND HEALING

PART I

THE KEY TO
LIVING IN HAPPINESS

THE KEY TO LIVING IN HAPPINESS

About the True Origin of illness

First and foremost, it is important to realize that it is best for humanity that no "dogmas" or fixed rules are established. It is best for us to allow Life to speak for itself: Truth shows itself and doesn't need "a name."

The time has come that man[1] learn to listen to that which Life asks of him from within, to that "voice of truth" deep inside himself, to that which "truth" — inherent to Life — wants. And that the Human Being now realizes that he has, in his own hands, the full responsibility for his life and shouldn't place it "outside himself." Yes, that his life lies completely in his own hands: that he will obtain INSIGHT into "how" life really functions, and that this will ultimately give him a yet unknown feeling of freedom and joy.

Then he will see and know how only he, the human being, can lead himself toward illness and misery, as well as toward health and happiness.

And hasn't he yet realized how he has lived "unconsciously" through ups and downs, convinced that it all "just" happened to him? Or was he convinced that this or that power "outside" himself determined his life? Now he will gain insight into the fact that every human being, unconsciously or consciously, "attracts" every circumstance in his life himself. And therefore it is good for him to tune in as consciously as possible to the Voice of Truth inside himself and lead his life as consciously as possible with trustful and positive expectations regarding Life.

In this way he will experience that "illness" or "recovery" isn't something that "just" happens to you — that illness is a signal, sent from deep within one's own inner life center, and that recovery occurs when one understands "why" this or that specific illness manifests itself, when one listens to what the Source of Life asks the human being to "change" in his existence. The more consciously the human being lives, and the stronger he tunes in to this inner voice of truth, the sooner he will "understand" his illness and the sooner the recovery can take place. At least, when he puts the "received insight" into action, when he truly psycho-emotionally, or on any other human level, corrects his course, there, where his Life-Core asks him to make changes.

Illness is just a "symptom" of something that lies much deeper

Yes, every illness is a "symptom" of something that lies much deeper; every illness, no matter if it is flu or AIDS, is a "signal" that something is going wrong on

---

[1] See the publisher's remarks about the use of the word "man" on page 8.

the deeper psycho-emotional level (that means going against the life current). Every illness has its origin in a much deeper level than the purely physical! It all germinates very deeply inside the human being and finally manifests itself in the body: the body speaks "a language." The body voices, brings out, that which inwardly is going "well" or "wrong." Illness has nothing at all to do with "guilt" or the "punishments of god"! The body speaks the language of that which constantly forms it, allows it to exist, brings it to life, and maintains it: the language of the Inner Life-Center or the Highly Individual Self-Core, the driving motor of Life . . . present in every human being!

Fundamental Healing
Insight and Responsibility

That which we call "Original Medical Science" is the science that searches for the true "origin" of illness and therefore considers the cure as a realization and understanding of the psycho-emotional cause on the one hand, and offering a solution to it, on the other. If cause and solution are being sought on the *true* level where illness germinates . . . *then* we can ultimately speak of *fundamental* healing. If one occupies oneself with only observation at the surface, however, one disconnects the deeper Human Content from the physical Body, and will never arrive at TRUE healing. One can, of course, temporarily fight "symptoms" and cure illness superficially separate from the Content, but sooner or later the Life-Core of the apparently "cured" human being will again develop yet another disease. This is in order that the human being will finally come to the realization: time to look deeper inside yourself!

There is a reason that you "get" *this* specific illness and not another — that it is not your friend, but "you," who are being infected with this or that virus. Yes, because on a deeper level — INSIDE YOU — there is a psycho-emotional condition that is ideal "fertile ground" for *this* virus! And your friend, who is not at all afflicted with this (unconscious) problem or this "psycho-emotional field," is therefore not being infected.

The same goes for all kinds of "illness": for instance you can only develop leukemia[2] — as a baby or as an adult — when the deep-rooted psychological field that is typical of this disease is present in you. Then your deepest life-center speaks the language of: "You have Leukemia, you have to solve something specific in yourself on a deeper level." Do it! And recover as a consequence. . . .

Never feel "guilty" about this, but understand in a warm and loving way the "why and wherefore." Never blame yourself, nor point at someone else because of

---

[2] You can read the text about the psycho-emotional origins of leukemia in this book.

The Key to Self-Liberation, Christiane Beerlandt © Beerlandt Publications

his "illness," but always remain in LOVING UNDERSTANDING toward yourself, toward others. Every human being is in a state of evolution, in his or her own way.

It's amazing how our Self-Core pushes messages "outward," manifests them via the body in "signals": SO THAT WE MAY CHANGE SOMETHING in our existence, in order to become happier people. Seen from this point of view, illness is *sometimes* a "necessity" — it forces you to consider that to which you may have been closing your eyes for a long time, or which you unconsciously didn't want to "see" in yourself. It forces you to look at how you, as a human being, hinder yourself from going through life in a TRULY HAPPY AND MEANINGFUL WAY. In order to bring you toward "True Life" — via a healing process which has to go together with essential inner changes that will "beneficially" alter your life!

Living according to Truth — from out of yourself — means Happiness and Health

"Truth liberates": every human being can work out for himself which path or life-philosophy gives him the most liberating inner feeling. Man may come to the realization that he has "free" choice between following the path of "Life-Truth-Joy-Love-Trust" on the one hand, and the track of "decline and death-delusion and appearance-lies-anxiety-lust for power-covetousness-doubt" on the other — a choice for Good or Evil. This choice, and the deeds that are in accord with it — will determine whether the human being ultimately will become "truly happy" or not. Therefore, it's important that man open himself up to "truth," to "goodness" — to Insight (becoming aware), to the Inner Heart (Love): all this in the full Belief that he, himself, can direct his own life, either toward misery or toward Joy! The more the human being becomes aware that *he* has the say over his life — as long as he is open to information of truth and "does" something with it — then the stronger and sooner he can make himself healthier and happier.

This book, therefore, offers you Information, without postulating any "dogma" whatsoever. On the contrary: this Information urges you as reader inside yourself and offers you facts about which you can thoroughly ponder, if you like.

Supposing man lived completely "according to truth." Then, he would be an extremely happy human being. *The goal is that we get tuned in more and more to that which "Life" itself wants inside of us — to that which we can call pulsations of truth within ourselves — so that we may become ever happier as human beings.*

If we evolve in the direction of what Life — in conformity with the deepest truth — longs for, if we connect ourselves with it and act accordingly, then we will not only become ever more harmonious with ourselves, but we will also see an en-

vironment (creating it consciously or unconsciously) that will correspond with the atmosphere of happiness deep inside us.

This is a fundamental law of life. A law of nature: Man, work Consciously on yourself, on your own happiness, intensely attune yourself with the Truth, with that which Life inwardly desires from you . . . then you will not only raise yourself toward more peaceful, intensely happier atmospheres, but will do the same for part of the world.

The Conscious Choice
Life-Force and Counter-Force

The Life-source, which is fundamentally powerful and eternally giving, bearing, and creating, has allowed a duality to come forth out of its womb, two movements that we could call "good and evil," "life-giving and deathly-destructive-taking," "Truth and appearance/lies," "Life-Force and Counter-Force." Here, the elements mentioned first are each time on the same line — the same goes for the last-mentioned notions.

Man has been given a free will in order to choose between Life-Force and Counter-Force (the anti-life-path). Only via experiencing this contrast between good and evil — truth and lies, life and death, joy and sadness — can the human being come to the realization of what TRUE LIFE means: a CONSCIOUS CHOICE is being asked for . . .

It's exactly through *confrontations* with lies and appearances, with sadness and death, that the human being comes to full understanding of the Value of pureness, of joy and of Life itself! That he can come to an awareness of *gratitude* because of the life inside himself. And this awareness of thankfulness then leads toward a greater feeling of Happiness, through which (be it unconsciously) happier circumstances in life are being created. Once a human being has made this fundamental Choice for Life, for truth and goodness, then he can start to build an existence full of happiness! Even though the voice of the Counter-force in himself might come to the surface once in a while, he has resolutely made his Choice, and now Life will assist him!

Be faithful to yourself, to Life

"Living according to truth" means that we listen to the deepest voice of truth in ourselves, to our authentic nature, to our Heart, to our *true* disposition. "Living according to truth" asks us NOT to listen to a small self-centered, superficial voice, a voice that takes into "account" only narrow-minded rational or external factors —

that which "should be so," or that which the human being absolutely wants to push through or sustain "at all costs," or the "current precepts of decorum and courtesy," or that which others or society expect of him while he ignores his own inner voice of truth, his heart — in other words the human being who sacrifices deeper truth and Life for "others," for "society," for his image, for desire[3] and greed, for wanting to please others, or for whatsoever. . . . Because this is self-betrayal, a betrayal with regard to Life. Here, we can quote the words: "Not my will, but Thy will be done." Not that what the small "I" wants may happen, but *what the great voice of the truth of Life inside yourself asks you.*

And you can realize very well what that means when you entirely open yourself up to Truth, with receptiveness and love. When you let go of "the absolutely wanting to have" and attune yourself to your *Being.* When you are attentively open to the signals on your path. When you let go of everything and everyone, letting them "be" the way they are. When you resolutely take your life in your own hands without stubbornly fixating on anything. When you listen to that deep Father-Mother-Voice (which is YOU!) in yourself: you, as a Nature-child who represents Life, tune in to the Good, to Truth . . . and you will see, sense — do what you feel you have to do according to this vibration of truth, and you will be happy. High morality is now inherently present. The human being who lives according to goodness will never "violate" his own nature, not even to please someone else, because he knows that he hurts not only himself — that Life itself is betrayed — but that by keeping alive a vibration of lies he doesn't help others either. In short: the world is not helped at all by this.

No one can "possess" truth, but you can attune yourself to the vibration of truth, the frequency of Life itself

In many books written in our world we can experience that they are not tuned in to the frequency of truth. There are "certain" things written that are in accord with the truth, but we must be careful with some writings that are completely small-minded-rational (cut off from intuition and feelings, from deeper knowledge), or are totally imagined (among others, in the New Age sector). These are not always written with bad intentions, but they are still misleading for humanity. Other writings are thoughtlessly "copied" from old (sometimes falsified) sources and are not understood the way they were "then" intended. Half lies, half truths: it is good for the reader to observe all writings *critically,* and especially to connect with *his own inner feeling of truth* in such a way that he can separate the wheat from the chaff.

---

[3] See the publisher's remarks about the use of the word "desire," on page 8.

This book has been written to offer information to people who consciously want to progress on the path to more joy and health. No one can "possess" truth, neither I nor you. Still, it is possible to connect yourself — while being completely honest with yourself — to what I call the "vibration of truth." In normal daily life this means: live always in total honesty with yourself — without lying to yourself, to Life; this implies doing certain things or precisely not doing those things, saying certain things or precisely not saying them, manifesting or behaving in a certain way, not lying to yourself or fooling yourself; not trying to escape certain things concerning yourself. Don't hold up a mask, but show your "I" the way you really are inside.

This is very important, and many people live "in lies" or "in appearances" without being aware of it (because they ignore the "signals" sent to them by Life as warning messages). The final result is that they make themselves sick and un-happy. Others lie to themselves very consciously. They are then not "faithful" to themselves, to the living voice inside themselves, to their own deeper, natural dis-position. They have betrayed themselves and are raping life inside themselves, with all the consequences.

A concrete example

"A" visits a certain person and after just a few minutes he feels, deep in his heart, in his total being: "I have to leave here! I don't like being here. . . . Yes, I'm doing this for my partner, or for this child, or for some host, or to please a sick person, or out of pity — but really deep inside myself, I feel how life calls to me: 'Go, get up!'" But what does this human being do? He lies to himself, sacrifices himself, thinks it is not proper, or that it is impolite, or not "dutiful" and . . . uneasily re-mains in his chair. The next day, he has a headache and nausea, he's itching all over, and his back is aching. . . .[4] This is because he wasn't in charge of his life, but placed certain things ABOVE Life, above "Living according to Truth," above Love for himself. Things like: "That's how it ought to be," Propriety, The unnatu-ral, artificial Rules, The Strict Duties (which curtail every natural freedom of a human being), Pity, etc. In so doing, he does not only lie to himself, but also to the person he visits! He places himself completely at the bottom and doesn't listen to his inner voice of truth. It is possible that another person in the same situation might feel good, doesn't force himself at all, so that it's not harmful for this other person to remain seated, as long as he feels that it is good for him. *It's important that the human being not place ANYTHING above his inner voice of truth, which is the voice of Life within him. This Love for oneself is something completely differ-*

---

[4] Read in detail about the psychological origins of these symptoms in Part II.

ent from "trying to force one's own will," or "egotism" or being ungenerous. On the contrary! Love of oneself and egotism are two opposite principles!

Compassion: with this, you don't help another person. You do help when BEING YOURSELF IN TRUTH. Do not suffer, do not suffer with others, but be an Example of Joy, of Honesty and Harmony: with this you also help others! If you are honest with yourself and act according to true Love for yourself, then you will stimulate others to search for Love of themselves and truth inside themselves. Even if there sounds a loud protest, it's only through honestly being yourself that you serve yourself, Life, and others! Don't live according to the conviction that life asks for sacrifice, that you have to violate yourself in order to please others. That doesn't help yourself or others to get one step ahead! In Love and Understanding you live "according to truth." And other loving people will understand you. And if your behavior is not being understood or accepted — in this example, when you stand up and leave — then you are dealing with a person who "demands" or "expects," in other words, "desires" something from you. This is not really directed toward Life! This person should start to search for self-fulfilment, for love of himself, for gratitude, and should learn how to let go (of person A)!

When you really feel inside yourself, when the living voice inside you comes rushing up, as it were, and says, "Go onward!" then get up from your chair, say good bye, follow this honest voice, and don't resist the inner truth. When you feel, "No, I'm lying to myself if I don't get up right now!" then don't try to stay glued to your chair because of rational or other ideas like "Tradition says it has to be this way," or whatever. Or because of lying to yourself, do you perhaps get "backaches" or "shoulder pains" that indicate you don't build your life on that straight-arrow, Honest Central Pillar of a Spine in you? Do you instead "hold on to" old habits that go against life (lying to yourself), and as a consequence do you feel heavy burdens on your shoulders?[5]

Moreover, when you remain FAITHFUL to your honest inner voice at every moment in your existence, then you do help not only yourself, but also others! When you live in HARMONY, with Love for yourself, and in this way listen to that voice of truth inside you, then you act according to truth and you send, perhaps unconsciously, energies of truth to others. In so doing, you unconsciously stimulate others to work on themselves. There is an interaction of honest energies. No matter how much the other person whines in order to hold on to you, or even emotionally blackmails you, do what you inwardly feel you have to do with Love for yourself. As a consequence, it's automatically good for the other person that you go away, even if he or she doesn't realize it. You cannot do "good" to others if you don't first act with Love toward yourself. This is the sounding of the bells of life: "Love your neighbor as yourself!"

Action according to Truth always causes a positive, energetic reaction toward yourself as well as toward others! *You stimulate the truth-energy in others by*

---

[5] Read more about the shoulders and the spine in Part II.

honestly listening to the living voice inside yourself! By placing nothing ABOVE this voice of truth. In this way, you help Life and the World along. Truth liberates yourself, but also helps others — when being confronted with your honest action — to live according to truth. . . . In fact, in this way this Love for yourself brings about a loving deed, also with regard to others, although they might not even be aware of it.

Be faithful to your True Nature

Another example: "living according to truth" means also *being Faithful to your True Nature*. If by nature you are round like a pumpkin or heavy and robust like a farm horse, but you think you should look like a string bean and you start to "diet," then you violate your nature, then you lie to your own constitution in order to answer to the exterior norms or rules of the society in which you live, a so-called slimness-ideal — or whatever medical science thinks it has to promote (wrongly) as being the only healthy way, (because it happens to be convinced of it, following the norms and indoctrinations of society). Here, too, the same rule applies: listen to your own nature, don't listen to those who think they know better. *True beauty, health, authenticity and truth lie on the same line.* Someone who is falsely thin through dieting, etc., will sooner or later have to pay for this lie against one's own "I." Sooner or later, this "false beauty," this Sham (it's a lie and therefore ugly) will crumble. What counts is to be plump or thin in a healthy way, small or tall, for the form is an honest reflection of your NATURE OF BEING. Things go wrong only when the human being begins to *doubt* his Power, his Mobility, his Natural Being. *No matter what your body shape is, when you live with the conviction that you are strong, mobile and healthy, then your body will grow in health.* Everyone will move through life in a way that honestly sprouts out of his nature of being.

It's the same regarding playing sports: if you do it while you don't really like it, against your nature, then you lie to yourself. Just FEEL, very deeply inside yourself, whether it is something for you. Especially listen to that voice of truth inside you. And even if you receive useful information from others, you yourself "know" best and "feel" best what's good for you. Don't just believe without question those who think they know, armed with so-called proofs and statistics regarding nutrition and health. These statistics were influenced, created and governed by the underlying convictions of the researchers. Running is good for whomever likes to run, biking is good for whomever likes to bike, etc., but as soon as it becomes a "must" or a "course of treatment," something is wrong. Then you listen to rules that are forced on you and possibly do not at all correspond to your true nature. Never do something that makes you feel: this is not in the nature of my constitution, of my inner disposition. Don't ask a "rabbit" to cut trees, and don't ask a robust, heavy forester to go jogging! *Do only that which you feel is in harmony with, and lies in the field of, your true nature.* (Read more about this in the chapter: "The Cult of the Exterior.")

Or do you eat things you really don't like just because it's so-called "healthy"? Then, you lie to yourself. Trust your nature!

Or do you pierce your face with holes, or do you bind your feet, or do you lace up your waist, or do you carry out other painful rituals because it's "the thing to do" within the tribe, the race, the country? Then, you place rituals, behaviors, external things ABOVE Truth, above Life. This *cannot* be! Dare to question everything. Arrive at love for yourself and know that *the ONLY true health and beauty can but go hand-in-hand with the truth.* All the rest is Sham and Glitter, fake and untrue, and sooner or later must be paid for with illness and deterioration. After all, lies destroy themselves.

"Signals" as road signs on our Path

Sometimes, we don't realize we are lying to ourselves, or that we are not completely on the right Track, not completely connected with the honest Stream of Life. Luckily, there are Big Signals and Little Signals that draw our attention to this!

It is necessary that the Human Being learns to live in the "here and now" in a Conscious Loving way, and learns to look at Signals on his life's path so that he can adjust his course where it is beneficial — first of all for himself and, as a result, for all of mankind. By "Signals" is meant: illnesses, emotions, circumstances that arise, occurrences, experiences, etc.

Less pleasant situations or painful Signals, like certain *illnesses, are there to show that we are more or less deviating from what Life in us intends. These Signals ask us to adjust our life's course in order to arrive at more joy and health.* And these signals don't just appear out of the blue. We — unconsciously — call them up ourselves. After all, Life inside us wants to bring us farther and farther along on the way to happiness. It is us, ourselves (be it unconsciously), from deep in our Life-Core, who call up Signals in life in order to make something clear to ourselves: You are on the wrong track! Correct yourself! So that you become a really living, happy, healthy Human Being!

Truth information

In order to write down my texts I tune in to truth frequency. I "call up" the texts in a concentrated way, after which the answer is received very clearly and consciously from the depths of the source of truth. Therefore, the calling-up and writing-down of this book — which includes the deepest psycho-emotional causes, the actual initial phases of about 900 illnesses — happened very fast. Within a time span of less than half a year, *The Key to Self-Liberation* was written. It has nothing to do with the observation of illnesses or sick people, nor with reasoning out or study, nothing to do with mysteriousness, trance or channeling, but with a very clear tuning-in to a deep inner knowledge. The human being has really no need for "guides, angels or extraterrestrials" in order to advance in evolution.

In this way, every human being on this earth can feel that fundamental, powerful life-source deep inside himself; in this way everyone has his talents, his possibilities, his specific task. It is, for instance, important that someone who has the talent to make furniture uses this talent in order to make people happy with solid, pleasant furniture. And when the baker who succeeds in baking delicious rolls thinks he *has* to come to a state of enlightenment by doing something else (although he experiences so much joy in his work) then there will be no delicious rolls on the shelf, and he is wasting his time with things that surely will make him feel "No, this is not my task." Life asks that every human being, true to himself, do what he feels he has to do according to heart and soul, in joy for his earthly "I." One task or job is not worth more or less than another. And every human being will open himself up to what his Living Self shows him to do or not do.

And all together, consciously living, good-hearted people, we contribute to the construction of a New World where it's good to live: here on Earth! It is better that we don't pay too much attention to the negative (without sticking our heads in the sand, however). Instead, let us bring building stones for that which is pure, honest, and New. Evil cannot survive: it ultimately destroys itself. Good will strengthen itself and multiply. *And Life revolves along in the frequency that connects best with its intentions . . . in such a way that, from out of our Living Self, we can know and say that the delicious-beautiful, the Good, will ultimately triumph on Earth.*

The meaning of life . . . is Life itself: the person who experiences his "I am" in the ultimate happiness to then share this with other people

It's of utmost importance that the human being, in his search for the meaning of life, for true happiness, in his search for "truth," dares to question everything — but really everything — that ever has been presented to him as being "truths" or "lies," whether through his upbringing, religion, political-philosophical, classical or alternative schools, etc. The ideal attitude of the consciously seeking human being is critical openness and "receptiveness" full of trust, while throwing overboard every "prejudice": he does not "just" accept anything without questioning — like a zombie — does not just discard anything in a prejudging way. Neither does he think anything to be "impossible." This is the most honest and healthy attitude of the human being in search of the "truth," of the true meaning of Life. A healthy, critical, though open approach to everything he hears, sees or reads.

It is necessary that, in his search for the purpose of Life, for the "truth," the human being is able to build on a fundamental, solid principle as the basis. There is one basic truth, one certainty, running as follows: "I-AM-HERE-AND-NOW." This conclusion, coming from the conscious living human being, doesn't need further proof. There is no basis "under" this basis. It's the Secure Basis of this human being who can know, feel, and be aware. Very important is this security: on this basis, the human being can build his life as an unshakable construction, in a never-ending growth-process.

Believe in yourself!

Here, it is very important that the Human Being come to a greater awareness of his "I," that he develop a strong "Faith" in himself, in his "I." After all, one of the greatest causes, if not often the deepest cause of misery and illness, globally as well as individually, is a lack of Faith in one's own "I." It's necessary for the well-being of a Person that he comes to a greater Faith in himself. Faith goes hand-in-hand with becoming more Conscious.

The human being is a living being . . . it is therefore necessary, in order to believe in himself, that he first and foremost chooses in favor of Life, believes in Life. And, finally, that he fully comes to the realization that he, as an "I," doesn't "just" exist here: every human being is the expression of one of the endless, profuse expression-possibilities of Life itself, and *every* human being has at his disposal highly individual, unique possibilities, *far* more than he suspects!

Every human being has actually formed himself within life's womb, however unconsciously, and from the beginning has always driven himself onward on the basis of an inner, unique disposition that grows and grows and grows.

Life has sought its path, ever further, and finally has put itself into the world of matter and has brought itself to further realization in "the human being." The human being is the result of a longing by Life to see itself reach a higher level of fulfillment, for which goal an alliance is formed, in a concentrated way, between the physical and the energetic, spiritual (consciousness energies) in highly unique beings. Man should realize that, inside himself, he has at his disposal all possibilities to function optimally as an autonomous and original being; that in himself he has all possibilities of Life in order to make himself into a healthy, happy being: as "himself," and not similar to anyone. The wonderful spectrum of the enormous diversity of people spread over the Earth.

There will be only misery as long as the human being allows himself "to *be* lived" in an unconscious way, and doesn't bring about CONSCIOUS changes where they are needed for his well-being: changes in his expectations and convictions regarding his existence, in his "passive" way of living, in his disbelief, etc. It's now up to the consciously living human being, in his shaped uniqueness, full of Faith in himself, to bring "Life" further along. It's up to the human being himself to unfold his energies, his possibilities, and to direct his life, full of confidence. We would say to everyone: "Man, take your life ever more consciously into your own hands, bring yourself to realization, believe in your own uniqueness, begin to search for 'truth,' and listen to that honest voice of Life in yourself."

Every Human Being has that choice: are you going to "allow" others, or exterior things, to rule you, letting yourself droop, living according to the conviction that life is a vale of tears over which you have no say? Are you slipping into a "depression," which by itself is already a signal that you need to change your course, that you don't consider Life completely "in accord with truth"?[6]

Or will you, on the contrary, start to live according to the conviction that you can make of yourself someone who takes deep delight in everything life offers, simply by listening to that voice of truth in you which teaches you that Life is something marvelous as long as you yourself contribute to its creation?

The voice inside you that gives you the most true joy is the LIVING voice, because real Life and Joy go together. Therefore, don't listen to that voice in yourself (thoughts, convictions, etc.) which brings you sadness, because this voice is called "lies" and goes directly against true Life.

Take your life in your hands, make something wonderful of it!

Do you notice that you become "sad" when you think of the past? Then stop this thinking and resolve, from out of the Present Moment, to experience the most beautiful situations in your life.

You create your future yourself, consciously or unconsciously

Every human being creates his life himself, consciously or unconsciously. You create your future yourself . . . there is no question of predestination, of fate or destiny, or of karma having to be paid off, of punishment, etc. The way someone's

---

[6] Read more about depression in Part II.

life, someone's reality, someone's future, unrolls, is the result of one's deep, embedded expectations, convictions regarding oneself and life. Are you convinced that you deserve punishment or that life entails suffering and victimization? Then you will experience sad circumstances and possibly "attract" an upbringing or dogmas which confirm your deeply embedded expectations of life. And why are you convinced you will have to encounter punishment and suffering? Because you are convinced you are a "bad" or "sinful" person? Then it is to your advantage to start seeing yourself as a good human being and live accordingly . . . drawing a line through the past. Then you will attract beautiful life circumstances and joyful experiences.

Know: *you can start every day with a new, clean slate, whatever your past might have been,* as long as you have the honest, sound intention to be good, to do good. However, as long as you remain convinced that you have to do "penance" for sins from a "previous" life (part of life) then you deviate from the Voice of Truth inside you which represents Life; this voice just wants to stimulate you to start again as a Good human being, NOW, today, and no longer hurt yourself because of possible mistakes or feelings of guilt from the past. So, stop burdening yourself with karma and original sin. "You as you" can, indeed, start anew every day, in goodness from out of your heart.

The word "sin" we can describe as a negative conviction that you have put upon yourself and on the basis of which you have begun to live and act. The most important "sin" mankind has put upon itself is: Doubt in the "I," in one's goodness, in one's abilities to create one's own life.

A doubt which often goes together with a kind of discontentment, dissatisfaction, unthankfulness. Doubting "whether happiness on Earth is possible"? This conviction is so deeply ingrained in humankind, from generation to generation through the ages, that we can really speak of "original sin." A deeply rooted conviction of Doubt that has already inflicted many wounds! It's time now that the Human Being, in thankfulness for his existence, in Contentment regarding his "I," no longer Doubts his ability to create eternal Happiness, his divinity, his Goodness. If he eliminates this self-degradation, this deadly *Doubt Virus,* then he will no longer feel the urge to fill himself with greed, desire, militancy, apathy — then misery, war and illness, and finally physical death will disappear. In other words, the "fall" of mankind (as described above) has indeed been a painful transition, but has its value for Life if the ultimate result is "The Faith in one's own Power and Goodness." If suffering and death are once and for all banned to the past. If Grateful Contentment triumphs regarding one's own existence! The resurrection of Life in every good Human Being on Earth: for ever. Eternal happiness on Earth is possible if Man believes in it and lives according to truth, to Love, in a Conscious way.

According to your experiences in Life you can detect which deeply ingrained convictions regarding yourself and regarding life you were born with; why you unconsciously attract certain situations (possibly again and again), situations of the same nature. This doesn't "just" happen by accident. Situations, events, emotions, but also illnesses, are being called into life by your "Living Self" in order to make something "clear" to you; in order to make you realize where you as a human being cause yourself pain, where you lie to Life inside you.

The deepest living and life-giving principle inside you (which we call the "Living Self") constantly sends out signals; because Life wants to bring itself further along, via your existence as an Individual Being, in a highly unique, honest and positive way. In other words: YOU as "I"-THE-HUMAN-BEING want to bring yourself, in a highly unique way, further along the path which will lead you to an ever-greater consciousness, to happiness. That's why the Living Self sends you signals again and again! Especially if something happens that goes directly against life. Then your Living Self sends you signals. Look, then, at these signals. Do not try to nip them in the bud; after all, looking at and understanding these signals can bring you, as a Human Being, a big step further!

The future is not "predetermined"

Sometimes we hear people say: "Everything that psychic has predicted has happened." If the future is not predetermined, how then is something like this possible?

The answer is: by NOT believing that the future is "not" predetermined; by living according to the conviction that everything in the future is predetermined, and that one cannot change it anymore. The "fortune teller" doesn't see "THE" Future of the person concerned, but sees the person's expectations as they are projected toward the future "by that person's convictions." When these convictions (especially of an easily influenced person) are, in addition, accentuated by the "predictions" of the psychic, then it's not so surprising that this person — who, on the basis of his convictions, creates his own future — will create a future that coincides with the predictions. The psychic then helps to "determine" a certain future. The important thing we can say here is: the fortune teller (without it being his first intention) makes the person aware of the deeply ingrained convictions that dwell inside him.

For instance, a pregnant young woman came to tell us that "a certain psychic" had predicted she would bring a handicapped son into the world, and that her marriage after two years would run aground. And that everything "he" had predicted to one of her friends had come true. Her fear was great. After we explained to her how "predictions" work, she determinedly started to take her life (and future) into her own hands. Living according to the conviction that NOTHING negative needed to happen to her, because she lived according to goodness. She banned from her being every "negative" conviction regarding fears that had to do with the birth and marriage problems. The negative predictions about this person *NEVER* came to be!

Regarding "predictions" about world happenings it's not difficult to pick up certain *unconscious* "streams" that dwell among humanity and "to see" a future on this basis: however, when the Human Being (as part of humanity) arrives at unexpected new Insights, and on the basis of this brings about *Conscious* changes, *then these unconscious lines "turn" as it were in a new direction! Then, no single prediction about the future will come true anymore!* Then, reality makes, as it were, a "curve" that no fortune teller had foreseen. THE FUTURE really lies completely open. Therefore, it's of utmost importance that we, as Human Beings, become aware of deeply ingrained convictions in ourselves, in order to transform all of them into happy, optimistic EXPECTATIONS of the future! Every human being will experience that which he consciously or unconsciously has created *himself.* Therefore expect THE GOOD . . . and live accordingly. Don't get into a panic when certain less-pleasant circumstances or symptoms pop up as a "signal": look at them and make adjustments as needed. Believe in it . . . and everything will work out fine!

Illness as a Signal

Illness is not something that "just happens" to be unalterably spread over mankind, as a result of which some are met by good luck and others by misfortune. Illness is a symptom — from the flu, to AIDS, to decline, to death — a signal that your Living Self-Core sends as a warning in order for you to thoroughly realize something, and to change your existence. To make you become "aware." In other words, you are doing something that doesn't run completely in the direction of "Life," because of which life cannot completely and optimally stream through you. Depending on how and in which way you need to adjust your life-convictions and deeds, you will develop this or that ailment or illness. Depending on what kind of "deviation" from Life you maintain in yourself — thoughts, convictions, emotions and actions that go along with them — you will attract this or that illness.

So, for instance, someone who has developed a throat infection has not listened to the voice inside him which asked for an honest expression of emotions, asked for autonomy, for emotional independence from others, and especially for him no longer to bottle up sadness and anger, which often go together with desires and demanding things from others, with feelings of rejection. Imagine that someone doesn't at all listen to the "signal" of throat infection and that this throat infection finally disappears, with or without medication — but surely without working on the psychological causes of throat infection; the infection disappears because the psycho-emotional causes have "eased off" or are being suppressed (but are not fundamentally resolved). Then this person can after some weeks or months develop the same illness, or perhaps bronchitis[7] . . . Why? Because his Living Self now sends out an even stronger signal in order for this person to finally reflect on the question of what Life really wants of him. Imagine this person allows his bronchitis to heal just by taking medicine, or by whatever alternative "treatment" on the outside, *without working on the true psycho-emotional cause, Origin, of this ailment. Then his Living Self again will send a signal, possibly even stronger than bronchitis . . .so that he finally might listen to himself, to the "why" of this illness, of this signal.* And we, therefore, should not be surprised that Life ultimately brings forth illnesses like pneumonia, cancer, etc., as signals.

Because man is often so blind and stone-deaf, keeping himself ignorant — because man regards illness just as a symptom (at the most calls it psychosomatic), because man never looks deeper into the *true* causes of illness, into the *true* origin (there, where the illness originates, there, also, originates the healing process!). That's why Life itself sends new illnesses again and again, illnesses that are ever more difficult to "suppress" or "heal" with medicines . . . so that Man might finally start to look deeper into the true meaning of the signal called "illness," and so become aware that illness as a symptom, as a signal, is there to show the Human Being another way, indicate a better life . . . a life that connects with the stream of truth and therefore with more joy, freedom, happiness.

Illnesses that are more and more difficult to heal, like AIDS, are for the human being to really start to think now, in a healthy, conscious way. He needs to realize *that the fundamental "healing" of AIDS or whatever illness doesn't happen on the level of medicine, but on a much deeper level!* The human being, *every* human being, has his own healing process in hand, as long as he dares to look at the reason, the true causes of why he has attracted this or that illness. Once he has understood this well, he can recover from this "signal," this symptom, this illness, by putting into practice what the signal (illness) asked of him, by bringing about changes in his life.

Mankind, and also "medical science," may and can no longer neglect these signals from Life itself, from the human being himself, if it wants to progress! When will medical science begin to search for the "True Origin" of illness so that we can call it "original," and "truthfully exploring the depths"? Still, there are already numerous doctors over the whole world who are enthusiastically responding to our work and often tell us in delight that "it really does work that way!" Doctors, care-givers, and laymen who are searching for "truthful information," for

---

[7] Read more about the throat and about bronchitis in Part II.

"more in-depth information," and for "true healing." The time has come that educational institutions and universities make room available in order to arrive at deeper insight into the true "origin" of illness.

Trusting your nature. Convictions. Immunity.

It's very important that the human being "lives from out of himself," that he believes in himself, that he honestly dares to be himself. But how many people put this into practice? It has been taught to the human being not to trust himself, his nature. "Don't go outside without a scarf or you will catch a cold." This is a conviction that indicates a weak self-image and a lack of confidence. And reality is a result of this conviction. Someone who goes outside without a scarf and doesn't believe at all that he will catch a cold, won't catch a cold. However, if in the following week it's comfortably warm, not even a breeze, not at all cold, but this person at that moment is psychologically very hard and cold toward himself, living in a rather deathly way, without warm feelings, as if wearing a mask . . . yes, then he can "catch" a cold, regardless his "trust," because the psychological field is very attractive to this specific virus! This person will heal himself from his cold by breathing warm life into himself, by coming home closely and warmly to his inner heart, and his Trust will *very* quickly help him over it. The same or similar "scenario" we can quote for every illness.

Because the human being doesn't believe in himself, in his immunity, in his natural powers . . . he becomes susceptible to an illness such as AIDS, which gives a literal translation for the paralysis of the immune system. Now the human being, mankind, begins to mistrust its own nature even more! Because, who can still trust his nature if the immune system can be paralyzed by a virus just like that? It becomes a whole vicious cycle that the human being has to break through if he wants to purify himself from all the disasters in the world of illness. Medical science, science in general, will have to study the true causes of illness in a very honest, open, conscientious way. Without doubt, when the necessary apparatus will be available, it cannot but find that *every* illness in its essence has its origin in convictions (do you believe in yourself, in your immunity?), and in the nature of the psycho-emotional field of the individual who calls up a specific illness as a signal . . . so that he might free himself of the underlying causes.

But the human being often places his "life" in the hands of someone else, a healer, a doctor (and doesn't realize he can heal himself). This is also because he allows his opinion to depend on the judgment of the doctor or care-giver, who themselves are often stuck in a short-sighted conviction-pattern. But truth-information will ultimately push through.

The most important task of the care-giver/doctor is to show the sick person the Core of the matter, the *true* cause of his ailment, stimulating him in the faith of self-healing (which doesn't mean that medicine as a remedy will have to be discarded right away; read more about this in other chapters).

Fundamental solution

Man, believe in yourself and work yourself out of this pernicious cycle of self-doubt!

It doesn't matter if you take medicine or not, if you follow classical or alternative ways of healing, make use of acupuncture or take allopathic pills — all this doesn't have to be "bad," but it has nothing to do with the CORE of the matter, nor with the ESSENTIAL SOLUTION of your illness. It can give you a kind of temporary balance, of comfort, a feeling of "being cured," but *real* healing can only take place when one "works" at healing on a deeper level at the same time as the "treatment" — or without treatment, depending on one's conviction. There, where the illness once started, on a psycho-emotional level — on the level of convictions and emotional depths — when a solution is offered for the *real* cause of illness that lies hidden *under* the physical. By looking precisely at the nature of the physical symptom (illness) and understanding it, then we can arrive at such a permanent fundamental healing. This can only happen when the "patient" *opens himself up* to this true "cause and solution." Because then, after all, he has to take responsibility and begin to do it himself! It is much easier to take "pills" without working on the deeper causes. And this doesn't *have* to be done (working on the fundamental causes), except that the human being will have to realize that his Life-Core then soon will send him a new illness (or another signal), in order for him to finally begin to heal himself and make himself happier in his CORE.

You don't just "accidentally" become infected by AIDS or whatever illness. For instance: two people, one of whom carries the AIDS virus, can have sexual intercourse for years, without the other person becoming infected. This is because this person doesn't carry the inner psychological field that is susceptible to this AIDS virus. We see a totally different "psychological pattern" with the flu virus[8]: when one person in a group of twenty only "infects" four of these people, it just means that the psycho-emotional field that is sensitive and susceptible to the character of the flu virus is present in these four people.

We have seen many people who have healed themselves from cancers, tuberculosis, rheumatism, etc. Certain ones took medicine during this psychological development process (healing process), but others did not at all! Healing demands

---

[8] Read more about AIDS and flu in Part II.

you look closely at the reasons why the Living Self has attracted a certain illness as a signal for you. Healing demands a solution for the underlying psycho-emotional causes: healing forces are being stimulated as a result, the immune system is being fired up, and consequently the human being also heals on a physical level. And whether the human being takes medicine or not depends on where his conviction begins and ends. If he is strongly convinced that he can do without, and psychologically does what he "must" do, then he will heal in that way. However, if there's anxiety, or the person does not dare to be without medicine, chemotherapy, operations, or whatever, then it's best that he does make use of these things. But, a complete and lasting cure depends only on psycho-emotional evolution! Swallowing medicine, or not, is actually of minor importance, but every person has to decide this according to his own feeling and convictions. We simply want to say that we have seen numerous cases — that it can be done without "help" from the outside — as long as the human being arrives at Insight into the true cause of his illness, "works" at it, believes in himself, in his self-healing energies, and this course of action doesn't go against the conviction-pattern and the will of this person. Every person has to decide this for himself.

And no matter if it's about an ordinary cold or AIDS: it's always about "signals" from the Living Self. If one has understood them well, then one can thoroughly work on the solution and in turn the healing. This is, actually, the only *true* healing, the only *true* medical science, the one that deals with the true causes of illness-symptoms and pulls them out by the psycho-emotional root. The result is that "illness" disappears. The "signal" coming from your Living Self was understood, and the necessary changes were brought about. This is true healing.

The person's convictions play a very important role. Imagine that someone heals himself from a severe ailment through — as he expresses it — following a very severe and sober diet, or by taking this or that miraculous herb or medicine. Then, on the one hand, this is the result of this "diet" and these "herbs" or "pills" interacting well with the SYMPTOMS of the illness. On the other hand, it's the result of the fact that there is also a back-up from the strong conviction that asserts "This diet and these herbs or pills are going to heal me." And the person heals . . . apparently! Another person with the same ailment, who follows the same "healing method" doesn't heal at all from the "symptoms," because his conviction doesn't back up the healing process. But, in reality, neither has been "truly healed," because they only look for the solution OUTSIDE themselves! Sooner or later the Living Self will send a new, possibly more severe, illness to the person who heals himself solely on the basis of help from the outside without looking at the real psycho-emotional causes, an illness for which diet, pills or herbs don't work anymore. This then happens in order that he will start finally to look at the deeper, *true* cause of his illness, in order that he will become CONSCIOUS, in order that he will

TRULY bring himself to healing and therefore to a greater harmony with Life itself!

Therefore, never ignore the message from your Living Self! *And whether or not you take medicine or herbs, whether or not you let yourself be operated on — always do what makes you feel best. In the meantime, don't forget to work on the REAL REASON for your illness. In this way, you will come to TRUE (inner!) healing. Therefore, as a result of this, your body will no longer have to attract any other severe signals.* In this way, the illness can disappear just as well without medicine, without operation, without diet, etc. (How many cases of so-called miraculous healing have we seen in the last years!). But, if you have the feeling that you cannot do without an operation, then it is best to follow this conviction; *then, in love, allow this operation to happen. In the meantime work on the fundamental cause of why ever you attracted this tumor or whatever, and then . . . your Living Self never again has to send such an illness to you. Because you have "understood," because you have changed your life in the direction the illness asked for.* And, possibly, you will finally become convinced that you have everything inside you and don't need to use medicine, herbs, diet or whatever, again! Believe in yourself, in Life, in those very deep life-forces in yourself; love yourself and don't close your eyes to the Insight into the true cause of a certain ailment. In this way, without help from outside, you will finally heal yourself of minor and major ailments, if they still would happen to appear on your path. But don't feel guilty when you still need medicine! This is not "bad": read further about this subject in a subsequent chapter.

With illness as a signal, always question yourself: *"why" THAT illness, THIS ailment?* (Read in Part II about the specific cause of why you have this or that ailment.) Don't ignore it. Look at the minor signals, like headache, sore throat, finger wounds, etc. — so that your Living Self-Core doesn't have to send "bigger" alarm signals to you later on.

A good example is *eczema:* if you don't listen to what this skin ailment wants to tell you, and you suppress it with creams, pills, or herbal products, then we sometimes see how the same person who was, allegedly, "healed" from eczema, now starts to suffer from asthma.[9] If you don't bring about the psychological changes the signal "eczema" asked for, then your Self-Core will call up an even stronger signal to force you to work thoroughly on yourself and so bring yourself to fundamental healing. There, where eczema, among other things, calls you to greater awareness of your spacious energy field, asthma will even more strongly reflect how you experience yourself as anxious and empty. Therefore, search for your Fullness, the broad space of your being, etc.!

---

[9] Read more about eczema and asthma in Part II.

You don't *need* to suffer pain.[10] *Pain is a signal* the Living Self sends out to make it clear that you are allowed to take up your space in a fuller, larger, and more loving way, and that you are "hurting" yourself in certain areas! And, as a result, you attract pain, accompanied or not accompanied by an illness symptom. *Work* at the deeper cause of this pain and illness . . . and, yes, if you have the feeling that it's necessary, take a painkiller. Life allows this — on the condition that, in the meantime, you work on solving the causes of this pain! If you don't do this, then you are just suppressing, ignoring, the "signal" that your Living Self sent you in order to urgently bring about changes in your existence. Listen to this! Be gentle to yourself, but go onward, bring about changes where it's necessary!

And then, — as we have seen in practical life, when someone has gained insight into the psychological cause of his pain and needs few, or no more, painkillers — pain will just disappear if that person does what life asks of him, for his own well-being and transformation.

The same is true for *anxiety and depression* (read more about this in Part II of this book): the human being can do without medicine, but possibly he temporarily takes a remedy even if, in principle, he can do without it and has everything within to immediately make a turnaround that will cause every anxiety, panic or depression to disappear, as long as he believes enough in himself, carries love for himself inside and shows willingness "to change." But, in reality, we see that certain people need some time to get rid of old resistance, to find a new track, and then it isn't "bad" or "unhealthy" to temporarily find a remedy in this transitional phase. One doesn't have to have any feelings of guilt about this, as long as one doesn't misuse remedies: here, too, it means that it's only good and justified for Life in you . . . when you at the same time work on the true psycho-emotional solution, when you bring about necessary changes in your convictions, your actions, etc. — when you "let go" of old things! If you are convinced that you can get by without remedies, so much the better!

No matter how you do it, arrive at honest, true healing, via the faith in yourself. Resolve those fundamental, psychological causes so that happiness and harmony will become an ever-greater part of you.

Emotions as indicators

"Emotions," too, are signals from our life-core. Also, the less-agreeable emotions need not be considered negative, but should be considered important indicators.

Do you feel *sadness?* Then this means that you deny an important part of yourself, of your existence as a Human Being, and that you insufficiently acknowl-

---

[10] Read more about pain in Part II.

edge your worthiness and your creative forces, the thankfulness for your Being! Listen to this . . . and help yourself. Believe in your inner greatness and offer yourself love. Life within you wants nothing more than that you are in constant "JOY"!

Don't forget: a certain happening in your existence is, in fact, only the *"occasion"* for a certain emotion, such as anger or sadness, to come to the "surface." Then, it seems as if the cause of your anger or sadness lies in those happenings! No. *The "cause" lies much deeper:* solve it deep inside yourself. You have already carried a vibration of anger inside you, and as a result you have attracted a situation in which you get angry, not the reverse! In this way, happenings and your emotional reactions to them, can reveal anger, anxiety, sadness, and feelings of guilt — or whatever emotion — that are still to be found in you. *The circumstances you unconsciously attract are only a result of the emotions already existing inside you.* Look at them and bring about changes in yourself so that you come to a greater harmony within yourself.

When someone gets into a fight then it's because the fighting spirit and the aggression were present in him beforehand. It is not the mocking laugh of the other person that brings up his fist — this is only the "occasion" — it is the deepseated feeling of anger, powerlessness, anxiety in himself, the auto-destructive mocking laugh toward life in himself. These are the True fundamental *Causes* through which he attracts such a situation and through which he begins to fight and furiously uses his fists.

Is there still *anxiety* dwelling inside you? Then once in a while you will attract situations which will "give" you anxiety. Know, then, that anxiety is a signal from your Living Self to make something clear to you. "You have to adjust your life's course in order to arrive entirely upon the path of life and happiness." Some examples: do you give yourself too little love? Are you suppressing your formidable life energies? Do you constantly sacrifice yourself for others, or do you cling to them? Are you only living on the superficial periphery of yourself? Are you constantly keeping your thoughts in negative spheres? Or are you on the track of discontentment, greed, and desires? Then, anxiety will be awakened in you . . . in order for you to realize: in this way you can never make yourself happy; this path leads to death instead of life. Therefore, be thankful that your Living Self-Core makes you feel anxiety in order for you to become conscious! As soon as you have solved the basic cause of anxiety, in love toward yourself, then you will no longer attract situations which will give you anxiety.[11]

Hatred. Every feeling of hate toward others finds its roots in hate toward Life itself, in the inability (or resistance) to UNCONDITIONALLY love Life and Yourself with regard to form and content. Therefore, don't put conditions on life. Experience your unique, beautiful Being in Total Love of Self, in thankfulness for Life itself. Hatred toward Life also means that you feel discontented and un-

---

[11] Read more about anxiety in Part II.

thankful, because you don't have or can't get "this" or "that" the way you would want to. However, if you arrive at unconditional surrender to "Love for Life," and "Love for yourself," then you tune in to the vibration of BEING, and no longer to the wavelength of WANTING and desiring. Then the current of life can flow, unhindered and happy, through your veins. This happiness for who you are, for the fact that you are allowed to exist "as You," without placing any other conditions on life, results in you attracting circumstances that make you happier and happier!

Also, with regard to *traumas:* you mostly place the cause for your misery in some happening from the past, whereas that happening was already a result of an inner "atmosphere." You then have attracted unpleasant situations — be it unconscious — in order to look at the deepest cause, the "why." Why, what energy field lives in you so that you have created such situations in your life? (Read, for instance, the chapter regarding incest and rape in Part II)

When you arrive at absolutely clear insight regarding this, then you will look at the past with different eyes and will no longer place in others the cause for why this happened to "you," but will place it *in yourself* (even though the behavior of the other person can't be justified).

You will bring about changes in the PRESENT, and ultimately you will look at the past in a detached, liberated way. In this case, it doesn't make sense to keep stirring it up and follow reenactment therapy for years. A spontaneous outlet for emotions is, on the other hand, natural and healthy and belongs to the psychological digestion process: no matter whether you are alone or with friends, or whether you have a good understanding with a doctor or therapist — ultimately you have to, and can, do it *yourself.* You are certainly allowed to have a healthy communication with someone, with a care-giver. You can pick up interesting information here and there, through teachers and books, but ultimately you, yourself, remain your own "professor." Count on yourself, and know that the solution of *whatsoever* problem is inside you! You can do much more than you think, independent of "help" from the outside — which doesn't mean you cannot have helpful talks with others without, thereby, falling into a position of dependency. It's important to allow yourself to express certain emotions, to let them flow out, very spontaneously, and not bottle things up. In a next phase you begin to search for the "why," for the causes of your discharging of fury, sadness, hatred or whatever feelings. The deeper *causes,* the roots of these emotions, you always find deep in yourself; the circumstances, happenings, people — these can only be *"occasions"* through which these emotions "surface." In this way you can lovingly allow yourself "to be," "to evolve," to better understand yourself. It doesn't make sense to stimulate emotional discharges in a forced way.

Live from out of your heart and trust your nature, your feelings. Consciously be your own Leader! Count on yourself. Heal yourself: all the possibilities are inside you!

Life, itself, doesn't want anything more than to allow its "emotion" of Joy to flow through you without being hindered . . . so attune yourself to that life-giving source inside you, listen closely to the signals on your path, and — full of trust — go onward! In this way you will get there for sure!

Desires

"Desires" as signals, if you look closely at them and understand them, are also a way of bringing yourself into greater harmony with Life

The earthly human being is naturally a wonder of power and fullness and vitality. But because he doesn't believe enough in his power and fullness, he has created all kind of authorities and powers outside himself, which have to replace, as it were, the powers and values that he denies in himself.

The human being who believes in his own powers and lives from out of himself, autonomous and full of love, experiences himself as a "fullness" and feels the true joy of life flow through him. Inside himself, he has disposal over all the possibilities of making a paradise of his existence on earth. When, however, through a shortage of faith in himself, he projects his powers, his contents, his possibilities outside himself . . . there comes about a feeling of missing something in himself. The human being no longer feels "complete." True joy no longer flows. Deep inside the human being lives that longing to (again) have that feeling of "fullness"; he starts to long for what he misses inside himself, because he has placed it outside himself. Desires represent, therefore, a longing of the human being who doesn't experience himself as "complete," a longing for a state of "completeness," for a state of joy that he naturally can experience in himself.

According to that which we desire, we can find out *what* we still keep outside ourselves, what we miss in ourselves to feel complete. An example is the urge for power. A person who's plagued with this has little or no power in and over himself; this urge will diminish according to how much that person develops power over himself.

When desire is directed toward money, then we have to look at what money symbolizes. This person has to deal with his self- respect, with the *true values* inside himself.

Something more about power and powerlessness. Certain people who posses special gifts (like bending metal objects without touching them, performing magic tricks or materializing money or gold, or changing or moving objects in an inexplicable way, or healing illness symptoms through magnetism) often feel they are called to say "it" to others. They bind others to them and feel good in this position of power;[12] of course these sect leaders attract people who want nothing more than that someone else, preferably someone they look up to, will lead their life. In this way, power and powerlessness meet each other: both sides hold on to each other in a situation that is not exactly directed toward life! The only thing these magic-makers prove is that the human being has much greater ability than he suspects.

Magnetism and so-called paranormal gifts are not always parallel with the state of awareness and the degree of love present in a human being. So, there are stupid and loveless "leaders" who gain power by showing off some of their tricks or by charming others in a sweet way. In the meantime they need to realize that their longing for power and leadership is a signal from their Living Self to strive after more power and leadership over themselves. The "followers," on the other hand, need to realize that they'd better break with a conviction and feeling of powerlessness, that they only need the faith in themselves in order to step healthily into life in all freedom and joy. Often, certain charismatic people keep others in their grip in a subtle, emotional way. We cite here the well-known words: "Ye entered not in yourselves, and them that were entering in ye hindered. . . ."

Therefore, we repeat again: *mankind, believe in yourself, in that formidable life-power that is present in your inner source, your core; believe in your highly unique individuality, in your ability, and take your life in your own hands! Don't follow anyone but yourself. If you like, enter into dialogue or relationships with others, share your love if you like, but never lose mastery over yourself, over your life. Make something beautiful of it, you as the masterful, loving leader over your existence.*

Your Living Self

Every human being is born within/out of the womb of Life. (By many, this life source is called God.) In EVERY human being there is a fundamental Life-Core present which "wants" (by an inherent drive, wanting to see itself fulfilled) nothing more than that the human being attune himself to True Life: that he will bring himself further along in life, and grow, create, produce, evolve, blossom, and in this way make Life *itself* progress. In this sphere of life there exists no (self-) degradation, no death, no drawing back or in . . . only giving life and life-growth. We call this element, this life-stimulating power center in the human being, the Living Self-Core: present in every human being in a different way (because every being forms itself from within in a highly unique way), but there is always one common point in all: as individual manifestation of the fundamental life-power (the 1 detaches itself from the 0, is born as "I") moving itself forward in the direction of Life.

---

[12] It's obvious that not all "miracle workers" act with negative intentions; things are put strongly in the text only because there are so many abusive situations.

The Living Self-Core wants to place itself, as optimally as possible, in a specific, individual bodily form that is appropriate for this or that person to allow to live — experience, develop in an infinite way — his life, his task, his talents, his enjoyments. An honest manifestation in "matter," in the body. *The Living Self* then represents the total human being, who as "content in physical form" truthfully exists as a "living Unity" and longs to "Live"! So, the Living Self that is you, YOURSELF, as far as you are tuned in to that true Life-voice according to "content and form."

The soul center, "deepest self," or Living Self-Core places itself in a REAL, honest and pure, physical body, not in a Sham body; this is a false body that is created by the Counter-Force in a human being — the "Deadly" force; a body that is artificially built up, inwardly molded, manipulated in order to want to please, seize, impress, draw in, have power, seduce, attract, etc. If a human being identifies himself with this "mask," then he gets completely lost, distancing himself from his *true* Essence, and anxiety and panic can come to the surface.

So, every human being can listen to the honest Life Force in himself or . . . to a kind of Counter Force, an anti-life atmosphere. Every human being has to make this choice: "happiness" or "misery" are permanently linked with this.

You can either connect yourself with the atmospheres of the Life Force or the Counter Life Force, the Anti-life force that works against, blocks, or would like to kill life. If you attune yourself to the Life-stimulating atmosphere inside yourself, then you will automatically grow, will transform instincts into awareness powers, and begin to live more consciously in greater love. And if you sometimes *make a mistake* — listen to the atmosphere of anti-life — then you will immediately attract signals that will indicate that you are no longer on the track of Life.

You are "you" with your awareness-content, with your highly unique nature in the physical body that is you and which you form from out of your living Self-nuclear-force. The body in Unity-alliance with the content: an intimate contact, a joyful feeling is the result.

Automatically, when the human being connects himself with the true voice of Life in himself, he won't sink to "lower regions," to a sheer animalistic, instinctive life, to greediness, etc. In this case, he will ultimately no longer experience anxieties and sorrow; after all, he continues to search ever further for his inner Greatness; he unfolds his potential powers, his abilities, in goodness. Finally, he bans every illness, all suffering, even death. That's the ultimate goal of the life-giving Power Sphere that is present in every human being.

Illnesses are signals of our Living Self-Core, to show us that we are not yet completely connected with Life; if we evolve further, listen to these signals, and do what life asks of us, then the ultimate illness (the physical dying) finally will no longer be needed at all as a signal.

There's always the possibility present in the human being to listen, on the one hand to that which we call good, noble, high-minded, connected with true Life, divine, the most beautiful and loving elevated spheres, a pure consciousness level unsoiled by maliciousness or greed . . . pure values of being, etc.: the voice of our Living Self. On the other hand, the human being can roam in the spheres of what we call darkness: the egotistical, vain, undirected toward Life level, the deathly and demanding, self-denigration, the image-oriented, the small "I" which misunderstands and denies itself in its greatness, remaining stuck, doubting goodness and truth, in spheres of destruction and self-destruction, of decadence and death.

The human being always has the CHOICE to ennoble himself, to attune himself to the first voice inside himself (it isn't literally a voice one can perceive, but rather an inner sphere or state of being). This voice directly connects with Living according to goodness and truth. It is that in the human being which connects with the powerful, Living energy-flow. We call it The Living Self, because it is so totally in harmony with Life itself. When the human being tunes in to this Choice, to these spheres that are directed to life, then he experiences true Joy and Love; then he opens himself up to signals and new information which will show him farther on the path of Life without end.

What matters is that the human being opens himself up to this voice of truth, this voice of Life deep inside himself. And, if he cannot "reach" it very well, then that is because he has fixated too much on the exterior of his being, on his outer appearance, or started to "think" too much — for instance, no longer feeling — or because he was completely convinced that there was nothing left under the superficial layer of the human being, under this "thinking above all, and maybe feeling and sensing a little." He has strayed from his inner being, from his vigorous, driving, vital force, by focusing too much on the "outer world," on appearance, on image, on others. He has closed himself off from his inner riches.

It often is asked: "But how do I reach my inner 'Life-Core'? I can't make any 'contact' with it." Many then begin to search in an anxious and panicked way for "something" that should be there. No!!! That's not really how it works.

First and foremost, you experience that *your body,* if not being manipulated to gain power over others (through seduction, drawing in, attracting, impressing others, etc.) is an honest manifestation of the Living Self-Core! If you experience your body, feel it, see it, *feel* intimately and lovingly connected with it, then you *are* actually (in this body) "your Living Self"! Of course, there are "unconscious regions," but you don't have to direct yourself to them. You know that your Living Self, according to soul and body, is being driven by a fundamentally strong "Life-Power-Core" inside you. For the rest: *tune to your HEART,* to Love, to giving to yourself — and, as a result, also to others — to intense and sincere receptiveness to what Life inside you asks of you (and, of course, to *doing* what life wants you to do), to feeling your earthly, living body. Then, everything will become clear to you through what you feel, through the signals you encounter on your path. Feel your heart, love your body, because in this orientation toward life "YOU" *ARE* YOUR LIVING SELF! Even if you cannot reach certain "underlying" regions, this isn't necessary at all! Direct yourself deeply inward and, there, profoundly sense *your warm Content;* don't get hung up in "outer" spheres (how am I being perceived?) but *live* spontaneously from within. Be who you ARE!

Let go. *Live* joyfully, *live* according to your heart, to what you feel, your intuitions, using your common sense. Follow the signals on your path, trustfully, not fanatically — and then you know that you *live,* that you yourself are your Living Self at body and soul level. Your Living Self is not something that is hidden very deep inside you; you don't have to dig a thousand miles under the sea! Tune in to your heart, to love, feel your skin, your honest body . . . the Word of Life was made "flesh": this is real, living flesh. Open yourself up to that which the inner life wants of you . . . and you will feel it. Just OPEN yourself up to what you see, hear, and feel, and to what the energy in you that is tuned to true life (your Living Self) attracts as signals on your path. And, if that powerful Life-Core in your being, drives and directs you further and further, don't then fight *against* it. Go along with yourself and never abandon life in yourself by clinging with your superficial small "I" to certain things or people or false values. Listen in all honesty to what inner life tells you, to your heart. Let go, and go further onward in an eternal, happy growth-process!

Finally, Mankind, take up your Inner Kingship!

We don't *allow* ourselves to "be lived" by "Energy," by this complex totality, by this bulwark we are, by the 1001 rich facets in us, but we Direct ourselves *very* Consciously. We don't have to "comprehend," know, all that goes on in deeper, more unconscious layers of our Living Self. But we may realize that the Potential in Powers is enormous; this asks for Leadership! Allowing that, under the impulse of Love and Insight, animalistic, instinctive energies transform themselves into noble, highly human conscious energies, directed Creative powers. The "male" and "female" aspect, in balance, united under the supervision of the Conscious leadership of a loving "I."

A being-open, in receptivity to the unconsciously living content and wisdom deep inside us. Ever keeping the balance between heaven and earth, between spirit and body. The brain will function optimally, and its capacity regarding "knowledge" and "awareness" will grow when the human being takes his place Consciously at the head of the Living Unity he is.

The Crown on the Living Self: the human being as Master over his existence in wisdom and in love. He rises above the narrow-minded rationality and listens to the *true* wisdom that lives inside him. Every human being has the ability to do this as long as he doesn't begin to "cling to" or "greedily fixate" his "thoughts," or his "emotions," and is attuned to the truth-frequency of Life. He lets go, and allows himself in all spaciousness TO BE, taking up his task as Leader over that multitude of conscious and unconscious Life-energies in his being. He makes his way in trust, and he *knows* that everything will be all right.

To survive or . . . to live!
Physical immortality?

The human being has been living for so long with *the conviction* that he has no other choice than eventually to die. You can ask yourself: and what if the human being no longer lives according to this conviction? It is a fact that Humanity knows itself to be imprisoned in the "web of life and death" and that it has created consoling perspectives to escape from this concept. And then came the answer, from the very deep source of truth, the most beautiful I ever "heard" — described under the title New Days.[13] The path to physical immortality now lies open to the human being who is open to it: however unbelievable it might sound, it's about a choice and the consequences of that choice, *the consequences of reversing deeply ingrained convictions.* Physical transformation follows that inner choice, inner transformation. *Every human being is free to believe what he wants and to determine whether or not he will make this or that conscious choice.* Here, we can only say that this liberating philosophy creates completely new, joyful perspectives, and once you are on this path of "Life," it will strengthen and enormously uplift your faith.

The Divine Image

Most people on Earth pray to a certain "Divine Image." Because mankind did not believe in itself, it has projected its power and forces in divine images outside of itself. From the divine image we see, we can deduce what values this person or this race embraces. The human being really created his gods according to his deepest longings (or according to his greatest fears): so, too, has the human being who highly regards Love and "expects" this love also from others created a god who represents love. In this same way, the human being who admires toughness and power, militancy and courage, has created a god in this image; he always expects trials of strength and only feels good in battle. Thus, in the human being who cre-

---

[13] The book *New Days* is already available in several languages.

ated a god which has to be adored, celebrated, and praised, there lives the longing that he too might be acknowledged and adored by others, just as he approaches his god . . . . but, in fact, he has a need for self-acknowledgment. Thus, the human being has created an immortal god because he, himself, actually would like to be immortal (and deep inside himself he knows that he actually is); this indicates the deep longing to break through the age-old pattern in which he keeps himself imprisoned: "having to die." The god who demands obedience and metes out punishments indicates that in fact the people who adore this god also expect obedience from others, and otherwise would possibly mete out punishment. But they, themselves, can also have the feeling that they are treated in the same way by their fellow men and — because they are hard on themselves — fear a kind of punishment.

If we use the term "god," then it would be preferable to regard this as "LIFE" or "LIFE-GIVING SOURCE" out of which everything has come forth and still comes forth. But we don't have to place anything or anyone "above" ourselves, or project outside of ourselves, because by doing this mankind immobilizes itself in powerlessness, and Life doesn't mean powerlessness! On the contrary. The more consciously you begin to stand in Life the more you will notice that you, and only you, consciously or unconsciously, lead your life, have it in your hands. There isn't a Fate or Commandment at all that stands above your head and will tell you what is good or bad!

　　　　Live in Thankfulness . . . for Life inside you, in Love toward yourself and Life, in helpfulness toward Life, follow the signals on your path; your inner living — or divine source, if you want, will show you the way. But it's up to you to take your place, solidly and self-aware, at the head of your ship of life. Listening to the language very deep inside you, listening to and looking at the signals your life source attracts. Redirect, adjust your course and go on ever further on that path of happiness.

All the people in the world who are good of heart and honest, thankful for their existence, Loving, and of pure Faith (in themselves and in Life!), can meet one another on the same wavelength. Here, it no longer matters what "religion" they practice or have practiced. Within the blissful "House of Hearts"[14] every good human being is welcome, a true "encounter" is possible, because one no longer "hides" behind a system. Here dogmas, doctrines, no longer count; truth speaks for itself, shows itself in The Act of Life. Here, churches, mosques, temples, and other houses of worship no longer fight each other, because every Human Being lives from out of his Good Heart, because one now realizes that such struggles for the sake of religion were just "alibis" in order to get rid of deeper, ingrained frustra-

---

[14] Read more about this in the book *The Twelve Gates of Prince Sirius* (not yet published in English in 2003).

tions. Now, *all* buildings can be opened — for Life, for True Love, and for all people who don't place anything or anyone above this Heart. An encounter between "Life"-friendly people with built-in high morality, by which peace and faith in one's own ability to make something beautiful of life go hand-in-hand. After all, every feeling of powerlessness (and as a result urge for power), every defensive or offensive (war-minded) behavior, disappears with this deeper "Knowledge" of the "Ability" in every human being to create one's own life, directed by "Goodness" and by "Faith" in that fundamentally strong, pure, Inner Divine Essence.

Love

Do you love Life itself? Have you chosen to firmly say "yes" to Life on Earth? Then, within this scope you can also love yourself; after all you offer yourself life, in thankfulness, and that is the most beautiful thing you can do. This *Alliance with Life* indeed consists of *unconditional love for yourself.* Sheer, pure, intense Love-of-the-Self on a Body and Soul level: the way YOU are, unique and irreplaceable, authentic in form and content. You radiate this love of life, this joy for your existence, this love for your "I." It's about a state of "being." You allow your heart, your thymus, your brain, to be filled with thankfulness and love of Life and for your "I." *Then, it is honest and good to share this Love with others.* Then, you will also be able "to give without expecting something in return," unconditionally . . . without bartering: "I give you this if you give me that back!" The latter is, of course, not love. But if you live according to pure, self-radiating Love, and give with your heart, you will automatically experience encounters with others that are full of love. A generous, happy, radiating state of Love simply attracts similar vibrations toward you: don't give in order to possess, to obtain, but *give* out of Love for yourself, for the Life Current inside you, in thankfulness for existence itself, for your existence, and for the existence of other good people . . . and you will turn yourself into a happy being! You will radiate this happiness to others, who then also will be stimulated to search for love and thankfulness for life, for love of themselves; others will be confronted with their hate or self-hate; they will be stimulated to resolve this in themselves and to transform themselves into a pure state of love.

Mostly, the human being is born with certain "expectations" and "instinctive" tendencies. He has to develop love inside himself. Although in some people this inclination is naturally more present than in others, many people again and again "expect" everything — in the first place from their parents. It's good that a young person soon learns that "giving" means "life and happiness," and that seizing, demanding, expecting only brings sadness, anger and a state of unhappiness. He needs to learn that he can take good care of himself — that he can offer himself love, in thankful contentment for existence, for what "is" there in his life; that it is necessary and good for him not constantly to want to possess and possess, falling from one discontentment into another, because desire creates new desires again and again. If things go wrong here, then later on he will project into a partner relationship the same demands and expectations and how his parents reacted to his behavior. The things that were not corrected in childhood are later on presented again as "lessons of life."

Therefore: love for oneself, allowing the full heart to blossom, thankfulness for just being "allowed" to live on earth, this attitude, this Feeling . . . makes it possible for this child or grownup to attract beautiful situations . . . which then make him even happier. It's a path of life full of joy, without end.

Love of Oneself versus Egotism

Love chases away every anxiety. LOVE FOR ONESELF is a great necessity for solving every problem. This has nothing to do with greed, with vanity, with egotism or image (these are accomplices of the counter-force of life), but has to do with true LOVE toward one's own total "I."

Living in total, warm unity with yourself means allowing yourself to truly LIVE and no longer remain stuck in sadness, anxiety, old patterns that once again will lead to suffering and death.

You offer yourself the Greatest Love. You don't expect it from someone else.

You don't have to go and live on an island, alone and far away from all life. On the contrary, enjoy; pouring out pure nectar to yourself! Feel like a god in the earthly paradise and make yourself warm, comfortable, cozy. Do only what you feel you have to do from YOUR HEART. No longer listen to that dark voice; offer yourself a conviction of joy: be convinced that the Good is stronger than the Evil and then Evil and darkness will disappear by themselves from your conviction-sphere. Offer yourself the most happy, loving energy.

*Love means **giving** . . . to yourself! And, as a result, you can also give to others.* As soon as you begin to ask, to demand, to hold on instead of to give, anxieties and dark, obsessive convictions can plague you. So, let go . . . give yourself Love. When you are tuned in to this high Love toward life and toward yourself, no anxiety can bother you anymore. For, life and love don't allow anxiety within the borders of your "I."

Don't you acknowledge yourself? Do you pull yourself down or do you consider yourself just as a limited, small or ugly being? Then you don't yet love yourself enough. Then you may be anxiously holding on to old patterns, to the primal mother womb, to people or things outside yourself, which makes a free life-current impossible. And *then* your Living Self sends you anxieties and panic to point this out to you: COME INSIDE YOURSELF, in your wonderful EARTHLY BODY; love yourself, no longer push yourself *away!* Don't flee from your true self, don't flee into thoughts, in the "spirit," don't cling to old patterns, to "drugs" or to other people. And, if you listen to these anxieties without running away from them and replace these anxieties with faith, Love, pure love for yourself, strongly coming INTO yourself, in your body here and now, with both feet on the ground, fully present in yourself — then anxieties will ebb away.

The mother and the father are INSIDE you. Don't deny either one, but lovingly integrate these primal powers inside yourself. Count on yourself; offer yourself Faith, Trust, and Love. Acknowledge your worthiness as a human being, your deep inner worth, and love yourself the way life has given shape to you: you *are* in your body, the way you are at its best. Don't desire to create — out of thirst for power — another outer form; be thankful and content in love toward your body-form which is an externalization of your inner, unique nature. Throw overboard every power-norm and seductive manipulation. Don't draw toward yourself, don't be like a suction force that absorbs others, but *give.* Fulfill yourself. Don't put DEMANDS on life, nor on yourself, but listen to the language of Love and then *give* to yourself, letting go of everything and everyone, also the old, compulsive patterns. In this way you become a fearless, happy human being.

The light of real LOVE FOR YOURSELF chases away every dark conviction, because true "love" will no longer tolerate sadness, suffering, or death to be present in your existence. So intensify this Love and be convinced that no single power is stronger than *this,* since it goes hand in hand with Life, with Truth, and even can bring Life constantly further along.

Living in relationship, love, and happiness

Work on the relationship with yourself, first arriving at pure Joy about yourself — only then can you experience pure Joy in the relationship with your partner.

Relationship is *giving,* not demanding. You don't *have* a partner, you *are* a partner.

You, yourself, attract EVERY situation, good or bad. So make something beautiful of it!

Do you have the feeling that the other person doesn't love you enough? Then this means that you insufficiently love yourself. Offer yourself more warmth, more love!

If you seize and hold on, you will be seized yourself, by anxiety, sadness or, for instance, an obsessive urge for sex.

You can say or discuss certain things — for instance something that is on your mind — but then you let go of it. You don't demand, you don't expect ANYTHING from the other person. You give, you speak and you let go of your partner. Then you come very close to yourself, ever closer, in profound contentment with yourself.

Thankful Contentment for life inside you. This thankfulness, this Love toward yourself, warms your heart. You say "yes" to life that is in you. In this harmony, this joy about life in yourself, you will AUTOMATICALLY attract these things and human friends with whom you will go on the path toward "the earthly paradise." Certain friends from the past might disappear from your life, because they are not on the path to life. Dare to say "No," when you feel so. Go to certain people when you, yourself, feel like it, not because "someone" expects it from you!

In the feeling of thankfulness circumstances change; problems solve themselves — if you stop blaming others, stop having feelings of hatred or resentment, because your partner doesn't want to "fulfill" your longings. After all, with this discontentment, desire, this criticism toward others, you don't get anywhere; you will only make yourself sick. This "wanting to get something out of the other" lies on the path of illness and death. Therefore, let go of that other person! Come very close to yourself and transform hatred into love, criticism into thankful contentment for what IS there! And you will see how life rewards you; you become warm, comfortable inside, and relationship problems, too, solve themselves. On the basis of your love for yourself, everything that is good for you will happen. Let go, don't seize, don't grab, don't blame others . . . and turn inward. *Give,* talk things out, and let go, staying very close to yourself, which also makes it possible for your relationship and love toward the other person to grow.

Stand on your own basis. Live from out of yourself. Stay faithful to yourself and at the same time learn to understand each other. Let the past be a closed book in order to be there for each other in the present, shaping yourself in a New Form. Not selfishness, but love. Not losing yourself, but a strong concentration on your own basis. Two people who live on their own strong basis can meet each other as equals. Everyone has his shortcomings, his strong or weak side to work on. Therefore, never point your finger at someone else, but always work on yourself. Then things will go well.

Don't lose yourself in someone else, because then you will be on the path toward death, where also blinding intoxication, empty romance, and sex without love belong. Therefore, be faithful to yourself. Don't do anything you really feel you shouldn't do, not even to please the other person, because then you lie to yourself, with that you don't help the other person either. Only the truth endures. . . .

Therefore, choose to live in Love, choose truth on the highest level. Work on yourself and, again and again, let go in order to discover yourself, down to the roots!

 The Key to Self-Liberation, Christiane Beerlandt © Beerlandt Publications

Leave the other person free, loose, because true Love is without Ties. Don't suffocate each other, give each other freedom. In this freedom there is faithfulness and a deep alliance.

Wherever you are, no matter how much distance or time separates you from each other, in your heart you are always together. This alliance has a strengthening effect. In this happiness, you go on with YOUR tasks, and your partner with his/hers. You are thankful and content because you are . . . in Life, because of the relationship which is allowed to be, *this* relationship which is best for you.

And you trust your Life and let go. In this way joy can flow through you. And you FILL yourself only with yourself, although your heart can feel full with love for the other person. But first and foremost you have to love yourself, very deeply. Only then can you exchange this love with your partner. Otherwise you would do things that go against your own nature, and sooner or later this will take its toll.

Power-struggle is bad. No one is worth more or less than the other. Don't elevate yourself, do not "tell" the other from above. You, too, have your faults and shortcomings. Always keep talking and living on an EQUAL level with each other, and calmly say what you have to say.

Don't try to bind the other person, to hold him/her tight to you, to pull him/her toward you; this is use of power. Give with your whole heart in joy . . . then everything will go well. Things go wrong when you end up in the lane of discontentment, disgruntlement. Therefore, be glad and thankful for the Life inside you and for that which *is* there. The rest will come at the right moment. Life will give you at every moment what is good for you! Don't seize, don't grab, don't demand, because it isn't always that which you think is good for you that is best.

From out of gladness, the thankful contentment with your own Being — all happiness comes to you!

You can really never feel anger, hatred, sadness BECAUSE OF someone else (a situation, an occurrence), even if it seems that way; this only means that these emotions are still deep inside you and need to be cleaned up if you want to be happy. Does a certain situation cause you sadness or hatred? Know, then, that you have attracted this situation as an "occasion," so that you can solve the "cause" of this sadness or this emotion in yourself. So that you will come to pure joy and thankfulness for your being.

Your happiness depends on you. So, come to warmly loving yourself in thankful contentment with life; then life will finally reward you. Come, in warm love, close to yourself; then you can "give," not "expecting" from the other person, but fulfilling yourself and making yourself happy, so that you can share this happiness with your partner, in truthful partnership.

"Life, I am thankful that I AM" — and, in this feeling, you know that everything and everyone will come on your path the way it is good for you . . . so that finally you will be able to live eternally toward greater happiness. *Therefore, let go of everything and everyone outside yourself, turn inward very deeply and be thankful. Then everything will happen that is good for you and for your happiness.*

About Love, Sexuality, and Power

It's important to realize *that sex is not love, and love is not sex.*

Two people who love each other very much can, within the language of the heart, under the warm mantle of love, meet each other in sexual intercourse. But it is not a must. Certain people don't at all feel like having sex, and then it is not necessary. It's very possible that a conversion, a transformation of energies, comes about so that primal creative forces express themselves in a different way than through sexuality. It's very possible that people also enjoy life in a completely different way than through sexuality. He/she who doesn't feel like this form of exchange doesn't have to bring himself/herself "into question"; follow the signals which your Living Self-Core sends you, makes you feel, and trust in this. By this, the human being needs to keep following his own Nature and stay faithful to what his Living Self makes him feel.

When sex becomes an addiction,[15] then love no longer counts: here, it's about the human being who is overflowing with creative forces and wants himself to be born, wants "to be" more and more in matter, and intensely longs to extend himself, in autonomy and self-assuredness, not in dependency (and as a result, addiction) upon someone else. He will make use of all his inherent energies in order to reach a higher and more powerful level inside himself; he will have to become "master" over his life, over himself; he will not adore anything or anyone outside himself, but will give shape to his inner heart and to his great, wonderful "I." Then, in this self-acknowledgement he will no longer want to "fill" himself with others, no longer want to fill his feeling of emptiness with the other person. He now fulfills himself, he finds himself, and in this condition of self-fulfillment and love for himself, he can, without being addicted, come to a physically tender and/or sexual relationship with someone else.

AIDS, for instance, also is a signal for mankind to not instinctively, like animals, without love, get involved with "sexuality." Life asks that we allow these primal forces in us to flow from the HEART under the guidance of LOVE, in creativity and as an expression of love. And as long as we just "allow ourselves to be lived" by uncontrolled urges and passions, we follow the track which completely runs away from "life." Therefore: guide yourself to your own Heart and then, as master over your own life, do what you feel you have to do. You as a completeness, experience that which is most beautiful in yourself, because of yourself, and either can or not, in physical form, bring this into expression with the other person.

---

[15] Read more about sexual addiction in the chapters about sexuality (See Part II).

The Key to Self-Liberation, Christiane Beerlandt © Beerlandt Publications

It's this Love that counts, and whether it is between two men, two women, or between a man and a woman that doesn't matter. We should not forget here that EVERY human being carries IN himself the female and male aspect.

It's so important that someone who doesn't want sex, not do it; even not, for instance, just to please the other person, because then he/she lies to him/herself, and this will take its toll sooner or later — for instance he/she then unconsciously will attract the signal "bladder infection" or "fungal infection."[16]

A Sham Life promotes illness and death

When a human being consciously or unconsciously develops and forms his or her body in order to gain "power" (mostly) over the other "sex" (through attraction, seduction, etc.) then this implies a movement of drawing in, like that of a vacuum cleaner. This is the image of dark death, which wants to get the other person in its grip, swallow him, and drag him to a deep dark hole. The story of the spider and its web, the fly is being eaten up. Men who are being dragged along in this way by the behavior, and certain physical manipulations of certain women, have to come to the realization that they allow themselves to be persuaded by "death"; that they attract this situation in order to finally "see through" sham and Death, in order to ultimately break with it and choose in favor of life, of love. Power and Seduction have NOTHING to do with love and life. (The same goes for the tough man who tries to impress a woman). Every man/woman does well to realize this. Do you still behave as a being who dresses, acts, applies certain plastic surgery, or shapes your body through diet in order to develop attractive powers? In order to have more power over the other person because you answer more to the current norms of beauty? Know, then, that you play along with death and that in reality you are extremely ugly. Therefore, become who you really are, dress yourself in clothes that you like (that your *real* Self likes), that are comfortable on you, in colors you like, but never do something "to enchant," "to charm" someone else, to be regarded as "elegant," or "tough" or to look "cool," because then you use your self as a Vacuum cleaner, then you weave a Web like a Spider in order to catch a fly. But whoever digs a pit for someone else will ultimately fall into it himself. This power-game only lasts for a certain time, and it ends in illness, decline, and death. Why? Because this whole game is built on death and not on the basis of life — on taking and seizing and not on giving. He who sows death, ultimately kills himself.

In all parts of the world there are prevailing fashion trends or traditions and habits concerning how to be regarded "attractive": this is about SHAM, not about real beauty. Because true beauty originates in the Heart and flows along with the truth. Truth is Life, is *giving* in love. All of the Sham World will sooner or later

---

[16] Read more about these illnesses in Part II.

fall apart; at this moment it is true that individuals and small groups of people are already being confronted with this: that the game of power and attraction can give brief sexual pleasure, but it is followed by hell and decay and misery and ultimately death. And that this kind of pleasure is NOTHING compared with TRUE ENJOYMENT . . . there, where two people let true Love reign and give to each other (also physically, sexually), without a question of drawing in, seduction, and swallowing up, addiction, false "beauty," sham forms.

It happens that people who, by birth, already have the conviction that they want to have power over others have sold their souls to the devil, so to speak, and, be it unconsciously, form a body, a face, etc., that perfectly answers to the prevailing beauty-ideal in the region in which they are born. As it is their desire to be adored and have power over others, they cultivate a so-called "attractive" body in a state of Sham Beauty. But their soul-core, their heart, their love-kernel, is "absent." And to those who are tuned in to true life, these masks are hideous, reeking of death; one "looks through" the game of the representatives of Lies and Death. These "people" and their "Sham Beauty," then, are being adored by those who are also attuned to false beauty ideals, who also allow themselves to be dragged along by the current norms of beauty. But this fairy tale always has a fatal ending, because it is built on lies and death. Certain people act "cool," others constantly smile engagingly and "sweetly"; they entice like the Lorelei or like a fragile elf. All life-force, all honesty, has disappeared from them; we only see a mask, a sham form. The distorted human being; the weak Eve's image, the tough Adam's image. Both types have strayed off the path called Life and Love and are holding each other in a whirlpool that pulls them down to the deep, to death.

Don't allow yourself to be led to the land of death.

Being nice, smiling . . . is not the same as "To LOVE"

Being nice, *"the smile"* is mostly *a mask,* a camouflage, because often there is no warm heart, no real joy present. There are so many women who are smiling all the time . . . . Or, if we are talking about people in a male form, with "charm," "charisma," or as tough, indomitable supermen. . . . There are so many forms, so many sham images — and their heart is cold or absent. Tests of the Living Self: how well do you see through "the devil" in yourself, in others? How well are you connected with your heart, with true beauty, with honesty and authenticity . . . or do you, too, lie to life, doing your utmost to shape your body the way it has to be in order "to catch" others in your web? Then, you play with death. Do you constantly smile sweetly, automatically, like a puppet, or do you show yourself tough and strong, forever shaping your body in a "seductive" way? Then, you are an accomplice of Death, and your life will end sooner or later in "hell" (here on earth). However, if your "laugh" is an honest expression of your Heart, then everything is okay.

So: choose the path of Life, of Giving, of Love, of Truth, of authentic Beauty: BECOME WHO YOU REALLY ARE. *Live from within, not according to the eyes of others* — then you will reach love and harmony with yourself, and only then can you Enjoy the Utmost in soul and body, meeting the Highest Form of Happiness in yourself or in a relationship. Because, as long as you kept roaming on the path of power and seduction, you could not — and can never — experience that high level of enjoyment, that higher happiness which grows endlessly. You then just kept stagnating in a kind of excitement or pink dream-atmosphere, which doesn't reflect one billionth of the enjoyment of an exchange with a partner that grows from the root of Love!

You just kept roaming in a phase in which one gratification and one desire was immediately followed by the next . . . an endless "filling" with something that would never be able to offer you true happiness and full enjoyment. So, if you still discover in yourself something of this power system, or discover it in people you become infatuated with, know then that this world of Power and Sham ultimately will completely destroy itself. Grow in LOVE, in AUTHENTICITY, in pureness and originality. In this honesty with himself every human being is good the way he is and this truth . . . brings Happiness!

The Cult of the Exterior

A PLUMP or THIN body, TALL or SMALL — in the eyes of Life, all this is of no importance — it is all BEAUTIFUL and HEALTHY, as long as the Human Being manifests his True Inner Nature.

In a world where slimness is represented as "beautiful," there is an urge for power that wants to suppress the true Fundamentally Round Female Aspect (the way the earth is round), to make it subordinate to the structurally more bony, colder, rigid male image. It seems that fashion designers (and those who slavishly wear these designs) hate and totally want to suppress in themselves, and in others, the primal, round femininity and the corresponding Forces, Potentials, Talents and Emotional wealth. A deep primal anxiety lies hidden under this, only to be solved by fully integrating into themselves the true, original, female aspect of life. Then, Life will blossom in them; then, true happiness can enter and anxieties will disappear.

Flesh and fat[17] are not ugly and not unhealthy. Flesh and fat are symbolic of power and energy! There's nothing wrong with a big belly — which symbolizes a rich Content and makes us think of certain Far Eastern fortune symbols which are presented that way. But, as in some other societies, in Western society the instinctive greediness and sexual organs are of prime interest, and love, the fully rounded

---

[17] Read more about the meaning of fat in Part II.

giving, has been trampled upon. Only sexually pointed and attracting cavernous beings are allowed to exist: in order to pull in, in order to pin themselves into others . . . in order to fill their own "chill emptiness." Bulging organs, tight clothes, but especially no belly . . . because that doesn't belong in the world of desires, of pulling in and seizing. The diet industry and sex exploitation are afraid that . . . Love might rise above Sex. A question of "money," isn't it?

Above all, they don't know that physical sexual enjoyment only gives a real feeling of Fullness when experienced out of Love, not out of seduction, "suction" or addiction.

"Dead flesh" is the body of the person who artificially keeps himself/herself skinny (because he/she thinks himself/herself "too fat"). Through diet, through operations or inner manipulation — all of which comes down to misuse of power — one molds the body: it is (negative) power flesh. Of course, the same goes for the person who thinks himself/herself too skinny (here or there) and wants to "thicken" himself/herself in an artificial way.

"Living flesh," a living body, is that body which is honestly shaped from within by the person who eats what he is in the mood for and doesn't "mold" his body in order to "catch" someone else; this human being lives in love, his body is love, is healthy, is true beauty, stout or thin, small or tall.

The greater part of humanity has strayed from heart and content. The human being clings to outer appearances — to "What do I look like?" — to stability outside himself. He doesn't believe in his inner divine power, in his ability to autonomously make himself happy in a self-aware way. He allows his life to be dependent on whether or not "he possesses" — perhaps this might be about material possessions, but it can just as well be about such and such a body, or this or that "partner" he has an eye on. The ideal of slenderness has, in the 20th century, become very fashionable in many parts of the world: everyone should be "skinny." One fools oneself thinking that this is the only healthy way of being: it's absurd. The ideal weight exists, yes, but it's different for every person. THE INNER NATURE OF A PERSON WISHES TO PLACE ITSELF IN A MATERIAL COUNTERPART. *If you are thin by nature, because of your inner character, then your nature wants to place itself in a thin body. If you are naturally round and robust, then your nature wants to place itself in a powerful, round, plump body.* And this doesn't mean that you are ill. *BE CONVINCED THAT THE SHAPE OF YOUR BODY ALWAYS GOES TOGETHER WITH POWER AND MOBILITY. NO MATTER WHETHER YOU ARE THIN OR PLUMP, LIVE IN JOY, ACCORDING TO YOUR TRUE NATURE . . . AND YOU WILL BE HEALTHY!* Don't at all allow yourself to be fooled by the Cult of the Exterior, which has lost every element of truth; don't allow yourself to be fooled by the drug industry and the doctrines of dieting-to-lose-weight. These want you to believe that you are unhealthy if you are heavy. This is not true.

"Yes, but I can't walk up three flight of stairs," sighs a man. Why should this man walk up three flight of stairs if he feels it's not in his constitution? Nor does an elephant do what a chimpanzee swinging on vines does. Nor does a tortoise do what a hare does. A farmer's horse is a farmer's horse, and a race horse is a race horse; we cannot compare them with each other. Don't ask a race horse to pull a heavy cart; don't ask a farmer's horse to run lots of laps. Fat is not unhealthy. (Read about this in Part II) Fat definitely has its function: it's a wealth of energy, warming, and holds substances inside which, when needed, will be released in the body. It matters that you organize your life in such a way that your actions, your movements, etc., are in harmony with your true nature. Don't force anything! And if you live according to the conviction that you are good the way you are — unique as "you," in your body, chubby or thin — then you will attract an environment and life circumstances which, in a good way, lie in the range of your nature!

In the research that has been done into osteoporosis,[18] it has been confirmed that this condition occurs much less in robust women than in slender women — meaning those slender women who "artificially" keep themselves slender while their inner constitution intends them to be robust. The result is all kinds of bone fractures and hip replacements, etc. What matters is that you belong to YOURSELF and become yourself, believe in your inner power . . . no matter if you are thin or plump. Your ORGANS and your complete bone structure will accommodate themselves in a way that is necessary for carrying YOUR highly unique body. We have seen many examples of heavy, healthy people, more than 95 years old — healthy, because they ate what they liked, and therefore needed this food in order to keep a balance between the body and the spirit. They didn't fool themselves into believing that being heavy was unhealthy. They felt and knew that being heavy goes hand in hand with power and mobility — as long as you are inwardly convinced of it, and as long as you live according to truth.[19]

Most people don't honestly place themselves in matter anymore — not only because they want to answer to the prevailing external norms (I want to be considered beautiful and perhaps be adored, to have power), but also because the entire medical world has begun to fool itself into believing that being heavy means one is unhealthy, and being thin is healthy. (This is not the case in all parts of the world.) In practice (the writer herself is robust, very strong, round and healthy) we have seen so many people who are heavy and healthy, at ninety, a hundred, or older — because they never listened to certain doctors (i.e., they never allowed their words to frighten them) who would say, "Mr. or Mrs. you are too heavy, you will get heart ailments, etc." The "fortune tellers" (certain doctors) make a big mistake here, but after all they have been "taught" this way, and statistics prove "it." Well,

---

[18] Read more about the psychological origins of osteoporosis in Part II.
[19] Read more about this subject in other chapters of Part I.

statistics don't prove anything because they are influenced by the convictions that lie behind them. Furthermore, many heavy people only begin to have heart problems because they live in a society where they are described as "overweight," condemned, blamed, and are walking around anxiously, taking pills, following diets, etc. In short, they don't dare be themselves anymore, and they become sad, no longer believing in their authentic beauty, in their power and mobility. Ultimately, they fall ill. The truth is: an *ideal weight* by itself — with all sorts of charts of height, weight, calories, etc. — *does not exist*.

The human being with his "rationality" has strayed far away from wisdom and clear insight. He wants to change a round orange into a thin bean sprout and the other way round, and doesn't at all listen anymore to the language of the inner nature of the human being. *Content and Form in Balance, in Harmony with each other — **that** means health.* So, it cannot be otherwise than there are healthy plump and healthy slim people walking around on this earth! Every human being is unique, and that's what medical science forgets, as it has strayed so far away from nature.

It's even *necessary* that spirit and content, consciousness and matter remain in Harmony and Balance: those with a strong energy field, very strong creative powers, and full of emotionally talented abilities, require a heavy, robust, strong body as a counterpart. Put them on a diet, and they will fall ill! It's a dangerous game society and science play, and the whole business ends in numerous young women dying from anorexia.

Anorexia originates in a person who wants power via a thin exterior, who wants to be considered beautiful by others — instead of offering herself love and allowing herself to grow and expand the way nature in her wants it. One wants to please others, to attract all the attention, and ultimately one receives visitors in the hospital, lonely, because eventually the "previous boyfriends" fall away, for embracing a skeleton is not exactly enjoyable. In this way, a life filled with sucking in attention and power ultimately ends very sadly. Therefore, we cannot repeat it too many times to everyone: become who you really are; don't compare yourself with anyone; don't listen to the herd-mentality of a superficial sham-world. Follow only YOUR DEEP LIFE CORE, your HEART, the voice of truth very deep inside you. Allow your body to be an honest manifestation, powerful and healthy, of who you *really* are. This truth means health, joy, and beauty.

Food and Health

Live in thankfulness, enjoy in thankfulness, eat delicious food in thankfulness.

When you are hungry, eat what you are in the mood for at that moment, *because your soul-core indicates to you via this taste what food product you now need most, according to soul, psyche, and body.* If you are in the mood for an apple, then don't eat a pear. If you feel like having chocolate, then eat it.[20] Do you not like salads, nor whole wheat bread, but do you prefer white bread and steamed red cabbage? Well then eat that! Do you like potatoes? Then they are healthy for you! *There's only one condition connected with this: live according to "truth" in your daily existence (and also listen to the language of the food product; bring into practice what food urges you to do).[21]*

The human being has lost trust in this natural taste. When you always eat what you like and live according to Life, then you will grow toward the bodily shape and body weight that is ideal for you. And this can be 110 lbs. as well as 310 lbs. You will then stay around this weight, and in this shape, because it is the ideal reflection of your vibration field — and that's good! That's ideal in order to achieve and keep an optimal state of health. And, whether you should lose weight or gain weight — whichever shape *really* belongs to your Content — that you will find out if you always eat what you are in the mood for, without forcing yourself. As long as, at the same time you live according to Life, not according to Sham, not according to the conviction "that you are not allowed to be who you are." *You can eat what you like, on the condition that you LIVE ACCORDING TO LIFE, experiencing yourself as a worthy person full of love, living with the conviction that you are powerful and mobile.* It speaks for itself that someone who doesn't live according to life — and for instance sits entire days dreaming in front of his TV screen — ultimately brings himself into a state of sleep, creating an immobile body, and his organs will become ill. But the opposite is also true: the person who forces himself every day to do sports and run, while his inner self says "stop," will make himself sick. Therefore: listen to your inner voice, to your taste, eat what you are in the mood for, trust and do what life asks of you.

Very important: every food product you long for — and which your body and your psyche therefore have a need for because they want to bring themselves into greater harmony and health — *every food product speaks "a language" which you have to listen to.* For instance: someone who longs for a tomato has a need to bring his joy outward in an extroverted way, not hiding himself in an introverted way. As, for instance, milk chocolate says: deal with yourself in a soft, warm, flexible, loving feminine way, don't dig in your heels, etc., etc. . . .

In the book *The Horn of Plenty,* the meaning of several hundred food products is explained, called up according to "truth." *In this way, you can learn to understand yourself better according to what you like to eat, and you will become more conscious of what life asks of you.*

---

[20] Except in case of certain illnesses: read more about this in *The Horn of Plenty.*
[21] Read about this in *The Horn of Plenty.*

The Western world (especially since the second part of the 20th century) is convinced that flesh, fat, and roundness go together with weakness, illness, and immobility. Nothing is less true!

Only that person becomes ill, (no matter if he is thin or heavy) who doesn't live according to life, doesn't live in joy, in thankfulness for his Being — for instance, he *who is convinced "that he is immobile,* that he is weak or limp." As a result of this conviction, a certain person, for instance a thin person, will develop an illness and end up in a wheel chair. Another person who's heavy won't be able to get out of his chair anymore. But both examples have by themselves nothing to do with being thin or heavy! The true cause of the immobility is the conviction one carries within . . . and according to which one lives. Therefore, we'll see two people who both weigh 100 lbs. and one of them will be as healthy as can be and the other ready to collapse; in the same way we'll see two people both weighing 330 lbs. the one going through life powerfully, dynamically and very strongly, and the other one is sad, slumps in a chair, considers himself sick, and can no longer stand on his legs.

So eat what you want and listen to the language of nutrition. Feel strong and powerful, mobile and beautiful, no matter if you are heavy or thin, and don't mind that stupid Cult of the Exterior. In other words arrive at the truth, at true beauty, at Living Power, because the human being doesn't know anymore what that is! Life never fixates itself on the outer form, but forever grows from within. . . .

It speaks for itself that someone who already has "diabetes",[22] which by itself has nothing to do with being heavy or thin, should not right away start eating loads of sugar, but first needs to solve the psycho-emotional causes of diabetes in himself in order, then, to gradually eat sugar again, as the pancreas begins to function better under the influence of the psychological changes being applied.[23] We have been able to follow this course of events with certain people who cured themselves of Diabetes.

Eating a lot when you are hungry is healthy. Don't confuse eating a lot with "gluttony" or bulimia. Gluttony is precisely the result of the human being constantly stopping himself with the intake of food, because he is wrongly convinced that "eating a lot" would be bad for him (unhealthy, or not good for "the figure"). In other words, he denies himself a certain food product or permission to eat a certain quantity of it. Because of this, his Life-Core will sooner or later force this human being to take in what he refuses to give to himself. Then, at a certain moment, he or she can do nothing but suddenly throw himself/herself upon the Food, emptying the refrigerator. If this person also has a "feeling of guilt" while eating cer-

---

[22] Read the chapters about sugar and sweets in *The Horn of Plenty*.

[23] Of course, all of this needs to be done in consultation with your doctor/therapist.

tain food products, then the brain "refuses" to send a signal of satisfaction, because of which gluttony is stimulated. That's why *the* cure for gluttony or bulimia says: EAT WHAT YOU ARE IN THE MOOD FOR, as much as you want, *without* feelings of guilt. You will then eat A LOT, without being a "gluttonous person." Eating a lot when you are hungry, without feelings of guilt, is healthy! Then, you just take in what your body and psyche need. Eating a lot has nothing to do with "desiring" or "greediness," but with maintaining or promoting health and harmony.

Certain people can eat very much (yes, also fats and sugars) and always remain thin. Others eat the same amount of the same food and are heavy. Because the form is the expression of a very specific nature. Being heavy or (honestly) thin is never a problem: as long as you are convinced of the fact that your body is powerful, beautiful, and healthy, no matter if you are heavy or thin. The problem only comes into existence when people *"think" they have to begin to worry* — when they "think" they have to "look" this way or that, or that eating a lot is unhealthy. Nothing is more untrue! Gluttony only comes to be as a result of the fact that you don't dare give yourself what your Being asks for. *Thin or heavy, become who you are!* Live according to the conviction that you can trust your taste. Eat what you feel you have to eat, what you like to eat, without complexes, without feelings of guilt, *living according to the conviction that you are Powerful, Mobile, and Healthy*. Live according to Life! And disregard the Cult of the Exterior!

Finally: why should we merely live on "light" alone, saying "no" to those delicious foods which life offers us like a Horn of Plenty? *Thankfully* enjoying — and knowing that *if* it would/will be good for man and humanity to "no" longer eat, then this *would* happen as a "matter-of-course" phenomenon, without difficulty or effort. The fact that there is famine in certain parts of the world doesn't require that the "rich" countries "fast" or live on "light" alone, but it asks for a total revision of, and becoming aware of, "how things can be done differently." One needs to look at the fundamental cause and the fundamental solutions in order to make it possible to bring about changes.

Heredity?
The genes: a dynamic system

A human being is not "just" haphazardly born somewhere. He is born to those parents and in that place in the world where his Living Self-Core directs him. And then he attracts — be it unconsciously — a genetic heritage, which he needs in order to work on himself, as a reflection of that which symbolizes him. But, *there's no question of things being "predetermined"!* You have brought yourself here, within this family, in order to show yourself a "mirror" of certain things you want to solve in yourself so that you can make yourself into a happier human being.

There's a kind of genetic pattern — *a predisposition* — in every human being, but he remains free to develop these patterns in whichever direction! Genes, cells, etc. are not "static," predetermined elements. They are in constant agreement with the psycho-emotional movements in the human being, with the underlying evolving conviction-field in man. And, therefore: *genes are also "in movement," susceptible to evolution and changes.*

Say that you, as a young man, are born with a "father" who has a heart condition, and you, too, have it . . . and someone says "that you, too, will die when you are forty, just like your father, because it's hereditary." You don't have to believe any of this; look up what the "heart"[24] is symbolic of, and you will see that the heart among other things asks for absolute love for yourself, joy for your existence, and especially no sham, no false appearances, no hardness, no image-striving, no exaggerated thinking with regard to feeling. Stop all this, and live in a gentle, honest, sensitive way toward yourself. Imagine the young man has seen his father living in a hard way, an image-striving way, and decides to take another path — what happens then? *Together with his own psycho-emotional changes, the genes, the cells, also undergo a "change of form" — yes, simultaneously; matter, the material, the physical, is constantly being influenced by the spirit, by consciousness, by thoughts, emotions, expectations. So, thanks to insight and the bringing about of changes in the psycho emotional field, genetic patterns change . . .* and the son, in our example, does not have to develop a heart condition and die early. On the contrary, the hereditary heart condition can redirect itself; the heart can regenerate and begin to experience itself and move in a completely different, healthier way.

We can produce numerous examples just like this. Did your "mother" or your "grandmother," die of cancer, and are you, as the daughter, afraid that you will develop the same illness because of "genetic inheritance"? Then, look at what cancer[25] symbolizes; bring about changes — in other words don't live at all in the same way as your mother and grandmother did, understand the true reason that caused their cancer finally to break out. Thanks to the changes you bring about in your life, the genetic pattern, too, will alter, and you will never get cancer. This is the liberating message of self-healing: you can do much more than you think, much, much more! Many examples in the world have repeatedly proven this to be true.

The Labyrinth and the Way Out

In all kinds of myths and stories, in old and new writings, profane as well as religious stories, the image of The Labyrinth, or of the "being lost" is brought to the fore. And that tells a lot about the experiences and convictions that dwelled among

---

[24] You can read this in Part II of this book.
[25] See Part II of this book.

mankind and still are dwelling among us. The motif of the Labyrinth, of searching and not finding a way out. This image of The Labyrinth has come to be in the human being and stayed alive because he kept looking for "true Life" and "true Happiness" OUTSIDE himself. In the past (and still today), he has conceptualized and walked a multitude of paths in order to find Life and Happiness outside himself, but they were all dead-end roads. Man carries within himself the memory of many roads that all end up in death.

Still: the Living Self wants to show the human being the Way Out, like the thread of Ariadne; the path to True Life, to Liberation. Indeed, many fairy tales and myths — which are, after all, a reflection of that which lives deep inside mankind — also tell us how the human being himself ultimately finds a way out, no matter how critical the situation he was in.

The only true way out will always be there, where man again finds himself, believes in himself and *knows,* very deep inside himself that he, himself, can build his life in freedom and happiness. That nothing or no one above or outside himself can break down and threaten his life, that he *himself* attracts all — yes all — situations in his life, consciously or unconsciously. The more conscious a human being becomes of this, the sooner he can deal with, and make an end to, the feeling of being stuck in a dead-end labyrinth. He will find, INSIDE himself, the thread of Ariadne and the path to Life without an end, to Freedom.

Concepts from the past such as "the fall of man" can be seen in this way: during the incarnation process — the birth of mankind in the earthly dimension — one has fallen into the wrong convictions, not (or no longer) believing in one's inner, divine powers, in one's goodness and ability to take one's life into one's own hands and building it into something wonderful — yes "the fundamental doubt." The result is a desire to find stability in all kinds of powers and forces outside of oneself, a desire to fill oneself with things or people from the outside, with covetousness, anxiety and greed . . . straying away from one's own Fullness. Mankind didn't recognize its own loving greatness (anymore). Mankind lost the contact with its Living Self-Core, with the True Life inside.

The path to Ultimate Happiness, to eternal life without suffering and pain — yes, finally to physical immortality, the way life actually means this to be — this thread which leads us out of the labyrinth where mankind for so long has kept itself shackled, is the language of our own supreme Living Self, of our Inner Heart. And to show us this Way, our Living Center sends all kinds of Signals on our Path, to make CLEAR to us: THERE lies the way to liberation, THERE you go wrong, or here you go right, ALTER YOUR COURSE, etc. We just have to follow this "thread" to the way out, and this can be done by being open, by looking at and listening to that which the Signals in and around us can make clear — and by no longer doubting the good outcome.

Signals, luckily, are being constantly sent to us, or even better: we call them up ourselves (mostly unconsciously) from out of our deepest Living Center; in this way it is made clear to us what Life in us wants, what is best for us. Signals can be positive or negative. In both cases they serve as INDICATORS that show us where we are right or wrong. Next to the language of *illness* and *emotions,* which are very important signals for "where we have to change our course," there are also the ordinary *everyday happenings* — apparently "just accidentally" happening to us, but nothing is less true!

When, for instance, a light bulb in the house pops, then this indeed has something to do with the material and technical side of things (the bulb was perhaps very old, etc.). But, still, you will see that this happening didn't just "accidentally" occur *in that place, in the presence of that person, at this certain moment.* It's always about a synchronicity, things that occur at the same time: on the one hand a light bulb that pops or lightning that hits, a glass that breaks, etc., and on the other hand "a happening" in the human being himself, in his psyche, his head, his total being. Why does this or that just happen NOW in a human life?

The energy that is too hard, sometimes too structurally cutting, the holding-on to old patterns and not being open to the stream of spontaneous, emotional, renewing energies: *that's* what the signal, "a light bulb pops," wants to say. It becomes a serious notification when, during a certain period, many bulbs in the house pop. Then, no longer be hard to yourself; learn to relax; don't think so "hard" anymore; don't stay tense within old structural habits; free yourself from old thinking patterns.[26] Understand this "signal" of the light bulbs; change your way of life, and in this way you can, for instance, avoid heart palpitations.

No matter if it's about a flat tire, a theft, a car accident, a fire in the house — or whatever — it tells us SO MUCH about ourselves. We have seen that even the greatest skeptics — those who didn't believe anything of it — when they read the texts about the "signals" that were of relevance to them, they confirmed in astonishment that this situation as described in its psycho-emotional meaning was indeed "true" for them. We, therefore, advise the reader to not simply believe anything, but neither just reject anything. A healthy, sensible, thinking person first reflects, "opens" himself up to investigation, and doesn't reject things beforehand. Only afterwards does he draw his conclusion. Many people seem to be afraid of a deeper truth, of the language of Life itself which "speaks" via signals. However, it's a pleasant, educational path to walk, without becoming fanatic. Does something attract your attention? Are you forced to look at something — for instance, you break a glass twice in a row, or you lose your wallet — then think about it, just reflect for a moment: why does this happen to me now? Read, if you like, the explanation for these happenings in *The Signal Book,* or try to figure it out yourself.

---

[26] You can read about 300 signals in *The Signal Book* (Signals on Our Path. The deepest meaning of life-happenings). At present (2003) this book is being translated into English.

Very often we have seen that, when someone "understood" the *true* reason for "losing" an object, and was prepared to bring about the necessary changes in his life, the lost object almost immediately was brought back or found. There are examples of how wonderfully life functions, and how beautifully we can learn to understand it and guide it ourselves.

Nothing happens to you "by chance"

Occurrences, phenomena or illnesses that happen to you, are not "just" there all of a sudden; they don't come falling from the sky, nor are they being sent to you by one or another force or god. You, yourself, attract everything in an energetic way.... All happenings and phenomena are there as an externalization of something that happens on a deeper level: in your psyche, your emotional life, in your conviction-and-expectation pattern. In this way man creates his life, calls up situations himself, good and bad. Mostly, this all happens unconsciously, which is why people say "it happened" again to me. One simply is not aware that everything is energetically connected (under the surface of what we can observe with our senses), and that man constantly creates his reality according to his own expectations and psychological patterns. If he becomes aware of this, then he will realize that things don't happen to him "just like that," then he himself will take his life in hand. He will then be able to look into himself and solve the deeper causes of certain unpleasant circumstances that are affecting him. He adjusts his course so that he doesn't have to encounter yet another (greater) Signal which makes the same thing clear to him, but with consequences that are much worse.

So, the human being, if applying what the Signals make clear to him, will ultimately encounter only joyful happenings on his path. Man becomes *conscious;* he realizes, now, that only he can change his life, adjusting his course in the direction of goodness, truth, and happiness, so that nothing sad has to meet him anymore. This, then, is one of the most deep-seated convictions that man has to deal with for good: that he is born in order to suffer, that it cannot be otherwise than for a human being to encounter unpleasant circumstances on his path of life, that he would not be able to take his life in his own hands and incline it toward constant Joy. If he breaks with this lie in himself and listens to the Signals on his path, then he will experience how he will see ever more clearly in life, how finally his Living Self will no longer attract any unpleasant signal.

Fatalism will only play a part in your life as long as you believe in it. Everything has a reason for being: observe it. Don't close your eyes to the road signs, the Signals on your path. Take your life in hand and guide yourself ever further along: fatalism no longer exists.

Occurrences, illness, etc., are like Signals; always ask yourself "Why"? and then correct your course. "Why is there an electric short in my house? Why that flood, that earthquake? Why does my left foot fall asleep so often? What's the reason my bike got stolen? What's the reason I have attracted this?"[27] In this way, if you already look at the smallest signals, you no longer have to attract the larger signals. If, however, you refuse to listen to the message of small signals, then your Living Self will send you ever-greater signals — negative, serious happenings, illness — so that you finally will realize: I am on the wrong path, the path that leads to suffering and death. Change your course! Look at the causes of these Signals and solve them in yourself, so that you will reach one step farther on the path to more Life, more Joy!

What about astrology?

It is not the stars and planets that determine our lives. At all times, we have our lives in our hands.

Stars and planets all have their own "character," just as everything that lives has its own meaning, its own nature. In a birth chart (or horoscope) you can read with which convictions you have come into the world; *a horoscope does not reflect who and what you are in essence, but it reflects a whole world of convictions and, perhaps, behaviors that are a result of these convictions, which are deep inside yourself.* So, astrology is not meant to predict the future or to be dealt with in a superficial way, but it offers an interesting *Mirror Image* of the human being's convictions at the moment of his birth. It does need to be said that there exist several "levels" in human evolution, and therefore we have to deal with it in a very careful way. Still, this study of Stars and Planets in your birth chart is of importance if it's about finding the "thread of Ariadne." This information, after all, can help you more quickly get out of the Web in which you have held yourself imprisoned. For this reason, I have called up the deepest nature of 231 stars (from Sirius to Castor, etc.), and also the true meaning of why someone is born with the sun in the sign of Scorpio, Gemini, Capricorn, Leo, Sagittarius, etc.[28]

As long as Astrology is being used and studied in order to lead man to "liberation," everything is okay. It's miraculous what characteristics every one of

---

[27] Read about this in *The Signal book*.

[28] Read about this in *On Earth as in Heaven* and *Liberating Astrology* — *"The deeper symbolism of the Sun in the signs of the Zodiac."* At present (2003), these books do not yet exist in English versions.

these stars carry inside them, and if one calculates a "star mirror" for a person,[29] then it's just as miraculous what philosophical psychological messages (signals) certain stars have to tell human beings: a colorful, instructive world!

Also, "numbers" represent much, in a very compact, symbolic, concentrated way, and the wise human being opens himself up to it as well as to the symbolic values of stars and planets, of plants and animals and — not to be forgotten — of all the people around us. The greater the receptiveness of a human being who wants to know and search life more deeply, the easier will wealth and wisdom develop in him. But, remember: *it's neither the stars nor the numbers that "determine" your life. They just are "mirrors" or signs. ONLY YOU have your life, your future in hand!*

Illness: the body speaks its own language

The body speaks the language of our deepest Self. The Key to healing and growth is true Insight into the psychological cause of illness or pain. What we refer to as "illness" and pain are symptoms of inner disharmony, indications of the fact that something is not being realized — that something is not consciously known about one's own well-being. A psychological change must be brought about to cure the disorder. The correct insight about this must be acquired; practical application will follow. Neither classical nor natural medicine offer *true* healing because they overlook the psychological correction which must be done in order for the body to heal itself in an autonomic way. Take away the psycho-emotional cause and the symptom disappears: that means *true* healing.

Yet, classical or natural medicine can be used in a transition phase, in certain developmental stages of illness, or in moments of crisis, and won't have a negative effect on the human being if, *in the meantime,* one works on the true psycho-emotional cause of the problem, of the illness. (Read about this in the chapter: "Heal yourself with or without help from the outside.")

Infection and contagion

Infections are (at the physical level) caused by micro-organisms: by viruses, fungi, bacteria. These organisms are constantly teeming in, on, and around our body, even when we are healthy. We are by nature immune to "contagion," to "developing illness" from one of these elements — immune to whatever negative influence by whatever organism. Earth swarms with thousands of types of bacteria, which by themselves are all harmless.

---

[29] The "Star-mirror" — which stars make an aspect with certain planets in your birth chart?

Certain people can be in close contact with contagious diseases for no matter how long or how intense, and still they will not be infected, while others will get sick right away. It does not matter if we are dealing here with AIDS or a simple flu. What is the real cause of contagion, of infections? How do we stay healthy?

Certain feelings — i.e. anxiety, aggression, anger — thoughts, and convictions activate that specific virus inside you, touch that specific body part of yours that best corresponds with this specific dislocation of your psyche.

When people with similar soul-states (for instance inferiority feelings) meet each other, then they will be more susceptible to "infecting" each other.

Your unconscious and conscious longings, your thinking patterns and your emotions, your convictions and expectations of life — these determine your body cells, your organs, your glands, your hormonal changes; determine your susceptibility to contagion. True contagiousness is to be found in your own psychological pattern, in the transfer of negative convictions from generation to generation, from father to son, from doctor to patient!

Becoming conscious of the endless possibilities for growth and healing in man is the only true Step which Medical Science needs to take.

Heal yourself: with or without remedies from the outside?

Without remedies from the outside.
This CAN BE DONE . . . many have shown it: by solving the true causes of the illness, the psycho-emotional center cause by which the illness was able to come to be. Read the sections in this book that are relevant to the symptoms or illnesses you are "plagued" with — read attentively, and come to an intense realization of the "why," to INSIGHT into the reason why the illness could grow in you. Then, read the incentive to the solution (mostly the italics) and put it into practice in your daily life. One person needs more time for this than another; in one person there's stronger resistance, or a more chronic process going on than in another person. Everyone brings about healing at their own tempo, in their very own way.

If you are convinced — consciously or unconsciously — that you cannot heal yourself without using medicines, then you *must* use them. This won't harm you! Only you — not I, the author — are responsible for yourself, for your healing process. The way you recover depends on your convictions and insights.

With remedies from the outside.
When, in a certain stage of transition, in a certain stage of psychological or physical development, or during a "moment of crisis," one calls upon medicine or other

remedies from the outside, then Life inside you finds this to be fine. You are allowed to make it easier for yourself; you don't have to suffer pain, and you are allowed at certain moments to use remedies from the outside, ON THESE CONDITIONS:

1) *That in the meantime you work on the TRUE causes, psycho-emotionally, which brought on your illness.* If you don't do this, it means that you are just using medicine or methods — whether classical or alternative methods of treatment — to suppress Signals that your Living Self is sending you in order to make something very clear to you: changes need to be made Inside you, in your existence. If you ignore these "symptoms" and just heal them with natural medicine or allopathic methods, without in the meantime working on the deeper causes, then you are not *truly* healed. Sooner or later, your Life-Core will send a new illness to you — so that you now begin to work on the *true* cause of your illness symptom. The purpose of your Living Self is ultimately to bring you ever more strongly on the path of true life, in truth, toward greater happiness! Therefore, listen to it, no matter if you use remedies or not.

2) That one doesn't become *dependent* on the remedy in such a way that — in a prolonged process through which a sort of *"laziness"* develops — that, finally, you might lose all faith in your own self-healing powers. At that moment you might have to check yourself, depend more upon yourself, and *strengthen the faith in your inner self-healing abilities!* After all, healing methods from the outside remain only "remedies" that have nothing to do with the CORE of the problem. They can "assist" you for a while, but in the end YOU heal yourself fundamentally, "in the core." Medicine can only be called a temporary "remedy" and won't do it instead.

3) *That, in the meantime, you understand that you give yourself this remedy "lovingly," but that it is really you who will heal yourself.* After all, you can take whatever remedy, but the healing only will be true and definitive if you "inwardly" work on yourself and adjust your course. Then, it is not the remedy that will have cured you — it was and is only a help. You have then healed yourself! As *Master* over your life, you have given yourself an aid, (the remedy), without feeling "addicted." You have given it to yourself in love, and you stop giving it when it is good to stop.

No matter whether it has to do with allopathy, acupuncture, aroma therapy, diet therapy, homeopathy, etc., these can be considered as artificial interventions from the outside, by which one actually doubts the self-healing nature of a human being. The Living Self can, for a while, enter a state of confusion by these applications, because it precisely had sent these physical and psychological signals in order for the human being to bring about a change in himself. This change is necessary to grow again toward a total condition that is more healthy than before. If one forces this with whatever application from the outside, then one replaces the self-healing nature forces with a surrogate.

But! . . . One can solve this inner "confusion" by *communicating with one-self in a loving way.* When a person is afraid, uncertain, or convinced he cannot be without remedies from the outside, then — in loving communication with himself — he will feel and know, in and through his deepest self, that it's accepted and understood in his deepest Life-Core that he temporarily uses natural or classical remedies. Yes, it's permitted, but it is not necessary, and ultimately the aim is that the human being finally feels his life-process no longer needs any remedies at all from the outside.

Numerous people become cured, without remedies, from all kinds of illnesses, from the most innocuous to the most serious; others feel they have to make use of remedies. One's own conviction, one's own faith, is what counts here, and it's important that one listen to this.

Therefore: this book does not say: "Throw away all medicine and other remedies." It shows you the true, deepest causes of illnesses, and that an illness is only truly "healed" when those causes are resolved, with or without remedies.

In principle, it can be done without remedies, as many have already shown, but here, you should do as you feel and not be hard on yourself. If, during a difficult period, you feel you need a calming pill or herbal tincture, then take it. Be gentle to yourself . . . ON THE CONDITION that in the meantime you work on the causes of your "depression," "nervous breakdown," etc.[30]

That person who *truly* knows and feels: "I BELIEVE, I can and will heal myself without remedies from the outside," will indeed be able to bring this into realization — if this is his autonomous decision, and not "because he read it in *The Key to Self-Liberation* and wants to try it out." For such things are felt and resolved deep within one's "I." *Here, every human being needs to accept his own responsibility and know, feel deep inside, whether he is ready for this, without building upon other people's theories while doing so.*

All the cells of your body are constantly being influenced by your emotions, your thoughts, your convictions. If you have complete confidence in your body, then every cell, every element of your body, will feel good and will execute its task optimally. If you doubt yourself, then you disturb this perfect functioning of your nature.

Do you foster distrust regarding yourself? Are you convinced that you are not really able to heal yourself? Then, you slow down a natural flow of energies; then, you neglect the message of your Living Self. Minor illnesses ask for a minor,

---

[30] Consult the relevant chapters in Part II.

The Key to Self-Liberation, Christiane Beerlandt © Beerlandt Publications

but not unimportant, change in your life. Don't suppress them "right away" with remedies. First of all, try to find out "why" you have a headache, throat ache, stomach ache, or infection. After all, if you immediately suppress these symptoms with medicines or think you have no other choice than, for instance, to build up your immunity via herbal extracts or homeopathy, then you don't really believe in your Ability, in your built-in, innate, fundamentally strong Immune System. (Read more in Part II under the category "AIDS.") Then, you make yourself totally dependent on remedies from the outside, while everything you need is inside you.

Immunity is inside you: an illness, no matter which one, disappears — the body recovers naturally — if you take away the PSYCHOLOGICAL CAUSE. Your body indicates what has to be changed in your life in order to live in greater Happiness and harmony. From this perspective, illness is a blessing; but being sick is not *necessary* for evolution! No one has to suffer: you, as a human being, have everything in hand.

Insight and ignorance

Our deepest, or true, Living Self-Core, this immortal Self, is the wellspring of our existence. It directs our life. We may depend upon it absolutely, without anxieties. It leads us to an earthly existence if we carry that longing inside us. We are born *there,* in that milieu, with these life circumstances which best give us a reflection of our inner convictions or our expectations for our life. We are not born here or there out of a "conscious" choice: nobody, after all, would then be born in miserable circumstances. A sad environment at birth or a handicap does not indicate a "punishment from God," nor does it indicate a "Karma" that one deserved as a consequence of so-called bad deeds in a previous life. It simply indicates the web in which we are psychologically imprisoned. It simply indicates the convictions deep inside ourselves. If it's our conviction that we are poor victims or sinners, who are only allowed to suffer and do penance — unable to take their lives into their own hands in a self-aware manner, but think that life should be put into the hands of one or another god or of a Destiny — then we unconsciously choose a sad, powerless, slave existence. Misery in the world is the consequence of a shortage of Insight and an abundance of "Unconsciousness." That's why mankind has every reason to lead itself toward "Consciousness"!

The kind of life we are living, the illnesses we "get," are a consequence of our inner convictions and psychological patterns. In proportion to man's increasing consciousness of his responsibility, of his possibilities to create his own life, a new world can be born.

Life is no "coincidence." Nothing "just" happens. Yet nothing is "fixed," nothing is predestined. Science already knows that energy and matter are interchangeable; but it is forgotten that all energy represents "a kind of life-consciousness." The conversion of energy into matter actually happens by the inner driving force of this "life-consciousness" that lies behind it. Our body exists thanks to the inner "Life-Consciousness."

There is no hell, not here, nor after death, unless we create one ourselves, by anxiety, by our frustrations and by our negative imaginings. Illness and misery — in the world, and individually — are caused by the fact that we are cut off from our Living Self, from our imperishable nucleus.

Deep within us rage negative opinions about ourselves: do you think yourself inferior or bad? Then your Living Self will send out signals via the body (for example, migraines[31]), then it will also attract situations in life which mirror your convictions (for instance a father or a partner who belittles you).

Never condemn others. You have attracted to yourself, albeit unconsciously, certain people and circumstances that present a looking glass for your inner convictions. Change your opinion, your philosophy of life, and the convictions about yourself. As a consequence, the circumstances around you will change. What illness do you have? What does your body tell you about yourself? Did you, albeit unconsciously, call up a "fall," and are you stuck with a bone fracture? Then look hard inside yourself: you want to break out of something, you are rebelling! Etc. . . .[32] Discover the true cause.

The body is constantly being formed by the Living Self: if we trust in our Source, then we allow energies to flow freely, also the healing powers. Immunity means trust in our Source, which constantly holds growth and health. It means going along with the flow of your life, trusting in the Inner Power, in self-authority, taking joy in your existence, feeling love for yourself. Knowing that this divine nucleus, this primal urge for life propels us onward, again and again, in spontaneous creativity and unlimited mobility, leading us to an ever-greater fulfillment, consciousness, raising the value of our life.

A surrender to our Living Self, self-creating life, a balance between common sense, the rational mind on the one hand and the intuition and feelings on the other hand. Such a strong faith in immunity, in the possibility of having our health in our own hands, that no illness can penetrate. Fears disappear when we trust in our Self, when we realize that we can create our own existence; we will not Want

---

[31] See the chapter about migraine in Part II.
[32] See the chapters about bone fractures in Part II.

or Force happenings to take place, but we can call up these happenings in our life which are the best for us and for our fellow man. Take the rudder of life solidly in your hands!

Don't confuse "positive thinking" with "desiring in thought" or "wanting to grab"

It is self-evident that it is better to think positively than negatively. Yet, neither thinking positively nor visualizing positively nor looking in the mirror every day and saying, "I become better and better every day" have any positive effect if deep inside yourself there exists a contrary conviction, such as, "I know I cannot do that; I was not born to be happy; I do not deserve it; I am undoubtedly a nothing, etc." You may stand in front of the mirror as much as you want and say, "I am beautiful, I am strong," but if you do not solve the deeper cause of your sadness and your illness, and you remain convinced of "I am weak and ugly," then positive thinking has no purpose.

True creation happens, first and foremost, via the elimination of negative, unconscious convictions and expectations regarding yourself and life. This will enable you to create your life in a self-aware way, on a positive basis.

When you think positively — "I *must* and will have that job. I *have* to be accepted by this firm." — then you may think as much as you want, but if this job is not good for you at this moment, then you won't get it. In this case, don't force things! Don't desire (grab) with thoughts! On the contrary, it is better to say: "I am convinced I will find the most ideal job with regard to nature, time, content, and place," and the rest you leave open. No fatalism, but a positive creating, and being open at the same time to what is best for you. Yes, just open yourself up to everything that is being offered: you look in newspapers, you talk to people who don't simply appear on your path "by coincidence." For the rest, have faith in your Living Self, in your inner computer, which knows well what's good for you, and this is not always what you (Here is meant: the thinking, desiring "Little I") WANT.

Are you sick, then you'd better ask yourself: "What is the cause of my illness?" "Why does my Living Self send signals?" It doesn't do any good to scream, "I Will and Shall get better," when in the meantime you don't understand the meaning and the language of your illness. Listen to your body; ask yourself for a psychological explanation, and you will attract circumstances which are a result of your call to understand your illness. Solve the psychological problem which lies behind it, and your body will heal through the recuperative forces of your Living Self.

Also, concerning money and material possessions: it's of no use to direct your thoughts particularly toward this! Let go! Trust, and know that life gives you at every moment what's good for you.[33]

Create Your Own Life

Wish, long, produce thoughts, express your wishes, call it up, very consciously, and wait trustingly. Meanwhile, your surroundings alarm you when you go wrong, for you also have "attracted" these surroundings. Or, your body will tell you via signals or via an illness where you are wrong, for it is your living Self, which uses your body as "language." Do not resist what your body or circumstances tell you, and go along smoothly to where you feel your Self is leading you. Let go where you feel you have to let go: a sign that something new in your life will be born. Your Living Self, "you" in fact are it, listen to it; an ever greater Unity will result.

The melting together of Man and the divine in him will give rise to a more Self-aware being, who is taking his life and his body in his own hands. It will lead him to still unknown perspectives, to a new body, and if he wishes to earthly immortality[34] and exploration of other worlds.

Children

Man is born with certain expectations, certain anxieties, certain hopeful outlooks on life. Man will ever be born *there,* where he will find a reflection of his negative as well as positive expectations and convictions regarding himself and life in general. He manifests himself in his body in a unique way.

Children are no one's possessions, not the parents' nor the mentors'. They belong to themselves. Therefore, give them to the life in themselves.

Children are not "just" born anywhere. Their Living Self-Core brings/drives them in this direction, to those parents, in that milieu — where they will receive a good "mirror" in front of them. Here, with this genetic, basic material (which in evolution is susceptible to transformation), in this environment and these people as mentors. This is a point of departure on earth which the creature — be it unconsciously — has attracted on the basis of its convictions, its expectations regarding life, its nature. Life circumstances reflect what the child inwardly is "stuck" with.

---

[33] The true cause of "financial problems" can be solved "at the core," (read about this in *The Signal Book*) and doesn't ask for a positive "calling up" of money!

[34] Read more about this in *New Days.*

The baby, who is born with a certain psychological problem has "come" to these specific parents in order, via confrontation, to give at last a solution to its problem.

Babies and children are very easily influenced by, and very sensitive to, psychic signals which are being sent out, be it unconsciously, by people with whom they have close ties. Let us take throat infection as an example; we will find the same psychological cause, and perhaps will find it even stronger with the mother and/or father. Here, angry, powerless, fearful emotions should be resolved by mother/father and child. *There is no question of guilt here, for the child was born — with a certain psychic problem — to precisely these parents, so that at last, via confrontations, it can solve its problem.* The parent, in her or his turn, can evolve by comparing him/herself to the reflection that the little one is for him/her. Mother resolves, for instance, her powerless anger and thereby helps the baby and herself by bringing about changes in her inner situation via clear insight and by putting this insight into practice in her daily life.

One needs to emphasize *that the deepest cause of the illness always needs to be looked for in the psycho-emotional state of the child itself.* Although the stronger the tie between parent and child, the stronger the factor of influence from parent to child on the psychological level. The more independent the child becomes, and autonomically it grows, the more this factor will disappear.

Do we hereby ask whether the "system" mankind has created — the "bearing of children" (mostly going together with painful labor), bringing "powerless" beings into the world, beings who, if not fed by the parents, would die — do we ask whether this "system" is the most ideal? *Would it be better to create a world where there is no question of dependency, powerlessness, pain — ever and again starting "anew" on a quite "unconscious" level?*

House pets

Pets receive the positive as well as the negative electromagnetic radiations from their "master." They are very sensitive to the alternating changes in the emotional world of their masters. No matter if it concerns a dog, a horse, a bird, or a cat, they will be a reflection of that which is in disharmony in you. Does your dog hurt in his knee joint? Look in this book, then, under the section about the knee, and you will find the psychic causes to be present in yourself, as the master. A message from the dog to its master. Listen to these natural messages and make the necessary changes in your life. In this way you help each other. What has been said before about "children" can also be applied here.

It is often said that dog and master "resemble" each other; and that is so. It is not an "accident" that a pet with a specific character ends up with you! Yet, as with children, the CAUSE of the illness always lies in the being (the animal), itself. The master, or educator, never has any "guilt" regarding his pet's illness. He can, however, positively influence the healing process by bringing about changes in himself, as the educator. After all, it is not for nothing that he "attracts" the situation of his house pet having an ailment, as a "reflection" of something in him that is in disharmony.

Awareness and Responsibility

Our body, matter, exist only because of and thanks to the inner Power source, which can be considered to be the motor of our life. The individualized spirit which reveals itself in matter. It is necessary that we grow toward more self-awareness, to a stronger Faith in our possibilities, to unconditional Love for ourselves; that, like proud commanders of the ship of life, we know an immortal nucleus lies deep inside us, sending us signals when we deviate from the right course, so that we can redirect our lives, in a Conscious way.

We are not subject to unconscious urges, to unconscious passions, we do not let ourselves "be lived" . . . whenever we do not wish so, whenever, with the Conscious "I," we direct our deep natural feelings in the light of a future which we ourselves can build. We are not victims unless we doom ourselves to it.

The world will stay full of misery if we do not believe in our own creative power, if we keep on waiting for a rescue from the outside, if we keep on pointing the judgmatic finger at others. The building of a beautiful planet, without illness, without war, starts with self-investigation. To make others conscious begins with becoming conscious ourselves.

Be the master of your body: heal yourself. Build up the intense Love for yourself. Believe in yourself and be open to the *true* causes of your illness; be patient with yourself and keep going onward, full of trust; in the meantime bring about the necessary changes in yourself step by step. Life will assist you!

Building an Earthly Paradise

Life has placed "spiritual awareness" into "Matter," and by so doing has given birth to the planet Earth, to the Human Being. Thus, Life has established the basis for further growth — for possibilities which ultimately will result in a paradisaical situation.

The Key to Self-Liberation, Christiane Beerlandt © Beerlandt Publications

It is via the Earth and the Human being that Life wishes to develop and expand itself in the richest possible way. We shouldn't be looking for paradise outside the earthly spheres, in other dimensions, even if they penetrate throughout our earthly spheres: we as humankind are allowed — beginning with "Life in Matter" as the secure basis upon which we can build — to create a paradisaical sphere. An ideal, beautiful integration within our "I" of "spiritual awareness" and "physical experience" here on Earth!

Let us make an eternal Alliance with Life, everyone individually, making something supremely wonderful of it. Life counts on us, and we as human beings have the responsibility of bringing Life itself to further fulfillment "according to living perspectives."

Happiness lies in our hands: a possibility of "creating" given us by Life, crystallized in our Living Self, full to the top with faith and love-energy. In *this* person — who indeed attunes to "True Life" in thankfulness for his "Being," as "I." It's up to this Human Being to DO it, to work on the Building of a Paradise: in himself, on Earth. Don't wait for someone else, for "something" else. You, conscious living Human Being, believe in yourself, and do it! For Life, for the Earth, for Yourself, for all loving People.

Thankfulness: the Key toward Life in Happiness

And . . . have you lost your track for a moment? Do you not see the sense in things anymore? Then tune yourself to THANKFULNESS again . . . for YOUR BEING, because you are *allowed* to be a Human Being on Earth. Acknowledge your unique being, your worthiness.

In this vibration of thankfulness, Life itself will help you — Life deep inside you, because you have connected yourself again with this wavelength which *gives* life and brings happiness.

Therefore: *"Thank you, Life, that I exist, that I am allowed to 'be,' as 'I' on Earth!"* In this way the opening is freed for the flow of joy in your being, so too for the wonderful happenings which you will, and can, encounter on your path, "not just by accident," very soon!

PART II

THE KEY TO
HEALTH AND HEALING

**Psychological cause of
and solution for illness**

&

**Psychological symbolism
of the parts of the body**

A

VITAMIN A
Deficiency, insufficient assimilation of

Like a frightened little child, you psychologically draw back into a hiding place. You are afraid you can't handle everything; you feel powerless, unable to get a grip on anything. You experience yourself as a face, sometimes as a mask — content seems absent: "Who am I?" You suffer, and you consider yourself a victim. You are convinced that if you absolutely stood up for yourself, you would immediately receive a "punch" in the stomach. In fact, you feel sad and incapable. You prefer to follow instructions from your environment, from your partner, than to live from out of your own nature. Finally, having deviated from your "I," you no longer clearly see your life situation — your original goals — and the personal aspirations you once had. To be able to handle this life, to come to terms with your feelings, you produce extra energy: we are dealing here with a waste of energy, as it were, because you are not living from out of your own deepest source. A matter of Transformation!

Your batteries can only be charged by your deepest living Self, which functions as the highest electrical power center. In other words, recognition of your own worth and precious Content stimulates the production, assimilation, and storing of Vitamin A. Look at yourself! Don't flee from yourself. You are not small. Open your eyes to your reality. It's only your negative, self-undermining thoughts that waste your energies and nega-tively influence your life. Truth you find inside yourself. No one else can offer that to you: live from out of yourself! Do you no longer have a vision of your original self? Then stop listening to others, and stop trying to live according to the rules, demands, norms, and structures that others burden you with. By following sclerotic patterns that are rusted-stiff, you alienate yourself from your Self, which is ever and again asking for growth and enlargement. Direct yourself toward your intuitive source, and then you will really begin to "see." Look beneath the surface, and then you will discover that deepest living Self, an inexhaustible guarantee of Power and Immunity, psychologically and physically. A clearer view of your creativity — your creative possibilities — in order to bring about changes in your life circumstances, individually or collectively.

THE ABDOMEN

Psychological correspondence and Ailments, in general

The Abdomen: you open yourself wide to what Life has to offer you, like a wide-open Dish antenna, directed to the living space. You open yourself, in receptiveness, to that which Life wants to offer you. In thankfulness, in happiness for what you are "allowed" to receive. This pure joy, this happiness "to be allowed to receive" from Life is incredibly great. Here, the Revelation of Life itself can come in. Then you turn deeply inward and cherish the golden treasures inside yourself, which you have been able to receive from the womb of life. You cherish that which is most holy, deep inside yourself. You cherish your "you-existence." You only expect that which is beautiful, delightful . . . and you open yourself wide for it with the heartfelt, true *smile of happiness* on your face.

You don't want to "posses"; you don't grasp, don't want to fill yourself with people outside yourself, but you just open yourself to that from life which is most beautiful and continuously flows into you. You realize, you are conscious of, the wonderfulness you are allowed to be, as a Human Being. Without grasping, all that's good is given to you "by itself." The golden experience of Life itself, the experiencing of yourself in a positive, emotional, happy way, the thankfulness for this. You don't want anything more than this, don't long for anything more than this simple "Being," the existence in all Greatness, in all Simplicity. The intensely warm presence close to your golden Content. The Angelic Human Being knows his place between heaven and earth and welcomes everything that's beautiful inside himself. The abdomen is a wonderful power field, which — if the human being loves himself and life — bathes in a thankful, golden energy field.

Depending on the kind of energy — the capacity for openness and receptiveness and for cherishing the golden energy flow — your abdomen will have this or that form, large or small, stout or thin. Be yourself, in thankfulness. Don't make your content smaller; always open yourself up in receptiveness to that which Life wishes to offer you, and then experience the bliss of the earthly-heavenly existence, in happiness, with satisfaction. Your thankful presence, near to your being, your content.

Things go wrong with the abdomen (e.g. pain in the stomach) when you don't open yourself up to life and life's construction, but deny your worthiness, deny your content, and pull yourself down in a destructive way, placing demands on life, being ungrateful,

living in anxiety because you close yourself off from Life and Love and the awareness of happiness.

Don't close yourself off; don't destroy yourself; don't deny your inner riches; don't place demands on life; don't make yourself unhappy. *Open yourself wide to Life and be aware of your ability to embrace all the beauty that Life wants to offer you.* You actually give it to yourself as long as you open yourself up to it. Don't pull yourself down; don't doubt your worthiness; don't turn your back to life; don't say "no" to what life wants to offer you; don't withdraw; don't shrink.

Expand in all directions, from earth to heaven, and allow to come in what wants to come in, what can help in your life's construction — in the direction of Growth and the Awareness of Happiness because of your life as "I" on Earth, angelic human being!

Hernia of the abdominal wall

A "stop" sign on the path you are now following. Stop! To the burdens of a job, a relationship, a life situation — which actually don't suit you. Your strong "I" has too little grip on your life: you blow with the wind in a certain direction, although you feel that it is time you chose your life-course *yourself!* You work, or slave, along — with what goal? Emotionally, you are weak in this unauthentic life-situation. You steel yourself to hold out, because you feel weak and too powerless to build up your reality yourself. You do what is expected of you. Or you choose a job that lies within the expectation patterns of your parents, your teachers — but it doesn't really sit right with you. You take a partner and marry because that is how it is supposed to be; you express yourself in words or deeds with which you inwardly don't much agree. Change or revolt do no good, or so you think; therefore, you remain indecisive. You go on in this direction until an abdominal hernia tells you: break with or stop this! You have to live YOURSELF.

Be faithful to yourself! Don't bring yourself into a needlessly tense life situation in which you neglect yourself. Now, come into contact with your deepest Self. Step out of this illusionary situation and go in THAT direction which you sense to be honest, straight, and liberating. Come to true awareness of your "I"-worth and create your life from out of your deepest longings. No longer follow the paths of the past — they don't get you any further. Let go of the relationship that is not good for you; let go of a situation or function that only demands tension and pressure. Now, stand on your own feet and choose, independent of external influences, what is truly good for you. Then there will be relaxation, and you will carry burdens lightly, with a peaceful feeling.

Pain in the abdomen
Stomach-ache
(See also Intestinal cramps, and Abdomen, in general)

You are bursting with potential, but you don't see which channel to send your energies along. Anxiety — you doubt yourself, doubt the direction you have taken — you don't really get a grip on your situation and don't trust life completely. Afraid of "evil"; anxiety about "death." Afraid to do wrong.... Unsure, unsafe. What will happen? You see things mostly darker than they are; you expect ghosts or an angry teacher in your classroom. This takes your breath away; you can't go on anymore; your normal flow of energy is being broken — in nervousness.

Be awake and alert: in reality. But don't be afraid: believe in the Good and this will reveal itself to you. Realize yourself!
Anxiety creates phantoms, unrealistic thoughts. Stand with your feet on the ground, and in self-assured openness now allow your energies to turn in all directions. Become free and open, with creativity! No one can have any say over your life unless it is you, yourself. Trust the process of life;

only the facts and happenings that you have called up yourself will occur. Therefore, consciously become master over your life and build it in faith, with the knowledge of your possibilities.

Little children with stomach-aches sometimes don't feel secure enough with parents who live in anxiety and are themselves unaware of their human possibilities. If they put more trust in themselves and in the processes of life, then this can favorably influence their children's stomach-aches.
(See also the category Anxiety, and the texts about children in Part I.)

ABSCESS
(See also Liver, Anus, Jaws, and Teeth)

Tightly wound energy within a restrictive framework: energy produced by frustrated feelings and thoughts. You dare not — or cannot — let your positive energies flow freely. On the contrary, you often develop anger, feelings of vengeance toward others. You appear stiff or cramped to the outer world, while you dare not let your inner creative energies flow in a supple way. Unsure with regard to yourself, you suppress your natural aggression, and then you suddenly try to reach too far or too high. Too quick to get to the top, you only feel anxiety about falling off. Don't build a life that is a reaction to your own uncertainties or to the humiliations you have endured.

Don't spew out your frustrations on others, neither openly, nor silently.
Why prevent your own breakthrough? A breakthrough based on self-trust! Let yourself go, open yourself, liberate yourself. Systematically clear the way you wish to go and then proceed! Don't project things onto others. You, yourself, are the cause of your experiences. Step out of your dark circle of thought into the light of Joy! Active Self-realization.

ACHILLES TENDON
problems, inflammation
(See also Tendons, in general; Feet, and Inflammation, in general)

Inwardly, you feel too empty: "Who am I really?" Sometimes you feel just like a pack animal that is called upon to carry the burdens of others. "I am but a. . . ."

Your attention is distracted by minor business instead of by important business. Do you live too externally, too superficially, too much directed toward materialistic society, toward achievements? So, finally, you strongly question yourself with regard to the contents of your real self. Possibly, you appear self-assured in a certain role or in a certain position, but where are the values in yourself which are not bound to time or place? In other words, your true certainties. In fact, man has but one weak spot by which he can lose every immunity — when he loses contact with his powerful, divine Self. As a consequence of this feeling of emptiness, you might suddenly come out of your corner in a sharp, aggressive way!

Do you not acknowledge yourself completely? Then others also will only partly appreciate you. (Because you this or that. . . .) So you sometimes feel used and insufficiently appreciated, hurt. Self-doubt: you consider yourself vulnerable when with others.

Experience and live through your totality. Dare to bring your own feelings and opinions forward; respect yourself. Don't frustrate yourself. Determined self-assuredness leads to healthy action and creativity. Don't doubt your deepest powers, and live from out of your Self. Grounding! Don't get too caught up in details. Don't live toward outer self-affirmation, don't force yourself. Always stay faithful to your nature, to your feelings.

Stand, steady and autonomously, self-assured and immune, on your own two Feet! Banish false values. Be flexible with yourself.

ACROMEGALY
caused by excess growth hormone production

You are afraid to step into this life. You experience "being born" as if it were a chilly landing on the North Pole. You feel an immense, silent, sadness and pain; you are convinced that others will hurt you again and again. Many people suffering from acromegaly will "feel" left behind by, for instance, those who raised them, will feel deprived of all warmth and love, even if in reality this is not true: the cause lies in the convictions themselves and in one's basic trauma. You *let* yourself "be lived," dependent on others. You, yourself, don't get a grip on anything, and therefore you bite like a vampire into something or someone and cling to them, and so you go beyond your own structures. Out of fear of being cold and being nothing.

When you give yourself warmth, others will give you warmth. Draw yourself into yourself, don't drown yourself in others. Discover yourself, apart from others. Don't run away from life: come, finally, with both feet on the Ground. Others hurt you only if you are born with the conviction that "they" will hurt you. Break through this vicious circle. What matters is that you draw REAL growth into yourself, not only structural growth. Dare to fully submerge yourself in life. Now, quietly develop your structure and give your feelings and thoughts a free existence within it; don't cling to form and matter, let your essence freely develop now and direct your life yourself.

ADDICTION
(See also Alcohol, Nicotine, Sex)

Being addicted to alcohol, drugs, sex, ciga-rettes, etc., are but the CONSEQUENCE of being addicted in general. One is a Slave, one feels like a slave.

One is not Master of one's existence.

One doesn't experience oneself as a strong, independent, and free man. There-fore, one finds oneself addicted to having the Acknowledgment of others, to being loved by others — addicted to acknowledgment or attention from others, from society or friends. One doesn't really live FROM OUT OF ONESELF, because one ignores one's worth, because one doesn't give acknowledgment, love or attention to oneself. In this way, one makes happiness dependent on the behavior of others. One seeks for the Meaning of life Outside of oneself instead of, first and fore-most, giving oneself the Right just to be one-self — in Joy, in Worth.

One pushes oneself away.

Because one doesn't believe in oneself, one cannot (or will not) experience the Joy of one's own Existence: one flees from oneself into the Substitute — into the replacement of joy by a stimulant, such as alcohol, drugs, sex, trophies, etc.

In this way, intoxicated, one experiences Pleasure.
Just this "getting wrapped up in the other person or thing" is so stupefying, so seduc-tive; but it is Self-destructive because it draws one out of oneself: an Emptying effect until death. Yet it is a hopeful thing that this "longing" is really a Longing for Life, but one has the feeling that one will not succeed. Because there is this Longing for Life, there is also a solution for every addict, if he wishes.

Insight into the true solution is necessary: he or she IS able to realize this Longing, and FREE from one or another substance or per-son he or she CAN experience this Joy in Life — because he or she IS worthy, because he or she IS a human being who can be loved. . . .

Except: he or she should no longer expect anything from another person or from a sub-stance, and he or she will have the ability to finally experience his or her life worthily and joyfully, in an autonomous way.

When one resolves this ORIGINAL AD-DICTION, then the consequences of it — al-cohol, drugs — will also disappear. As long as one has not solved this original addiction, it makes no sense to stop drinking or smok-ing. If one works on oneself, however, by no longer having to be dependent (or addicted) on the approval, acknowledgment, or love of others, of society, or of a partner — and if one finally offers all this to oneself, stops one's self-doubt, then this self-appreciation finally will lead to MASTERY over one's own existence.

Here, one will enjoy the enjoyable, but will say "stop" when one wishes to do so. One will begin to create one's life oneself.

ADHD
attention deficit hyperactivity disorder
hyperkinetic child

Inner powers, emotions, natural energies, are constantly being restrained. You hide your-self, as it were, under a thick coat — a sec-ond personality, behind which you anxiously conceal yourself — afraid as you are to be overmastered by the enormous powers in yourself. The surface hypermobility is only an outlet, an escape from yourself. You ex-perience yourself as "split": On the one hand, feeling imprisoned in your own nature, experiencing yourself as vulnerable and wanting to hide behind a second "coat," you would like to slide out from under it all. This is because you feel unstable on your basis (as if at any moment your structure can collapse); this is also because you have no Insight into life, into yourself, nor into the how and why of happenings; and this is because you feel insecure and don't know at all *what* direction to take, experiencing yourself to be on unstable, uneven foundations. On the other hand, feeling oppressed in this situation, you want to escape from your own inner steam. You are afraid of these unconscious, sometimes strongly aggressive powers in yourself; you don't live with both feet solidly on the earth; you live in realms that are too ethereal, in insecurity; you don't trust your own nature. You constantly hold yourself back; you feel held back by others. Sometimes you would like to pull down structures, break through, but it is only a further escape *away* from your inner, personality essence. You feel unsafe, and you protect yourself by, on the one hand, hiding your deepest emotional powers, and, on the other hand, by escaping in all possible directions outside yourself. But none of this solves anything for you. Children who, in addition to all this, are being torn by an environment in which mother and father contradict each other, have an even more difficult time; but they have attracted this situation themselves, precisely because the inner division had been already present in them before. The insecure child will be on guard, inwardly aggressive, because it has no clear View at all and no trust in its nature or in life. Searching, fleeing, agitated; not daring to look inside itself or to stand still for a moment and think.

Such children have a need for a large psychological space in which they can experience themselves freely. Creativity, music, etc. — that which is being felt from within; tasks which are experienced from out of one's own Essence, with which they will be totally involved. So that they will find themselves again "within rooms"; so that they might discover the safe Basis within themselves. Searching one's own heart; a con-frontation in the mirror. Giving them the Insight that they exist firmly, safely, and securely in themselves; that they themselves create their lives; that safety is not to be found in the outer world; that they don't have to flee from the powers in themselves; that they don't have to "protect" themselves, neither against inner emotions and energies nor against the outer world.

Making an end to unreality: waking up out of the nightmare, out of things which are not there. Common sense and awareness; a solid concentration, in the body, of consciousness: this can come to be when self-assuredness, trust, and a feeling of safety are present. Taking away, via insight, anxiety about feelings, about life. Staying in the here-and-now, in oneself, so that aggressive powers no longer restlessly escape. Enjoying the sweet and the delicious, candy and beautiful colors; no restrictions in this area! Believing in the sweetness and beauty of life itself. The child needs to trust in that firm basis of its nature; no anxiety any longer about the Self and its powers. Freely surrendering to its nature and energies thanks to knowing itself to be safe in itself, thanks to daring to be unified and straightforward. On the basis of inner sureness, push through to the outside in a powerful, dynamic way.

*   *   *

Too great a power-pressure of spirit on body, of thoughts and head on the body. Enormous *"SPIRITUAL baggage,"* which mostly presses on your life with too much power — symbolism of the number "eight"; *content of thoughts which press too heavily and darkly on top of the physical body. Yet, those energies in the spirit/the head then all of a sudden do look for their "channel," their way downward;* a current from above downward, into your body, into the "EARTH," as it were. Toxic substances are also diverted downward. In a negative sense, it could be that you pollute or poison your total body with dark energies that are powerfully planted in your brain (negative convictions/thoughts).

It's often difficult to make a connection between head and body, as if you distance yourself from your body by a long, narrow connecting road (via the neck), *as if you consider the physical inferior "to the power of the spirit."*

It's very important to come to a complete *"integration,"* in totality, of your being, no longer placing yourself above or outside your body. To look at yourself *as an earthly human being, something beautiful and wonderful — and definitely don't distance yourself from material life, dwelling away from your body, critically and in cold arrogance.* Do you say "no" to your body? Would you rather have been born into another body, perhaps in a female, or male body, or perhaps into a more "spiritual" body? Perhaps you would have preferred to *stay completely in "the spirit,"* and not be incarnated on earth? Consider this well inside yourself and draw your own conclusion! Do you *really* want to live? Well, then this can only happen on Earth, as a divine human being in the matter of your body, heaven and earth in warm harmony united; then descend into your body in a loving — not in a self-poisoning — way. Don't spoil the atmosphere in the cells of your body which are begging for warmth, life, LOVE from you! Don't lift yourself above the earthly part of yourself but acknowledge the wonderful luxuriance of it: to be allowed to live, to be allowed to be from head to foot in matter, on earth! Turn yourself toward *that which is Good in you;* no longer turn your back to yourself, to an aspect of yourself! Descend into *your body,* down to the roots — in a heart-warming way!

Filled to the top with energies and creativity, which you actually keep under tense pressure inside you like a dark bomb — dark, because you don't provide yourself enough with friendliness and love and warmth. As a result, you perhaps expect this from others and look at them in anger when they don't give you what you desire. YOU WILL HAVE TO GIVE IT ALL TO YOURSELF: that happy, optimistic outlook on yourself, on your body, on life. Free yourself from dark energies and transform them into cheerful, creative action!! Sometimes it really looks like a bomb is about to explode: *a time-bomb which you yourself have in your hands.* No longer allow any time to pass; *don't allow dark emotions-thoughts-energies to ferment inside your being, in your intestines, your richly filled abdomen, but believe in the beauty of your human existence* and arrive at a rosy perspective on yourself, on life. In this way energies will be able to flow happily through your being.

Do you sometimes feel angry with life, because of yourself? Do you somehow feel disdain for that which is earthly, considering it to be "lower"? Earthliness is not at all "lower"! Without earthliness Life can't do anything: via your descent and your acknowledgment of the magnificence of the "earthly," of your physical presence, you will arrive at a way out of this labyrinth in which you have kept yourself imprisoned and from which you unconsciously want to get out! You have no single reason to cultivate dark energies inside yourself and keep them going; don't fool yourself. Every human being is unique and has his highly individual reasons to be born here on earth. Take up your task, your being, in thankfulness and you will see what noble promise Life holds for you!

Don't hesitate, don't tarry — stop defiling yourself with dark thoughts, Plutonic, deep black convictions. *Give, produce, only that which is lighter in your thoughts, and descend into your entire body with these happy thoughts and convictions.*

Perhaps you can't go on anymore; you are at your wit's end. *You would like to break out,* but you don't know to where. Know that the solution doesn't lie in ESCAPING FROM YOURSELF, but in the TRANSFORMATION of yourself, in a sincere acknowledgment of your being: you will find a treasure of gold in that inner world of yours, in the earthly body that is you. *Manifest yourself in full force and let the darkness disappear from your thought world. Replace it with lighter convictions.*[1] And especially: discover your HEART — love chases away anxiety and restlessness. Your HEART IN YOUR WARM EARTHLY BODY. Listen to that loving, angelic center in yourself.

Don't denigrate yourself; don't break down life, but bring your creative forces above water and do something with them. Create. *Do, at any time, that which you feel you have to do.* From deep within yourself *you know that life really holds "Light objectives,"* and as soon as you think, see or make things too dark or too heavy, you actually tune in to the frequency of death and lies. Therefore, bring yourself close to yourself, get in touch with your TRUE, happy, living Self. Stop breaking down yourself, life, that which is earthly, or other earthly beings, and lovingly turn yourself toward true Life inside you. Make things warm and comfortable for yourself; experience the comfort of being allowed to be inside your body; a wonderful, delightful happening.

Get rid of your feeling of *floating, lonely, on an endless ocean so very deep — and jump on land.* Look, YOURSELF, for Happiness: only you can make yourself healthy and happy! Leave that old alley, that dead end, and allow yourself to be born in a new form: *on EARTH in your body! Don't keep floating above dark waters;* leave that old sea and now CHOOSE life on earth. Say YES to it! *It will be wonderful, warm, full of love and light, sacred, delightful, and happy. Only then will you be able to find your inner rest. Out of this inner rest you will be able to go through life in a dynamic way, no longer feeling restless, because you no longer run away from complete integration with yourself, from a complete choice for life on earth,*

from demolishing the dark, spiritual power pressure. You see and think and feel: yes, here in my body, it's good to be on earth. *Walking with both feet on the ground,* realizing that a human being is able to create wonders as long as he chooses to be himself, in the powerful union of his spirit and body. Yes, you can do it; you only have to believe in it and do it.

Place yourself on the side of Love, of *giving* and doing good, not of desiring, "wanting to posses," doing evil. Only in this *atmosphere of Love* can you find *rest!*

Therefore, open your heart in Love . . . to an existence in your body; don't look down on yourself with power, nor on others, but live out of thankfulness for "being" on earth and for your specific gifts.

The feeling of "there's a dark bomb inside me which might explode" disappears like snow in the sun when you take away the negative, dark point of view that occupies your mind; when you stop floating in the spirit; when you replace the power grip on yourself (and possibly on others by asking for attention) by lovingly giving to yourself — by being warm, heartfelt, open to other earthly people, who in their own way all represent a marvelous aspect of Nature and Life.

Life is wonderful *inside yourself,* and Paradise can be established on Earth, out of light and happy convictions. *Therefore, no longer pile up inside yourself any emotions or dark, hateful or arrogant energies, but transform them into happiness, thankfulness, and respect . . . for yourself,* for that which is earthly, physical, for every human being of this earth who is attuned to life and goodness. No one is worth more or less than another. And you too are good: in your own way, as spiritual content unified in your body, no longer rejecting yourself or others in any way; not "drawing in" or "attracting" others. You now take good care of yourself.

---

[1] Read the symbolic meaning of the Grapefruit in *The Horn of Plenty.*

You have understood the signal of your living self-center!

Energies now flow freely, very joyfully and *constructively*. Your feelings are being directed now from your *warm heart,* from which you had *separated* yourself in the past. Now you discover that in this healing of yourself, in this love toward yourself, you no longer have "to fill" yourself with (or escape into) people or things outside yourself (like television, computer games, attention from others). You take care of yourself in a warm way; you give attention to yourself, present, close to your total body: there's no longer any distance between your spirit, your thoughts, your mind, your head — on the one hand — and your body, the earthly aspect on the other hand. You no longer poison yourself with dark convictions via the power of your mind. You call up your spiritual energies in order to let them flow through the Nature of your Body in a joyful way! *"White Master" over yourself, but not worth less or more than someone else — unfolding your energies powerfully and harmoniously:* that is beautiful and unique. You *create* new things, are in a state of *friendship* with others, without allowing any *competition or power and criticism* in your existence. You now exist as a *unified force,* in the Nature of your total being, loving and energetic, original and creative, *giving* and sharing with others.

You have driven out of yourself the "little devil" that powerfully poisoned itself in a dark and self-willed way, and have changed it into a kind of delightful, "holy enlightening love energy." The angelic human being, walking around on EARTH with dignity, doing good for others.

*   *   *

Your head filled to the top with brooding thoughts, emotions. You chew and ruminate inside *your head,* with your jaws, your teeth. You nervously, confusedly, insecurely, look for a way out, a solution, but it seems that you don't get anywhere at first. You seem to have to look for an *escape route,* because it becomes too hot in your head, and you are convinced that the escape route lies in a flight outward. Driven by a feeling of: "I have to do something, I have to work myself out of it." But you don't see that the solution actually lies in an inner reflection, exploring your own depths, no longer directing your head toward looking for an escape route in an "outward" direction. BECOMING AWARE of these things will transform the instinctive "hothouse effect" in your head ... so that you can find rest inwardly. Therefore, no longer run away from yourself. No more searching desperately, but contemplating "yourself" and all that accumulates inside you, and why. You will realize that all this isn't necessary, that you get nervous and excited by constantly turning your mind to that which you think you have to do, to seek, to find "outside" yourself. Let go of everything ... and turn toward your own wonderful depths: start to communicate with your own content, with your heart, your inner source.

What will you do? Sometimes an inner conflict; not knowing very well *what* to do, where to go. You are angry, but on the other hand you can't blame anyone: you have to lead your life and not expect anything from others; inwardly you unconsciously know this. And you want to realize yourself; you might be angry about your own feeling of powerlessness, being stuck and unable to efficiently go onward and do things right away. Nervously running in place: *how* will you do it? How will you realize yourself? You don't *see* it right away. You keep hold of a lot of things, store much in your head. You have a hard time swallowing things and letting go, because of anxiety and restlessness. *Holding on to things, not really daring to make the leap into life as "born as 'I.'" Also, and especially, because you are convinced this has something to do with achieving something or doing something outside yourself, with trying to get somewhere, having to "have" or to "obtain" something. The necessity for awareness: realizing yourself means self-contemplation and having self-esteem, inwardly becoming restful because of the richness in yourself. No longer wanting to flee, no longer looking for a way out: the SOLUTION you will find IN yourself!*

Unconsciously, there's a great need for "clarity," for *"clear insight,"* perspective within clear, structural lines, a cleansing of old passages, but at first you don't know how to begin, as if you are afraid to make a mistake by letting go, by going on, by purifying. You *can* go onward, but you don't dare take the step right away: because you think you have to make the "step" outside of yourself. A kind of stage fright which will disappear when you realize that you can find everything within yourself, that you have to make the big Step toward, and IN, yourself. That *there,* everything will become opulent and restful, that there you don't have to get agitated and won't "need" anything but this.

In certain cases you possibly sacrifice your "I" to circumstances, situations within family or social connections, instead of living first and foremost, once and for all, as "I." You keep yourself *"hidden"* behind a mountain of arguments, possibly behind people, behind family, behind drawings or whatsoever. These are only excuses for not having to spit out or swallow, let go, and go onward. Therefore, trustfully turn toward a new path and let go, with ease; don't be afraid, everything will be fine, as long as you don't bottle things up, frenetically holding on to things/people outside yourself. Quietly go onward and know that nothing will happen to you, that nothing negative will hit you, as long as you rely on your inner protective angel! Don't get so excited: you don't have to prove yourself outwardly at all; you don't have to achieve or realize anything for others. LET GO AND COME HOME TO YOURSELF. From this inner point of departure, where it's good to be, you will be able to unfold yourself harmoniously, in a

consistent and steady way. You no longer escape, no longer hide in *false behavior* in order to conceal your anxieties; *you no longer run away in a certain "behavior" that you "are" not (for instance teasing others, acting like a clown, etc.).* You no longer anxiously/nervously walk back and forth in order to not let yourself "be known." You know that you are good, that the solution lies in the acknowledgment of your wonderful being, of your trustworthy basis, and in letting go of everything in your environment. You as you, honest, straightforward, no longer running away from your *true,* reliable inner "I"-basis. Turn to your depths and bring out your feelings and thoughts in an honest way. Don't look for your happiness and fulfillment in the world around you, but experience the happiness about your own existence and *then* develop your energies in a spontaneous, lively, "natural" way: true, authentic, no wearing of masks, not hiding your true "I." You as "you," pure and original. From out of that fundamentally deep Center of Security that is inside you.

ADRENAL GLANDS

Psychological correspondence and Ailments, in general

Every conscious or unconscious thought, every emotion that moves you, brings about activation in the glands, and thus also in the adrenal glands. Depending on what mental or emotional experience you have, a specific change will occur in hormone production.

It is our consciousness essence which directs the body, and not the reverse. By bringing about a change in our emotional and thought world, we will find again a balance in the hormonal household that had been disturbed by influences of negative convictions. The adrenal glands, which produce several important hormones, are firstly a reflection of Balance (or imbalance) in the human being. Of the harmony between the so-called female and male — between the soft, caring, receptive being-there, on the one hand, and the active, self-assured, achieving power, on the other hand. Yes, to achieve an optimal functioning of the adrenal glands, one must strive for a balance between earthly physicality and spirituality, between the emotional elements and the mind.

An emotional or mental imbalance can be kindled by hormonal disturbance. This hormonal disturbance, however, was caused by your negative thoughts, expectations or emotions! The adrenal production of hormones will become disordered when your feelings, your thoughts, have stimulated it. (see also: Cortex, Medulla)

ADRENAL CORTEX

Psychological correspondence

Adrenal glands represent the feeling that everything is being taken care of, that you can live in a carefree manner. Everything is strong and sturdy; let us jump high and far with all our powers. Action! Manifestation! An active power of accomplishment, impelled forward by enormous, radiating, joyful energies! You believe in your own richness. In full trust, you go into battle for your ideals on earth. In flexibility, you blow off steam, flying like a free bird — peace and joy because of the soul-conscious impulses that can permeate you with happiness because of existence itself, which constantly grows, in Motion, outwardly.

Insufficient activity of the adrenal cortex; hypofunction

You think you are weak; you might hide behind clouds. You are not really here. You aren't really participating in life. You think yourself to be but a nothing, inadequate, impotent, unable to do much. You are unable to blossom like a part of nature, like a flower.

Self-suppression because of anxieties. Fear of deviating from "habits."

Suspicious, you feel threatened, on guard. Scanning things, seeking, but you don't fight; you pull back when there is trouble! Over-accentuation of Structure, form. Sometimes the sense of responsibility is so great that one fears one is unable to handle it; one compensates by building structures in an exaggerated way — at the expense of CONTENT! You don't trust your own content, your feelings; you retain your talents and energies in the bud, shutting them off. You sometimes experience a contradiction between, on the one hand, your unconscious longings — your natural desires — and resistance to your own nature, on the other! Thus, you put a "stop sign" up, out of fear of natural self-experience. In this way, not only are physical enjoyments hindered, but so too are an extensive range of activities. Eventually, you feel cut off from your body. An imbalance arises in the relationship between (more) spirit and (less) matter — being truly conscious in the here and now. In this way, energies cannot adequately do their work in your body.

Spontaneity; emotional unfolding; suppleness! Action! Handle your conscious energies with mastery, for true commitment in life. Feel the powerful presence of your Soul-essence course through every fiber of your body. Enjoy physical activities! Liberate yourself from anxieties and trust your deepest Self. No longer lock yourself up; come back, take part in life, on earth! Sincerely express your feelings: truly be yourself! (See Anxieties; Cortex, psychological correspondence)

Overactivity of the adrenal cortex; hyperfunction

Exaggerated aggression, often toward yourself; blaming, feeling guilty. Self-hatred, looking down on yourself. General anger. An enormous energy-development, exertion — often in a negative sense: just wait! You are panting, full of angry thoughts that storm your mind. You put your potential energies into the ground while you rant and rave in powerless insecurity. For the most part, you appear outwardly proud, sturdy, and strong! You safely put away your gentle interior: you are afraid of your gentler feelings. Because you dislike yourself, you might critique others negatively. Much pain, sadness, and disappointment lie hidden behind the bold mask of aggressiveness. Anxieties pursue you as if you were a wild beast.

Quietly take the time for yourself and for your gentler feelings: expose this beautiful aspect of yourself. Don't be ashamed of it. Don't be too hard on yourself. Look now to see what sadness is hidden behind your aggression. Immerse yourself in a sea of restfulness. At a steady tempo, develop your energies, your creativity. Realize yourself, without too much haste. Cherish the little child inside you, which you are. Be kind to it. Come to true self-trust, and not to a show of tinsel for the outer world.

Addison's disease
(See also Adrenal Cortex, insufficient activity of)

"Help! I'm being tortured and tormented; I'm being used and ground to bits!" Panic-like anxieties. "I want to go away from here! They are going to kill me." Absolute tension. "I'm just a poor victim. . . ."

Put a stop to your foolish beliefs: don't make yourself into a poor soul. If you stamp yourself as a victim, then this will be also confirmed by external situations to which you then can say: see that! Do you, however, consider yourself to be a respectable person? Then you will not attract sad situations!

Take up your total space as an individual and liberate yourself. Elevate yourself above all those inner threats and become master of your situation.

ADRENAL MEDULLA

Psychological correspondence

An inner flame which burns constantly and steadily radiates a quiet power. It gives assurance that nothing can happen: don't worry about anything. Threats around you? This can do no harm; "I am here," a quiet presence inside yourself — security, safety. Peace, balance, harmony.

Ailments of the medulla, in general

Profound anxiety, mortal fears, by which you might be overwhelmed as if by a heavy flow of lava, as it were, against which you can do nothing. Self-destruction: because of fears, you take on an aggressive, boisterous attitude. Especially in feelings and thought! You fell on your nose. . . . With an aggressive desire for power, you will get even with them! You are far too much "spirit" in your head, and too little present in your body; nor do you stand with your feet on the ground.

Very quietly, harmoniously, self-assuredly: "I am." Relaxed in your nature. Balance, tranquility, rest . . . grounding. (see Medulla, psychological correspondence)

AEROPHAGIA
swallowing air

Anxieties. You feel pushed back by an indefinable threat. You hold your breath, so to speak. Inner powers — creativity, aggressiveness, sexuality, etc. — are strongly developed inwardly, but really not fully expressed in your being. You hold back timidly, in anticipation. You don't really take up your space; you let your life be dominated by others or by a so-called threatening something in whose clutches you could become caught: this can involve very concrete negative situations which you dread, but likewise this can involve an imagined threat (imaginary illness, a monster, etc.). From an emotional perspective, it indicates that you feel as if you are caught in a chaotic tangle of yarn. It indicates insufficient self-awareness and trust in your Self. You allow your life to be directed by that which your anxieties call up in your head. You allow yourself to suffer needlessly. Do you think that "something" can take possession of you? Are you afraid of those deepest powers inside yourself? Do you think that something very bad lurks inside you?

*Allow that resolute, male power to break through! Acknowledge this sun in yourself. "Here am **I**." Don't give the negative and the anxieties the right to exist! Take up your space yourself. Allow spontaneous energies and emotions to flow through freely, and work with them in the building up of your life. Know yourself to be safe upon the extremely sound basis of your immortal Self. Nothing can happen to you, nothing is more powerful than you, yourself.*

Don't be afraid of these deep feelings and these powers in yourself; don't push them away, because pushing them away only leads to anxieties. Make use of these potential powers to create your own existence. Open yourself up to that inside yourself which is the most beautiful; know yourself to be safe, and feel at ease, in your living Self.

AGGRESSIVE BEHAVIOR, EXAGGERATED

You want to prove to yourself that you are the first, the greatest, the best — because you are not at all convinced that you have any value! In actuality, however, you condemn yourself for the most part; you are often very hard on yourself, an iron hand on the back of your neck. The exhaust valve is aggression. You feel anxieties and don't quite know about what, but you think you have to be on guard. You think you constantly have to take into account that something is threatening. As a child, you pick up these unconscious tension fields from your parent(s). You think you are allowed to exist only between these or those restrictive structures, which are pointed out by yourself or by your upbringing. Suppression of your full nature will lead to exaggerated self-manifestation or aggressive action when it comes to those whom you use as your projection screens. Aggression, often shown toward those who supposedly prevent you from being yourself. You develop an exaggerated type of aggression because of suppression of your nature and of your natural, spontaneous aggression. An expression of powerlessness! Do you consider yourself to be just a devil? Then you will behave like a devil!

Nobody limits you unless it is you, yourself. (However: silent quarrels, tensions, suppressed actions of the parents — the child will reflect this via a burst of passion.)

Don't suppress your spontaneous way of expressing things, even if you are angry: don't be afraid of this! Unexpressed emotions will come to an accumulation of energies which will finally burst. Don't be afraid of these deep emotions and powers inside you: express them, live from out of your nature. It doesn't matter whether you are first in line, but dare to be your SELF. Be milder to yourself, without prejudgment. You are full of energies; indulge in them creatively, as only you can feel it. Do you hurt others? Then in fact you hurt yourself at the same time. Do you feel so small and afraid? So fearful? Look now for contact with your own fundamentally strong basis! The real powers are inside you: because you aren't conscious of this or refuse to acknowledge these powers, you become aggressive toward others, powerless and (self-) destructive.

AGING PROBLEMS
(See also Part I, Physical Immortality?)

You don't really live from out of your heart, from out of your deepest Self. You don't acknowledge the authority in yourself. You live the way you are "supposed" to live; you adapt yourself to the norms and habits of society without really questioning them. You allow yourself to *"be lived"*; you don't direct your own life. You place yourself in a Role: you place the power, the Authority, outside yourself.

Do you worship a system, a being, a person, an authority outside yourself? Do you still know who YOU are, independent from the outer world and from your role models? Who are you really? A false ego, an outer Face? Did you live for money, image, accomplishments? Or do you not believe in the individual, divine power of every human being, of yourself? Do you emotionally cling to others? Anxieties, sadness, feelings of guilt, powerlessness. . . .

You don't dare to build upon the autonomous basis of your Self. You direct your life too much toward others instead of first trusting the security within yourself — instead of first offering yourself Love. You doubt that it is possible for a human being to create his own life. Do you live within the limits of a structure that is too tight and too tense, where no room is allowed for personal spontaneity, for natural impulses, for creative ideas? Do you just toe the line, wearing a wig to conceal your true "I"? You don't live from out of your inner being, but instead live for the eyes of others: how hard and unfriendly you are to your own nature! Don't devalue your individual worthiness any longer. Take hold of yourself and create your life in a self-aware way! Don't live tomorrow, but Now. From out of the now, let go of the past and the future. Eternal, youthful Now — be. To do this, it is necessary that you be faithful to your deepest Self; here there is no room for sadness and tears. Feel that power in yourself; trust, don't worry, because if you wish

to you can build up your life positively: a path which does not have to lead to death, to an unconscious state of being. Become master of your existence: what will happen is what you expect to happen.

Wipe away your tears, take up your scepter, cherish yourself in love, be proud of yourself, become conscious of your creative possibilities; no god or devil is more powerful than the divine Self of a human being. Transform yourself unto a higher level; don't ruin yourself any longer.

Consciousness powers feed your body. Direct them in a positive, rejuvenating way by being convinced that you don't *have* to age with problems. Your body will listen and will react to your inner convictions regarding your existence.

Joy and trust offer power and health; sadness and doubts break down! You only "age" and die when you are convinced that it just has to happen. Embrace yourself: take up your eternal space and allow "spirit and matter" to find *this* way that is necessary to seal an eternal living alliance. Surrender to the Now, to life, to joy, and know that you are Now eternal. Here, there is no aging, no death.

Growing old, in age, yes, but there is no question of "problems" accompanying this. The eternal youth! And the body takes on that form which the life within you thinks best. Don't attach yourself to the accepted norms of "how" a human being is supposed to "look": Nonsense! Just be yourself! Live from out of your Heart and be happy.[2]

AGING PROCESS,
HIGHLY ACCELERATED

You don't really participate in life, here and now; you float with dreams and thoughts to all possible times and places. You stand, as it were, outside the earth. With a panoramic

---

[2] Read, if you wish, the book *New Days*.

power of imagination, you are one time here and then again there; you flee and fly with your thoughts to wide spaces — without borders, so to speak — while you, yourself, are immobile here in life, with stiff and wooden feelings. Your energies don't concentrate in your body; your powers don't bunch together in matter — a spiritualized, Neptunian presence on earth. You are really so afraid to completely incarnate; fearfully, you seize the hand of those who take care of you. In this way, you will be dead before they or your parents die: a measure of self-protection, because you don't believe in your personal powers. You put conditions on life for you to participate in it, because you don't dare to stand on your own feet. You already dream about your death and your grave; you refuse to fully experience yourself on earth. You would rather flee to unearthly spheres.

Develop self-reliance, live for yourself, in independence. Know that your are safe in your deepest Self, in your Consciousness-power. Allow the spirit to fully live in matter: direct your body with your conscious spirit, become master of time, of your earthly existence. Build up trust in yourself here and now. Safeguard yourself — don't allow your thoughts and your consciousness to flee from your body again and again, so that it "runs dry," withers, and ages.

Give your body the protection of a spiritual consciousness, which makes itself complete master over the body. Feel your feet burning on the surface of the earth; open your senses to intense earthly experiences; feel your natural aggressive powers come through, and don't resist them. Dare to let your emotions come through, and outwardly demonstrate them; don't withdraw to a dream island.

Develop love of yourself. A concentrated participation in earthly life.

Allow the Mars powers to burst through and destroy the Neptunian dream-sphere.

It is necessary to experience the Space in yourself, to open your lungs wide, to inhale life in deep breaths, and to feel how your brain is being nourished by powerful consciousness energies.

The parents of such children should instill the conviction in these children (and in themselves) that certain "giftedness," or phases of intellectual development, are not bound to a certain age — for these children are often way ahead of their age in certain areas. In these children there is an (unconscious) conviction that a certain giftedness can only be used optimally starting at a certain age, so, in order to be in accord with their "talents," they create a body that "radiates" old age much faster than normal. In fact, these people live with an unconscious conviction that they can only use their talents to the utmost at an age which, "normally viewed," is not achievable according to the dominant conviction system. In this way, they bring death, as it were, much too soon upon themselves.

AGORAPHOBIA
fear of open spaces

You don't utilize your own psychic space; you find yourself unable to really live. Underestimating yourself: in the "field of life," you consider yourself to be less than others: unable to fully explore life joyfully. Fear of totally losing yourself ("Who am I?"): you hold on to something, mostly to somebody. You prevent your own "I" from fully coming through, you limit yourself. You allow yourself to "be lived" too much by structures, by the influences of (dominating?) loved ones. You feel you are being forced in a certain direction, and that you are unable to go in any other. You resign yourself to it, but the problem manifests itself via a phobia. Do you feel yourself to be powerless, sucked dry, lonely, without love? You were born with these feelings, and your upbringing confronts you with your deepest problems, which now have to be resolved. The space of your total "I," the experiencing of your inner Self, the Powers which are at the foundation of your existence and which always allow you to grow through all your lives, the ability to create your own Life according to your wishes — become CONSCIOUS of these things.

You are not an insignificant little pixie that just happens to walk here on this earth. First, there was your divine conscious essence, from which you have created your personality out of flesh and blood. Via over-accentuating your intense doubt, you have unconsciously attracted an environment to yourself in order to solve your deepest problem. So go and seek yourself and explore your space. "I am." (see Part I)

True love gives, does not need, is not dependent, but creates independence. So be good to yourself and build your life upon inner wisdom; feel safe inside your self. Begin searching for your deep inner Self, which never deserts you. Systematically build up your structures from this personal foundation, not from the views or way of life of others upon whom you were or are dependent.

AIDS
(See also Part I)

Your self-doubt, your self-negation, blocks your natural immune system. You refuse to wear the Crown of a worthy Human Being: you flee, as it were, from yourself. Do you perhaps feel a pitiful being, ashamed of yourself? You feel suffocated by, or cut off from your own emotions — a feeling that mostly was built up in your childhood. You condemn yourself. You feel you are bad or guilty. You will not or cannot experience your sun-center, and you possibly flee into sexual relationships to Compensate for your

own so-called insignificance. This leads to anxieties, feelings of guilt, and alienates you even more from your own Essence. Someone else can never fill your emptiness. You struggle with feelings of powerlessness; you feel suppressed or tied down. As a child you possibly experienced your self-authority as being very insignificant, subordinate to a more or less dominant authority. But don't look for the CAUSE (and solution) of your problem in situations from the PAST! After all, already as a newborn you stepped into life with feelings of Doubt regarding your own mastery and your own Power and Immunity. "As a consequence," therefore, in the past you attracted life-circumstances, and now "AIDS" (albeit unconsciously) in order to become Aware of this deepest cause! In order to deal with and end this feeling of Inner Powerlessness. Once and for all. Now, solve the real cause of AIDS! Through Transformation . . . not by stirring up mud from the past!

Humanity wishes to liberate itself from fear, powerlessness, and lovelessness. Through AIDS, one discovers that Trust in oneself, Consciousness-power, and Love are the true medicine for the psychological causes of misery in the world. After AIDS, the world can look completely different. With this remedy, one will cure AIDS. Medicine can be helpful, but no therapy or drug offers the TRUE and definite cure: the true vaccine is present in every one of us, except that it is not being used. Love of yourself. Belief in the power of your consciousness and in the healing influence on your body this will have. Don't block your healing process by doubting your possibilities. It is only because of one's conviction that AIDS ultimately "must" lead to death that this then happens. You recover from whatever illness if your convictions, your longings, and your Belief in your "I" lead you to healing.

Now, finally, be born in yourself: accept yourself as you are, acknowledge yourself, and warmly appreciate yourself. Cherish your body as if it were a small, loveless child who still has to learn to walk and to grow, but who this time feels *"welcome"* as a precious bit of divinity. Allow it to become conscious of the healing energies which constantly flow from its deepest essence. Trust this Self, have faith in the healing mechanism of your nature, and it will heal you — if you truly want . . . to live? Don't paralyze your immune system by rejecting your worthiness and your right to love! Considering the psychological causes of AIDS, it is to be expected that the illness was first found in population groups that considered themselves most discriminated against.

Free yourself, en masse, of the feeling of being victimized, and lovingly appreciate yourself, as a highly unique Individual with a specific nature.

(To resolve your problem, read also Part I, and the chapter about the Thymus gland.)

Born of a mother with AIDS

You came into this life as a baby with fears and sadness, with the firm conviction that you possess little worth. You don't know where you are going, and you anxiously hold on tightly. It was not by accident that this baby was born here. To solve its own psychological problems, the baby attracts (unconsciously) a mother with similar problems. If the mother comes to Belief in herself, to "I"-consciousness, and to a warm feeling of security in herself, then the baby will automatically also experience this. It immediately receives all self-healing signals from its mother.

ALBINISM

You have come into this life to deal with a negative emotional situation. You constantly have had the feeling that you are not allowed to exist. You have denied yourself too much. You think you have to flee. In your heart, you escape into a fairy tale world of elves and gnomes — for you have always felt like the ugly duckling. Small, at the mercy of harsh stares from others. You feel "strange" and "different" from others, you don't really belong with other people. . . . Therefore, you put on your fairy-tale clothes. You may also play the funny clown in order to camouflage your inner self-doubt. You have allowed your life to be too much determined by others. You have paid homage to the sad conviction that "hell is other people," and with that you locked yourself out.

Actively intensify your self-awareness! You have excluded yourself: your body is the reflection of your deepest thoughts. On the other hand, you bear witness to the originality of Nature: the rich variety of unique beings on this earth can only be fascinating. Everyone is welcome. So, don't close yourself off. Now, consider your outer appearance as a unique manifestation of YOU, and no longer as a manifestation of a "duckling" that considers itself ugly but as an individual person: "I live — with my feet on the ground — spontaneously, from out of myself, unique, authentic!" Not in ethereal realms, nor in a dream, but in natural Reality.

ALCOHOLISM

Lack of true love: you have to give true love to yourself! You consider yourself powerless, dependent, frustrated, worthless, inept, or inferior. You discard yourself like a used rag. You are born with the conviction that your aren't "worthy" of love, but as a consequence you may attract an environment in which you will know little understanding or real love.

You don't see the real sense of your life; you would rather lose yourself in a relationship, or in alcohol. Lack of self-appreciation: you feel too weak to build your life upon your personal basis, according to your specific nature. *You don't really live from out of your essence,* from out of what you feel inside. On the contrary, you live too much according to the norms of your parents, your surroundings, of society. You *alienate* yourself from yourself, from your feelings. You try to satisfy the expectations of others, but in so doing you betray yourself. This cannot go on, because you are YOU. No one has to satisfy the norms of others, no one is more or less worthy than another. You too little realize the worth of your unique being; you drown your Self in extreme *self-repression.* Feelings of *frustration* only become worse by doing this. You feel your are not able to exist independently, because you don't believe in the worth of your unique being.

Possibly, you feel enormous respect for people who, on a social or intellectual plane, are highly developed; meanwhile, you forget your own potential. Your "I" asks to be allowed, at last, to be acknowledged as an autonomous, independent being! No longer lie to yourself about being *Powerless:* you, yourself, ought to give yourself the love, understanding, trust, attention. You are your father and your mother. Your "I" cries out for acknowledgment and for love: give them to yourself. (Urge for *Power* and aggression are but a consequence of powerlessness and self-repression.) It is not alcohol, in itself, that is your problem, but the self-negation, which is at the bottom of the problem. Don't be hard or judgmental with yourself.

You must not stop enjoying the pleasant things of life. You can enjoy food and drink: when you resolve the true cause (this self-renunciation), then the exaggerated urge to drink will disappear. You don't have to punish yourself by discarding all pleasures in your life. Dare to *enjoy* the pleasurable without, however, *fleeing* from yourself! Love and appreciation of yourself will allow you to enjoy life without alcohol being an addiction any longer. While working on the "cause" of, and solution to, your addiction, it

may be useful for a certain period not to drink alcohol at all.

Mostly, alcoholics are sensitive people who — especially because of their sensitivity — are able to explore not only their rational qualities, but above all those areas inside themselves that lead to true wisdom: intuition, creativity, imagination, artistry, etc. Neither worth nor wisdom lie in a diploma nor in an important position with a lot of "external" authority. We often are dealing with people who are increasingly alienated from themselves in a society where they don't feel at home.

They don't realize, however, that it is not they who might have something wrong with them, but something might be wrong with society! A society in which people become estranged from their intuitive Self, from what they *feel,* a society in which value is exaggeratedly attached to things such as material possessions, outer accomplishments, etc. The alcoholic *unconsciously knows that he possesses a broader and richer aspect within himself;* he knows the solution lies inside himself, and therefore addiction is only an intermediate phase — the transition from feeling like a nobody in the world to the realization of one's unique worth independently of others. *Discover your richness.* First and foremost, you need yourself: *no longer run away from yourself.* Are you different? Then experience that difference. Every human being has the duty to listen to his unique nature. *Dare to trust your feelings, your intuition,* and don't cling to restrictive rational structures or to ready-made rules to which you believe you must answer. Let your true nature come through now. *No longer block your feelings. Live your unique Life to the fullest, the way You are, as a Complete Human Being. Don't hide yourself away. Don't try to meet the expectations of society or of others.* Acknowledge your inner kingship; don't deny your unique, human possibilities, by which you — with your sensitive nature — are perhaps much closer to the essence of true life than are those who outwardly seem to lead a perfect life, which inwardly is sterile. Experience yourself as being "complete," and then you no longer have to "fill" yourself. Acknowledge yourself as worthy and don't let any regulation hinder you being yourself: there is but one law of life, and it is called Love. When you finally *love yourself,* you will also be able to experience true joy together with others.

ALLERGY

Allergies, in general

Allergic to yourself or to an aspect of yourself. Allergic to your spontaneous intuitive energies: afraid of letting yourself go, of surrendering yourself to Life, to your Nature! Afraid to be totally yourself; afraid to totally experience your nature as you really are. Why do you not find yourself good enough? What do you dislike in yourself? Your nature? Sexual desires? Or do you not like your body? These, in fact, are consequences of an original dislike of an essential, natural part of yourself. In this way, you ultimately hinder yourself from fully enjoying all the sensory pleasures of Life. Your senses rebel and demand a complete appreciation of your own Nature! Possibly, you focus too much on certain things; you concentrate on a few points in your life and neglect the rest of your possibilities. Unconsciously, you blame yourself for this. It makes you want to cry! Because of the fact that you don't totally acknowledge your Self, you give more importance to the being of another — a partner, a child — than to yourself; which again can lead to irritation or to allergic reactions to the other (and vice versa). Or: you are in search of Shiva, or a guru, or a spiritual system or idol — looking for something *outside* of yourself. You live too superficially (above/ outside of yourself, as it were), and you

avoid the responsibility of daring to experience your personal life unto its essence. Being allergic means an inner revolt against your own superficiality or negation of your "natural, sensitive BEING," a call to come to TOTAL INTEGRATION, to come to an intimate reunion with your Feelings, your Heart, your earthly body, your true Nature.

Total self-acknowledgment and realization of all your possibilities! Dare to fully experience yourself. Nothing is bad or ugly in you: it is simply about your own convictions. Let your energies flow freely, so that no exhaust valve is needed. Go to the Essence of your being, go and seek your depth. Don't play hide and seek with yourself! Develop intuition and higher energies. Enjoy your sensual perceptions. Stop this self-blocking. Seek no longer outside yourself: discover now your inner richness, the beauty of your Nature, your wealth of feelings, your "body-heart."

*   *   *

Allergy breaks through: for too long you have grasped, held on to, things (or people) outside yourself; now you are forced to let go, to come *"close" to yourself.* You no longer can escape from yourself. You tense up: "Help, I can't come close to myself, let me hold and grasp onto things or people outside of me!" However: the sooner you let go of that which is outside of you, the better. COME INTENSELY CLOSE TO YOUR-SELF, INSIDE YOURSELF, and don't cry for what's not there. After all, sadness indicates that you now may come *to full acknowledgment of yourself,* that you may cherish yourself in love, that it's about time *that you find yourself, that you fulfill yourself with warmth.*

Do you sometimes feel like you're only a cold insect (with many legs so it can grasp things outside itself), like a *wooden horse* that has to carry burdens but can't enjoy its own "existence" on earth? Do you see your life as just being something boring, senseless, monotonous? Then this is precisely because you are *"cut off"* from your heart, from your "feelings," because you don't experience, or don't experience enough, *joy for your human body of flesh and blood.* Present inside yourself in a too cold and stiff way. Why experience yourself as a wooden board? You are not an animal, but a human being who is capable of experiencing true joy; but then you need to connect yourself with the vibration of thankfulness: thankful for your being, for being in your body on earth, for being able to live, without attaching any condition to this. Just "BEING" in happiness about Life, about yourself. *A total experience from your heart, from your feeling in your nature, in your body:* there lies the solution! An exciting happening: that's you. *And you connect yourself with the inner dynamics, with that warmth of life, with that happiness and respect for yourself, for your life!* Don't maintain an Ivory Tower.

Originally, a "refusal," a stagnation by holding on, not really going on; "No, I will stay here!" you think, like a duck that is brooding over its eggs. It *pushes others away with sharp needles (aggressive and rejecting). It wants to go on brooding and keep what it "has," while it would do well to realize that it has to come into its BEING instead of existing only by holding on and possessing things outside itself.*

Until it is forced to get up and begin to live itself, to let go and go onward.

A self-penetration, a self-destruction: if you don't go onward; if there is this stubborn refusal to let go of that which you are holding on to, and there is refusal to acknowledge yourself and experience yourself, in totality, from out of your heart and pleasure.

You won't get any further as long as you keep things and people in your *"grip,"* possibly with power — doing so because you can't get enough of a *grip on your own life,* because you are *not present enough in yourself (your body, your heart, your feelings). Now surrender* — *to yourself, to life.* Not

grasping and holding on, no longer filling yourself with things from outside yourself. Open up that grip and *offer yourself freedom. Let go of everything.*

Don't think you know it all, but open yourself up to information and take from it what's good for you. *Lead your life in a simple, natural — although masterful — way, without arrogance,* without pedantry, without wanting to tell someone else what he should do; *don't live from an elevated place . . . distanced from yourself.* Let go: come very close to yourself now, and the poison will leave you by itself.

A confrontation with yourself, which is meant to completely release your grip — and begin to discover, to acknowledge, yourself in the totality of your being, in *fullness.*

Allergy to bee or wasp stings
(See also Allergies, in general)

Instead of "radiating" your true Self outwardly, you withdraw within yourself; you'd like to slip away through the back door. With feelings of inferiority because you don't find yourself worthy to manifest outwardly, you'd like to escape — if need be, through death. You put others on the throne and push yourself away. Do you not fulfill the expectations which you, yourself, or your parents have required of you? Do you not measure up to the norms which society everywhere honors? Do you find yourself to be stupid or ugly? Negative thoughts about yourself poison you: spit them out. They are lies!

Values and possibilities are different for everyone. Realize your special nature, and radiate your worthiness, in openness, outwardly. You are blind because you don't live from out of yourself, but under the authority of others. Take off the blinders and discover your unique being.

Allergy to certain foods
(See also Allergies, in general)

You anxiously keep yourself pinched closed. You block normal energy-circulation. Nevertheless, you surge with accumulated energies. You are a barrel full of creative pressure and natural, aggressive deed-power! But you feel so tied down; "you cannot"; you feel restricted; you dangle there like a victim. . . . Allergic to a "complete life" for yourself, to "fully living"! Allergic to yourself, your full-blooded, earthly incarnation as an "I."

As a result, babies with this feeling of frustration possibly become allergic to the hand that holds them (sometimes too tightly). Often, too, the mother doesn't dare to completely be herself: babies then reflect this frustration. In this case, the above-mentioned causes — as well as the causes mentioned under the heading Allergies — also need to be solved in the mother, even if she doesn't have a problem with allergies.

Don't suppress your energies, dare to fully experience your nature and accept every part of yourself. Go on in self-certainty! Trust your Nature! Don't hold yourself back. Let it all flow through, these energies! Open space for the baby, and also liberation of the parents.

Read more about food allergies in "The Horn of Plenty": are you allergic to a certain food product? For instance strawberries, chocolate, etc.? Then, the food product is "symbolic" of that to which you are allergic!

Allergy to cow's milk

The cause of an ailment such as a baby being allergic to cow's milk lies in the psychological nature of the baby concerned. But often this ailment serves as a "mirror" to the parents. (read about this in Part I)
The text below is therefore directed to all concerned.

An aching for further, for more (outside yourself) . . . for a way out. . . .

Unconsciously, you feel locked up; you want to escape from a system wherein you experience yourself as a prisoner, escape first of all from yourself. But life forces you to stay on earth here and now, and prevents you from fleeing toward the clouds high above. You don't very well know what to do: descend or rise upward? A feeling of being "stuck"; rescue is being sought, a yes, a no. "What shall I do?" A doubt, wanting to escape but not knowing how. You still look at the world, at things too much from "the outside," not understanding, not being able to immerse yourself in things, to comprehend other people; as a result you can't grasp things at all with your rational way of observing everything from the outside.

A very strong pistil, as a center pillar, is ready to shoot up as a flower . . . but is still inhibited, held back, is forced to turn IN-WARD, to come close to its feelings, first going to its own roots. A feeling of suffocation is the result. You will have to come to the realization that you first need to "descend" into yourself, come very close to yourself, to your earthly body of flesh and blood, that you may/must stay within this established triangle on earth. Then you will feel free. And that is the purpose of this signal: that you come to the realization that you can make yourself "free" at all times, as long as this freeing doesn't mean running away from yourself — on the contrary, a total integration into your Nature, into your body of flesh and blood, brings true freedom.

So, no longer feel "imprisoned" in your own body on earth, don't force anything, stay very close in and near yourself. No longer AVOID yourself. Look at yourself, give yourself all the attention; love your body and enter it completely and lovingly. Come home to yourself, so that there no longer exists any distance between your spirit and your body.

Possibly you hide behind an attitude — even instinctive and animalistic in extreme cases — or in an attitude that has been socially taught to you. This is the herd animal, not the individual human being you are suppose to be! Possibly fixated on narrow femininity instead of experiencing in yourself, as a human being, the *primal female force,* no matter if you are born as a man or a woman. You ache and desire for things outside yourself; you would "draw in" things or people, but do everything but "become yourself in Fullness!"

Self-destruction; you constantly hurt yourself, as if you are mad with yourself, with life, with being the substance of your body. Arrive at love for yourself! Love yourself the way you are, unique and like no one else. Don't strive after social norms. Transform instinctive forces into creative loving deeds and leave that which is instinctive-animalistic completely behind. Go onward in healthy Pride about your Content, which places itself honestly into the Form. Don't follow that which is marginal in yourself, but place yourself in the center of your being. You are not a number in a line! You have to develop yourself as a Human Being; you are not an animal.

Do you feel life as a torture? As if you are placed on a torture rack? Then this is the result of your conviction that life is a painful affair, of the fact that you don't truly and consciously come to yourself, to your body, in love. Possibly you behave as someone who does penance, as an infidel, as a martyr. You don't believe (or not enough) that you, yourself, have your life in hand. You still look for salvation and rescue in leaving life, a rising up again in the mist of "nothingness." But Milk tells you: go onward on your "new path"!

Enlarge your space: rise up as a Human Being and realize yourself in all your broadness! There are no burdens to be carried. No longer live according to this conviction. Not even your body is a "burden." *Be grateful that you are allowed to be in matter, in your body on earth!* Don't turn away from it! Throw from your shoulders every "alleged"

yoke, every negative conviction regarding existence on earth, and come in love to yourself. Live according to the conviction that it is wonderful living … in yourself … on earth. Don't want to flee to no man's land, to the empty mists of death.

Get a strong hold of the reins to control that mass of energies in yourself; become master and turn the steering wheel in a new direction, full of self-assuredness, one direction … that of LIFE! You, yourself, have it in hand: therefore take a hold of it! Allow to flow from you wonderful, primal female energies that create and give birth; let it come out of you, let it be born out of you. Don't hold anything "back," don't stop anything, just let it go, just let it happen. Many products stream, as it were, by themselves out of your body. Get rid of the animal and allow the human being to know his/her creative powers. Know how to enjoy life in a wonderful way. Thankfully enjoy delicious meals, for instance, and surrender to this complex enjoyment of existence.

Yes, thankfulness, being happy that you are able to use all your senses in this delicious enjoyment, also of the little things around you. From this feeling of thankfulness for being on earth, in your body, for being able to enjoy what is there in existence … you will attract circumstances in life which will bring you much joy.

However, *from the feeling of discontentment and wanting to escape from yourself, from earth, you will attract situations which will give you the feeling of, "There's nothing doing around here; now I am not even allowed to drink milk," and so on. Therefore, first get into intense contact with yourself, in extreme thankfulness for your being-in-matter on earth, so that being allergic to that which "milk" symbolizes[3] can go away: don't flee from yourself, but incarnate firmly and full-blooded into your body and go onward on the newly entered path!*

---

[3] Read about the psychological symbolism of milk in *The Horn of Plenty.*

Hay fever
allergy to pollen

The allergy to your own nature, to your disposition, is being projected onto the grasses. You tie down your hands and feet! You keep yourself anxiously closed up, frustrated, but filled to the brim with possibilities, clogged up and bottled up, like a stuffed tomato. Feelings are being restrained. You don't trust your own nature, are afraid of it, or you feel inferior and don't dare show yourself or express yourself the way you really are. Perhaps, also because of fear of the reaction from the outside world.

The way you sneeze out the pollen, so also do you sneeze out your gifts, your nature, your talents. Are you ashamed of yourself? Do you think you are no good and have to hide your "ugly" aspects? Self-suffocation; holding in energies which want to come free. A feeling of insecurity in yourself doesn't only make you look for a hold outside yourself, but also hinders you from leading a new life. You hold on to an old pattern, to a system that is rusted, sclerotic, and too strong. Full of complexes, refusing to evolve. The way you are anchored to an inner pattern that is too stiff — in this way you also tie yourself to the pattern of the hay fever season.

Dare to experience yourself totally; acknowledge your content and develop your possibilities. Don't rust, but allow all energies to flow freely. Dare to experience your Nature completely, and no longer confine yourself! Accept yourself one hundred per cent and be proud of every unique detail of your specific being that can't be replaced by any one. In the first place look inside yourself for that which is beautiful, and no longer close yourself off. Free yourself from this

isolation. Explode, burst open like a tomato[4] in that full Joy of your Being!

Allergy to house dust
(See also Allergies, in general)

You consider yourself dirty, ugly, or bad. You constantly condemn yourself, and you want to force yourself into all kinds of twists just to feel accepted by others. You feel as if something dark is stuck to you, as if something unspecified, but devilishly big, eventually will drag you away. These are unconscious anxieties. You hold on to your emotions, sadness; you feel outcast, not good enough. Because of your inner self-rejection, people also really might begin to shun you; you are asking for it. Irritation and criticism toward yourself, and projected toward others. Often, you have difficulty respecting your body as a beautiful part of nature. Moreover, if you find that even some little piece of dust irritates you, then realize that you are extremely given to fault-finding, to critical self-judgment! Do you not love yourself, your body?

Accept yourself as good and human. Your body is also a part of you. Look with respect upon yourself, upon your nature, at your particular uniqueness. Acknowledge your intuitive wisdom. Get your feet on the ground and be realistic: you are the one who locks these elements outside yourself. Now, communicate in peace with others. There is a collision inside yourself. Nothing from the outside threatens you: you unconsciously fear profound feelings, which you suppress. Let your CONTENTS come to life, don't fixate yourself on outer forms! Allow your NATURE to live, don't limit yourself to structures. You can live life to the fullest, you are not dirty or bad: these are merely your convictions.

---

[4] You can read more about the psychological symbolism of the tomato in *The Symbolism of Food — The Horn of Plenty;*

ALS
amyotrophic lateral sclerosis

You experience your life as a path of penance. "A beautiful life? That is certainly not for me". You are convinced that nothing delightful is meant for you. You think others will hurt you, torture you, but in fact YOU are so self-destructive! You give yourself little or no value. Unconscious feelings of guilt cause you to endure a "punishment." You find it self-evident that others also would punish you.

Your life is built on negative prejudging regarding yourself. See clearly! Bring change to your pessimistic convictions, to these Lies. Where does this denigrating self-delusion come from? Throughout your life (or lives), you have built up "guilt and punishment" as a necessary evil, : "I, humanity — evil, worthless. . . . What sense is it to experience joy when we are 'evil' and powerless?" Have you, in this life, attracted parents who once again reinforced this philosophy in you? Punishment, suppression? Liberate yourself, now, from this web of unconscious Lies: every human being possesses goodness deep inside his Life center; because of a lack of insight and loss of contact with his own divine self, he began to be dashed upon the waves of an endless sea, no longer conscious of his origin, nor of his Ability to build up his life, to create — as he wishes to do. He therefore experiences himself as being powerless and fearfully delivered to the mercy of Fate or of one or another power outside himself.

Become aware of your own Power center: seize your life in your own hands. Your body listens to conscious impulses from your brain, to unconscious convictions. Therefore, expose suicidal convictions, putting them on the table, and give conscious orders
to restore your body. First, the thought; the physical form follows. Experience the joy of your eternal existence! Live according to the knowledge that your life no longer has to be a path of suffering, and that you deserve happiness! Your body will react to this.

ANKLE

Psychological correspondence

It represents the flexible giving of direction and the taking of new turns; yourself giving shape to your life — not letting yourself be dominated by others, but instead depending on your own Authority. Proving yourself, manifesting yourself independently, without letting yourself be too strongly influenced by others. Solid reliance on yourself, not on others.

Seeking your own way and following your intuition, your inner Self.

Becoming one with yourself, the rest that results from it, flexibly changing direction in your life. Because of an intense contact with your deepest essence, you are not afraid of your feelings.

No umbilical cord or other ties that oppress. Daring to turn a key, choosing a certain direction so that potential powers inside you are allowed to blossom. Bring out that which is most profound inside you; don't remain immobile.

Ailments, in general

Do you remain under someone's wing? Do you hide yourself? Are you too weak, too pliable, too yielding? Perhaps you have let yourself be sat on for too long, have let yourself be dominated by a powerful person. Or, do you keep on living, suppressed, in a system, in a job, in a direction that doesn't fit your true nature? Sooner or later, you will come to the end of your strength and you will blow off steam or feel cheated and will react aggressively! Perhaps then you will push others away from you. You have bottled everything up for too long! You feel cheated and tied down in a compulsory system, or by a person, and now you burst.

You explode; you will no longer let yourself be ruled by others, and you will begin to determine the course of your own life! Sometimes, however, it happens that certain people tyrannize themselves and, under pressure, push themselves into a certain direction or structure, of which it would be better to let go.

Cut all limiting ties; determine, in love and freedom, the way which is best for you! Don't doubt your own authority — your worth, your possibilities — and build only on your inner leadership. Flexibly turn in the direction that presents itself clearly as the only right new way, and no longer hold on to a stiff, old pattern. Ask yourself for advice. Bring about changes where necessary. Don't "twist" your personality (nor your ankle); feel the strong Essence inside yourself!

Edema of the ankles
swelling caused by
the accumulation of fluid
(See also Edema, in general)

You stay in one place, standing still: you hold on too much to old feelings and oppressive thoughts. You constantly worry, you go in circles fretting about things.

Your thoughts fixate mostly on the same matters: you hold on to this, no longer really coming to action, to mobility. You carry a cross instead of living joyfully. You sleep, sit, and rest; you brood and feel deep sadness about matters you would like to force.

Stop your limited thought-circles, throw open your life and trust! Dare to let go of everything and count on your intuition. Live, do, act, trust, go on, action — rise above the

narrow-rational. ***Feel*** *with your senses and enjoy. You are good as you are, don't run ahead of your time, and live fully in the now. Take another direction now: cast away all somber thoughts and needless burdens from the past! The sadness you feel comes out of yourself; outer circumstances seem to be the cause of your worries, but this is only a fallacy — not having to acknowledge your own Authority, not having to begin to lead your life in a Self-aware way. Without dwelling any longer upon so-called limitations, throw away this backpack, and go on!*

Experience the joy of yourself; sadness and worries will then disappear. Fix your thoughts on the essential, on life, joy. Somberness and self-destruction are lies. Love yourself and allow tenderness into your heart; let your feelings now flow freely. Don't block your life path with stupid brooding. . . .

Ankle sprain

You depend too little upon your own basis; you don't see everything clearly — what direction might you take? You go to others for advice instead of listening to your deepest Self. You feel yourself to be somewhat clumsy or stupid; you exert yourself for a certain something, but you aren't really involved in it!

"What shall I do now?" You don't know what to do with your possibilities, your energies. "How will I make use of them?" Too weak a grip on your life, too little backbone. Your own "I" is not present enough.

Stand up straight, come to a clear overview from above: you determine your life, don't allow yourself to "be lived." Choose your direction resolutely and don't allow yourself to passively just dangle there or be directed by others. Be strongly present inside yourself; realize your worth!

You place too much Authority in the Outer world, and often this goes together with:

"What impression do I make? What do they think of me? Beautiful, handsome, tough, perfect, adorable, quick, or exceptional?" In a certain sense, we are dealing here with an "exhibition," a show, in which you like to get a certain grip on others, so that they might approve of you, etc. Let's compare this with the following: you look in the mirror of a makeup box to see if you look good enough; you powder yourself a little where you think it's necessary: the mask that — according to your opinion, your norms — camouflages "flaws." You want to appear at "your best"! But, in the meantime, inhaling the powder takes your breath away: you cough and suffocate yourself, as it were, by fixating too strongly on the "exterior" of your Totality. You care too much about how you are supposed to look according to expectations you have adopted or according to indoctrinated norms.

"Mirror mirror on the wall, who is fairest (best, toughest) of them all?" In this way you not only immobilize yourself, but you also maintain power over others. You are wrapped up in the exterior; perhaps you dream away into the outer "ideal" image, into THE MIRROR IMAGE.... "How beautiful, how successful, do I appear to myself, to others?" You too much inhale, as it were, the stench of a world that is directed toward death, toward superficialities: the mask that crumbles, and the content that is denied and therefore cannot keep living. The MASK of SHAM asks to be removed for good; acknowledgment of your true "I"! Don't get wrapped up in your mind, in the dream, the ambition, in the achievement.... Don't imagine yourself to be the Prince or Princess of one Kingdom or another, because in this way you reign over a kingdom of death! The "layer of skin," the mask — the exhibition, the show, the achievement — disappears, and nothing is left over.

The sphere of transience, of polishing and making yourself shine, or of being the sportsman of the year, getting the highest prize for this or that, but forgetting that truth lives INSIDE you, forgetting that achievement and sham are completely directed toward "death," that there is a CONTENT inside you that awaits acknowledgment! You don't realize, or don't want to know, that in this way you place yourself on the death list. Fortunately, your Living Self calls a halt to this! Life asks you to turn inward, but you linger on the SUPERFICIAL EXTERIOR; this exterior becomes more and more a reflection of your inner self-betrayal, so that finally there's nothing left inside, and on the outside we can only see a layer of cellophane, neatly manipulated according to the norms of "this is how it's supposed to be" with regard to honor, (false) beauty, stupid achievements, etc. Doomed to die, because it has not grown from within, from the Heart. So: now choose Life or Death. Also, regarding sports or achievement at work or in whatever area, if you connect your happiness with achievement or with approval from an outer, superficial world, then you will be cut off from your Living Content, and life will call you to a halt.

BE YOURSELF, FROM WITHIN.

Don't for a moment consider how you look, how you are perceived, or how you must behave to appeal to the outer world, the public, others! Narcissus drowned in his reflection in the water. Don't want to be the first, the best, the most beautiful, the quickest ... because this is NOT LIVING! Now, IMMERSE yourself in your Content, your Essence, and know that *there* lives the real beauty, that *there* truth is to be found, and happiness! *Now, stand solidly on your true, basic center, your true Life Core,* don't build your life on superficialities, outer appearances, sham beauty, achievements, but *live from within.*

Break with death, which just wants to build a mask on the outside and forgets about the living content. Break with the cult of the exterior[5] and connect yourself with *the main*

---

[5] Read more about this in *Large, Beautiful, and Healthy.*

road of Life! *Take a radical turn toward Truth, toward the Heart, toward Content, toward true beauty, toward True Life! Break with everything that has to do with sham, superficialities and therefore with death.* It speaks for itself that with this inner Transformation you also have to bring about concrete changes — turns (symbolic for the joints[6]) — in society (work, family, relationships, etc.). But the most important deflection is still that from death to life, from superficiality and sham to truth — from sham beauty and achievement for the sake of others, to "living from the heart, in true beauty, from within, honest and straightforward." *Take a turn there, where you feel deep inside you have to turn: follow the sign called "LIFE."* What does this mean for you? In what way are you practically and concretely going to live a life in which every trace that reeked of death is now being destroyed?

Don't resist taking a complete *"turn"* when necessary. Very deep inside yourself, *feel* where "truth" begins and "sham" stops to exist . . . and in a consistent way bring about *changes* in your life. Listen to the truthful NATURE in yourself and break with every artificial pasted-up facade. The former leads you further and further toward life, happiness and health; the latter leads to decline. Which do you choose? *On the one hand, stand solidly in your deep roots, and on the other hand, supplely go along with what true life asks of you!* Don't offer any resistance to this; listen to those signals on your path that you yourself attract, and that ever and again make clear to you: there is the main road, in that direction you can make a step forward. Therefore, connect yourself well with this truthful energy in yourself, and comfortably glide through life. Don't be disturbed by what others say about you or expect from you. Live life on an honest basis, from out of yourself!

---

[6] Read more about the symbolic meaning of the joints in the relevant chapter.

ANKYLOSING SPONDYLITIS

On the one hand, you are full of pent-up aggression. In powerlessness and sadness, you would like to shake someone, as it were, or beat someone; on the other hand, you let yourself droop under heavy emotional burdens and dark thoughts: "There is nothing to be done about it anymore." You collide in communication; possibly, you appear distant or aloof, critical or chic; but inwardly you are fearful, emotional, vulnerable. To protect yourself, you take on an outward attitude that is too artificial or unauthentic. You doubt your goodness, rather believing in the blackness in yourself, so that you camouflage yourself and possibly put on a show for the outer world. You swallow everything, keeping yourself anxiously closed up; warm, powerful energies are not really being used; you accumulate aggression. You have the feeling that others don't allow you to evolve further, that they pull you back by the collar, but it is you, who don't listen to your nature, who don't give in to your true feelings. On the one hand, you'd like to crawl away fearfully, because you don't really dare to stand on your own feet, because you would rather hide behind a partner, behind a life-situation, and because you don't at all feel supported by your own Basis. On the other hand, you feel chewed up by others, like the core of an apple, so empty and so far away from yourself; the lack of power to be able to live in an independent and genuine manner leads to frustration, to inner reproachfulness of others, to difficulties communicating with others. You are afraid of that which is deepest in yourself — afraid emotions might overwhelm you detrimentally. It seems that a constant threat hangs over you; you trust neither yourself nor life. Heavy burdens weigh you down; you don't see a way out.

You would sooner give your attention to the burdens of the past than direct yourself to a new future.

Know that you are safe and protected in the warm stable of your deepest Self. Free yourself of those pessimistic, unrealistic thoughts: you are master of your existence; you are able to create your life according to your own longings. No longer look backward, but resolutely go onward on your path now. Surrender to your true nature; you are always protected inside yourself. Come to honest and open communication with others. Transform aggression into creativity. Stand solidly on your own feet, no longer doubting your powers and your worth. Productivity! Enjoy! Letting go of needless emotional burdens. Live from out of yourself, toward personal ambitions: realize yourself and don't follow in someone else's tracks; no longer block your progress! Self-manifestation, self-realization!

Self-satisfaction and peace within will lead to joyful, spontaneous contacts.

ANOREXIA NERVOSA

This disease receives ample treatment in Christiane Beerlandt's book "Large, Beautiful, and Healthy."

People suffering from anorexia nervosa have to solve a Power Struggle inside themselves. When, in their lives, they meet certain situations of "power-and-powerlessness," then it is the result of this inner power struggle. It's as if the wicked, cruel dictator in himself wants to kill the little child in his soul. Self-destruction.

Healing from anorexia nervosa means:
This person lets go of others and no longer expects any love or attention from them. He

now gives himself life and love. He nourishes himself because he loves himself. He allows life to be inside him. He doesn't make any demand on himself or others. He considers himself good and beautiful, the way he IS. Now, he/she doesn't want to assume power over others with his/her exterior, nor to use force to get attention for her/his little personality.

ANTHRAX
splenic fever

Compulsively, with aggressive thoughts, you are focused on something.

It *must* and it will be! Insane fury, sometimes vindictiveness, constricting your own neck; putting hard and merciless laws and structures on yourself (and sometimes also on others.) An extreme strictness, the voice of Saturn, an exactingness. Emotionally being fixated or obsessed: emotions take possession of your thoughts.

You don't dare to enjoy, or to experience your more gentle emotional nature.... Sometimes it's a question of a frustrated urge to achieve.

Turn yourself toward the child inside you; make bendable wood out of metal!

Look inside your brain content: to what degree have you been misled by certain philosophical lawmakers, by severe mentors? Why are you embittering your life? For it is you who has attracted a certain environment as a result of your inner severity. So don't reproach others.

Use your common sense in a relaxed way and free yourself from indoctrinations, which are a result of your own convictions.

Accept that which is gentle, warm, loving, spontaneously childlike, that which is natural inside you and let go of your obsessive thoughts! Find rest in yourself. In love to-

ward yourself, trusting your divine core, build up new ideas and live from out of your heart. No longer be so hard on yourself; live flexibly; become aware of this self-delusion and pull yourself out of that straitjacket.

ANUS

Psychological correspondence

To give ourselves the chance to transform ever further, it is necessary that we "let go" of the old, that we are thankful for that which has enriched us. Our experiences — that which we have taken up, digested, and from which we have assimilated the essential — now demand, on the other hand, the letting go of the superfluous in order to make room for the new. When we don't cling anxiously to the past, nor to things or persons from the present; when, in love, we produce our fruits and gladly share with others this continual growth; when we dare to say goodbye to emotions such as anger, anxiety, and sadness — because we unconditionally trust in the Authority of our Self — then the anus will relax. Letting go means, psychologically and physically, a virtuous liberation, especially after a period in which you have retained too many emotions and dark thoughts. This spontaneous liberation will then cause diarrhea, especially when it comes to an abrupt turnaround from tensely holding on to relieved releasing.

Do you anxiously close up? What do you not want to let go of? Do you inwardly feel so unsure that you fearfully hide your feelings, bottle up your emotions, poison yourself by accumulating negative thoughts? When you angrily stop up the natural channels by which feelings and thoughts can be externalized, aggression can turn inward and cause destruction inside yourself. Do you have a hard time letting go of something or someone or of a certain situation?

You don't produce in order to let your fruits rot on the tree, but in order to joyfully share your bounty with others. You feel steady on your foundation; you feel safely connected with the earth. You easily take leave of that which has been digested within you so that you can evolve ambitiously. Daring to enjoy the earthly experience. Or do you not dare to trust your nature? Can you not let yourself go in joy and flexibility? The old, the time-worn, has been burned; you again can give birth to something new. Surrender to your nature, so that there will be no question of anxieties, of tensions. When you come to a clear and broad insight, you will be able to more easily let go of all old norms, structures, and laws. It can cause you much pain and misery before you can let go of something or someone. You can stubbornly and doggedly hold on to things or people; a painful process of letting go. Or: you stand solidly with both feet on the ground; you believe in the Authority of your Self; you sow and reap, in freedom and trust.

Anal abscess
(See also Abscess, in general)

Hesitation and stubbornness, anger regarding something you should better let go of!

But with your thoughts you keep beating around the bush — you can't cut the knot, so to speak, nor draw a line between the present and the past.

Being totally stuck; with stiff tenacity, you fixate your thoughts on facts which you consider impossible to let go of.

Now, trust your intuition, let everything flow away. Don't stay put; resolutely fire off your liberating Mars energy and don't let a single fact, a single thought, dominate your life! Clear the way for new avenues — if you hold on to things, this is not possible. Produce, be fertile in thought and deed. Stand still no longer, open up and let yourself grow.

Anal chapping, fissures

You experience yourself as vulnerable and weak. You are holding on too tightly and are closed up — to protect yourself, to defend yourself. Out of fear and because of having too little faith in your Self, you refuse to solidly stand on your own feet and go on.

You experience the world as hurtful and hostile; you carry yourself as if you are stalwart and strong, but really you feel like a victim. To satisfy others — to be able to hold your own or to appear favorably to the outer world — you would strain yourself, would fit yourself into a structure that is too tight.

You are hurting yourself by holding on to a situation in which you don't feel good.

You may trust your feelings, don't be afraid. Let your own nature exist freely; dare to express your opinion. Evolve, slowly if necessary, at your own pace; expand your life broadly, take up your space calmly; your place is as worthy as that of every other human being. Feel yourself safe; relax on your strong basis.

Don't go out of your way to please others; first of all, accept yourself as you really are. You don't have to force yourself! If everyone would be in harmony with themselves, the world would be a paradise.

Anal fistula
(See also Fistula, in general)

You hold on tenaciously to things and people, you feel tied down and limited in your movements. You stay closed and don't totally reveal what you really feel; you stay partially hidden. Inwardly you feel anger, wrath, you believe in the wicked, in unconscious dark powers which also are to be found somewhere inside you — so you think. You fill yourself with black thoughts. You pull and suck things toward you, again and again, instead of giving and radiating. Dark remembrances of the past instead of cheerful projections of the future. Inability to truly communicate lovingly in the present.

Let go of your dark feelings and thoughts regarding the past and begin with a clean slate. Be convinced of the goodness that dwells in every man. Don't bottle yourself up, digest all your emotions, and express the way you feel. Discover the beauty in yourself, and then you will experience joy in true communication, then your bad thoughts will dissolve.

Anal itch
(See also Itch, in general)

You feel irritation, dislike, sometimes disgust, regret, anger concerning a happening from the past. These feelings are possibly directed toward a partner: maybe you feel aggrieved, hurt, or, for instance, irritated by sex without real love, or sex without your feeling like it. You place question marks on happenings from the past. Shall you feel guilty? Maybe you feel ashamed; you'd like to put on a mask so that no one recognizes you — You feel sad, nervous; certain facts keep haunting you. You don't have a very clear picture of it. You feel pursued by it. Doubts: Did you do right? New energies are ready to be born, even though you don't very well see which direction you will take. You intensely feel the need to let go of the old.

Show understanding, come to a clear insight in yourself; digest it, shake it all off and let the old make way for the new. You can but grow, evolve; concepts such as regret and guilt don't exist in this process. Don't doubt yourself; believe in your goodness; let go, and now go on, toward another phase.

Anal pain

You "tighten" yourself, are hurting yourself, because you think you deserve it. According

The Key to Self-Liberation, Christiane Beerlandt © Beerlandt Publications

to you, the past proved how bad you are or can be. You think it is too late to make good what you have done "wrong," and you willingly suffer punishment. Also, possibly, feelings of guilt tied to sex. You prevent your longings, your joyful nature from flowing freely. You prattle and talk much, perhaps, but in fact you keep hidden that which is deep within you. After all, you want to please or satisfy. Also, because of this, you can close yourself up too tightly and release nothing that you think will be condemned or will not fit into the framework or the wishes of a person who is dear to you. You have kept this up for so long — this self-punishment — now you can't go on like this anymore.

Open up, in friendship, acknowledge your inner beauty; "guilt" and "badness" don't in fact exist; everything is growth or resistance. Stop hurting yourself, and gently offer love to yourself. Don't constantly pour water into the wine; don't live for the expectations of others, don't close yourself off: communicate honestly and openly, take up your space, and express the way you feel! Only in this way can you evolve — and not only you, but also your partner, child, or friend. Be faithful to your own nature and let everything flow out freely from you.

Piles, hemorrhoids

Pressure and counter-pressure: a deep longing to liberate yourself from being "oppressed." You are afraid to swallow everything and let go: thoughts, emotions, experiences from the past, possibly also material things or a job. . . . Here, it's all about holding on to something that actually isn't good for you, holding on to something that stops you from further evolution. Perhaps you are angry or feel wronged — a negative energy conversion, which requires volcanic liberation. You possibly restrict yourself by holding on to values that are too structured, too

materialistic, or simply are external values. How are you keeping yourself prisoner? Which norms or facts prevent you from being yourself in all freedom?

Trust in this longing to be yourself without limitations! Let go, and stand in the center of your world instead of giving this place up to dark feelings. Experience the NOW in all freedom: let the past be a closed book. After all, there is no question of anything being "determined" by the past. Change your life, if you wish. If you feel anger, it's the result of your own powerlessness. You have, after all, unconsciously attracted into your life the situations or people with whom you are angry. Learn from this and go on, more consciously now. Let go of the thoughts and feelings which don't give you joy, and direct your own future, on the basis of new convictions. Clear the way that was blocked by self-obstruction.

Pinworm infection

You are bursting with productive energies, but you bind yourself and close yourself up. You allow things to be done to you, letting yourself "be lived"; you don't really live from out of your heart. It seems you put yourself behind bars because you don't believe in your real worth. You therefore don't show the way you truly feel deep inside; you'd rather wear a mask. You have no perspective of yourself; you don't get a grip on your life. Inner confusion of feelings. You stagnate in the mud of the past, not really open to new experiences, dragging yourself forward in the tracks of the past. Fuel is not really being made use of: Mars powers are being restrained. You experience yourself to be a wretch, doing what you have to do — your so-called duties — but you don't believe in your Self. You don't allow real, authentic experiences — no joy — into your life. You have the feeling that others could chew you up like a bone.

Powerful self-realization! Being conscious of your worthiness; knowing yourself to be safe and protected in your own being. Like a bull, barging ahead on earth, and putting the "enemy" to flight, away from your territory. Realizing the power of your consciousness; determining the borders with regard to others. Satisfying yourself; daring to enjoy beautiful and delicious things. Being open to new experiences. Transformation. A strong "I" makes itself comfortable, takes leave of the past, and builds a beautiful future for itself. Daring to confront yourself and placing yourself a step higher! Take up your space.

ANXIETY
(See also Part I)

Anxiety is a *"signal"* from your living Self-Center to stimulate you to come even more onto the path of LIFE, to make some correction inside yourself. In the first place: arrive at greater LOVE FOR YOURSELF (your content, your body). Second: BELIEVE in that immense power-center that is inside you.

Third: become AWARE that you have your life in your own hands (read Part I).

And ... don't live too much "in the spirit," in the head. Anxiety tells you to stay very close to your Living "I" Being, to your body on Earth.

You deny your personal mastery, the power you have over your life; you hope there exists something higher, something mightier outside yourself — even if it is but a rescuing angel that might offer you eternal safety and protection. You look for, or place, Authority and Security outside yourself. Of course,

you cannot feel safe this way, and you have anxieties. You are not aware of the central Power Source inside yourself — your always-trustworthy and always-present inner Essence, which can only grow and cannot be destroyed, not even after physical death.

The fundamental question: "I am, so can I also *not* be?" Those who only partly use their brains and who try to give an answer to this question in a merely narrow, rational way, will not get very far. You will find yourself standing out in the cold if you close yourself off from your deepest intuitive Self, from the basic consciousness that lies behind three-dimensional existence and constantly feeds our present body.

In the case of an airplane going up into the fog and the pilot no longer remembers his point of take-off or his final destination, it is evident that he will be anxious. The mist can be lifted by tuning in to your deepest inner Self and trying to see how your life develops as a consequence of your deepest convictions and expectations of life. Do you consider yourself worthless? If so, you will attract circumstances that will confirm this. Do you find life beautiful? And do you think you have the possibility of directing life in a direction that for you is joyful? The consequences of this conviction will not remain at a distance. Or do you view life as a stupid, accidental happening? Do you not believe in the devil, but probably do believe in Destiny or in a God in Heaven who will arrange everything for you? No. All sorrow and misery in the world are a consequence of humanity being "unconscious." Man is not aware that he, himself, does not allow the world to evolve into a paradise! This is because he doesn't believe in his own fundamental goodness and doesn't realize how he, Himself, can consciously direct life by changing his convictions and thinking patterns!

Does he believe in a new earth of peace and happiness? If so, then it will be there. At least, if he lives lovingly, according to goodness. Do you believe you will see Satan after death? Then you will see him. Man is able to create the objects of his anxiety. You can be blindly seeking outside yourself for some hold, afraid that at any moment death may come upon you. You feel full of sadness and tied down to an earthly, almost senseless, existence.

*Become aware of your possibilities, of the power of your creative consciousness! Have faith in your Self. Don't **let** yourself "be lived"; direct your expectations toward something beautiful and good and then let go of your wishes — don't reach for them. What is good for you will be there at the right moment. Via LOVE FOR YOURSELF, you will make contact with your deep, eternal Essence, or soul. You are a life magician who determines his own life when he but believes in his power of creation. Know veneration and respect for your Divine Being. Accept, in thankfulness, life itself. No one dies and no one gets hurt if he has not first pushed himself in that direction. Your convictions, your thoughts, and your longings determine your life, your future. Our earthly globe is not an accident! All matter, all living beings, are constantly being fed and created by the consciousness power that lies behind it. Why anxiously call up negative happenings when, with responsibility, action, and love, you are able to CONSCIOUSLY push your life and that of mankind in a beautiful direction?*

APATHY, LISTLESSNESS

You *let* yourself "be lived"; you don't really live from within yourself. You don't manifest yourself the way you really are, don't live consciously, but rather mechanically — following a role model, or behaving the way you are supposed to according to certain so-cial or family norms. It is simply supposed to be like that. You are cut off from your feelings, from your inner power source, out of which you could draw all your energies and life-motivation. Energies can no longer circulate. You no longer really believe in these inner powers; you feel powerless and weak. You doubt the worth of your life; perhaps you are of the opinion that you have to carry the heavy loads of others. You don't acknowledge yourself and just exist — You don't see the sense of your existence. Possibly, painful experiences of the past make you take distance from your own deepest feelings, fearing the anticipated pain. If you live in fear because this or that might happen, or because you don't believe in a fascinating existence that is without misery, then you no longer allow yourself to surrender to the full Life, nor to any feeling, nor to joyful moments in the now. Closed off from all emotions, you can no longer experience even simple happiness.

Have no fear of truly living! (see Anxiety) Tune in to this strong energy source inside yourself. Recognize inside yourself the play of passive and active. Confront yourself in the mirror. Respect yourself and take care of yourself! Arrive at Action from out of your longings, from out of your personality. Do what you wish deep in your heart to do.

Again make contact with your deepest essence and feel, experience, enjoy — with all your senses! Spontaneously play your life! Rediscover the earth beneath your feet, here and now, your nature. On the other hand, stimulate your brain: mental activity, your personal thinking power, giving form to life in a creative way. Come completely into yourself, seize life, and make of it that which makes you personally happy.

Again attune yourself to the frequency of THANKFULNESS for Life, for your "being" the way you are. Gratitude leads to pleasant sensations and happenings!

APHASIA

**inability to speak properly or
to understand language, due to
cerebral disease or damage**

Deeply buried aggression. Tensely retained sadness. Feelings of being sacrificed on an altar by others. Nervousness. With these convictions you come into the world. These manifestations, and also the attitude of others toward you, are a consequence of the original expectations that came into the world with you. Powerlessness. As a consequence, you would passionately like to possess, dominate, and have power over something or someone. You experience deep anxieties that your own foundations will be undermined. You feel at the mercy, as it were, of something powerful that comes from your deepest unconsciousness, something you suppose to be much stronger than you are. Therefore, you "grasp," hold on too much and for too long, and you stick, as it were, to people and things. At last, you push everything away. "I can't go on any more; I don't want it any more." Powerless anxieties. Dread of transformation; not trusting the transforming powers; fear of your own deepest feelings. You don't have a hold on it.

Trust your own nature, your intuition, your flexibility, and come quietly to yourself. Don't try to tensely comprehend everything with your mind. Experience this harmony in yourself; your personal terrain is naturally "safe," and built upon a fundamentally strong, central basis. No one can penetrate here without your asking for it. Nothing can undermine you if you don't desire it consciously. Don't hold on to anything; regularly let feelings go. EXPRESS your sadness, your anger, your anxieties. At last, you will see that these emotions are not based on anything but your distrust of your own deepest "I." The only strong basis, finally, is love for yourself, which makes all feelings of

anxiety and powerlessness disappear like snow before the sun.

APHTHAE

Because of fear of the reactions of others, because of fear of losing your safety, you don't say what you want, you are not what you would like to be. You don't express yourself fully the way you would like. Aggressive thoughts, sadness, nervousness; you are urgently in need of rest in yourself. "I just can't go on any more." You can't hear it any more, and you close your ears; it makes you angry. You are extremely sensitive, and you experience sudden nervous outbursts, which you immediately suppress. You take certain facts too seriously, because you have lost your contact with your deepest source. Your deepest inner Self is not afraid, is full of faith, but you don't tune in to it. On the contrary, you are afraid of your personal unconscious feelings, which sometimes seem threatening to you. Therefore, you don't let these intuitive streams flow through. As a result, you only play your outside role, anxiously. Sometimes, you even have the feeling that deep inside you are bad, or that you have done something bad: feelings of guilt. Inner collision: on the one hand, much repressed energy, many wishes, and an urge to manifest yourself; on the other hand, you don't trust your deepest Self, and you block the flexible circulation of energy toward the outside. Unexpressed criticism and accusation of others can be the consequence.

No wasting of energy, nor misspending of time: take things in your own hands! Action! Trust your nature, your flexibility, your intuition. The wisdom is in you. It doesn't matter what you have been branded with from the past: start a new life NOW, and realize your personal development. "Guilt" does not exist, but ignorance and evolution do. Your criticism of others is mostly your own self-projection; look inside yourself. Feel safe in yourself; stand up for your true self! Keep things in perspective; consider life as a process of growth and give your "I" all the opportunities. Externalize!

LACK OF APPETITE (FOR FOOD)

You experience yourself as being lost: "What shall I do now?" Not aware of your unique being, you feel like one of those so many people who are swallowed up in an endless mass! You let yourself be sucked up, absorbed — by your partner, your mother, your father, or your friend, by someone who is stronger than you are. This is how you experience it. This way you squeeze yourself flat. You idealize others and tighten the noose around your personality. You don't let your lungs breathe freely.

Sometimes you really have the feeling that this other one — or a certain life situation — holds you back from really living. It is, however, all about not acknowledging yourself, about underestimating yourself, about a feeling of inferiority — the feeling "I cannot live and they can" — about sometimes sacrificing yourself for others (which never has to do with love). These situations will go on for as long as you allow them into your life, for as long as you are convinced of your powerlessness! Others seem to have Power over you, because you refuse to place the power inside yourself. You push yourself to the side, you hurt yourself, sometimes uselessly exerting yourself, going against the stream, if only to get a grip on something. You punish yourself, don't allow yourself to live, keep on leaning against death. Sometimes there is even a mistrust of others because you mistrust yourself, because you don't acknowledge your warm, living heart, and you consider yourself to be bad and "poor."

Perhaps you seek affirmation in others, but as long as you fail to acknowledge yourself, they will not offer you true love. Don't allow yourself to be taken advantage of, but acknowledge your worthiness, give your deepest Self complete trust, and dare to live!

Know yourself to be safe and protected in yourself: for that, you don't need others at all. So, don't grasp at others; don't ask/demand their attention. The small, sensitive child in you looks for a strong father, a loving mother: don't seek them outside yourself! Therefore, allow yourself to flow in the direction your Living Self shows you, and don't fight against it! Take a strong hold of the rudder; you can go in every direction the wind blows as long as you don't fixate yourself on a handhold that is outside yourself. True joy flows into your life only when first you place the autonomy fully inside yourself, no longer dissolving into your surroundings or into others or into one or another philosophy. You are you, unique, on your own feet, independent, full of possibilities — Don't let yourself slip away; get a good grip on yourself and affirm your personality. Don't let yourself be eaten up by others any more, by vague spheres; also, don't parasitize others. Bite into "Life"! Bounce on its springs! Be aware of your value; no one can take your place. Stop underestimating yourself. Put all power inside yourself now and only surrender to yourself. Only you can truly take care of yourself as father, as mother, as teacher.

ARMS
(See also Skeleton, fractures)

FOREARMS

Psychological correspondence and Ailments, in general

How much do you open yourself up to yourself? To others? Active participation in life:

resolute action. Holding on/letting go. Balance between left and right poles (feelings, intuition — mind, logic; see also the category *Body Halves*).

Do you close yourself off in self-protection? From experiences? From communication? Or are you totally open and allow yourself to be overwhelmed by happenings, contacts with the outer world? If so, you might emotionally lose your balance! Can you no longer take it all in? Is it all too much for you? Let go; close yourself off a little. First build up your own solid basis. Only then can you powerfully radiate outward instead of absorbing everything. Only then can you welcome others without having them disturb your private terrain.

The contrary can also be the case. Do you hold yourself back from completely blossoming, and from fully experiencing and engaging life? Possibly, stubborn opposition, resistance; you writhe against it. You cannot let yourself go, cannot really relax or be open to totally new experiences. "I don't want to."

When it comes to arm problems, we often speak of an attitude of dubiousness: yes/no? What shall I do? Insecure tension; accepting or pushing away?

Are emotions running away with you? Does your self-awareness no longer have a grip on your emotional life? Or, on the contrary, do you think you have to banish everything that has to do with intuition and feelings? Balance is beneficial.

Open yourself up in freedom. A healthy self-awareness explores itself, others, and life. On the other hand, it does not throw itself away. Take care of yourself, of your innermost worthy "I"! Don't let yourself be carved like a piece of wood. Roll up your sleeves in order to do things freely, happily, and come into action. Let go of whatever hinders you on the way to evolution. Don't carry needless burdens. Give yourself what

you are entitled to. Give others what they are entitled to. Sway your arms in a supple way and direct your life in a healthy balance: give/take, feelings/reason. "Let the children come to me." Come to the essence of your life core, and that is: a joyful, loving, spontaneous game, like that of a child.

UPPER ARMS

Psychological correspondence and Ailments, in general

Protect, cherish, care — clasp to your heart, embrace — be able to contain.
The heart gives warmth, love; the shoulders radiate power, will, and self-awareness; from this triangular energy field strong energies of consciousness flow to the upper arm. These are the angel wings of a human being: the ability to protect yourself and others lovingly. The ability to rise above your problems and embrace everything from a panoramic level of consciousness and to know *what* to let go of.
More than do the ailments of the forearms, the ailments of the upper arms indicate that one tries too much to embrace, hold on to, pile up — and that one is too anxious, too unsure. On the other hand: resisting, pushing away, not accepting. Wanting to embrace too much, more than is good for you. Do you really, absolutely, want to add this or take that, too? Maybe it is to satisfy others that you take your task and responsibility too broadly. In fact, you don't trust yourself and the life process enough. Out of fear of not being able to keep your grip on situations or people — fear that something might escape you — you try to keep everything under control and therefore sometimes try to get too much power over people, projects, situations, etc. You in fact doubt your own possibilities. Perhaps you feel too weak and powerless. "It" escapes you. You offer resistance, and you are in pain. Does your feeling of safety stand or fall with that which you accomplish? Do you therefore want to get a medal? Is

your self-assurance dependent on the praise of others? True security lies in your Self! Don't let it be dependent on others. Because you give yourself too little credit, you might "fill" yourself by spoiling, coddling, caring for others. By doing this, you forget your Self. Self-reliance and independence lead to true love of yourself and of others. Otherwise, it is all about "need."

Perhaps here we are talking about fear of failure, unsureness, having to choose between two paths. Choose resolutely the path that is in harmony with your nature.

Do you push something away from you? Something you have had enough of? Look, then, and see if it is a reflection of a part of you that you dislike. Resolve this resistance and integrate. Perhaps you don't want to hear or see it; you shut it out! Look at it!

Dare to say No, with Willpower! Dare to bring your feelings outward. Be gentle to yourself and speak up when something is too heavy for you: let go. Never try to get a hold on, or power over, others, for that is but a sign of lack of belief in the power you have in and over yourself. Acknowledge your own possibilities. Direct your life, resolutely and calmly, from out of your heart. Give and radiate instead of attracting toward yourself. Trust in your deepest divine self drives away all anxieties (see Anxiety). Follow, quietly, your own tempo, without forcing.

ARMPIT

Psychological symbolism

Trust in the original powers of your nature. Enthusiastically, in self-realization, you bring hidden energies outward.

You go straight ahead, unhesitatingly, externalizing your intuitive or instinctive

powers dynamically, playfully, and strongly motivated to live.

One's inner contact with primitive powers — the economical, the cautious, the careful (the "female" aspect) — brought together with the active power — self-assuredness, the energies that turn outwardly (the "male" aspect). The place of meeting of that which comes to us from the outside with that which finds its way from the unconscious to the surface, to the outside.

Ailments of the armpits, in general

You force your nature; you absolutely want to push something through that is not good for you: you insufficiently trust spontaneous growth. In this way you are hurting yourself. You suppress these natural powers, your healthy, aggressive energy. Fear. Or you allow yourself to be led by primitive emotions, by the sexual, instead of you — in a self-aware way — leading your nature. You are too absent in yourself, or you are going against the stream. You refuse to follow the external signs which your deepest Self has called up in order to make you evolve further. You don't listen to your intuition, your nature.

Follow the signals from your deepest Self and flow along with the course of the most natural stream. Don't violate yourself; let go of that which is not good for you. *Don't remain closed up, but sing out your joy!*

Openness toward your Self, toward the outside. Know yourself to be safe in your Self. Do you keep yourself fearfully "hidden"?

You are *you:* calmly manifest who you really are.

Lymph node swelling in the armpit
(See also Armpit; Lymphatic system)

You cut yourself off from your nature, from your emotions; you don't really live here-and-now in your body. You float and think, fret and speculate in thoughts; the most un-pleasant, fearful, worrisome images occupy you. You don't keep yourself to reality now, because you flee *away* from that which is earthly. Unreal thoughts can distress you be-cause you don't trust your earthly Nature. You feel stuck in a situation or in problems with a relationship, but you don't realize that the cause lies inside you: that you are not *really* connected with your body, with your earthly being: you flee into spirit and thoughts; you are Afraid of your emotions; you think you have to protect yourself against them. Considering the hidden char-acter of your armpits and the primitive power current that is present here — which is con-stantly being supplied by your Living Self — these glandular swellings indicate in part that this primitive stream of energies and emo-tions is being suppressed by you because of fear for yourself and fear of those deep pow-ers and feelings in your nature. This also means a suppression of intuitive energies, of productivity, of female aspects in you. This suppression can lead to compulsive emo-tional outbursts or to sexual and other com-pulsions.

On the other hand, this all indicates con-cealment of emotions; you close yourself up, anxiously conceal your emotions from the outer world. This can lead to problems in a relationship. (Don't blame the cause of this problem on the relationship; it's the conse-quence of your inner state.)

You don't really believe in your own powers; you feel too weak, too limp; you would allow yourself to be hurt, allow your-self to be "intruded" upon by others. You try to shield yourself, but because you don't really believe in yourself, you cling to things and people outside you and remain stuck like a caged bird that dreamily gazes into the distance without progressing. Because you are afraid to throw yourself completely into life, to emotionally engage yourself in your existence, you'll possibly behave as if your emotions don't exist. Possibly, you hide them behind the shield of the perfectly spiri-tual, holy, or intellectual being — who ap-parently has no problems. Your emotions dwell under a glass bell jar. You don't con-nect with that original inner Source deep in Yourself; as a result, you don't allow your-self to deliver original, creative work. Possi-bly, you live like a parrot, or like an intel-lectual monkey. But, still: emotions and imagination will come to the surface without you being able to avoid it.

Enter the "earthly" realms: remain, here-and-now, with your feet on the ground, within space and time, without going beyond your boundaries and taking flight. Break down those barriers regarding your emo-tions, regarding others. Feel that wisdom, that intuition, the female productivity, the free emotional flow in yourself, and give yourself total freedom in this. Nothing about you is threatening unless you suppress your emotions for too long. No longer carry those worrisome burdens in your head: trust!

Build, in a self-assured way, your earthly existence; be creative, productive; don't hold back any spontaneous emotional flow. Ex-press yourself, free yourself, take that glass helmet from your head and come to open communication with your nature and in your relationships. Don't dream, but do! Let go of the unreal, of that which causes anxiety in your imagination. Feel those inner powers and use them in actual self-realization. Don't hinder the circulation of spontaneous energies; give free passage to emotions. Be close to your body. Be clear and sober in your thinking! Dare to trust in your deepest Self.

ATONY
sickly slackening of the smooth muscles of the intestines, stomach, uterus, etc.

You don't have yourself totally under con-trol: you no longer really direct your life from out of your consciousness power. You succumb to certain facts (or to life) in a fatalistic or resigned way. Your body is separate, as it were, from your spiritual being. You no longer really live. Nevertheless, you are full of electricity, energy; you feel uneasy in yourself, but you don't let it all come through. You don't express it. You don't take the straight path! You constantly look to others, perhaps with inner reproach. You'd like to force everything, change everything into different directions from the way they now are going. But the only thing you are really doing is accumulating feelings. Your energy, your warmth, are held back and locked up in a container that can give way under this burden. Perhaps you direct yourself too much toward the material structure of life; you don't allow the real warmth of the Heart to radiate enough.

Direct your energies with your Conscious "I." Draw from your power source, don't block it. Don't cast your light on others; allow the light to radiate out of you. Express the way you feel. You are bursting with potential powers; don't lock them up or direct them toward wasteful activities. Follow your heart and consciously build your life. Go straight ahead: overcome hindrances and go on with willpower.

myself to be nothing." Because your own authority is not yet recognized by yourself, you want to justify yourself, sometimes to excuse yourself to others, perhaps afraid that someone will point a finger at you or accuse you. Finally, you perhaps live only for how others see you. You want to accomplish something or to please others outwardly so they will confirm that you are okay. You want to be liked because you don't like yourself, and are even alienated from your Self. One often says of these people, "They are egocentric, pretentious," while in fact they are actually wondering about their "I" and are always searching for themselves.

Let your own character break through. Be faithful to your nature. Build your life on solid structures, on your own basis, not on those of others. Hold on firmly to yourself: what you feel matters most, not what others think or say. Don't be a slave of the norms of other people. Your life is good and beautiful if you independently build it up according to your convictions and longings. Pay attention to yourself! Being in harmony with yourself, without having to force anything, you will automatically attract those people who will be in harmony with you.

EXAGGERATEDLY WANTING THE ATTENTION OF OTHERS
"wanting to attract notice"

You feel locked up inside yourself, for you don't experience your "I" as being rich and self-fulfilling. Possibly, you then run away from yourself, nervously, from here to there. Though searching for your individuality, you still feel small and dependent. You don't find yourself one hundred per cent all right, and thus you look for affirmation from others: "Do you consider me okay? For I think

AUTISM

An autistic person believes too little in himself, *condemning* himself to failure. He comes into life with a feeling of being shut out, of being a marginal person, a beggar, an unrecognized artist who lives in an attic somewhere. Nevertheless, he is full of ambitions, talents — but the feeling of incapability and the fear of being *hurt,* cast out, or devoured by others, causes him to *shut himself out.* From the urge to protect himself he builds a strong wall around his personality. Inwardly, he is *fastidious, critical.* In his thinking patterns, he develops himself into a perfectionist; in his thoughts he is always busy realizing his ambitions, small as they might be. But he doesn't get anywhere with this perfectionism regarding himself, certainly not when he already feels himself to be so incapable: "I know I can't do it." When it comes to these *critical standards* he places on himself, he fails completely: "I am horribly bad and not worthy to really live fully." Indeed, others might only reinforce this. He locks himself behind high walls. In this way, he gets the *attention* he so longs for, and does so without being condemned for his bad aspects — for is he not sick and unreachable?

By being a mirror for the suppressed problems of the parents, the child can allow the parents to evolve. The parents can allow the child to evolve by not trying to flee from the psychological situation, but by resolving it in themselves. The *fears,* the conviction, that they, themselves, don't *meet certain requirements* in order to be good human beings.... The fear that the world is, in fact, an unsafe place in which to exist.... All the above-mentioned causes also need to be considered introspectively by the parents (*self-criticism, self-demolition,* etc).

*Hospitality, warmth, security: for yourself, for others! Anxieties are the reason a child doesn't dare to **truly** come out of his shell until everything is safe. At that moment, it is best that one let him come out by himself. An attempt by the autistic person to communicate — even if, for instance, it is only asking for a cookie when he has not had solid food for far too long. The turtle only shows its head when it intuitively feels it will be safe, that people will not consider him an ugly worthless being and crush him. Because after all he doesn't approve of himself, he is sensitive to judgment and criticism from the outside, and he hides.*

It is therefore of absolute importance that the autistic person can develop his special talents without hindrance or criticism from the out-

side. In this way, he can start to eliminate self-criticism and self-destruction. Without those who raise him having to go along in a kind of power-game that is being set up.

Indeed, autistic persons are often "specially gifted" in one area or another, but question their own worth too critically, even break themselves down. They give themselves, and also their surroundings, this lesson of life: *everyone may and must experience his own unique Nature without attaching "norms, demands, or expectations"* to human development. There happen to be several ways to be "gifted" that our Western society does not understand (yet). It is of extreme importance for the autistic person to know that — because of his unique Nature — he is "welcome and accepted." Being allowed to FREELY be himself, and yet still be "safe": still, first of all, he will have to GIVE this to himself ... and should not expect anything from others. Thus, he can respect his own Worthiness; thus, the "static" he has built up with regard to his own "I" — in a critical, disparaging, condemnatory way — can be resolved. Only if he has esteem for, and awareness of his Worthy "I" can he come, without fear, into Contact with others.

AUTOIMMUNE ILLNESSES
a group of illnesses by which antibodies are produced against one's own tissues

You should unburden yourself from heavy loads, let go ... but you don't; even if it makes you lose your balance, even if you might collapse under it, you still try to hold on to it. Even if it all weighs as heavily as a stone Menhir, you won't let go!

With pressure, with power and force, you absolutely want to push this and that through. You don't take pity on yourself. You oblige yourself: you MUST do this or that. You are actually merciless with yourself. You act like a hard, iron tyrant toward yourself. Possibly, you attract certain people in your surroundings — be it unconsciously — who stimulate this attitude in you, who hold a mirror before you because they, too, are battling with this psychological problem. But the cause of the ailment lies in you. You are mercilessly destroying yourself. STOP!

Now, become gentle and good toward yourself. You'll stop obliging yourself to do, to perform this or that, to persevere, to achieve. . . . Stop the PRESSURE, the POWER PRESSURE on the living child inside you.

Let go of everything . . . and learn to explore LIFE itself . . . in happiness about life itself . . . about beautiful nature . . . where "You MUST" doesn't exist, where no single flower has to satisfy the demands, the duties, and the enforced rules of a hard, life-crushing voice in oneself. Allow yourself to take on the same natural way of growth as the flowers in the field! No single tree, no single bird, no single person can blossom and grow up healthy if this hard, demanding, forcing dictatorial voice thunders in his soul. A flower that is forced to grow in this or that direction, to take on this or that form — because the voice inside it refuses to listen to its inner heart — will immediately wilt.

It's up to the human being to live in harmony with his feelings, his heart, his nature — and not force, not have ambitions for, a certain growth-pattern. It can be the "Striver," the tyrant, the unrelenting severe voice in himself that suppresses the natural gentleness of his being. With anger, hardness, severeness — grimness sometimes — man forces himself in this or that direction . . . and he will only be content if he satisfies these demands! He demands this or that from himself. The child in him suffers! His happiness completely depends on those demands and obligations he puts on himself, on the burdens he makes himself carry. But *true* happiness, life itself — allowing himself to live freely without the least pressure — that, he doesn't know. And no matter if he

has to achieve by pleasing others in one way or another — or by shining in one or another area, or by HAVING to carry the heavy burdens he has been carrying for such a long time, or by dieting in order to satisfy a certain physical ideal instead of taking in those foods his nature asks for, or by obtaining a diploma, or by doing duties and carrying burdens for others while leaving himself in the cold — it all comes down to the fact that he HOLDS ON to a way of living, to certain things that he knows he should have let go of a long time ago. He refuses to let go.

On the contrary: with an iron hand he directs his life, forces himself into structures which have a self-destructive outcome because they leave no room for LIFE itself. It seems as if he is punishing himself, as if he doesn't give himself the right to live if he doesn't live in THIS or THAT certain way. He does NOT LISTEN to the call of his constitution, his nature, but keeps on trying "to satisfy" — he goes on in a hard, sometimes merciless way. And if he attracts teachers/people in his life who seem "severe and merciless," or who crush every natural thing underneath an artificial structure, then these are only mirrors of his inner condition.

The cause of autoimmune illness lies in himself. He has the opportunity to totally reverse the course of this illness by completely changing his attitude toward life, by beginning to respect other values than the ones he has treasured so far.

The process of self-destruction can be reversed.

The human being calls out loud — so to speak — with lungs that beg for LIBERATION, for OXYGEN, for an "I! will LIVE from now on! And open myself to that what LIFE in me asks. I no longer do that which I made myself believe I SHOULD do."

Man will make open space for his own large, natural being . . . without complication . . . without attaching any kind of conditions to this. He allows himself to become happy without having to carry burdens. Man will have to choose in favor of his original Nature first and foremost; he'll free himself from the oppressing straitjacket of obligations, of duties and of carrying burdens. He'll push through with force from his deepest Essence and say: "I ALLOW myself to live . . . I no longer FORCE myself to blossom in this or that direction. I stand up for my true nature, which until now has been suppressed, again and again. I offer myself all the free living space. I throw open all the windows. I no longer crush myself; I no longer allow that which is most beautiful in me, my living heart, to be crushed. I no longer allow myself to live in this self-fabricated pressure cooker. I BURST open like a chestnut bud and THROW OFF EVERYTHING that, until now, I've pushed upon myself with power and force! Life means JOY, in the first place, and out of thankfulness for BEING I follow the most flexible path, no longer attaching any hard, ambitious urge to it.

I no longer refuse to let go of that which weighs 'heavily' on me. I become a loving, gentle mother to myself; I am no longer a hard tyrant with regard to myself; I no longer hurt myself. I now let go of everything. Hardened body tissues become soft. I allow my own 'I' to come through so that the cell tissues begin to regenerate. I no longer destroy the tissue of my own natural 'I.' I don't destroy my heart with hardness: I no longer punish myself. I now live with the conviction that I have the right to love, to a natural growth, and I ban from my life every POWER PRESSURE and 'urge for self-destruction.'

I allow myself to blossom, to BE, in the fullest sense of the word."

B

B GROUP VITAMIN
Deficiency, insufficient assimilation of

You live too much in the "spirit," in the air, instead of with your feet on the ground in the here and now. You are absent in yourself; you think that everything just happens to you, and that you cannot do anything about it. You consider yourself to be someone who has been hanged, someone at the whim of destiny, in the grip of people or of circumstances; you don't *truly* see reality, and the connections you see between things are out of proportion to reality. You might take things out of context and make big things out of small details. You feel anxious, nervous; you are not "aware" of what is happening. You sometimes experience life as if you have a rope around your neck. You don't trust your deepest Self, and you are trying to force things: you absolutely want to push certain things through, even against the flow — or against your intuitively knowing better. You are not really standing on your own solid footing; you consider yourself clumsy, incapable of.... For that reason, you might force things, for that reason you anchor your life in structures that are too narrow. Others tease or hurt you in your weak points: because you are unstable on your footing, you quickly feel hurt and angry! Reproach and constant stress. Your brain does not find rest. You become more and more oversensitive, and you no longer at all turn to your own powers; you feel inferior, or you are allergic to a part of yourself (to your body, for instance). You feel limp and can no longer partake in the joy of life. Your heart asks for more space and love, for recognition of your Self!

Put your feet on the ground, here and now, in your body. Be aware, here and now, of your power, your presence, your certainty. Dare to trust your living Self in flexible self-assuredness. Feel the balance between mental and physical experience. Be completely aware of the animating presence of your Consciousness in every cell of your body. Become conscious of your powers to create: you can direct your life toward your longings. Fate does not exist! Nothing happens by coincidence. You have unconsciously called up everything that happens in your life: now direct your life Consciously. Trust in yourself; fretting is not necessary. Don't take all your powers away by denying these possibilities! (See also Anxiety)

BACK
(See also Spinal column and Skeleton)

Psychological correspondence

Knowing yourself to be strongly supported within yourself; self-assuredness; flexible power; the proud, pure bearer of a beautiful Self-awareness. That strong aspect inside yourself that carries the small child; that aspect which, like a pillar, can also help support others.

Feeling yourself to be good and strong within your Self.

The spinal column: the freedom to be able to turn flexibly in all directions, a flexibility which is only possible through the feeling of safety and support within your structure. A loving pliability, a suppleness, to give to, and to support, yourself and others.

UPPER BACK

Psychological correspondence

Communication with ourselves, with others, in warmth or in coolness.

Protecting wings, as it were, with a radiation of power and love, protectors of the heart; a solid central pillar which carries our head proudly.

The upper back has a powerful capacity of carrying emotions. Processing, working out feelings: allowing your feelings to flow through freely, but still keeping them in hand. Making yourself master of your emotional world on the basis of the inner wisdom of a worthy, self-aware "I." Feeling comfortable in your powerful nature, in your body.

The intense presence in yourself: "Who am I? What am I worth?" Knowing who you are, feeling yourself strongly tied to your inner Self. That part in ourselves which pricks bubbles, which deals with vagueness, with uncertainties regarding yourself, regarding your relationships. A powerful contact with our deepest Self leads automatically to flexible contact with others. A clear view of ourselves leads to a clear, open relationship with others. Love for yourself opens your heart toward others.

How much do you feel protected and warmly taken up in your Self? Do you welcome others, or do you experience relationships to be a burden?

Ailments, in general

You don't warm yourself, are too stiff, don't really live from out of your sun-center; you doubt your worth. You long for love and for support from others.

You aren't really Open, not to yourself, not to others; you block yourself. Are you not really in touch with your heart, with your deepest Self? Are you unable to warm yourself with your love? Do you feel unloved? Or do you not succeed in truly making intense contact with others? Do you not have a perspective on yourself? On the relationship? What heavy emotional burden can you not work out? Tension.

Communication problems. Holding on to feelings, longing to be cuddled in the warm arms of love — but you are not really convinced that you are worthy of being loved. Do you feel lonely and cold? Being confused and powerless in yourself, you might sometimes try to seize power over others. In this way you play with fire. Guardian angel becomes devil.

Or are you too hard and too cruel to yourself? Do you not allow gentleness or love in your life? Do you live too much in your head? Do you neglect your physical pleasures? Know that others just react to the convictions you carry within you. Do you think yourself to be unworthy? Do you think yourself to be unable to share love with others? Then you create the distance between yourself and others.

Freely move, flexibly allow your feelings to flow through, without blockage, toward your deepest Self, toward others. Let the bow not be strung too tightly.

Dare to manifest yourself the way you feel inside. Be aware of your worth as a human being, and allow the warm powers to flow freely from your heart center. Enjoy life with your entire being; don't only live with your head. Open your arms, welcome yourself. Fly with your own wings, full of self-trust.

MID-BACK

Psychological correspondence

Represents the flexible undulation of our existence, the freedom to let go and to go on; an active dealing with impressions and emotions. We find ourselves to be spacious, very broad, when we dare to continuously evolve — when we open up our consciousness to all corners of our existence, to others.

Knowing yourself to be taken up in the All as an individuality; a safe feeling within your Self. Feeling yourself to be at ease amongst the mass of people; everyone having equal rights.

Coming to an overview of the multiplicity of details in your life. Mastering any situation, no matter what. Enjoying the panoramic vista you have when, in *self-awareness*, you gain mastery over your Life. An unlimited feeling of Freedom.

Ailments, in general

You hold on to the past; you go around in circles. You fixate your thoughts on facts that are long gone. Emotions are not being worked out — on the contrary, you blow them out of proportion; you keep on brooding. You get angry.

An indefinable feeling of anxiety; sometimes you feel pushed away by others, but in fact it is you who pushes others away from you. Sometimes your conscience gnaws at you, and you cannot forgive yourself for certain matters. At other times you impatiently and irritably turn against others. You stagnate your own evolution, refuse to go on, imprison yourself. You feel threatened.

Don't hold yourself back any longer, and let go of everything from the past. Everyone needs experiences to learn lessons from them; but if you get stuck emotionally on certain facts, then you ravage your health. Unload, let the air out, purify yourself, go on! Feel yourself to be warmly taken up among people and offer them the warmth of your heart. No longer feel threatened and fearful; you are good as you are, safe in your deepest Self. Free yourself from this suffocating atmosphere, be gentle to yourself, and place yourself above every situation in life, like a Master. In a self-aware way create a new, original life. Allow your feelings to flow freely, feel yourself relax, and come to

restfulness. Let it all slide off your back. Live in the here-and-now; look farther and enjoy the broad space inside yourself, your possibilities for self-development. Action! Self-liberation. Take your opportunity and your right to begin again, today. Drink from the cup of peace!

LOWER BACK

Psychological correspondence

The primally strong Basis lies within your Self.

The belief and trust in your inner power center, your deepest Self, allows a powerful fire — an orange-red energy as it were — to radiate and rise within your total being: *"I" am.*

The proud presence in your body, the absolute feeling of safety.

Independence, self-assurance, standing sturdily with both feet on the ground.

Transformation of primal powers and emotions into higher consciousness. Peace and security in the sanctuary of your inner self.

Ailments, in general

Is your fundamental feeling bad? Are you convinced that you are bad or devilish? That you cannot trust your nature? Are you afraid of that which is deepest inside yourself? Anxiety. You look to others for refuge. You cling to your mother or to friends, to matter or to outer appearances. Your existence, your security, stands or falls depending on these secondary things. You ignore your own Basis.

Money worries, the loss of a friend, of material things, no acknowledgment in your work, not being admired for your outer appearance or for your productivity: this can lead to complaints of the lower back. You place certainty outside yourself.

You conceal yourself; you don't dare let your sun, your self-certain "I," radiate; you feel small, insecure, attached; you ignore your worth — you are not proud of yourself at all. Because of your self-doubt, you block powerful creative energies. Then again, you can get angry because of this feeling of attachment and insecurity.

Emotions can pile up; possibly, you defend yourself in a very aggressive way because you feel threatened. You give others too much power. Do you feel hurt in your weak spot? Do you feel hit on your insecure point?

Because you don't really depend on yourself, do you anxiously flee from certain situations?

Don't be afraid any longer; don't doubt yourself. Don't doubt your worth; let powerful energies flow through freely. Don't block your self-realization. Flexibly deal with your emotions. Know yourself to be safe and protected in your deepest Self. Feel this primal, strong Basis; say goodbye to the old. Resolutely build a new life, in full self-trust. Be proud of your unique being, develop your possibilities. Don't let yourself be intimidated by others. Believe in your Living Self and make use of the possibility of *Self-creating* your existence. Your happiness and your safety don't depend on factors from the outer world! Be faithful to your nature and dare to be yourself, without hesitation. Care for yourself; don't always ask another, but listen to your inner voice.

Don't sit still, don't stand still in evolution — don't look backward: continue onward and develop all your talents.

BEDWETTING

Anxiety, a feeling of powerlessness and helplessness, fear that something or someone stronger and bigger than you will crush you. No faith in your Basis. In certain situations this can indicate a fear of the strong authoritarian power of parents or mentors. But, essentially, we are dealing here with one's own dismal feeling of not being safe; fear of the

jungle, of chaos — where all perspective and frameworks are lost; in other words, you feel your Self to be so insignificant and defenseless. You are in a dark tunnel and don't know where you are going. You are like a small bird in a wooden cage, feeling imprisoned, looking up in awe at totem poles outside yourself, but suspecting that at any moment this authority can hurt you and gain power over you. Of course, you become extremely sensitive to punishments and other restrictions. You trust too little the power of your own identity. Delusions and anxious fantasies only make things worse now. A child, in its purity, strongly experiences it when parents grasp for power in order to obscure their own powerlessness: the child mostly reacts to the anxieties of the parents. When the parent liberates himself or herself, then the child will be positively influenced by this. A tense daytime life leads to a relaxed outlet during sleep: a letting go of negative, soiled, accumulated emotions. . . . It's a good thing that this negativity can be eliminated.

First of all, put the child at ease: it is good that nature eliminates its sadness and pent-up tensions, like dirty smoke through an exhaust pipe. Don't place a "warning device" in the bed of the little one: by doing that you play ostrich and only heighten the tension. If the child is already able to comprehend a little, then talk about it. Tell him that fathers are not powerful bosses (if need be, adjust your attitude as parents), say also that the teacher in school is unable to trample, destroy or threaten the Powerful little Soul in the child — the Soul which ever and always grows and is safe in himself. Tell him that he may peacefully trust the inner Angel-core that lives INSIDE him — his divine leader, who will guide him in every way, even if he, himself, does not yet see a solution.

Don't tell him about God high above him, one who is yet another boss, but tell him about the extremely strong "I" within him, which is just as strong as the "I" within his father. Tell him parents are here to offer love and to guide in this love: to help him see clearly, help him share with others, help him to take up his responsibility so that later on he will be able to live among people as a joyful human being. The child longs for a safe haven where there is calm, security, peace, and gentleness. It is necessary that parents resolve their anxieties. The real feeling of loneliness can only be resolved by the child through grasping the small reins and directing himself toward a real goal, small as it may be, and by feeling himself to be peaceful and safe upon his own basis. The warmth in himself. Optimistic joy of life for parents and child! Do. Realize plans. Powerfully go onward, Action; don't sit and fret about unreal things; create your life, seize it!

BERIBERI

A strong longing for self-manifestation is being undermined by feelings of fear, of being imprisoned, powerless. An overwhelming feeling of being completely stuck: you experience yourself as a victim of sad circumstances. Your feelings of sorrow increase and rise beyond you; you even become afraid of these emotions. Mortal fear. In order to stay ahead of death, you might destroy yourself. You anxiously hold on to your feelings, not trusting them to flow freely.

You refuse to come outward. Your self-aware "I" has no authority over your accumulated sadness. Out of sheer necessity you would cling to something or someone. Self-destruction, suicide. Many people with these negative convictions ("I know I have to suffer"), and with the same self-destructive feelings of powerlessness, are born in miserable circumstances in those regions where beriberi, among other diseases, can be one of the symptoms of such convictions. Psychological solutions need to be considered in group settings.

It is necessary to acquire a clear view of mankind and of its possibilities for creating other life circumstances (See Congenital; Born in Miserable Circumstances). Truly becoming aware of, and gaining insight into, the causes of the situation. Coming to a firm awareness of inner safety and, with strong willpower, setting up an organization, constructing a plan together with others. Knowing it is good to let the emotions flow freely. Change your conviction that you were born in order to die as a victim. With love toward yourself, make a one-hundred-and-eighty-degree turn regarding your life expectations. When inner convictions about life are inclined toward an optimistic view of life, then changes ALWAYS follow, however unlikely they may seem. A first small step will be the beginning of revolution for yourself, for your race, for your total environment. The matter of the earth — desert, wind, water, storms — are a manifestation of consciousness energies. On the basis of love and the positive wish for transformation, propel onward life and the nature around you. A population group that has always lived in poverty and experiences itself as martyr of the world, doomed forever to remain in poverty, will not create change. As a group, convince yourselves of the contrary, direct energies in a totally different way, on the basis of opposite expectations, and outer circumstances will change. Become aware of these of these powerful, creative possibilities! Evoke life instead of death.

BITE WOUNDS OR STINGS FROM ANIMALS

Bite wounds from dogs, cats, . . .

Dogs, cats and other pets react very sensitively to your psychological radiation. You aren't bitten just by chance. Your psyche leads to this happening. You feel threatened by something indefinable, by a shadow behind a chair; you don't see very clearly, nor into yourself either, everything blends together, you cannot get a grip on anything. Because you don't believe enough in your own goodness, you are afraid of a kind of dark power, of a hand that might come from above and seize you and destroy you. But this is about your anxiety, about insufficient trust in your own divine Self. Outwardly, and with your rational consciousness, you can think clearly and can radiate goodness with your heart, but unconscious deep emotions of fear and sadness — "I feel so small, helpless." — grab hold of your sunshine in a black claw. You feel imprisoned in a dark tunnel, where you cannot do anything; you are afraid of the hour of truth. You consider your inner Power to be bad and dangerous! Unconsciously, you tell yourself that you, therefore, have something devilish inside, something you had better strongly suppress! Clearly, this is a problem of "seizing power — being in the power of"; being scared of letting your own Powerful, Mighty "I" come through completely! A true suppression of the strong possibilities in yourself. One often doesn't see clearly: on the one hand, having power over oneself, and on the other, having power over others. Of course, it is fine if the former condition fully comes to be; but the latter is not wholesome for either party. Nevertheless, it happens that — because of the feeling of powerlessness and the suppression of the Power that is in the Self — power is being wielded over others: more anxieties and feelings of self-rejection arise from this situation, even if one is not aware of it! You are afraid that if you would let all your energies and powers flow through, you would be dragged completely into a whirlpool without end: you mistrust your Nature and you experience the cosmos as being full of powers or forces upon which you have no perspective. In other words, you are putting actual authority outside yourself!

Acknowledge the mastery within yourself and quietly look with your eagle-eye upon your life and your world. Nothing outside you can threaten you if you feel inner peace and self-assuredness. Place the power within you, and in this way the dog will not behave like a substitute for your own Power. Power is good when you place it fully within yourself and don't use it on others. Don't let yourself be seized, and don't seize others. Let your action-power break through in full potency! In a flexible, resolute way, not on the basis of suppressed fears and exaggerated aggression. Determine inside yourself this marked-off structure, where nothing or no one can come in uninvited; your power and solidity safe inside yourself. The certainty that the boundaries of your terrain are not being violated finds its true basis upon the gentle, loving feelings directed toward yourself. Are you afraid of a so-called sinister aspect of yourself? Then, this is but a sign that you insufficiently know and love yourself. Accept your totality now; you are good. Just because others have constantly blamed and have underestimated you, that doesn't mean you are "bad." These are just deep, deceptive convictions within yourself. Acknowledge your warmth, your beauty, your power.

Bite wounds from fleas or lice, in general

You feel you are stuck in a structure that is too limiting; your energy is not being used correctly and burns away on the spot. You *cannot* get *away,* cannot at all be yourself the way you want to, and you are feverishly searching with your head, your thoughts, for a way of saving yourself from this frustrated feeling (unconsciously, inner nervousness).

As for children:

You feel so powerless, in the grip of the powerful teacher who is standing before the class on a pedestal; you don't experience the teacher as a "guide who helps you learn how to live and be creative," but rather as a Boss, who is always telling you what to do. Your eyes are fixed on the kindergarten teacher — or another authority — but meanwhile you are searching with confused, irritated feelings, groping in the darkness for your Basis. . . . The sun above you, as an authority, scorches you because you cannot find your own sun-power. Feelings, emotions, free expression, are being suppressed by a structure that is too tight; certain schools are like an artificial safety net, with a life philosophy that is too narrow.

Are you, as a parent, too hard on yourself? Are you imprisoning your nature, your spontaneity?

Free your NATURE! Don't suffocate yourself in smothering structures. Adults will transform to a self-awareness, with inner feelings of pride and safety. Transformation of thoughts; life is a free choice, with all the creative possibilities. This awareness will have its influence on the younger generations. No one has to feel bitten and imprisoned by an authority or in a system — as with a flea from which you cannot escape. You may feel powerful within the protecting mantle of your own strong being. Societies and school systems which are too much directed toward restriction and power will destroy themselves. Guidance, yes, but not at the cost of stunting the nature of a human being.

In order for people not to burn away where they stand (the bite), it is necessary to have a balanced appreciation of, on the one hand, the emotional, the intuitive, the creative aspects, and, on the other hand, that which is rational. All these beautiful energies: no longer throw them as pearls before swine nor as blood before lice!

Bite wounds from insects

Not everyone in the same room will be bitten by an insect: depending on their psychological situations — and as a consequence of a specific physical condition — one person will not be bitten and another will. The following situations enhance the chance of insect bites.

"I, poor, small victim, don't have a grip on my life; I'm vulnerable." You look upon life as if it were a chess game, black-white; and the moment you don't pay attention, you are beaten. You radiate mistrust, insecurity, suspicion, and fatalism. You feel cold and oppressed in life. You consider yourself to be *but* a poor creature. You don't take up the space you should; you even feel unworthy. You consider yourself to be locked out. You feel hurt when others speak sharply to you; you experience the world as an aggressive war game. Possibly, you flee from it or escape in "dreams."

Look upon life with a balanced mind: there are always aspects of Light and shadow. Begin to appreciate the sunny sides of life, also within yourself. You will begin to create life more positively. Don't fixate on the negative, on the aggressive. Feel safe, accepted and protected within yourself! Others, insects, will hurt you if you are convinced you have to be a victim. Take up your scepter as a worthy human being and don't close yourself off in an imaginary inferiority complex. Cheerfulness, security in your own being.

Mosquito bites

One needs to understand the upcoming text in a strong or weaker sense depending on the severity and the amount of bites, and whether one has or has not received an "infection" through mosquito bites

You keep yourself somewhat white, limp, passive-weak, openly directed toward the Neptunian clouds on high; you don't stretch out your neck at all. On the contrary, you'd rather draw your head in between your shoulders, not really realizing your full worth and your range as a human being. The human being, a small, humble, and inferior being, not very capable? This is how you feel after all; you don't integrate yourself into your inner greatness, and you stay in the background of yourself. As a result, you think yourself possibly very little and/or ugly. You make yourself believe anything — you flee toward higher, more ethereal, spiritual dwellings, away from earth. You don't really participate fully in the earthly existence of your "I"; possibly you think you're not worthy of it; you don't descend completely into matter. Sometimes your legs almost give out, white and pale in energy. You have no "resistance" anymore against the negative, because you don't bring your spirit into your body, because you keep yourself somewhat uninterested and absent regarding your earthly existence. You don't take any responsibility for yourself; you just feel cold and empty here on earth; you have no idea about the inner richness inside you, about the warmth in your heart. You seem to say "no" beforehand to taking yourself completely into possession. As long as you don't bring yourself into "life" as a human being, you actually follow the guidelines that lead to nowhere.

The solution is — BE! *Take your life powerfully in hand! Become fully aware of your BEING. Wake up out of a passive, apathetic dream state; come to the belief or awareness that YOU, in your great divine human state, have your life in your own hands; BECOME PRESENT in yourself, in your body. Open your eyes clearly and concentratedly. Wake up! YOU — yes, YOU — are allowed to assume responsibility for your existence! Don't refuse. Shake yourself awake; descend — descend into your body and participate in it in a happy, joyful way!*

The negative isn't all that bad: everything, also the negative, which you (unconsciously) have attracted in your life, has had its reasons. Don't remain stuck, like a helpless *victim,* to the sad or shocking experiences of yesterday, or of the past, but enter the warm-cold waves of life and allow

yourself *to REALLY live in your body!*[1] REALIZE who you are — in your beauty, in your greatness — come to fruitful development and catch up with what you have lost. Come closer to your warm heart and unify yourself with your wonderful earthly body; *feel master over your existence; take possession of yourself, and don't rise up into "thin air," into vagueness,* Neptunian-spiritual, ego-absent, fleeing spheres. Give yourself, as it were, *a Martian "whack"* in order to bring yourself INSIDE yourself, powerful and resolute, and no longer run away from this! Yes, that's why you attract it, that darn mosquito making you get up, in anger, impatience, action (and "whack!" you swat at it), because it's precisely that which your living self-center wants from you. *Stand up as "I," solid in YOUR body; acknowledge your powers as a human being, your possibilities, and no longer make yourself smaller in any way; no longer flee from your body in the dream or in the spirit, because you will only make yourself impatient and angry about your own "escape route."* Stand up, come inside yourself, in your earthly body of flesh and blood, and say "yes" to your "being" as I-in-matter, as master over your existence. No sad little creature, no withdrawal anymore, no excuses: *with your feet on the ground, aware of your inner greatness, solidly incarnating yourself in your highly individual, beautiful, strong, physical earthly body.* "Bring this to realization or I will sting you!" says the mosquito.

Snakebite, poisoning . . .

An appeal from the Heart for Love. A sadness, a longing for warmth and gentleness. You constrain your feelings too much: they have no room to fully exist. Outwardly, you exert yourself in order to stand strongly and stalwartly, but inwardly you haven't really

---

[1] Regarding "warm-cold" experiences on your skin (the itching pimples), also read the symbolism of "Sour Cherry" in *The Horn of Plenty.*

found your authority. Life circumstances force you to be hard, but inwardly you experience a sensitive longing and a doubt regarding your masculine aspects. A baby who longs to be surrounded with motherly love. Therefore, you allow yourself to fall, jumping into the abyss. . . . You believe in death.

At last, be born in yourself: die and be reborn (symbolism of the number 13). Transformation! Shoot and kill your own powerless, dependent "I"; it was but a Skin which now can be thrown off; come to true acknowledgment of your powerful self, realize your independent worthiness. You are not a child without love: true love will now come out of you. Toward you, toward others. Don't expect, but give. Don't allow yourself to be poisoned by the adversary of love: the emptiness and powerlessness of death. Discover the Power in yourself! Turn toward true Life! Inner wisdom, love, and power will make you immune and will ward off circumstances in your life, such as snake bites.

BLEEDING, IN GENERAL

You feel stuck, unable to manifest yourself powerfully. This even leads to anger, aggression — deep sadness. You feel crushed, as it were, by others who are stronger than you, or by a punishing god, or perhaps by certain social icons, by comparison with which you are a poor, small nothing — at least, that is how you feel. You can also behave like a daredevil, because you don't attach any value to your life anyway. Do you look to false values, false gods, and do you go on in a frustrated, self-suppressed way? You deny the Authority in your Self. The blood, symbol of power and life joy, will then flow out of you.

Don't angrily walk away from life: stop! Clot your powers until they become a self-protecting energy, until self-aware mastery over yourself is achieved. Feel safe in yourself: control and direct all your powers or desires, in self-chosen channels. Arrive at self-worth! Feel at home in the warm, friendly sphere of yourself, and project this sphere outwardly.

Experience the joy of yourself; the more powers you use and radiate, the stronger you will become as a result. The more powerlessness and anger you build up, the weaker your situation becomes. Take the bull by the horns in a positive, creative sense!

COUGHING UP OR VOMITING OF BLOOD

Powerless fury, desperate sadness, which was accumulated for much too long. Because of experiences from the past, you rear up, angrily, furiously, but you keep your mouth shut, close yourself off. Often, very sad experiences from childhood are being pent up and stowed away. Self-realization cannot fully come through in this rotten soil. This anger and urge for battle rise up in your thoughts: in fact, this is a reaction to the pain you have suffered. You carry burdens that are *much* too heavy; emotions, through which you only keep on hurting yourself, often with feelings of responsibility toward others,. . . .

Peace, reconciliation. Gentleness to yourself! Be no longer so hard on yourself! Express your deep feelings and don't keep on digging deeper and deeper into them, for then you just make things worse. Take the little, lonely, sad child within you by the hand and calmly teach it to walk. . . . Build your life on the Now; don't linger in the past! Understanding for others makes hatred as well as forgiveness unnecessary. It is you who unconsciously has attracted circumstances in order to be able to make a decision and to go on.

BLOOD, HEART, AND BLOOD VESSELS

THE SYMBOLISM OF THE HEART AND HEART ILLNESSES ARE DISCUSSED UNDER THE LETTER -H-; CONSULT THE INDEX

Psychological correspondence

This symbolizes a warm, safe presence in yourself. An effervescent life energy is being propelled in the blood: longing, love, and joy for life itself, a dancing-free and light feeling — that is the blood. It is a direct physical manifestation of the urge to live and experience, an urge present in us from the beginning, already there long before our Consciousness-essence entered the three-dimensional system. A voluntary presence in the body, which, thanks to this transition, finally can lead to a New Body. Thanks to Conscious Wisdom and Love for oneself and mankind, man can finally evolve toward new forms. The heart and the blood circulation, together with the nervous system, the brain, confront mankind with its wealth of emotions, with its knowledge, with the possibilities of ever again evolving further on the basis of knowledge, creativity, and love: an interaction between Wisdom and Love in order to come ever again to a greater awareness.

The heart is a symbol for the absorption — the taking up — of emotions into our deep self, and for the letting go of other impressions. The heart is the basis which represents the authority of our individual feeling. The

original trust, our Power for firmly gripping onto the Earth and experiencing our Self-awareness.

The guarantee we give ourselves; the optimism which we either do or don't allow ourselves; vital growth in life: the blood, propelled by the heart in *one* direction, namely the direction of Life. If we block this faith, this joy, this light, warm feeling for ourselves, then we no longer nourish these physical channels, and they will no longer efficiently carry out their work: our consciousness, our feelings and thoughts, are the ultimate propelling force *behind* the blood. Also, the joyful, powerful "I" is able to transform the body unto immortality.

The heart and blood circulation symbolize life energy, the power, the earth-magnetism, and sun-warmth; they also symbolize the "I" that puts on its crown and places its kingdom inside itself, not outside itself. Symbol for mankind's irresistible urge to ever again push through, in love, to new paths. If a man stands still, his heart will stand still. Do you take love away from yourself? The longing for life? Joy? Do you think life is a hard battle, and do you enchain yourself? Then you are taking away all nourishment from your blood, and you will die. Feeling good, open-minded. "Everything will be all right. I can trust in this Powerful energy" — the heart, the sanctuary within you, which you ought to cherish. Your deep Self, which continually nourishes and goes on without you needing to *consciously* command it to do so; you can trust it totally and let go — the heart beats for as long as the "I" wants to live, consciously or unconsciously, on Earth. If man remains faithful to custom and programs himself to die around the age of eighty, then the heart unconsciously will follow this conviction. (See Part I)

Ailments, in general

Are you hard on yourself? Are you listening too little to your gentle feelings? Are you living under the pressure of a crushing structure which hinders you from breathing freely? Are you tying yourself down to a materialistic world? Because of doing this, are all higher energies being blocked? Does THINKING overpower your heart, your bodily sensation? You don't let your powers flow through! Because of not believing in yourself, and because you limit your own possibilities, you hang your head, losing the joy of life. You degrade yourself; you don't take the steering wheel of the car of life in hand yourself. Instead, you allow yourself to be led by others and their rules. Life becomes heavy and dark.

You go *far* beyond your powers because your inner power source is not being used. You have hardened your heart against loving yourself; perhaps you consider yourself as being too bad, too small, and you have everything except self-respect. Sad and dissatisfied with your situation. . . .

Does your heart ache because, in a relationship, you experience "power" and "sex" instead of complete love and feelings of affection?

Broken off, cut off within, from your own deep, warm source, which, because you don't believe in yourself and your life power, can no longer radiate toward the heart. Belief in a God above you, but denying the divinity in yourself?

Joy, love, gentleness, flexibility, openness. Discipline is good when it leads you on the path you chose out of free will and on which you feel at peace.

Break through your self-curtailment! Free yourself from negative programming. Realize your worth as a human being, your unique being! Spread your wings and experience the joy of your space, the power of Life, of your personal Consciousness-core, which, if you surrender to yourself, propels you ever again toward higher values and deeper feelings. Don't confine your heart: allow your emotions to flow freely. Don't fight against this life-urge, and don't drag

yourself down with negative thoughts: make good use of all your energies and create your life on the basis of a self-aware trust in your Possibilities. No longer self-suppression or self-condemnation. Love yourself, love life: life will reward you.

AILMENTS
OF THE BLOOD

Anemia

You look too much for support outside yourself. You hold on to life buoys. Not believing in your own powers, you consider yourself a weakling. Warm energies seek their way; feelings want to *live*, but they are nipped in the bud, sadly, led like a funeral procession to an isolated spot in the body: a solitary flush of the cheeks. These are the tears of Life, because you fail to appreciate Life, which is Joy. You think a lot, but you don't FEEL from out of your deepest longings! Sad, feeling no real life-motivation, following others — you don't achieve a real contact with your emotional life: a sort of absence. As if you are standing *apart* from life. You don't really belong, experiencing yourself to be psychologically marginal, like a refugee in a camp instead of in one's safe, warm home. Hesitant, pliable. "What shall I do now?"

Well, your body and your life are being experienced as a mysterious, strange, endless road — you don't know how or what. Powerless. You don't grasp the sense of living; you experience yourself as helpless and fearful and are looking mistrustfully toward the future. Tired: because you don't trust your deepest power source, because you don't achieve real love for yourself, because you underestimate yourself.

*Don't brood! Feel your body, your senses. See, breathe, smell, taste the beauty in life. Direct yourself inwardly now, and discover your warm Heart, which sends forth joy and power when, in acknowledgment of yourself, you are open to love and life. Don't look for support outside yourself; don't live the life of others, but direct yourself toward your longings, **feel** what you would like to do in your life, and begin with that. First of all, see with your eyes and not with your thoughts. Experience how sensory impressions can stir up your feelings and allow you to enjoy life in a joyful way. Choose in favor of your nature: it will reward you. Enlarge your life space in all directions. Spin the wheel of fortune **yourself**. Don't wait passively — choose, act, determine **yourself!** Descend into your body: come, and taste the happiness that every cell of your body radiates when you simply become aware of your unique worth. Instill your being with love and appreciation: the fuel for your body.*

Aplastic anemia
aplasia of the bone marrow

Anxious, on your guard, anxiety about being hurt. Powerless aggression, a dark rancor against life itself. You don't trust things; you experience life as if it were a masquerade, with masked, lurking powers, mysteries and threats. You, yourself, are also hiding behind a mask, playing a role to please the public, but inwardly you feel lonely, bored, dark, monotonous. You want to protect yourself from supposed "evil." On the one hand, you are on guard against dark powers outside yourself, and on the other hand, you might envelop others in your grip, in your Power, manipulating them, in order to make yourself feel stronger. In this way, you live untruthfully, play-acting, although unconsciously.

You would heroically go into battle for an ideal, for the good, against the evil. You'd like to outwardly manifest grand feelings, with aggressive power, but inwardly you

don't come into true contact with your deepest feelings, with your intuitive channels, with your heart, with the fire of your being. Your deepest essence is deeply stowed away, so that you are no longer in touch with your personal, true nature. You try to compensate for this empty, tenuous feeling of self-negation by manifesting yourself outwardly or by getting attention from others so that you might feel more at ease, more safe, and warmer. But you keep on feeling like a hung bird, like someone who is cut off from the Authority in himself. As a consequence of this, you are all the more vulnerable to the outer world's reactions to you. You think you have to protect yourself in an aggressive way because you ignore the masculine "I"-power, the true Sun-center in yourself. You place all power and authority outside yourself. You stand at a distance from yourself, living not really "ensouled," so that consciousness-powers cannot adequately nourish your body. Hard inner tension, resistance against one's own transformation.

Stand on your own feet, independent, trusting in your deepest Self. Bow only to the Authority in yourself and dismantle all false values and authorities outside yourself. Dare to express your feelings, and know that nothing inside or outside yourself can threaten you; confront yourself, therefore, with your deepest emotions, with reality. Don't dream, don't live in your imagination; reach out for yourself only, and let everything and everyone go. Become aware of your worth. Build solid structures upon your Basis; create your life in a self-aware way. Know yourself to be protected and safe in yourself. Look inside yourself now, no longer directing yourself toward the outer world: in yourself you will find the inexhaustible energy source of your life. Don't close yourself off from it; listen to your heart, and from out of your true nature bring yourself to realization — original, honest, fearless. Feel that inner flame, the fire of life in yourself, and allow yourself to live in peace and tenderness. Let the masculine and feminine elements harmoniously merge. A flexible attitude within the secure framework of your Self. Create space for enjoyment, for a smile, for joy!

Sickle-cell anemia

Your true being, your content, your powers, your "I" are all living, hidden, behind a screen. You suppress your true energies. You, YOURSELF, don't really come through; possibly, you function very well in a superficial pattern, talking and chattering up a storm. But where, really, are YOU so deeply stowed away? Why do you not truly live from within your deepest essence? Perhaps you imitate others — your stalwart father or perhaps a fashion model. Why live so artificially? You don't dare to manifest yourself as you *are*. You assume your Role: in the family, in school, or in society; you behave the way you THINK you have to be in order to seem "good" to others. For instance, as a child you "earn" the attention and love of your parents if you behave according to their life pattern. Sometimes, you identify too strongly with others because you think you are not good, because you consider yourself to be inferior. Finally, do you not know who you are? In the meantime, you restrain your personal energies, your creativity, your real feelings — you don't really dare to bring yourself outward. You sometimes hesitate: "Shall I or shall I not open the windows? Do I 'play' along, or shall I 'push through?'" Anxiety hinders you from expressing your emotions, your aggressive powers, but the pressure becomes too great. You no longer can hold everything back; you tensely retain yourself and your energies.

Unburden yourself! Blow off steam; allow sadness and anger to escape. No longer hold everything in. You are unique; no one will forbid you to be who you are. Don't be afraid of losing people by manifesting yourself the way you really feel: the ones who are

*your true kindred spirits will come to you. Stand up for yourself! Transformation: pull your roots out of this ground, which is not really your soil, even if it means home to you. Only when you send out your own roots will you really come home. A break with "false appearances"; a breakthrough of "authenticity." Discover your deepest longings, your feelings; no longer superficially live according to others. Throw the windows wide open and deeply breathe in life! When you turn, in all honesty, toward your "I" and dare to proudly manifest your own individuality without fear, then you will discover this profound joy inside you! Grow up in happiness, no longer keeping yourself underground: show yourself as you **are**.*

Disorders of coagulation of the blood

Powerless aggression! Because you don't get a grip on yourself, you might "grasp" at others or let yourself be dragged along by a "leader" or an "ideal" outside yourself. Your life is not (yet) really built on inner Authority! You allow yourself to be led by false values, possibly by a powerful image; you don't really dare to live from your true nature. On the one hand, you might conform too strongly to the ones whose love you have to earn, to the person you anxiously consider to be your "dominant" authority — by which you ignore your own gentle "I". On the other hand, however, you revolt: aggressive resistance! You seize others the way you feel yourself to be seized. Did you encounter "possessiveness" or "power-grasping" instead of love that cherishes and liberates? Are you now going the same way? Or do you just "linger" in the past, in the nest in which you grew up, without daring to stand on your own feet, without daring to realize your own Worth? You *let* yourself "be lived," and then again you feel angry because of this powerless inability to really be your SELF. You too much deny the intuitive, the "feminine" aspect, the gentleness in yourself, and possibly you hold on too much to outer values. Because of that, your real substance cannot come to the fore. Or do you try to prove yourself in superficial assertiveness, because you doubt your inner worth? You constrict your existence; don't allow *true* joy in your heart; you are too hard on yourself, or you allow your life to be led too much by someone else. Thus, you stand, too cold, too tense, at a distance from yourself. You live within a confined structure: as your blood flows, so too do your deeper emotions, your Nature, break through such structures and ask for acknowledgment and liberation. Possibly, you have fears of Authority, or you position yourself in a strongly authoritarian manner. In every way, it is your anxieties that hinder you from going along spontaneously in life on waves of joy and longing.

Transform powerless aggression into Action and Gentleness! Discover the gentleness inside you and place yourself on your Throne. Become yourself! Don't grab at others and don't allow yourself to be grabbed. Instead of "stopping" (or "stemming") the gentleness, the intuitively natural in yourself, you'd better surrender to these aspects, in relaxation: acknowledgment of your nature, of your true character, of your body, of your values. Integrate the intuitive, the gentle feminine aspects, into your existence. Come to inner rest; don't make yourself anxious about the outer world, but dare to listen to your heart. Allow higher consciousness-energies to flow through. Build up your life in joy, on the secure, safe basis of your deepest Self, not on false foundations. It is not the outer appearance, but the inner certainty that counts. You have attracted precisely these parents, or those who raised you, in order to be able to deal with certain of your psychological aspects — which you will encounter in them, as if in a mirror-image. It is you who has to evolve now, without blaming others. Put all power inside yourself, so that all frustrations will disappear. Feel at peace and safe in
your gentle, powerful Self. An autonomous, loving existence. Take good care of yourself and create, **yourself,** the joyful circumstances in your life: resolute self-realization from within, not seeking outward affirmation.*

Hemophilia
(See also Disorders of coagulation)

You are looking for love and attention, for acknowledgment from others, because you don't really welcome yourself into life! You feel powerless and unsafe in yourself. You'd like to charge full-steam ahead, with all powers and built-up energies. To prove yourself. But you *cannot.* An accumulation of frustrated and fearful thoughts are holding your mind under a spell. Loneliness. On the one hand you feel pain, are hurt, don't feel able to assert yourself, to let your energies flow outward; on the other hand, you inwardly make a fist, and revolt and anger grow because of this powerlessness! Powerless aggression. Burning anger and an intense feeling of being hurt. Because you don't really like yourself, you attract situations whereby you think you must defend yourself extra strongly — also with regard to love-relationships. "This partner belongs to *me*; don't touch!" Or, in your feminine, gentle feelings: "Don't touch my private domain!"

Sometimes, you turn away from life, close yourself off, to protect yourself against those who might hurt you, who possibly might have power over you, who could force themselves upon you. You feel threatened by another "authority," because you doubt your own. Do you attach too much value to the Outer world?

Possibly, a strong authority, a parent or an older brother, was considered to be a threat when you were a child. You have felt inferior to a scorching, sometimes really suffocating, Authority. Possibly, you have clung to a parent. This "illness" is drawn in with the mother's milk, and will disappear when you let yourself be "reborn" as an autonomous individual. A mother, who experiences emptiness and sadness in herself, will possibly bear a son who actually has to fight with the same inner problems. Because of this, both exercise a "compensating" but suffocating, influence on each other. The inner conflict — "holding on tightly, and at the same time longing for self-liberation" — is thus strongly present; the love-hate relationship toward oneself, toward the parent. When the mother resolves these problems in herself, it will be easier for the son, via this confrontation, to find a resolution for his inner emotional battle. The true reason for the problem should not, however, be sought in the dominating presence of the father, nor in the oppressive pressure of the mother, but in the son's powerlessness to realize himself as an independent authority. Your life energy flows away — fear of pains hinders you from truly *living!* Do you live too much toward the outside? Do you have a feeling you must do things? Do you attach too much importance to that which "another" demands of you? Do you not dare to follow your heart?

Acknowledge the inner Authority of your deepest Self! Enjoy life in deep draughts, and drink of it instead of letting yourself drain away. Self-confidence, self-awareness; faith in your Powers. Don't close yourself off; surrender to your gentle, emotional realm, but calmly mark off the limits of your terrain, within which you can completely indulge yourself, in all freedom, released from everyone! Love yourself unconditionally; determine your borders regarding others; don't smother yourself, but take up space and stand solidly on your own feet. In every man there flows a radioactive power: when, in love toward yourself, you acknowledge it, you can turn again and again to this power for healing. You are not powerless, but are a life-magician, if you want to be. No standing on the defensive, but building up. Transform aggressive powers into actual self-realization. Be kind and gentle to yourself; incline, flexibly, toward your longings. No longer be hard and angry, but acknowledge that Power over your life IN yourself, and

*bring it to realization! Just be yourself in a spontaneous way, no longer being tensely on guard. Dare to surrender to life; determine your direction **yourself**, and trust, without feeling obliged to do or allow certain things against your will. Offer the love which you so need, and don't, firstly, expect this from others. When you live in love toward yourself, you will attract those people who are good for you,— not out of "necessity," but out of Love.*

Don't let yourself be blinded by Authority outside yourself: acknowledge your self-Authority!

Erythrocyte sedimentation rate, elevated

You would like to realize and prove yourself as a human being. You *want* very much and would force things, pulling a cart that is *much* too heavy, until you are dragged away with it. You might do everything cautiously and with premeditation in order just to achieve that which, in your mind, is at the Pinnacle of your ambition, your aspirations. As one who is powerless, you want Power! Perhaps you only want to prove yourself to the outer world, or in order to be esteemed in your circle of relations. You blur your weak points and constantly live under stress. You look up to power institutions, religions, or systems, trying to fit into these artificial constructs and to apply their rules so that finally you might be able to sit on a (false) throne. Are you so afraid just to be who you are? Do you consider yourself just a nothing?

Become again a human being among human beings: recognize your "weak" points. Accept yourself as you are. Everyone has distinctive points: express your beautiful qualities and see the relativity of your minor aspects. Live with the fullness of who you NOW are; don't live in the future. Enjoy, and remain in your own shoes. Don't flee from yourself, nor from Life.

Blood poisoning

Overly passive participation in your life, you just sit by and watch. An inner conflict: "Shall I stand up for myself or not?" You invariably push something away; you don't want to see the truth about yourself! Stay, rather, in the old (blind) alley.... Do you not love yourself? You still do experience this conflict in yourself: you'd like to raise your fist and stand up for your rights! But you feel emotionally overwhelmed and incapable of taking hold of yourself and directing yourself where you want to go. You lack Self-aware authority and faith in your powers and possibilities to be the leader of your own life. You *let* yourself "be lived." That inside you which you neglect or push away raises its head in the form of poisoning. Do you behave as if nothing is the matter? Do you live superficially? Do you suppress sadness or pain?

So, resolutely arrive at action: offer yourself happiness! Now decide henceforth to seize the power over yourself; dare to observe your feelings calmly, don't run away from them. Observe them, accept them, let them flow through under the supervision of a Powerful self-awareness. Straighten up, come forward with all your energies! Allow love and strength to triumph in you. Don't hesitate, take up your space! Listen to your Nature: offer yourself true Life!

Purpura
small bleedings in the skin
and mucous membranes

You just sit there, moored to the dock. You run in place. You keep still, like a dependent baby, and in the meantime your candle burns away. Docile and virtuous, sometimes over-mothered, languishing in this situation, dominated by people or by bookish wisdom. Like a sheep, you follow others — you don't *really* live! You copy others; you do what

the teacher tells you to do.... Energies, healthy aggressive powers, are not being lived to the fullest.

Put out new roots and experience your own basis! True learning is to be found under your own feet. Allow all paths to open like blossoms to you! Don't force your spontaneous, natural energies into a pattern which is too rigid for you, thus blocking them. Throw open all doors and liberate yourself: live from out of your power center and don't restrain yourself, especially not by theoretical thinking or by an unnatural attitude to life.

BLOOD PRESSURE, TOO HIGH

Insufficient love for yourself, self-suppression. Unconsciously holding on, repressing emotions, often reaching back to experiences from childhood. You look, *thinking*, confused, for solutions, but you don't see it clearly. As an adult, as when you were a baby, you again and again look up to people, to systems, to authority outside yourself. Your heart becomes confined because you deny your own full Self-worth. You'd like to acknowledge your Sun-center, and you do exhibit it boldly to the outer world, but it is just an ostrich-like attitude of yours: sadness, feelings of inferiority, belittlements — possibly you were born with these self-crushing feelings, and you feel powerless and small, like a baby. You keenly would like to manifest yourself! One can speak here of an inner revolt against these unconscious self-degradations: blood pressure goes up. Because you cannot solve emotional problems by stepping beyond them and putting on the mask of the stalwart hero. Therefore, look into your heart: Why do you not love yourself as you *are?* Which elements in yourself

The Key to Self-Liberation, Christiane Beerlandt © Beerlandt Publications

do you condemn? Do you find certain feelings of yours "bad" because earlier conditioning has spoon-fed you that this *really* is not done? Are you so afraid of your feelings that you stifle them with all your might? Were you taught that emotions, feelings, and relations with others are untrustworthy and a threat for the human race? Or do you not trust your own deep emotional energies? Do you think they will pull you down in a whirlpool? Do you not dare to show your feelings for others? Do you not dare to acknowledge your own gentleness? Are you trying to camouflage yourself with a hard outer shell? You cannot really go forward and are running in place because you are not solving this problematic emotional situation. You will force yourself and will try to reach beyond yourself. Because you don't trust your emotional nature, because you deny your self-worth, you are becoming afraid of death. Anxiety.

*Don't flee, with unreal illusions, from the reality of your feelings. Dare to put your deepest feelings under the magnifying glass. Proceed slowly, building upon both poles: don't turn off the emotional pole to the advantage of the rational pole! You have already been thinking enough. Cherish the gentle, small feelings in you and don't follow cold, rigid examples — such as, perhaps, the examples of those who raised you. No one can say what is good for you, so therefore follow only your own heart. Dare to let these gentle, living energies of joy and pleasure penetrate. No longer keep a distance from yourself, no longer look at yourself in a destructive or severe way; make yourself welcome. Only when this duality has been resolved in you can you feel love that will drive away anxieties. Release the pressure on your life: that of self-negation and self-rejection. You have unconsciously attracted circumstances from the past because you have been under the conviction that, in your essence you are not worthy of experiencing joy and of being the way you are. This is a self-destructive atti-*tude, with all the consequences thereof. Be convinced, NOW, that it is very good to be the way you feel. Live!*

BLOOD PRESSURE, TOO LOW

You direct yourself toward everything and everyone outside yourself: you want to reach very far, far beyond yourself. You spread your arms open to the furthest extent, as it were, and embrace everything tightly. Specifically, you feel extremely responsible in life: also for others. You think you have to keep an eye on everything — yes, even having to be an overseer, required to punish others because they must listen to you! You are so demanding and severe with yourself that you can also be this way with others. You would in an authoritarian manner seize someone by the collar instead of occupying yourself with your own development. In an extreme sense of responsibility, you crow like a cock from high up in the tower; you straighten yourself up , sometimes arrogantly, to be able to take it all in. Out of fear that you might totally collapse, you present a stronger outward appearance than you inwardly feel. For, in fact, you feel small.

Come to gentleness and Love toward yourself!

Keep to yourself: fall back upon your intuition and come to self-expression from out of yourself. Dare to show yourself as you are, independent of others; don't crow on someone else's roof. Become conscious of your values. Communicate peacefully with others, without overstepping your bounds. Respect everyone's space and come to yourself. Let go of all burdens and dance into life! First of all, live for yourself! Because of the way you are, you are worthy; give the love which for so long you have denied yourself.

AILMENTS OF THE BLOOD VESSELS

Aorta, rupture

One is more dead than alive: a surrender to someone else, to a god, a teaching or a system, without really knowing contact with oneself. Everything lacks perspective and has slipped away; one cannot get a grip on anything. One believes very strongly in the dark, threatening aspects of life, because one's own inner power is being denied. One is not oneself, would rather wear a mask: a bird that ties his own beak closed; self-blocking; joy cannot be felt. One still lives impersonally, blind. With one foot in the living, the other in death, it is impossible to find enjoyment. Here, we are dealing with disbelief in the worth of oneself, in the significance of Life: one breaks with it.

Arteriosclerosis

Resistance, mostly unconscious, to real, psychological evolution. You limit your Being: for instance, by only letting the rationality come to the fore. Or: you identify yourself too much with that which your educators, your father or mother — or one or another indoctrination, religion, sect or system — have spoon-fed you. You cannot, or don't want to, come out from under this; you stick to it in voluntary imprisonment. So you live, constricted, narrow-minded — not in a supple way that is from within your deepest Self. Watchfully, anxiously, you stay cautiously within these or those borders, not deviating too much here or there, because, "Hey! That's just not allowed, or what would happen then?" In other words, anxious refusal to *self*-evolve, often hard stubbornness — not wanting to broaden your outlook. In this way, you confine your life to a dark forest of blinders that has narrow paths, and you narrow your arteries. You can develop an enormous reverence, but at the same time develop a fear of certain people or of authority outside yourself. After all, you experience yourself as being unsafe; you think you always have to be on guard for something bad that might happen. At last you let yourself droop completely. You no longer see the broad, beautiful stream of life. Your brain doesn't dare to come to full, joyful development; also, it confines itself within anxiety-ridden structures: trust in your deepest Self is lost. You don't at all dare to depend on your personal intuition, your inner "knowing"; the consequence is mostly a one-sided, purely rational approach to life. The attempt of your full consciousness to manifest itself is being hindered; the capacities of certain parts of the brain are never being exploited. You don't believe in your own broader possibilities.

As a human being, you have at your disposal a natural immune system against illness or accidents — if you believe in this Self. Your anxieties and negative expectations call up sadness and misery, which eventually lead to death. Joyfulness creates Life and health: open your arteries and acknowledge your mastery in building up your life as you wish. Don't shrink yourself, don't put your possibilities in the ground. Get rid of narrow-minded prejudices: they hinder you from living truly and fully. Be worthy of your own godly origin: the kingdom of God is within you! Your consciousness is open and unlimited.

Phlebitis
vein inflammation

You feel unstable, shaky, discarded. . . . "Who am I anymore?"

You experience yourself as "old"; you're not sure of your own worth. Unsure, with chaotic, nervous, brain activity, looking for something to hold on to! You see everything in a fragmentary way; your energy flows in fits and starts. You cannot get a clear overview anymore. Self-doubt weighs heavily on you and robs you of psychic stability. Life becomes a burden. Sometimes you get inwardly angry because of this frustrated feeling of unworthiness. Sometimes you lay blame on others, while it has to do with your own powerlessness.

Don't stamp yourself as old and worthless. You are as you've created yourself, according to your own convictions. Arrive at self-respect. Perhaps you've never done this? Depend now on your deepest Self, acknowledge your nature, feel the Earth and — above all — enjoy yourself and your environment! Straighten up and radiate in all directions. A human being is a natural pearl — without accomplishments, without special functions, without having to satisfy any social or outer requirement in order to be a beautiful individual — because he is Life. Life is: experiencing the joyful, primal power that floats through your being, now and in eternity. . . . Don't block this love energy by self-condemnation! Love yourself, and thus choose life, not death!

Thrombosis
local clotting of the blood

You are stuck; you live rather unconsciously, in your thoughts, in your spirit, than in reality, in the here-and-now. Pent-up emotions. Your personal powerful "I," your sun center, is being suppressed: you might experience this sunrise as a threat! You let yourself slouch; you think joy is not meant for you; you are even angry at your emotions. You too little believe in goodness, and therefore you don't radiate it toward others. With (self) pity, no one is helped. In powerlessness, you perhaps direct blame toward others, but it is you who does not allow any progress, happiness, in your life! Do you give yourself so little credit? You don't truly "live"! You remain too "impersonal," too Neptunian.

Follow, with self-awareness, your earthly path, and for once look upon yourself from a distance; keep your feelings in perspective and pull yourself up onto the bank: become master over yourself and feel your warm heart. Place yourself higher. No longer crawl. Flexible self-manifestation, releasing pent-up energies! Don't bottle up anger, but transform these frustrations into action, creativity! Contentment with yourself leads to joy. Allow yourself to enjoy! Live very consciously and allow your heart to radiate goodness: don't degrade yourself to being a sad little fish, without recourse.

Blood vessel tumor, angioma

You don't feel safe in yourself. You don't really choose a direction in your life. You don't dare to enter into earthly life. You stagnate your life. Mortal fears. Emotionally, you cannot handle things. You don't dare trust your own Basis. You are afraid of inner fire powers, of the responsibility of having to manifest Yourself as an Individual. It all is becoming too hot for you. Because you hold yourself back from growing, powerful "Mars" energies are driving inwards instead of being used as building blocks. You are afraid. The earth appears to you like a claustrophobic threat because you psychologically oppress yourself, because you don't see the reality of things concerning yourself: that you are an extremely strong being who is able to *self*-create his own freedom.

Pent-up aggressive powers are drawing together. You are afraid of your own Substance, of your inner emotions, of your powers.

Don't be afraid. You are safe in the womb of your imperishable deepest Self.

Know yourself to be protected, and build up your life as if it were a feast. Joy, cheerfulness, humor. Don't "tighten" or constrict yourself; feel your solid foundations and let yourself be free!

Give your feelings, your energies, freedom: use these beautiful inner powers in happy self-realization. Love and trust in your stable essence drive away all anxieties. Dare to surrender to that which is deepest in yourself. Nothing can threaten you: let yourself go, relax! Peace in yourself, peace with life.

Blood vessel tumors are often congenital: the above-mentioned causes and solutions will apply not only to the infant, but also to the parents, the mother.

The infant will find its rest and safety when the mother resolves needless anxieties.

Varicose veins

You bear heavy burdens. You feel as if you live the role of a victim.

You try to seize, to embrace, everything, emotionally as well as in the area of work, but you exclude a great part of your life! You don't really live in love toward yourself, possibly because you feel inferior, because you feel "obliged" to live in this way.

Your feelings tell you that you can't go on like this, but you ignore them. You feel too weak, too ashamed, or too slavish, too inferior, to bring about changes in this situation.

You flee from true life; you stick your head in the sand, because you have the conviction that you can't really be yourself in this life. You can't get a grip on yourself, on life, the way it could be more pleasurable for you, and you flee or despondently remain stagnating in an oppressed situation.

Anxiety about totally being yourself, about taking up your complete space, living a life that accords with your nature, that doesn't force or restrict you.

Also in pregnancy: you can barely carry yourself; you hardly dare to realize yourself; you feel "seized" by circumstances instead of creating your life yourself in a self-aware way on the basis of your longings; you now drag your feet, carrying even heavier burdens. You should urgently "run away," but even your survival instinct doesn't work

anymore because you don't really believe in your Power, in your rights to Joy!

You would like to stand up for yourself, but you think you can't. Possibly you were raised in an environment where the emphasis was placed on "being obliged" instead of "being allowed"; on "materialism and work" instead of "love toward yourself"; on the "weakness of the human being, of the woman" instead of on "inner Power"; on "severity" instead of "joy and gentleness." You apply that which has been taught to you: indoctrination doesn't do you any good. Your head, your thoughts, are in the grip of tongs. Because you don't believe enough in your Conscious, unique being, because you don't really lovingly accept yourself, you remain rather passive in this situation, in spite of the fact that you are in pain and feel sad. You don't do anything about it. You are too cold and hard with yourself.

Feelings of inability, a life full of tension. Your feelings aren't being respected, but are being subordinated to your "thinking." You don't allow your emotions, your spontaneous creativity, to flow freely. You reach very far; you do a lot, but you deny your feelings. Your heart, your joy, is imprisoned in the fist of "outer or rational justification"! Perhaps you blame others for your sadness, your being overburdened, but you are the cause of this. You throw yourself into your work or you concentrate on others instead of first and foremost looking out for yourself.

Allow your Self to "burst open" like a bud! Give yourself all the space you need! You will have to make a choice; a solution needs to be found. Free yourself from this factitious, restrictive life. Acknowledge the Fullness of yourself, of your existence. No longer put your feelings in a suitcase, till it bursts. Dare to live, to enjoy; unburden yourself. No one is a victim unless he dooms himself to it. Break with old habits and listen to your heart: in love, come to yourself; acknowledge your worth; no longer treat yourself like a machine or a slave. You are a human being filled to the top with possibilities and creativity; life is Joy first of all, but you force yourself; you cause yourself sadness and too much burden. Let go, bring about changes in your convictions regarding yourself, so that you will also attract other circumstances: Self-Respect!

Don't only build up your life with your rational "mind" or with your "duties": LIVE and discover yourself; offer yourself warmth and don't expect someone else to look out for your happiness. No longer allow yourself to "be lived"; step out of the deadlock or out of this "unauthentic" life. Show your feelings, show yourself truly the way you feel inside and don't hide from yourself, nor from others! Don't make yourself appear harder than you feel. Pull yourself out of that victim role and dare to enjoy! It's your inner convictions that cause others to react to you the way they do. If you think yourself but a mule, then others will treat you that way. If you acknowledge your inner beauty, your kingship, then you will encounter joyful warm people who will treat you with respect. Live more spontaneously and more intuitively; don't violate yourself. Get a hold of yourself, full of self-confidence, instead of wanting to "grab" for "work" or "others"; don't go beyond your limits; in a relaxed way turn toward your deepest Self and respect your nature.

Vasospasm
spasm, cramp of blood vessels

Refusing to go on joyfully, to transform. Although you overflow with ambitions, longings, aggressive powers and emotions, you hold yourself back so that emotionally you almost explode. You would like. . . . But you restrain yourself. You feel unsure; you hesitate, between two possible directions. You remain standing still. You dare not. You don't dare to externalize your inner powers. You don't allow yourself to grow, blossom, or open up. You hold on to emotions, still clinging to the past or to something or someone. It is better to let go now.

You have anxiety about the future; you call "letting go and going onward" a risk.

You hide behind an accomplishment, a job, an outer Image, a Trophy, but inwardly your feelings become rigid. You don't really listen to your heart; you are at odds with yourself because you don't offer your deepest Self any trust. Frightened resistance to self-realization. Then, all of a sudden, you might force things and reach beyond yourself.

*Close the door to the past. Don't attach yourself to material or outer so-called values, but in true Love direct yourself toward yourself. For too long you have been neglecting your heart and your emotional life. Life is joy and beauty, but you are walking right past it. Become conscious now of the treasures inside yourself, of your worth, of your unique possibilities, and no longer hold yourself back. Express your emotions now; use your inner powers in creativity, in experiencing your feelings. Make yourself happy. You decorate life the way you want it, so make something beautiful of it. Don't force anything. Evolve gradually, in a relaxed way, but resolutely let go of that which is superfluous in your emotions. Be proud of yourself and dare to manifest yourself instead of holding back. Feel safe on your fundamentally strong Basis and go on without hesitation. Proceeding on and **self**-creating your life means joy and evolution. Self-aware producing, daring to let yourself go without anxiety.*

BODY HALVES

The polarization of "left-right" is true today, but perhaps will not be tomorrow . . .

At the moment, one can (still) speak of specific psychological correspondences of the Left and Right halves of the body (See also

Brain hemispheres). With regard to this, the following is presently stored in the conviction-apparatus of mankind:

Intellect and intuition merge in the Oneness of our Self-awareness, where separation between left and right falls away.

Left half of the body
corresponding to
the right hemisphere of the brain

For the most part, ailments of the left half of the body indicate the emotional aspect.

That which is generally labeled as "feminine": receptiveness — flexibility — the emotional — the more unconscious regions — nurturing — tenderness — intuition — suppleness — Venus and the Moon — mobility, fitting-in, adaptability — abandon — maternal — receiving/passive — spaciousness, boundlessness — silver — the night — producing/giving birth.

This polarization is relative; at the moment, it is still true for almost all people, but tomorrow, perhaps, it will no longer be true. A constant interaction between "left" and "right" powers is a self-evident and continual occurrence: duality-unity. A healthy "left" side requires a flexible dealing with — and flow of — feelings, an elimination of burdensome emotions, of sadness. . . .

Good health also requires not going against the current, but flexibly flowing along with the tones of your deepest Self, without putting up blockades: follow your intuition.

A too-strong binding with or influence of a Maternal figure can be mirrored in a symptom on the left side. An imbalance caused by over-accentuating the left aspect in a man or woman indicates a lack of Conscious mastery over your unconscious life, over your emotional world: a preponderance of the feelings over the rational, of unconscious upwellings of emotions (for instance anxiety) over self-assuredness.

Right half of the body
corresponding to
the left hemisphere of the brain

That which one generally labels as "masculine: the "I"-awareness — sober logic, the rational — the active, the connecting — Mars powers and the sun — outer ego — consciously rising above your emotions — resolutely intervening: cutting the knot — strong, stalwart, solid — hard, sifting the wheat from the chaff — logical and analytical — the Father in yourself — the day — gold — spontaneous aggressive energies — warm red powers — marking off boundaries, defining clear demarcations — constructing — assertiveness.

A healthy "right" side requires a self-aware life course: in awareness of your self-worth, resolutely choose the direction of your life and grow upward from your deep roots. An exaggerated accentuation of "thinking," of the rational, without taking into account your intuition and your emotional life — being cut off from your deeper Source — leads to overburdening the "right side."

The sun shines above deep waters and illuminates a proud mountain in the middle of the lake: warm self-respect; rising above unconscious dimensions in yourself, a conscious mastery, yet rooted in our deepest soil — interplay of right and left. Daring to stand up openly for yourself, letting your Heart open up, not letting yourself be overmastered by your emotions, nor by others; an openness for growth, allowing that which is precious inside you to come to light, an integration of the secure, paternal aspect into yourself: this leads to a healthy "right."

BODY ODOR, EXTREMELY STRONG

Unsureness: you don't accept yourself and are afraid others will not accept you either; feelings of inferiority.

You feel rather threatened by others; anxieties! "Yes or no? Shall I dare?" Inner conflict; you might sweat from it — "No, let it be, I will withdraw." Strongly experiencing primitive emotions, unconscious powers: you don't really live consciously. As with the instinct for self-preservation: secretion of odors to keep others at a distance.

Hindering yourself from self-development; suppressed possibilities, talents.

Acknowledge your worth and become master over yourself: discover your particular possibilities and dare to come outwards in a self-aware way. No one else can threaten you: by degrading yourself and keeping your friends at a distance, you are but your own enemy. Integrate your feelings into the totality and dare to be more spontaneous; anxieties will disappear when you start to love yourself — why have you thus far repudiated yourself? Transform primitive powers into awareness.

BONE MARROW

Bone marrow is the soft substance of certain bones in the body, which produces the blood corpuscles. Ailments of the bone marrow, therefore, have direct consequences for the Blood (See Blood).

Psychological correspondence

Feeling safe and sheltered as a child of the "earth." Already in the mother's womb, a continual genesis of your human condition, a development of expanding energy fields, which carry with them power and joy. Life is eagerly grasped for, a strong urge for life shapes structure. The consciousness that was already there before becoming a human being propels and directs onward its irresistible longing for life; the bone marrow immediately converts these impulses into the manufacture of the "guarantors" of life — among others the fiery, radiant red blood corpuscles and the protecting white blood corpuscles. The bone marrow, therefore, symbolizes a feeling of safety, of power, and an awareness of immunity — of inexhaustible growth and extension of human existence.

Feeling yourself one with the flower children and, while amongst them, still being aware that you are boundlessly unique. The suppleness and free radiating powers of man, incorporated in a structure (skeleton). The longing of your consciousness, your life essence, which is asking to build up your existence, to blossom, and to place yourself safely therein. The bone marrow is like a seed, which, if well-watered with faith, guarantees total compliance with the longings of the deepest Self: a powerful growth of a secure life on earth. At the same time, it is also a translation of the Balance between spirit and matter, of the consciousness that is in every cell in the body and of how the body grows: instructed by our deepest inner Consciousness — the captain of the ship — the bone marrow responds to these commands. Commands which are based on longings, emotions, expectations — the urge for Life.

Ailments, in general

Have you no faith in this strong basis? Do you neglect your personal Self? The power of your Consciousness? If so, you pass on negative information to the bone marrow, which then is disappointed, although it was prepared to guarantee you a strong life. Why do you block this beautiful system with your thoughts and feelings of inability and insecurity? You feel a rope around your neck. You hinder yourself from blossoming forth, from growing, from creatively going through life. Needless anxieties. You seek too much safety OUTSIDE yourself, in a parent, a partner, or a teddy bear. You cling too much to others; you smother yourself and refuse to recognize your independent Self as *the* central power source! In other words, you simply don't call upon your secure axis, your bone marrow: therefore, it will not be active the way it should be, or else it will give a distorted image of the distorted relationship you maintain with your Soul essence! You close yourself up instead of radiating joy and freedom. You would rather endlessly run in place, doubting your possibilities; you are brimming over with potentialities, but you are holding them back and don't allow them to blossom: only your disbelief, or that of your parents or mentors — who influence you greatly — block you.

Stretch open wide; stop tying yourself down. Acknowledge your safe basis. Break radically with dependence on people or means that take the place of your original self-healing system.

Trust your nature completely, and this trust will reward you beautifully! You are you. You have yourself, and no one can assume this precious place. Nothing "just happens." Have you lost a friend? Is your world falling apart because of this? Do you say, "What do I have left?" As a human being you are unique and so worthy: build a new life upon your Self, and enjoy! Now realize completely that it is you who creates your life. Be open to the inner propelling forces of your Consciousness and let yourself be led intuitively: the only thing you really have to do is believe, trust.
(See Part I)

Bone marrow infection
osteomyelitis
(See also Bone marrow, in general)

Unconscious mistrust, even suspicion — especially of yourself, and also of life in general. You don't trust the solidity of your own safe little house! You are filled to the brim with energies that would like to blossom, full of potential, and you want to push through and live your powers to the fullest — but first you look suspiciously around, carefully and anxiously. You experience the pushing and stimulating power in you, a pent-up urge for life, which even tends to become aggressive because of this suppression — you are poised on the edge of your chair, wanting to make the jump into active life and — "Help! I can't! I feel so lonely! I don't feel safe. . . ." You pull back, and you would even go against the stream to pull back. Unconscious anxieties and emotions hold back the productive spreading of energies. You don't at all realize how your Self-awareness is the true Leader of the unconscious, even if you experience this unconscious as a vessel full of dark, yes, black, untrustworthy substance. You have to govern it all, hold it in or control it — so you think. You assign great power to the negative in yourself. You are afraid of being hurt and, therefore, do you not dare to live? You only hurt yourself. You are angry because you don't get the backing from a partner, a parent.

Nothing is negative in you, neither are your powerfully pushing energies, which wish to live in joy, but which, because of suppression, can be experienced as a threat. Trust the inner Essence in you — which you can consistently trust — and burst open in a fearless lust for life! Get your feet entirely on the ground, experience the balance of your consciousness in matter.

Enjoy spiritual as well as physical possibilities in your existence. No longer hold back the flow of energy; don't make yourself angry in this powerlessness, but break through! This powerful energy that wishes to come through is nothing less than Joy, than your Self's love of you, of Life. This power drives away all anxieties.

Surrender to it. In this you will find the only true buttress.

The Key to Self-Liberation, Christiane Beerlandt © Beerlandt Publications

BOTULISM

You feel yourself very slowly taken by the neck, by something powerful, undefinable. For a long time, you have lived with anxieties. You offer no resistance any more. You are defenseless against your dark emotions, your sadness, your deep anxieties. You feel helplessly sucked along in an enormous stream of negative energies, which are the result of your powerlessness, of your self-denial. You live for others, not really for yourself. You let yourself be seized and controlled by others: a dead-end street, which leads ever further toward emptiness — this illness shakes you awake out of your dream!

*Come into yourself and **give** yourself the life, the warmth, which you deserve. Don't **let** yourself "be lived" any longer: feel peaceful and safe in your nature. You will find shelter only deep in your Self. Your eternal "I," which never dies. Anxieties are needless. **Feel** your strong energies, allow them to come through with great speed: direct them with the power of your conscious spirit. Only you are master over your body. Stand solidly, with your feet on the ground; listen to the deep inner wisdom in yourself, and again bring rest and harmony into your disturbed and anxious life. (See Anxiety)*

BRAIN

"We are no victims of our brain. . . ."
(See also Hypophysis)

The "Living Self," the entity we are, this Spirit-consciousness, is the eternal, driving power behind the physical body we take on. It carries a computer memory, knowledge and insight out of the "past" — your personal past, and that of the entire cosmic happening. It bears your emotional memories, but above all also your personal conclusions and convictions, which you have formed on the basis of events and personal experiences. It bears the creating powers just as much, the possibility to grow constantly, the spontaneous joy of being, the longing for self-discovery via experiences in a physical existence. Individual and unique.

We mean here a very wide, open awareness. The activity, the power of the brain, is precisely a manifestation of this Living Self, which enters into the human, earthly existence. The brain is able to take up information from the personal computer of the Self, store it, and translate it outwardly.

Certain older parts of the brain, such as the brain stem, store primitive information and send impulses that have to do with the most primal needs of man: his defensive response to danger, his hunger, his compulsive instincts to preserve the species. . . .

The so-called newer parts of the brain, especially the cerebrum and the cerebral cortex, allow man, on the one hand via subtle patterns, to arrive at creativity, conscious emotional experiences, intuitive growth, artistry — and on the other hand to develop rational, organizing, logical behavior.

The evolution of man requires that we — in expanded Consciousness — increasingly use the as yet unutilized parts of the brain; that here and now we should, with our Conscious "I," increasingly acquire a "hold" on the ages-old, compulsive or unconscious stored-up habits or reflexes. We should transform these unconscious power fields into Consciousness. (See Menstruation, Sexuality; Dying, Part I)

The brain is governed by the Living Self, but also, thanks to our becoming more and more Conscious — through utilization of the brain, among other things — we are able to bring new information into our computer, information which can usher in a totally new evolution of mankind. In order to take our lives in our hands and direct them in the way that is necessary for the liberation of mankind and its suffering, we are required to become Conscious of that which, until now, was an obstacle to leading the Earth to joy — and we are also required to become conscious of that which has hindered every individual person from building up his life in the way that would offer the most happiness. In both cases it has to do with the following: the negative vision of ourselves and Mankind in general; doubt about ourselves.

We think we possess, deep inside, a sort of inescapable, dark "subconsciousness," and that we have no say in the matter. We think that a lot of "evil" — many suppressed emotions, anxieties, and aggressions — have become master over us. And we think that, because of this, we can do nothing more than look for a "pure" way via either wearisome therapy or wrestling with ourselves!

One is of the opinion that everything from the past has to be raked up again before one can resolve the sadness, the anger, or the anxieties of the Now. This is not necessary!

Regarding hypnosis: instead of letting yourself be put under hypnosis, it would be much better to obtain Conscious insight from the here-and-now, and reverse your negative expectations concerning your life. Be your own master and modify your convictions yourself instead of letting others do it (which after all will have only a temporary positive effect on you for the most part, because you would be letting yourself *be* directed instead of controlling the rudder in a self-aware way).

The more conscious your changes, the more effective they are. Your conscious adaptations are immediately received by the underlying Living Self, through which it will transmit new impulses and messages to your brain. As a result, and because of your altered convictions, you will attract totally different happenings. Altered feelings, thoughts, convictions, immediately input new data in your Self: in fact, these convictions, feelings, and thinking patterns work like a propelling motor. On this basis your body and your brain react, and your reality is being built up.

Are you convinced deep inside that you are a victim, one who always will have misfortune in life? Then your brain will send out impulses which will contribute to your future being full of misery. Change these convictions, however, and your brain will create joyful energy fields. The emitting and creating of a positive life happen on many levels. The brain is really like an intricate bunch of yarn, but it forms a perfect system. Via this system our Conscious "I" is also able to gain insight into our deepest Self, into our intuition, into unconscious treasures. We will use this organ to come continuously to further consciousness; left and right brain hemispheres have at this moment yet another function here.

Be convinced that you, yourself, build up your life, that you, yourself, attract all occurrences in your life: but do it consciously, and don't *let* it happen to you.

Open yourself up to your deepest "I," your Living Self, which is not locked up in your brain-structure, but *uses it.* An even-stronger unity between our Living Self and the physical form is at hand: the brain serves us as an intermediary in this evolution.

*At present, one can say that **that** part of the brain stands for this or has that function; but tomorrow it might be different. After all, the brain is a computer that constantly reacts to directions from our Living Self. When we input new data, yes, totally new convictions, then the Living Self will pass different impulses through to our brain. If we accept our* *divinity and our intuition as a deep source of knowledge, then other yet-unexploited brain canals will come into use. Then, our brain will evolve even further, will take on another form; certain parts might disappear or might fulfill another task, everything functioning in accord with our Living Self!*

New energies, also cosmic, offer themselves nowadays: these are only reflections, reactions to the altered condition of mankind's consciousness. The consciousness changes: the brain will accommodate itself to it.

The physical brain is a conduit for making our divine content known: via intuition, introspection, we pick up miraculous information.

Rational exploration of the world is good, but it needs to go hand-in-hand with this inner wisdom. Via our antennas — in the brain — directed outwardly and inwardly, we can evolve toward ever-greater Insight, in truth.

Brain hemispheres

The two hemispheres of the brain are cross-linked by diagonal connections.

For the time being, the left brain hemisphere still stands for those characteristics which for ages long have been labeled as being more "masculine": rational, sober, logically thinking, organizing, controlling, analytical, firmly sifting the wheat from the chaff. . . . The right hemisphere has, instead, a function in the area of intuition, sensitivity, the flexible, the unconscious. By itself, this has nothing to do with "male" or "female," but the man has more and more identified himself with the traits of "hard soberness," whereas the woman was allowed to be gentle and sensitive.

If one hemisphere of the brain would be taken away, however, the other would easily be able to carry out all the functions. In fact, this division into two hemispheres is a reflection of the deepest convictions of mankind: the duality of yang and yin, man and woman as opposites, etc. Furthermore: it

renders *that* point where he, the human being, separated and separates from his original divine Nature. Man placed the gods outside of himself, and he relegated woman and nature to secondary positions.

The intuitive, the divine, in himself was separated from his outer being, from the self-manifesting, active aspect of the Man. A schism — left-right.

That which is often most admired in a person — his or her rational, thinking aspect — is especially experienced via the left hemisphere, by both men and by women.

This polarization had its reasons and its usefulness, but the Unification of the human being within himself is imminent: an harmonious experiencing of intuition and rationality, without a separation between. If a person is open to this flexible unification of the intuitive (which can transmit direct information from the Living Self to us) with the rational, the conscious thinking, the organizing, then he will unify the "male" and "female" in himself, the earthly human and the divine.

LEFT HEMISPHERE OF THE BRAIN

Psychological correspondence and Ailments, in general

A primal potential ability, full of soft golden energies that are asking for a powerful and constructive building of your life, for being used in an active, creative way. Like the storage gland of a spider who is able to create a beautiful, artful web. Let it be the artwork of your life, not to attract or draw in others and devour them, but to build something beautiful for yourself! An enormous storage of Potential, fuel, energy, of creative possibilities that are waiting to be allowed to flow, to be allowed to serve, in order for you to start using them as a Master Human Being in a positive way. Not in an instinctive way, not on a low sexual level, but in service of the Heart, of life, of building something beautiful. Don't *let* yourself be seduced, but develop yourself with gentleness and, at the same time, with force and ability. Don't hang on to others, don't catch anyone in your web, but *give* life to yourself, and help life along.

Build, construct, do masonry, and work on your life. Not vague and absent-minded, not hazily Neptunian. No vague promises and far-away dreams somewhere in the clouds and unreality, nor lovesickness and infatuation, lifeless spheres, angel choirs, and non-existent elfin spheres: it is then the language of intoxication and death, of not living on earth. Don't let yourself slip away here, but anchor yourself solidly and deeply inside yourself; then impel all those energies toward development, and in this way you will never poison yourself. In this *actual, active, creative approach to your existence — very consciously and to the point, actively participating with responsibility,* not PILING UP your energies — it's impossible to poison yourself, nor harm others. At least not if you don't start to grasp, pull or draw others in.

You posses the ability to build strategies, to work out a complete plan, a big house, to elaborate a construction — this is all wonderful as long as you execute it in the service of Life, of your Heart, not in the service of instincts in order to "posses" as much as possible.

You need to build YOUR house of life; therefore don't pass over your limit, or life will call you a stop. He who grasps with black spider-power will himself be seized. Therefore, stay very close to yourself and constantly unroll, dynamically, your wonderful potential in the construction of your existence. Give to life, exploit all your talents, your powers, your creative possibilities, and don't tarry in doing this. Don't direct your outlook toward "How can I catch someone," or "How can I fool someone." Instead, know that you as a representative of the network of life may yourself contribute to this most wonderful, endlessly evolving artwork of

life, whose construction never stops: the symbolism of "8" in the most positive sense!

Now, bring yourself close, very close, taking yourself into the circle of life, as a Human Being, and fully participate in it. Don't allow yourself to live by your Instincts; don't allow yourself to run dry, nor grasp for things outside yourself, but take hold of *your Scepter* and lead your mass of energies in the right channels. In this way, you will grow more and more. Your *life's construction* becomes magnificent! You don't stop; you go on, and constantly give, without expecting, taking or demanding anything! You don't take a single step backward. You UNFOLD yourself by your deeds, in your work, in the development of your talents.

Symbolically, this indicates the correspondence of the testicles[2] which speak about the "female," productive, expectant aspect within the "male" structure. *The left brain hemisphere asks for active construction, a taking things in hand, a constant going onward, using your brain in a creative way in order to develop yourself and your life more and more, farther from the deathly spheres, away from the primal womb out of which you once came. When set to work in this constructive, creative way, everything will go wonderfully, and you will feel happy, not anxious.* When, however, you try to "think up" or "spin" something in order to provide against all kinds of things in an instinctive, rational way — instead of going onward, working, building, in trust — or to outdo someone else, or to get someone, catch him, then things go wrong. Then this brain hemisphere, the human being, will be swallowed up in the dark tunnel of death, which he had planned for someone else. This brain hemisphere wants to build, to contribute — in a constructive, logical way, and at the same time based upon a deeper knowing, an intuitive knowing — to the construction and development of Life, in and outside itself.

---

[2] Read more about this in the category *Testicles*.

The Key to Self-Liberation, Christiane Beerlandt © Beerlandt Publications

The human being has within himself the ability, the potential, and the Power to bring himself farther along in Life or to guide himself again and again in an old pattern toward death. It's up to him to allow the web (which he is able to build so wonderfully) to expand in the direction of *more life,* thus exceeding the borders of Pluto, while still remaining very close to his core so that he doesn't build anything that might lure himself or someone else (again) into the Trap. It is the spider web that never catches a fly but is built in order to be an ever-greater, magnificent image of life: golden threads with the dew of life on which life can establish itself, always, eternally, constantly.

The human being takes this *Power in a positive way.* Standing at the head of his existence, the scepter in his right hand, continuously building, he applies his forces as a Human Being, not like an instinctive animal that has to figure out strategies for survival. Placing his brain at the service of further development of life, without end. All talents and abilities in the service of this. Structures are powerful, clear, and transparent, like a framework for life, ever more. The human being who never stops creating — very structurally harmonious, in the service of further life expansion — is definitely getting out of the attracting primal womb. He no longer draws in himself, no longer catches prey, is therefore no longer swallowed up by it. Here, the human being makes an end to the physical death, if he so wishes.[3]

RIGHT HEMISPHERE OF THE BRAIN

Psychological correspondence

Supply you glide through life, bendable and flexible, with healthy pride. It all happens automatically, as it were; you "feel" how and where you have to be, go, or sit, what you have to do and when. You don't ponder it; in an intuitive way, you bring about what you feel you have to do. In this way everything also easily slides off you; nothing sticks to you. You don't worry about anything, and you experience life as being easy . . . because you "yield" — however anchored you are in your solid, thick roots — because you don't offer any resistance. Flexibility combined with skillfulness and being nimble in the way you move through life.

And if there's a problem, it can't last for long; you "know," "feel," a simple, natural solution for everything; you don't worry. And if one thing doesn't work, then you will find something else. A lively mind, a flexible back, not holding on to things that belong to yesterday. You go onward, agile and happy, full of trust, and without even once questioning yourself about your safety, because you are safe and strong in your own womb. You don't droop. You always go onward and never step back from the decisions you have made, except if life asks it of you. You bend . . . very easily: to Life, yes!

Ailments, in general

You are sharp, hard, cutting. You would cut your own skin, as it were. You say, "No." You refuse to go along supply in the direction of the wind of life. You fight against it, offer resistance. You hurt yourself in a hard, sharp way. You stand still and refuse to go any farther.

You tie yourself down, tie down your flexibility, that which we mostly call "the female aspect," the "dolphin mobility" in yourself. You allow it all to "dry up"; you don't allow yourself to play around freely and merrily in the sea of life. You force the dolphin inside you out of the water, out of the sea. You immobilize yourself, paralyze yourself. A refusal to go on, to swim on. Stubbornly, coercively, holding yourself back. A self-blockage, even withholding life

---

[3] Read more about this in *New Days.*

from yourself. Loveless, hard, unmercifully cold.

Therefore, surrender now in all flexibility to life inside yourself, to a free waterfall that guides you in a delightful way to earthly paradise. One with your body, gentle with your body. Strongly swimming along, sensitively and intuitively... GLADLY enjoying your existence in this life-space. You let yourself go; you allow yourself to be taken along by this stream of life, through the happy waters of life. You let everything be, everything go, and you know, you feel, that it is good.

Concussion

Where is your Essence? Your self-aware sun-center???

You are like a hollow barrel, filled with emotions, with "other(s)," instead of being aware of the fullness in yourself. Are you perhaps of the opinion that you *really do* live from out of yourself, that you surrender to your deepest "I"? No: you place the Sun, the authority, the center of your life, outside yourself. You are like a Full Moon, which can only give light when she finds herself in the rays of the sun.

In this way, you live artificially: you hold on to a partner, to another; you follow in the footsteps of that other so that you no longer go straight for your goal.

You look for rescue outside of yourself. A friend can be a drug for you, in which you totally sink away.

In this attachment you finally smother yourself, immobilize yourself. You feel totally squeezed closed, seized by the neck — you are dragged along. It seems as if you cannot resist.

For instance, a child can feel totally crushed under the authority of father or teacher; it doesn't truly believe in its autonomous worth.

You go along with (or follow) someone; you are afraid to be yourself, would run away from yourself. You feel safer in a situation

of attachment. Your head overflows with emotions . . . : by far, the "female" aspect dominates the "male" in you. In a Neptunian way, you flee (alcohol, outer image, . . .); you wish only to be held by someone else. . . .

You ignore your personal worthy content!

Have you been shaken awake? Take a good look at yourself: immerse yourself in yourself now and arrive at your Essence. Don't be afraid, no longer run away from yourself; make use of a beautiful balanced structure within: feelings, inner life, and powerful self-aware manifestation! Not the moon, but the sun is the center; so is it also with you.

No longer neglect the gold in yourself. Become conscious of your personal worth, talents, and possibilities. Only when you ac-knowledge yourself as autonomous and Worthy, independent of others, can a beau-tiful, balanced relationship with others come to be, without your losing yourself or suffo-cating in it. Thus, first arrive at this unifica-tion with yourself, no longer placing yourself below anyone. Discover this deep, beautiful reality of your personality: brain concus-sions ask for a transformation. Now draw out of yourself the most beautiful and deepest treasures.

Take pride in yourself and live with self-respect, trusting that everything which is good for you will come to you if you open up for it and if you no longer cling emotionally to people or things outside yourself. You are a sun: radiate and you will warm yourself and attract beautiful things toward you. Or, would you rather let yourself be burned by the rays of someone else?

Free yourself, enjoy, create your life **yourself.**

Brain embolism

You flee. . . . You feel totally stuck; you'd like to escape from life; you are already looking at that which comes after death — you are already occupied with death because here on earth you don't want to — or can't — go on.

The Key to Self-Liberation, Christiane Beerlandt © Beerlandt Publications

You feel too much like a child, dependent on others; you have much to ruminate (memories, experiences, impressions, emotions), but it's getting hard for you to swallow it all. Life becomes too heavy for you. ... You stand, as it were, not truly on your own feet; you feel seized by something or someone; you experience yourself like a fish in a net; it's as if you've been beheaded — you don't truly live from out of your center!

To avoid brain embolisms one will have to acknowledge and respect one's royal worth as a human being; open your brain to the light, to joy, and let your sunbeams be freed: a complete liberation from black thoughts and from a hopeless existence. Do you choose life or death? Don't live like a dead person; in freedom, choose and determine your life's path.

Don't be downcast; go onward in joy. Come again out of your hiding place!

Brain hemorrhage

Like a Jupiter, you would — with the best of intentions because you know best of course — like to regulate, arrange, and control things too much. Wanting to organize everything from above; you try to rise above everything. You embrace *very* much: work, relationships, children — you continuously envelop more, without once falling back upon your own Essence.

You go beyond your limits, as if your worth as a human being depends on the degree to which you do or organize everything for others.

For once, sit still by yourself, on *your* chair. Stay within your territory; trust your strong Basis: giving your full attention toward others is in part, self-delusory, resistance to evolving yourself, to discovering the worthiness in yourself, independent of others.

You don't truly live from out of yourself. You probably don't accept any interference from others. You definitely don't accept any contradiction.

"Take," you say to others; in this way you bind them to you, but you don't help yourself, nor the others. You give freely, but perhaps others "have to" accept it. If one refuses your energy, your help, then you are now thrown back upon yourself! Let go. No longer grow away from your own center; discover life within yourself.

Let go of your stubbornness; no longer look for "self-affirmation," but be aware of your Worth and simply enjoy. Don't be afraid to look inside yourself.

Or would you rather die than *really* Live?

Meningitis

Fearfully and furiously running away, fleeing. Inner aggressive powers press for a breakthrough, but neither self-realization nor anger find their way outward. A short circuit, caused by an overload of heavy, emotional thinking and thinking — without end. You fear you are "bad." You don't dare live according to your nature, your feelings. You are fearful of school, severe structures, church or an authority over you, afraid of being punished. At the same time, you are furious about it. You feel constricted around the neck. You feel bound at the wrist — "Let go of me!" You don't succeed in standing on your own feet and living from out of yourself: your true fruitfulness is being drained away, unused. Mortal fears. Guilt feelings. It seems that everything happens to you as if you have no say in your life, as if deep emotions drag you down to dark depths, and that you cannot do anything about it. Sadness; you are afraid of being unable to handle everything, because you live like an automaton, or like a chameleon which constantly adapts superficially to others and to its environment.

The alarm clock now sounds in order that you might find the true Authority in yourself. So that you no longer resist your own "goodness," your own creative possibilities.

Actually, you would struggle against the mother who feeds you because, powerless and angry, you are fighting for your own space. But you remain closed, so afraid of these deep emotions in yourself that you anxiously keep them hidden in your head, which is about to burst. As a matter of fact, you hide your total being, your nature, in order to protect yourself, and you do so as if you don't want anyone to see the way you inwardly feel, or the way you *are*. You don't know yourself; you are searching, but you don't trust it all. You firmly hold on to certain things because you are afraid it all might escape you: a sense of threat.

Perhaps you "prattle" away, but then only superficially, so that you keep yourself hidden in the depths, but at the same time can still win attention from others (and approval). For this reason, you adapt to the demands of your audience so that you ignore your own true nature. Emotions run over, you are in pain, you cannot handle it this way any longer.

Let the bow not be strung so tightly: release your feelings, let yourself go; emotions can never destroy you as long as you don't keep bottling them up. Express your talents, come to true productivity, place the mastery in yourself, demand space for yourself (in Love for yourself and assertiveness, without desires or anger); stand on your own feet now. Show yourself openly as you are, and struggle free: then you will no longer be angry with others. You are protected in your Self; know yourself to be safe and sheltered. Take a good look into yourself: you are good and unique, in your own way. Arrive at openness, clarity in yourself, and don't hide yourself. Channel your emotions and creative powers and work them out; don't bottle everything up.

Be proud of yourself; climb out of this emotional darkness – for you ARE not really if you dwell in this darkness. Deal with and make an end to negative influences from the past; live here and now in the true light of the sun-center within yourself. Nothing just "happens" to you: become master of your

own existence and in self-awareness create your life. Turn yourself toward life instead of toward death. Your life lies in your hands; make something beautiful of it. Bring in joy, and in this way manage your emotional powers and thoughts so they can serve as building stones for a new home.

Stroke
CVA — cerebrovascular accident
brain damage because of a reduction in blood flow in the brain, often with paralysis as a result

There is a kind of dividedness: "Shall I or shall I not let go?"

The end of the rainbow. A profound, unconscious longing to leave everything behind dwells inside you — to let go, with one cannon blast, of everything that's past, leaving it behind. (The solution here doesn't mean: escape from the earth; on the contrary, you, yourself, have to leave the past behind in this existence!) It's all about to explode . . . you have been keeping it in for too long. Therefore, let go of everything now, let it all explode, and get in touch with the PRESENT, with YOURSELF, your wonderful body. Look only at the cheerful things; darkness lies behind you, dark clouds have been driven away. Now, go onward. Have you tried to embrace so much that you almost started to strangle things, possibly in anger and frustration because of what has been done to you? Then let go now, let go of everything, and believe in your good fortune — as long as you let go, then this happiness lies in front of you!

A bomb is about to go off, therefore, let it go, let it explode. Spring from yourself, jump out of your egg; no longer immobilize yourself with pent-up energies; don't run in place; don't keep thinking in circles, but break through with all the Mars power inside you, allowing the old to destroy itself. Go on, uninterrupted. Don't get stuck with your thoughts on certain things (from the moment or the past), but allow these thoughts to constructively build toward something new!

Allow emotions to exist/go freely . . . allow the sadness from the past to flow away; don't hold your feelings back. Allow the excess to flow away, let them stream away. There will only be a flood if you hold them in too long. Water finds its way where there is least resistance: from now on handle your water of life, your emotional forces, in a fruitful, creative way.

Bring to the surface that which resides on the bottom of your being and allow that sea of energies and feelings inside you to swirl and foam! Bring above ground all that is inside you; expand, construct. Make something wonderful of your life! Get intimately in touch with yourself, with your body, and feel that joy that scintillates in your body; because you are happy with and about yourself, because you now see the sense of things again, now that you leave everything behind and turn yourself, full of faith, toward a magnificent future. Forget the old, and build up your life anew! Tune in to that fundamental power in yourself, to the inner life-source that feeds your body — which concentrates itself with full force — and experience that motivation toward Life in every fiber of your body! Reunite yourself with yourself again and no longer worry about the past; go onward.

Don't keep yourself at a distance from the Earth, but plant your heels solidly on the ground! Feel in touch with your body, your earthly ground. Feel that FORCE OF UNITY, which you ARE — soul power in your body — and take your place, highly unique like no one else in the world. Because you are very special as YOU. Make yourself happy, and begin again as never before . . . in happiness about your being.

TIA

transient ischemic attack
temporary attack from a shortage of oxygen in the brain (can cause, for example, transient paralysis or temporary loss of eyesight)

You experience yourself too much as empty, and you would like to pump yourself full of stuffing as it were, with thoughts, too. Your living Self-center calls a halt to you and urges you to turn the steering wheel of your life vehicle in the right direction: turn it 180 degrees . . . toward YOURSELF! You want to, want to, and do want to: go here and there, want this and that, but you run in place as it were, because deep inside a voice offers resistance; this can't go on any longer.

Stop! First, look INSIDE yourself, and only then go on. You can't drive on in the same way as before; you first need to look for that which is not really right. You may offer yourself all the chances now to investigate inside yourself. Why does something not go smoothly in life? Because first of all something has to be "realized." Possibly you don't understand it very well, can't grasp it completely: "What's happening now?"

Yes, now let everything outside you go for a while and calmly think about things. Look upon things in wisdom . . . and contemplate for a moment. Don't run on. The signpost is now directed toward your self: therefore, turn yourself deeply toward your own Central Content. Is there any question of "doubt"? Then the moment now has come to solve that deep-rooted doubt in yourself in order to finally arrive at absolute Certainty regarding yourself and your goodness, your autonomy, your Power. Contemplate yourself a moment. Calmly come home to yourself . . . sit down for a moment; turn deeply inward and there feel that safe, eternal basis in you. Know that you can stand at the Head of your life, in Mastership, but that this can only happen when you connect yourself with the *true* values of life, when you don't get stuck with things that are of no importance in life. Autonomy is being asked for. Calmly contemplate yourself a moment, without flying from here to there at the surface of life or letting your thoughts go all over. Come home to yourself again.

Time to come close to yourself, to look inward and go onward in a state of great Rest, without rushing yourself. Inwardly living restfully out of a feeling of certainty. Staying in the HERE AND NOW! Never running ahead of things because if you do, you will attract signals which tell you: return, don't run so fast, go back "to yourself"! In warm love and fully Conscious PRESENCE come to yourself!

Brain tumor

A summons from the inner Self for radical transformation! A life that cannot go on in this way.

It requires a radical break with the old life, with negative convictions about yourself, with indoctrinations from the past!

Aspiration to rebirth; a reconsideration of your life, putting a stop to self-destructive thinking and habits.

Perhaps you have constantly cut yourself off from your intuition or from your feelings and higher consciousness. Did you cling to the one-sided rationality, "the thinking," or to the superficial.... Reconsider your convictions: let go of all resistance and look for a solution with a complete alteration in yourself!

A new life, saying goodbye to the old! There is no middle course. The cause of emotional overburdening lies with you. (See Part I)

BREASTS, FEMALE

Psychological correspondence

The breasts symbolize, on the one hand, the safe sheltered feeling in yourself, and on the other hand, the self-aware, giving, radiating toward others. They symbolize gentleness, goodness, the maternal, cherishing aspect, being welcome. You can ever and again fall back upon this inner, nourishing source. The breast will give a healthy or unhealthy reflection of the necessary balance between give and take, between the "masculine" and the "feminine" elements. The "moon" pole represents the emotional, sensitivity, receptivity, intuition, the unconscious, the maternal; the "sun" pole represents the active-producing, the self-manifesting via thought and deed. Interchange between both poles leads to true productivity and growth. The balance is mirrored in the breasts, which symbolize the proud space of a woman, who in a self-aware way leads her emotional life in the right direction, in harmony with the rational.

Ailments, in general

You would like to feel free, but you feel yourself drawn along in a powerful stream of experiences, feelings, on which you cannot get a grip. This causes anxiety. Or, inversely, you *think* and *think* — you don't at all trust your intuition; you try, in an exaggerated way, to control everything via looking and thinking. You accumulate negative thoughts.

Or, do you completely neglect your emotional world? Are you acting as if it doesn't exist (any more)? Hurt? Do you hold on to everything with such an oversensitive, maternal solicitude that you have a bloated, suffocating feeling? A dominant, possessive demeanor? Do you manifest yourself as too strongly aggressive, suppressing the more gentle aspect?

Play first fiddle in your life: in a self-aware, powerful way. On this basis, your warmth and solicitude for others can grow in a balanced way. Give the death-blow to the overbearing moon (holding on to feelings and *exaggerated* concern for others), bore right through in order to arrive at your light, self-certain, sun-core! Radiate in joy; then listen attentively to your emotions. Allow yourself and others to live in freedom. Without suffocation. With the beauty of your creative talents, overcome all that is negative. Blow away that dark vapor of sadness of the past; allow new life-expectations to be born.

Breast cancer
(See also Cancer, in general)

How long will you stay pregnant: with pent-up emotions, with exaggerated concern for others? It is now time you be fully born YOURSELF. You pass yourself over! You cling to others because you have too little faith. Your deepest pain and sorrow from the past are the result of the inability to live yourself, to live for your own being. You grab, instead of letting everything and everyone go — anxieties. Perhaps you clutch to your partner out of fear: you insufficiently trust the life process. Thus, you suck everything in, including the feelings of others — to fill your emptiness. You are not yet aware of the power in your "I" to create and direct your life, *yourself,* the way you wish. Do you constantly walk around with anxieties about "cancer" or about this or that? Then you will attract this negativity!

You have unconsciously called up the cancer *yourself* in order to, among other things, make it clear to you that something in your life must change. Reverse your convictions to make them optimistic about the future, call upon your self-healing energies, trust in this, and let them take their course. Don't block them with brooding, fretting, and doubts! Do you now still live *too* superficially because the past has disappointed you? Are you cut off from your feelings? Do you hush up all kinds of things? Do you live in "false optimism"? Do you grasp for power? Do you and your friend smother each other in a relationship where you both forget that every individual demands "personal" acknowledgment? Love does not smother. Do you take a hard, angry, rancorous position toward the sadness from your past?

You will heal, one hundred percent, if you now erupt, one hundred percent, like a VOLCANO! That is to say: **speak** *about that which you have for so long kept hidden. Express your sadness, don't store up anything anymore, allow your feelings to flow freely; no longer be hard on yourself. Allow yourself to express yourself spontaneously, like a child, to weep, to show your anger: this will not last. But you have already piled things up for too long. The purification phase now requires a total liberation from your burdens: simply* **say** *this to the people who live with you. But stand up for your life! After a short time, you will feel how you, yourself, have activated this powerful, magnetic flow of energy in yourself in order to bring your body, step by step, toward healing! Stand up for yourself: no longer* **let** *yourself "be lived" through the lives of your partner, your children. Learn now, yourself, to enjoy; do things you like to do. In other words, begin at last to love yourself. No longer mope with your thoughts, your fretting: realize the power of your consciousness to direct every cell of your body! Negative thoughts and disbelief in yourself stimulate the cancer cells; on the other hand: full belief in yourself, awareness of your ability to reprogram these cells, will bring you to recovery. This is the reason you have cancer: now, you can teach yourself to feel how You, with your will, are master over your body, which simply obediently carries out your (previously unconscious, now conscious) orders! Bid yourself welcome on earth; be good and tender to yourself. Instead of "grasping" for the child, open your hands wide and* **give** *— to yourself and others. Radiate yourself outwardly; no longer hold yourself back: in this way, your cancer will diminish every day and be replaced by new cells created by your joyful urge for life! There need be no more, but also no fewer.*

Cysts, benign tumors, connective tissue growth
fibrocystic disease

You have no contact with your deepest intuitive Self, with your trustworthy basis; you place the Powers outside yourself and therefore experience yourself as anxious and powerless! You hold on tightly to all problems concerning love and relationships. You don't trust the life process, don't yet have insight into how you can direct your life via your creative thoughts and convictions. On the contrary, you have anxieties about yourself and about others. As if a constantly threatening undercurrent might thwart the positive course of your life. As a consequence, you grip too much onto everything and everyone — in order to feel secure. So that nothing might escape your attention, you begin in an exaggerated way to meddle, to protect or control. In this way you doubt your own proud worth as a human being; you then will let yourself be more easily drawn into a love relationship in which you lose yourself, in which you barely still live for yourself, or into a passionate relationship in which the other is being experienced as the ideal in order to compensate for your own insignificance. Your tremendous, joyful energies cannot produce healthy fruits because these energies are becoming lost in emotions, in worries, in sadness about the past, which you don't let go of. Your sun cannot rise because it is being sucked down by a (often unconscious) dark stream of anxiety, mistrust, and powerlessness. You don't see clearly. You again and again expect yet another problem — and thus, you build up your life in a negative way and call up negative happenings which cause you to "reach for power" all the more over situations and over people. Finally, you don't trust anything anymore and are either going to try to completely dominate others or you will collapse in an outburst of sadness. Perhaps you are anxious about your own hidden, deep stream of emotions, and you try to put everything under the control of the Thinking; doing this only takes you further away from your joyful, powerful Core.

You are waiting for a dangerous bomb to explode: there is no bomb at all! It is your suppressed, enormously creative and joyful energies, which, if you crush them, become threatening powers. These energies require a free breakthrough and trust in your intuitive Self. Come to the fore now! The way a child spontaneously plays its game, so silly and cheerfully may you live! Become aware of the kingship that every man carries within, if only he realizes that it is not one or another fate or god or devil, but he, himself, who determines his life and future events. Nothing happens without it having been self-evoked beforehand in the person! Convince yourself, first of all, that you and your fellow man deserve happiness: in this way, you will give happy occurrences a chance to come through, which until now you have hindered with anxieties! Swellings diminish and disappear when you let go of that of which these lumps consist: your anxieties, the past, your worries, your mistrust. Throw it open, let everything go; know yourself to be safe in your Self!

Mammary gland inflammation
mastitis

Perhaps you have already for a long time been sacrificing yourself for the sake of your children, your partner; or for a group, an ideal, a religion: you sacrifice your personality in order to crawl, as it were, into a task or an outer situation. You become swallowed up in society or a system in which you are totally stowed away. Outwardly, you might appear sensitive and accommodating or "dutiful," balanced and peaceful — but! Inwardly, you pay for this self-denial! You want to get out of this situation! Aggression! You are bursting with emotions, sadness, and negative thoughts (of rancor, even hatred and revenge), full of accumulated frustrations. You'd like to manifest your powers in deeds, to come to the surface, to become master over your anger and sadness, but you don't see how — you don't *really* break through! You have for too long subordinated your "I" to others or to certain situations: your "masculine" active powers, your self-awareness, now finally wish to come through freely.

*First of all, put both feet on the ground: sleep no longer; make your life into **your** life. Your aggression and emotions are the result of self-suppression that has gone on for too long, and of a lack of self-confidence. So, don't be angry with others. Realize that all situations as they exist now in your life have been caused by you, by your unconscious convictions — "That you must sacrifice yourself or must live in a situation that doesn't fit your true nature because you are **but** a servant." This is self-delusion. Be aware of your worth, give yourself love, and as a result you will not care for others or fulfill some artificial task just because you have the need for acknowledgment and gratitude! Then, from out of a self-aware, voluntary, and independent feeling, you will with pleasure enjoy your life, and with pleasure will be ready to help others: in self-respect, let go and also be aware of your place.*

Cracked nipples and breast-feeding difficulties

You believe too little in your inner worth; perhaps you outwardly appear majestic and kingly, presenting a false image, but inwardly you feel insecure, and you ignore the truth, ignore your inner content. You feel more or less anxious because you insufficiently appreciate yourself, bear yourself too little love; you think you have to be on the defense by "having to" behave in a certain way toward the outside. In this unsureness, you hold the little child too tightly; you very dutifully produce milk, but you hurt yourself in doing so because you consider yourself too much like a machine! Namely, you don't establish a *truly* safe, peaceful contact with yourself, and so you squeeze yourself out that much harder to at least be perfect to your baby. Actually, you'd like to feel free, take up space for yourself, but doubts regarding your own possibilities hinder it. Unconscious anxiety that something against which you have no defense might "seize" you; you are not yet completely, lovingly, present in your body, and now another being has a grip on it! It overwhelms you.

*Don't be too hard, too sharp, with yourself. Live from out of your feelings, in self-trust: no one can tell you what to do. Determine your life and lifestyle yourself. Are you "violating" yourself by breast feeding your baby? Then it is better not to breast feed. The real influence on the health of the baby comes from your emotional world! Love, trust, shelter are the most essential nourishment for big and small. Never feel obligated! Anxieties are totally needless: trust, give, and throw off your brooding. Do what you intuitively feel you have to do. Do you **really** want to breast feed? Then first of all cherish your own body, respect it, and know that it is your Consciousness that is master over the whole situation. Self-trust, with your feet solidly on the ground; every baby is different, every mother is also different. No nurse or girlfriend can tell you what is good for you both. Unconscious anxieties: your little one has chosen to be born with you: it is a matter of welcome and longing, not of threat.*

Oversensitivity of the breasts

Oversensitivity, sadness: your happiness, your joy, seem to be dependent on external factors!

An entire mountain of feelings, upon which you cannot get a grip. You let yourself droop in emotional weakness; limply, you allow yourself to be ruled by others. No trust in your own powers and possibilities; experiencing yourself as dependent and unable to take life in your own hands and direct it. You are too easily influenced by your surroundings.

Self-confidence! Let your inner nature say it: follow your deepest intuition, allow yourself to be steered by inner knowing and feeling. Trust in this automatic control system of yours, which always works like a sort of radar: dare to fly into life, like a bird, carefree, and without brooding or fretting. You cannot understand everything with your rational mind. Govern your life with your Self-awareness, make your wish-list, and leave the rest to the natural, creative processes, which react to this without the need for your conscious interference. True joy lies inside yourself! Mark off your terrain; only you determine your life!

Breast prosthesis

Whether a person has breasts or not — or one or three — what does it matter? It is of no importance. The human being urgently has to step out of his norm-pattern and begin to live from within, from out of the heart. Every human body is different and unique, good the way it is. Our world has set itself to fixate on outer appearances (one of the greatest diseases) and no longer knows true beauty![4] True beauty places itself in the form that is honestly shaped from the heart. Ugly is the form that is molded and manipulated in order "to look like . . ." Breast prostheses are not "necessary."

The female and male aspect are present in every human being, and THIS IS INDEPENDENT FROM ANY OUTER FORM. Do not want to "look like," but "BE" — like YOU, as who you *are* as LOVING HUMAN BEING, no matter if you have no breasts or many. This has nothing to do with the essence of life, nor with true beauty. Just be yourself, the way you *are:* live from out of your heart, and those who love you will find you beautiful for who you are, according to content as well as form, the way you are, with or without breasts, whether they droop or are firm. This is of no importance whatsoever, no matter what society says about it.

Don't betray your nature. Show yourself the way you really are, according to content and form. "Living according to truth" makes you happy and healthy.

True love experiences with a partner, true enjoyment in sexuality, has nothing to do with the fact of having breasts or how they might look. True love, intense enjoyment, and sexuality go much deeper than that. Only those people who create norms and make conditions and want sex without love, possibly cling to indoctrinations regarding beauty, but this path ends in death. So, be yourself, uniquely beautiful in your way; live from out of your heart and experience the love in your body the way you are, no matter what you look like. You are good and beautiful the way you are as long as you are honestly yourself, with one, two, none, or three breasts. This is not important for life and true love enjoyment!

BAD BREATH
halitosis

Having difficulty working out psychological problems: you hold on to certain emotions like someone who is a Cancer. Obstinately, stubbornly, you keep a hold; you want to be defiant and prove yourself strong. We are dealing here with an inner resistance that results in a lack of ability to assimilate or accept external occurrences or emotional matters. You form, as it were, inner poison, because you feel defenseless, indignant, or mistreated. Anger, powerlessness. Unconsciously, you might allow feelings of revenge to brew (only in extreme cases).

This requires an "airing" of yourself, a ventilation in order to purify yourself of negative feelings. Listen quietly, live in a relaxed openness, without feeling threatened beforehand! Feel strong and protected in your own

---

[4] Read more about this in *Large, Beautiful, and Healthy.*

power center and peacefully work out all the factors that work on you from without.

In love, GIVE to yourself, to others, being grateful that you "ARE." Be aware of your inner grandeur, and now look deeply into yourself.

BRUCELLOSIS

Enough! In fury, pushing away, with all power! "I'm allowed *nothing* anymore!" You cannot be yourself at all in the space that is allotted to you or in the psychological prison in which you are. With tremendous aggression, you break out! Revolt. A call, directed toward the outside: "Help me! Free me now from this oppressive situation." You don't feel yourself appreciated; indeed, rather you have the feeling of being not acknowledged by others. You refuse to accept this situation any longer.

Mark off your own terrain, take up your space and make everyone understand: this is my place; respect my existence. For this, it is necessary that you first of all become aware of your own power center. Be good to yourself, to the little child inside you. Don't take a hard, stalwart position; don't suppress your gentle heart. Don't lock yourself up. Make your fellow man understand that you wish to experience this psychological space for yourself, in freedom. Only when you acknowledge yourself will others acknowledge you.

BRUISES
(See also the relevant body part)

Fear of no longer having a grip on anything; you even don't feel you are truly in yourself: you are running away from your individual

worth. Suppression of your own power; frustration. You feel sorrow, emotions, but you would rather run away from them. Your feeling of weakness sometimes makes you angry! You put yourself under an Authority: "Don't we have to be of service, submerging ourselves in an anonymous mass of people?" Or, are we slaves of television, of laws that society has put on us? "Me, poor me; I have no say over myself anymore!"

We *let* ourselves be hurt, are martyrs, pity ourselves — whenever we are *just there,* static, bound like a slave in servitude, obedient, accepting that things are supposed to be this way: "What do I have to say? Nothing. My boss or my god, they know better and are allowed to punish me. . . ."

Liberate yourself! Live your life YOUR-SELF! Hold on tightly to your central Essence and truly stand on your own feet. Don't first of all live for the group, the club, the masses, or for others, but for yourself. Not in an "egotistic" way, but in full Respect. Servitude by which you harm yourself is not Love, but is self-denial. You can love others only when first and foremost you love yourself: stop this self-torture!

Base yourself on your own authority!

BUMPS

You cannot or dare not really be yourself; you save up all your potential energies, your talents, your range of possibilities. . . . Emotions and frustrations grow but find no way out. Considering yourself through the eyes of the outer world and in order to protect your image — or just because you don't believe in yourself or think you have to hide — you can kill your true, dynamic, fiery nature behind a mask of silent holiness (or sanctimoniousness?). You might sacrifice yourself for others this way; inwardly, you are straining at the leash, in conflict: on the one hand, powerful energies, and on the other hand, tensely holding yourself back. You feel powerless to go in the direction that is in line with your true nature, with your longing. It seems as if others are hindering you, but it is you who plays the ostrich, who holds on to things which it would be better to let go of. An inner collision, which can lead to a confrontation with the outer world: a hard, aggressive collision with situations — with things or people — is but the consequence of an accumulation of aggressive powers in yourself, powers which bring a strongly charged electromagnetic field into existence. Do you not live in inner harmony? Do you live in conflict with your true nature? If so, you will attract a "collision" with your surroundings. That which the outer world, your parents or mentors, long to have from you is in conflict with your own longings: there is a collision. You offer resistance to others, but also to yourself, to becoming who you are. You are not sure of yourself; you don't really feel safe in the Basis of your Self.

*Sail on another route, hold the controls tightly, and be faithful to yourself: cover the whole gamut of possibilities in yourself and no longer bottle up natural energies! Action, creativity, expression! Be yourself; accentuate your self-aware powers in the building up of an honest life without self-impediment. Especially don't be afraid of expressing your emotions, even to speak hard words or bang your fist on the table: these are natural human expressions which avoid accidents or larger disputes. After all, it is just suppressed, accumulated emotions which finally lead to physical violence. Experience yourself without frustration. But then look closely at **where** the cause of your anger lies (deep inside yourself) so that a feeling of Peace and power over yourself, peace with others — contentment regarding life itself — is ultimately the final result.*

BURNS
burning oneself

A form of painful self-destruction, which mirrors the image of someone who burns, suppresses, his creative energies, emotions, and self-realization. You burn from withheld aggression! A Peak of nervousness and/or anger. Powerlessness, revolt. You feel bound, held back, as if you can't go where you want to or can't do/have *what* you wish to do/have. You are inclined to blame this on others, but the true cause lies inside you! You'd like to stand up for yourself, but you don't do it, or do it insufficiently: this makes you extremely nervous and angry. The true cause? You lack Self-respect, love for yourself: you suppress certain energies, pushing away certain emotions, longings, and spontaneous impulses. As a response, you might make yourself nervous about petty things and exceed your limits when it comes to inner control of your nerves. You simply fly off the handle because of frustration! Your emotions spark into flames that require action: stand up for yourself, express your feelings and longings; the stored-up, unused energies in you grow too hot and ask to be freed. Perhaps you are angry with others, but this anger is simply a "diversionary tactic" to avoid confrontation with the truth regarding yourself: it is now time to turn this dormant aggression into an active, powerful development of your life. Don't live only for others, nor in a way that totally dissatisfies you. Come into your "Being" and abandon your "wanting to have."

No longer flee from yourself! Take up the scepter as a worthy being and realize that your nervousness and anger are, in fact, expressions of powerlessness because of the situation your are in. This requires a calm introspection. In what do you feel hindered? In what respect do you prevent yourself from coming to complete self-realization? Have you directed your anger toward certain persons? Look close at why you blame these persons, and for what, and you will notice that you are dealing with self-projection, or with an inability to express yourself to them in a healthy way. Are you angry with yourself? If so, you become angry with everything and everyone. What do you find so bad in yourself? Why do you not break through? Get rid of your feelings of inferiority or of being limited; and in rest and self-trust enjoy everything you undertake. Don't rush, not for anyone. Allow your total personality to develop peacefully, at its own tempo, without throwing up self-impediments. Don't resist true EVOLUTION; don't stagnate in ancient patterns that paralyze your true creativity. Let go . . . and go onward!

BURNOUT

You are "bending" so much that your knee joints are crunching.[5] Are you bending so deeply in life that you come to "nothing"? You hurt yourself; you are hard on yourself. A pent-up resistance. A persistence, no matter how many times you get beaten, no matter how many signals. You don't give up; you stubbornly go on, despite your pain. A holding-back and holding-in of energies, of information, of things that would be better if you did say them, announce them, express them to your environment. But you turn inward and hurt yourself, instead of stopping inflicting pain on yourself. You hold everything in; you *swallow* a lot, swallow everything, and you refuse sometimes to bring out words of truth. Why torture yourself in this way? Why be silent when you feel you have to speak? Do you sell your soul, your health, in order to "fill" yourself as much as possible with things outside yourself? So that you

don't really have to become yourself: afraid of being "nothing" outside your work, or outside the filling-yourself with others, with things, with people, with a job? Falling in a black hole, so to speak?

A kind of *stubbornness, resistance* to letting go, even if you suffer under it: "I don't want to, and won't, stop!" You shall and will *keep it up* until, as it were, you collapse under it. You commit treason on yourself, on your heart — not only out of fear of falling into a black hole if you don't do it, because you don't yet recognize the true value of yourself, and possibly you look for fulfillment in work, in earning money, in recognition through your job, etc. — but possibly also by "going on" at whatever cost in order not to be unfaithful to others, in order to save others, to help them (or so you think).

Know, then, that life asks you first and foremost to look deeply inward for the worthiness of yourself, not clamping onto things, no longer "filling" yourself with things that should give your life a kind of "purpose or worth." This can't be: look for the TRUE worthiness deep inside yourself, and let go where necessary, say "no" where necessary; stop where you feel you have to stop: always be FAITHFUL to yourself! No more stubborn persistence!

First and foremost, Love yourself. Only then can you do good for others. Doing good for others at the cost of yourself — this life cannot accept. Filling your time by working for others, for instance, and in the meantime not enjoying yourself nor taking time for yourself — life no longer can allow this.

You swallow, and you throw your head back; you take in, you let things happen, like a snake that doesn't transform. You can handle a lot, but now you have come to the absolute limit.

Don't refuse to stand up as a human being. Bring out your energies, speaking honestly; be yourself in words, deeds, and feelings, exteriorizing yourself. No longer hold yourself in. No longer swallow, but push

---

[5] Read the category "Knee" in this book.

forces outward; no longer fill yourself with things, work, people, but stand straight, as "I." Rise up as a human being and transform. Become who you really are and rise up from your old state of not yet really wanting/daring to be yourself. Take your place as you, completely; don't allow yourself to be filled with things, energies, people outside yourself. Straighten that solid skeleton in your being. Rely on that stalwart structure of your being and stand firmly straight, no longer bend low. No longer fill yourself with things from outside you, but now bring yourself to fulfillment; realize your fullness, your power, and live while being honest with your living essence. Or for you is it so difficult: *starting to fill yourself only "with yourself"? Is there an unconscious refusal to truly allow yourself to be born as a human being?*

No longer hurt yourself. Now direct your forces outward; come outward with all these energies in a giving way — to yourself, to others — no longer closing yourself up, making yourself smaller, opening your mouth like the mouth of a snake in which everything can disappear. *Transform! No longer draw in; no longer torture yourself; stop stubbornly filling yourself with work-patterns and certain things/people. Don't swallow things up anymore.*

Spit it all out for once and become purely YOURSELF. Stand up and go onward as "I," not like someone who thinks he has to constantly *comply, bend, crawl along with a system;* stand up straight, on your own feet, and now bring yourself to realization, separate from anything or anyone outside yourself.

Don't place ANYTHING above LIFE itself, and things will go well for you; then Life is with you. Don't place finances or achievements or honor above life. *When you are always faithful to yourself, life will give you what you need at any moment. First, let go; first, stand up for yourself, and allow yourself to be born in an honest way — "live!" Then the new things will come upon*

your path. Trust in this! Resolutely, get hold of your life, take corrective measures, and let go. No longer try to bend and comply in all directions in order to be able to swallow it all. Don't swallow anything anymore. YOU determine your life: organize it differently. Come close to yourself in LOVE; no longer poison yourself by taking in so much that you are NOT. Discover your true self; discard needless burdens, and offer yourself all the space for a *true* existence. Break with certain things where necessary.

Don't crawl, don't bend, don't fill yourself, don't force yourself. In all honesty, come home to your living Self and do only what you feel you have to do.

Don't live according to the *conviction* that life is a Via Dolorosa, a Mount of Calvary in which you MUST endure; stop making yourself believe this, and bring about change. Break that hardness toward yourself. Don't place anything Above life itself! Take good care of yourself; no one will do this for you. Or are you afraid to start searching for yourself, separate from your work? Trust, let go, and open yourself up so that all held-in, still-unknown treasures/talents/possibilities inside you can make themselves known!

BURPING, EXAGGERATED; BELCHING, REPEATING

Something overwhelms you, overpowers you; it is too much to digest all at once. You cannot completely comprehend something or immediately get a grip on it. You totter; you sense a certain instability inside yourself: an unconscious, nervous anxiety about being unable to completely maintain a hold on yourself. Seen positively, this symptom may be caused by a multitude of impressions and information which even appear very agreeable to you, but which disturb you because they bring new information you have not yet assimilated, digested or integrated into the content of your being. In certain cases, you feel out of control, in the grip of something others have said to you. When you are unsteady standing on your own feet, then doubt, being startled, or anxiety, will flare up much easier. Perhaps you feel in the grip of someone whom you experience as being "mightier" than yourself. Or do you just walk too fast, ignoring yourself?

Experience the solid central point in your living Self. Discover yourself, turn yourself inward. Look at possibly unconscious anxieties. Approach life with inner peace, with self-confidence. Don't be tripped up by your enthusiasm, come quietly to yourself. You have all the time in the world! That which is beautiful — life — doesn't run away! Trust: stay here-and-now, present in yourself, don't run ahead of yourself.

BURSITIS

inflammation of a bursa, i.e. a sac of fibrous tissue, filled with fluid, mostly near a joint (See also Shoulder, Elbow, Knee, etc.)

You are stuck in an endless, repeating pattern; it all seems senseless to you; you don't find real satisfaction in your task. Boredom in life. It all works on your nerves; you position yourself stalwartly and imposingly: you become angry with others; you'd like to work off steam with an aggressive word or gesture! You probably do much for others, and therefore you ask for recognition from them. An internal conflict in your thoughts, which are always colliding and storming in your nervous brain: will you, *yourself,* begin to live more strongly, for yourself, even taking a new direction if need be? Push others away? Or will you stick to the old way, let-

ting yourself be used by others? Aggressive doubt!

The true cause of all the above-mentioned lies in the frustration of not being able to experience yourself as you would like to. You think you don't have the right to live for yourself, or to enjoy, and you think you are not worthy of all this! Your head becomes hot from this glowing doubt: instead of bringing yourself to realization, truly manifesting yourself, you would like others to do what you expect from them. The angry urge for power you feel toward them is but a reaction to your own powerlessness to go straight ahead and choose resolutely in favor of yourself. You oppose resistance to certain matters or details that are of secondary importance. With your hard, dominating attitude toward yourself, you suppress all your emotions and also that for which you intuitively long. You are too severe with yourself, not really allowing gentle feelings of love. You will project this upon your surroundings. You lean on others, on a job or function — on everything but your own feet! Your thoughts are searching for a way out; you don't see how, you can't. . . . The propeller gets stuck, all flexibility has disappeared. You have put yourself in a completely blocked position.

No longer hesitate, go toward your goal, self-assured! Say or do what, for a long time, you have already felt you have to do: cut through the knot. Surrender to your deepest feelings, your intuition; no longer offer resistance to your inner longings. Enjoy yourself, enjoy life — in Love. Only when you learn first of all how to appreciate and love yourself and your life will you then joyfully take charge of every task or responsibility regarding others. So relax in yourself, don't trot ahead, stand still a moment and enjoy a glass of wine or the play of a bird on the windowsill. . . . Completely experience your nature, don't doom it to dissatisfied fretting and brooding; joy begins with the acceptance of the flow of life in yourself.

*Listen to this intuitive source in you and build up your life yourself. Don't **let** yourself "be lived."*

BUTTOCKS

Psychological correspondence

Symbol of the safe basis in ourselves. This secure feeling of always being able to rest in the shelter of your own haven. Powerfully being. Foundations. Though you might stray from your path, you are always the possessor of a dual security system by which you can again land safely in your self after a Fall. And when you are thrown upon the ground, look closely: Why does your security system begin to work? Why does the alarm bell ring? Often, the answer to this will be: "I don't trust my own, strong, powerful Self; I let my life be too much determined by others, etc."

Fully come back into yourself. Build a solid construction upon these foundations of rock-steady pillars! Don't look for fortune outside yourself. From your dreams, create a beautiful future. Don't *let* things happen to you. Steer your life yourself in the direction you want to go. Symbol for authority in yourself, for pride, and for a concentrated presence in your own being. Steady as a rock in the breakers: *that* is the strength of your inner Core, your power center, in which all emotions can collect and be worked out.

Ailments, in general

Feeble, self-negation, absent from yourself — anxieties, unable to get a hold on anything, drawing yourself back, quickly getting away, fleeing, doubting the Power of your Self.

A feeling of psychological castration. You feel yourself to be only a "piece"; you can muddle along through life being deaf, indifferent, or apathetic. . . .

Your head — your consciousness — has no power over your body; your balance is unsteady. Do you feel threatened by vague, dark powers, by the eyes or judgment of others? Where is your willpower?

You let yourself flow toward all directions and don't *truly* determine what your life is to be. Your are "stuck" in negative thoughts.

In order to have healthy, sturdy muscles as a physical foundation, it is necessary to be aware of the above-mentioned psychological correspondence. Thus, purge yourself from negative, burdensome thoughts and energies, and build up your life in a self-assured, active, powerful way. Concentration in yourself, in the here-and-now; no longer doubt your own possibilities!

C

VITAMIN C
Deficiency, insufficient assimilation of

Anxiety blocks all joy! Your life lies bound in armor. You live too mechanically. You dehumanize yourself by smothering your spontaneous natural longings and your enthusiasm under a dominating symbol (a Miter) of rational authority, no longer trusting in life, in the way in which it would like to stream freely. You hold on to so much, trying to keep everything under your control. It is so difficult for you to let go. Situations or people outside you are, in fact, a support for you because you keep yourself "empty." You don't realize your own worth and powers; perhaps you live too superficially; you are afraid of digging deeper into yourself because you don't at all feel able to create your own life yourself. You fear you would totally collapse if you gave yourself over to your spontaneous intuition, to your Nature, to your deeper feelings. Thus, you would rather live in "nothingness," and you will rust in your armor. You ignore your fundamentally strong Sun-center. You deny the spontaneous child in yourself.

Cherish your own deep energies and feed them by trusting in your own powers; allow your nature, your feelings, to come through freely. Don't mistrust yourself! Don't try to limit everything, to squeeze it within the controlling eye of your thinking. A healthy dose of common sense, a self-aware overview, looking at and understanding things from all sides: that is very good, but also give your emotional world a chance to blossom; trust your deepest living Self — which has a need for space and trust — so that everything which makes you happy can flow toward you. Mistrusting your Self only calls up negative events. Your energy source is inexhaustible if you don't allow it to dry up. So, make use of it: live, play, enjoy, feel, create — don't hold yourself back! Allow joy to stream through your blood; stop fearfully holding on to everything. Let go; relax; know yourself to be safe within yourself! Have nothing but happy and optimistic expectations regarding your life. Nothing happens "just like that". . . . (Read Part I.)

CALCIUM
Deficiency, insufficient assimilation of

You experience yourself as a victim, unable to take your life in your own hands. You don't build yourself up like a unified being, on a solid foundation; you seem to be dancing on a string, like a marionette, held together with hooks. You are so stiff; feelings seem to be separate from your structure. You keep yourself standing up, but you don't truly live in joy, in flesh and blood. You don't give yourself and others room to exist. You live cut off from your deepest Self, rather like a mechanical puppet, with several parts glued together: where is that central Pillar, your Self-aware "I," as a conductor of the totality? You lack solidity.

You don't at all feel yourself supported by your Self; you are dependent on others; you allow yourself to be hollowed out by others instead of experiencing your Fullness *your-*

self. You don't trust your intuition, and as a result you bring yourself to a state of anxious tension with nervous thoughts. Possibly, you tensely close yourself up within certain severe structures and rules, in this way not taking into account your specific, natural disposition. You don't truly live "ensouled," not really concentrated with your Consciousness in your body.

*Allow your nature to exist freely; offer your feelings the chance to circulate flexibly. Row with your own oars; place all authority inside yourself. Keep yourself to those structures which are naturally good, no more, no less. Don't stick oppressive, artificial structures and laws onto your life, but trust your intuition. Become aware of this solid, immortal Basis within yourself and **live** from out of your Self. A strong consciousness-concentration in your body, as a consequence of Belief in yourself, in your power and your worth.*

CALLUS FORMATION

On the feet, possibly chapped

Anxieties: you are afraid of your own feelings, your own nature. You don't have real trust in yourself, so therefore you follow a very limited path in a stiff way, and with blinders on. Self-limitation within structures that are too tight. It often takes your breath away. You don't truly take responsibility for your Life; you limit your path by not *truly* living yourself, but instead are a parasite on existing rules, laws, structures, ideas, habits, other people — you anxiously stay high above ground, afraid to feel the earth with your feet, and afraid to be obliged to come to a deeper confrontation with yourself, with your emotions, with your deepest nature! Thus you of course remain cut off from your basis, from your own nature: you don't trust

your spontaneous gifts, inspiration or creativity. You are afraid of them. Too hard on yourself, on your nature; you stand at a distance from yourself.

You look at others and you posses too little self-confidence.

No longer hide yourself away! Dare to crow with pleasure and, full of pride, experience your being unique! Come down, out of your tower, descend into yourself, into your body, and feel your true heartbeat, your nature! Reach out with your legs and arms in self-confidence; dare to look at your emotions in depth, bring them up and work them out! Finally, confrontation with your anxieties, your deepest feelings leads to transformation, advancement, and joy in your life! No longer flee from your deepest Self; there is no question of threat when you surrender to your soft, sensitive nature; put your life-mechanisms in motion and go on, aware of inner mastery! No longer walk on these hard carpets of anxiety: come on the earth with the REAL soles of your feet, feel yourself safe, sheltered, very close to your gentle Self, to your Body. Break through that distance, come to unity in yourself by working through and assimilating all your feelings.

On the palms

Your nature, your spontaneity — the healthy impulsive childlike, the playful, the free and cheerful — is only allowed to exist in a stern and stiff way, within the confines of a suit of armor, of a severe structure. Perhaps you are very sweet and friendly to others, but inwardly you are hard, stubborn, obstinate, in the first place with yourself! "No!" you say and you push the sensitive heart away. Like a little porcelain statue on a dresser, you are allowed to be beautiful, showy, prestige-minded or friendly, but you sit motionlessly! You shake off the little child in you, harshly and roughly. Are you so afraid of your feelings? Do you therefore cling to rusted, sclerotic structures, to stubborn ideas?

No longer ignore the cheerful-spontaneous, the child within yourself. Go flexibly along with your wishes and longings; go along quietly and no longer hold on obstinately to restricting structures, nor to outdated or false values.

This self-protection is unnecessary if you dare, in self-confidence, to manifest your own strong nature: dare to live, free yourself! Soften yourself and caress life lovingly, without anxieties.

CANCER, IN GENERAL

The deepest cause: you hang in life like a puppet on a string. You place the sun outside yourself. A surrender to something that is bigger and more important than your Self-aware "I" — or that's what you think. Being too little present in yourself, or hardly at all. Adoration or reverence for Authority outside you (instead of placing the Sun-center, the "power plant," in yourself) leads to estrangement from yourself.

You ignore your own self-aware, divine, creative abilities. You don't really live consciously, you allow yourself to "be lived" — by others or by your feelings, by your function or by influences from the outside, by a group, by an ideal placed outside you in which you put all your faith. This surrender, this absorption in the "other," this Neptunian LOSS of yourself, can only lead to death! The more you give the first place to a Sun outside yourself (this means pushing yourself into the background to the advantage of another person, group, authority, sect, religion, etc.) the more you will stand in darkness. Strange, dark cells take up the space of original "I" cells. Causes which play a role here — other than this self-negation — are of course the Anxieties, often the fear to live. You don't dare to fully take responsibility for your life; you flee, as it were, from yourself,

perhaps even believing that something more beautiful than Life exists (death).

The deep anxiety which makes you grasp even more strongly for Authority outside yourself. "Ah, who am 'I' anyway?" You think you need support from the outside to be able to keep on standing.

You flee into the Masses, or into a presence that is more "spiritual" than earthly human; at last you live like a Zombie, or like an Image. Your Self-aware, Powerful "I" is being denied: emotions and passivity have the upper hand. Especially sad experiences — also from the past, from childhood — don't leave you: you allow yourself to be dominated by these unconscious, pent-up worlds, instead of placing yourself above it all, observing your emotional burdens, letting it stream FREELY and working it out.... Pain, fury, rancor, hatred, disappointments — "What sense does it all make anymore?" — these all have truly come to dominate your life because you keep on bottling it up! Allow this ball of Misery to open up; give your emotions an outlet. Let it flow; speak and express yourself — every release is one less cancer cell. Are you so afraid of these emotions? Are you afraid to live your life to the fullest? Were you taught to stay inside a certain armor? How long will you go on still suffocating yourself in this unnatural straitjacket?

No longer stir up old problems; no longer brood and fret for days. No longer cling to something outside yourself (a business, a job, etc.) or someone (a partner, a child, etc.), as if your life depends on it. Everyone directs his life. Trust in this and let go of everything and everyone.

No longer allow yourself to be swallowed up in a swamp of emotions: deal with them. No longer allow yourself to get lost in the authority of others, in the ideal, etc. Observe everything from above, like an Eagle and become Master over your life, over your body. Your psyche, your thoughts and convictions direct the functioning of your body. Are you convinced that healing powers will destroy your cancer because you have the right to Live in Joy and Self-awareness? If so, then your body will react to these impulses and will recover, with or without pill or herb. Other conditions? Enjoy! Strive after Insight instead of brooding. Dare to live in the here-and-now, no longer in the past; acknowledge the Authority of your eternal, divine self just by believing in yourself. No longer be afraid of your emotions, fury, vengeance, passions, aggression — accept them, bid them welcome, experience them and deal with them; part from the feelings which hinder you, But experience aggressive powers as a positive presence for self-realization. Do what you like to do, come close to yourself, don't expect anything from others, from your partner — but GIVE joy and love to yourself: only then will you attract situations and people to you which/who will also bring joy and happiness into your life — if first you live a hundred per cent in and with yourself. Don't change others, but choose a new direction, Yourself. When you change in a positive sense, you will attract joyful situations; also good health.

These healing energies — call them up and replace all your worries with Faith in yourself. Then you also can, like a white dove, carry this new, true, message into the world: a human being has the power over his own life, his health, when he himself becomes Aware of it.

*   *   *

The feeling of standing on the edge, almost falling off, dangling on the hook, and it seems you can't climb up it anymore. Something bends/breaks; you would like to go back, grasp on again, but life now prevents you from getting stuck again in structures and habits from the past and asks you to unhitch yourself from where you have been holding on. It asks you to let yourself "fall," in trust, knowing that you will land ever and again with your feet on the ground (as if you have a built-in parachute), knowing that

something new is waiting for you. *Now, let go of old habits and systems!*

Under the skin, something rages and boils, like a beast growling in your stomach, but you don't make it known. You suppress it and possibly look at your surroundings in an angry, primitive way. You identify yourself with the rumbling animal voice inside yourself. As if you might be a growling lion in the jungle who considers himself strong in power and master over things and now is angry, feeling hurt because life doesn't give him what he wants to "have." Protest and dissatisfaction.

From out of a primitive, instinctive basis you might dress yourself with superficial decorations, with fringes and noisy pearls on the bare skin, dancing to the rhythm of the underground and instincts, dressing yourself up with jewels which also serve to intoxicate male or female animals. The rhythmic cadence puts a magic spell on many animals, on many animalistic people, and, if necessary, you also undress yourself in order to show who you are as a human monkey.

But *who are you as a HUMAN BEING, as a highly unique Individual,* separate from these habits, from the spirit, from the group? It's true that you like to be noticed, but what is added to this is your way of life. Not really sober and "fully awake" as a "human being," but whipping yourself up, sometimes intoxicating yourself in the rhythm of an animal. You don't have a true opinion of your own about something; you go along with, and turn with, the herd of your soulmates (no matter if this concerns the clan spirit, the work spirit, the science of your time, the religious or family sphere, etc.). After all, you don't have demands or expectations; you lose yourself in the group spirit and addict yourself to "the spirit," the primal spirit.

Going along, flowing along on those primal rhythms, you no longer find yourself. Do you sometimes shiver from the cold? That's just because you feverishly let your thoughts dance and search . . . but you won't find a solution as long as you stay stuck in this state of not-really-being-"I," the Human Being.

Do you cling to others, like a monkey to its mother? Then this is because you don't believe enough in your unique greatness and immunity as a human being. You are safe in yourself! You don't have to turn away so timidly from true individuality, from self-acknowledgment. You don't have to "hide" yourself (behind this or that, those or these), nor adorn yourself with frills and camouflage accessories. Show yourself as a human being and acknowledge your "I": don't be ashamed. Ban such desires and rhythms from your life. Recognize the rhythm of life itself, the one that is not intoxicating; the one that knows unexpected turns depending on the inspiration of your life-core, of your conscious "I" who chooses, "Yes," *consciously chooses* to do this or that, to go here or there.

You therefore no longer allow yourself to "*be* lived"/stirred up by compulsiveness, by impulses that don't come from your heart, your Feeling, your consciousness.

You do want to get to know yourself now, to become aware of your "I," separate from the group/society-spirit/masses, etc.! Let go of the old, and be reborn in yourself as a Human Being; no longer hold on to systems, to things outside yourself — in habit-patterns — but rise up as the Leader over your existence, in love and power, as "I," Consciously Awake in Life!
(Read Part I.)

living from out of yourself; because you keep yourself locked up within a circle, and it seems you are unable to break out of it; because you keep yourself "closed," and it seems as if the future makes no sense to you anymore; therefore you weep, therefore you hold on to many emotions, and therefore you cling to a partner or to children, to futilities. Sometimes, as a reaction, you also direct your aggression toward others, because you are filled to the brim with energies, but you don't succeed in using them in personal development. Perhaps it seems to you as if you have nothing worthwhile to do, as if you just go through life routinely, without real satisfaction. You are angry because you cannot get out of it. Possibly you inflate yourself from within by brooding and pondering, but with this you don't get one step further; you aren't really doing anything about it. The real underlying cause is that you insufficiently dare to stand on your own feet, that you make yourself dependent on others, that you don't dare live originally and spontaneously according to your longings.

Break out of this constricting armor! Total self-realization; allow this fruit, which you are, to blossom; acknowledge your nature, your feelings; allow energies to freely turn outward and create your future yourself. Put your own solidity and power in first place. Dare to look much further than at a dead, black wall; enlarge your vision and unfold your possibilities, enlarge your existence! Don't allow yourself to "be lived" by others, but dare to live from out of your heart and allow yourself to fully enjoy life.

CARPAL TUNNEL SYNDROME
numbness and/or pain in the first three fingers, caused by nerve compression at the wrist

Your life runs but through a narrow tunnel; you allow yourself to be limited by structures and time, by your feelings of powerless aggression. Because you don't succeed in truly

CARTILAGE

Psychological correspondence

To what degree are we faithful to our Natural dispositions? To what degree do we overburden ourselves, striving again and again after things which don't *really* fit us? The cartilage symbolizes growing in a supple way toward ever-greater Balance; an even distribution between working actively and pure Enjoying. It symbolizes the soft, caring aspect of ourselves; the limber, supple part that adapts and adjusts itself, that cares for our existence in relaxed flexibility and watches that we are supplely open to our inner Self, to our deepest "I," to our true nature.

The cartilage symbolizes the ease with which we experience our structures in life — only those structures which self-evidently come out of the spontaneous needs of our natural self, without imposing any limitation. Also, it symbolizes the ease with which we go onward on our path in life, proud of ourselves — not because of an external image.

It symbolizes pure instincts, led by a Self-aware "I." The impulse for life, the primal instincts of a human being to build his or her life on earth. The trust that we place in our "automatisms." (We don't have to question how our stomach functions; when we are hungry, we don't have to think about it, etc.)

Without fear, we put trust in our Body, in the impulses which our deepest Self sends through to us. The onset, the beginning of coming into our earthly nature; giving shape.

The cartilage symbolizes primitive, and also (sexual,) creative powers in ourselves.

It symbolizes the Contact Point between not only body and Consciousness, but also the loving contact between two people. In supple surrender to yourself, you can open yourself up in a tender way toward others. The experiencing of primal energies: sensory, sensual, creative, caressing; a cherishing of the corporeality, of our nature.

Ailments of the cartilage

Ailments of the cartilage will appear when we don't dare to trust in our deepest Self, in the primal powers that are in us, which constantly create and lead life toward greater fulfillment of itself. These ailments appear when we would rather believe in authority outside ourselves, through which we finally lose all contact with our life-giving source.

This causes a feeling of threat, and deep anxieties; a way of killing oneself, cutting oneself off from the regenerator — from our essence.

Living at the surface of existence, without truly deep contact, neither with oneself nor with others. A curtailment of those primal, necessary, and primitive impelling forces which give life to our earthly existence. Open yourself flexibly to all parts of yourself and don't block these powerful, creative energies in yourself! Come to relaxed mobility, without forcing anything. Acknowledge your Worth, place the Authority in yourself and build up your existence in a self-assured way, from out of your natural disposition — not according to the norms of others. Be faithful to your nature; don't ignore or violate it by carrying out tasks that go against your true nature.

If you fulfill a function, then be relaxed; don't let yourself be rushed by that which is outside yourself: determine your own rhythm; don't overburden yourself. Strive for a balance between work and rest; enjoy via senses and a flexible contact with other people. Be softer and more lenient toward yourself when it comes to going through with exaggerated work — or relaxing. Don't forget to truly LIVE; first of all for yourself, without stress.

CELLULITE

Cellulite is no illness, is not ugly. It might as well stay there. It does, however, want you to take the following psychology into account.

You feel like a squeezed orange: in powerless fury you'd like to seize — take to yourself, possess — that which you lack inside you, namely love. You feel hurt and sad, unable to build your life energetically. You are looking for attachment in your relationships because of your lack of self-confidence. You think that you can get from others the warmth and love which you are not giving to yourself: you condemn yourself to being an inferior, dependent child.

You consider yourself to be ugly; you build your life too much on outer factors in order to camouflage your inner insecurity. You take a tense, forced position, but you don't really take action; you let yourself be ruled by others. You are but an apple, and so one is allowed to eat you: self-degradation. You don't allow yourself to enjoy freely; you'd like your body to "shrink."

Now take your life in hand in a self-aware way and experience warmth, love for yourself. Cuddle that teddy bear, which you are, and allow it to grow up in the safety of your Powerful self! No one can take your unique place; acknowledge your worth, then others also will respect you. Don't throw yourself away; discover your talents; stop running yourself down: become aware of the higher energies that wish to break through and that are waiting for the moment that you acknowledge your mastery. Now build up your life according to your wishes. Powerlessness and aggression will transform into strong creativity and experiences of beautiful feelings, which you have for so long denied yourself. You are worthy of it! Be YOURSELF, don't fixate on the external! Allow yourself to expand where it's good for your well-being, soulwise as well as bodywise. Cellulite does not have to disappear. Also, don't try to become "slim" when your Nature is to be well-rounded.

CERVICOBRACHIALGIA
restricted mobility of the neck, with pain which radiates to the arm or hand, possibly coupled with numbness and prickling in the hand

You keep yourself so stiff, you play a role; you live "angularly" without suppleness; you direct yourself tightly, as if in a strait-jacket,

toward superficial matters. You cut yourself off from your heart, from your emotional world. You don't live really consciously! Like a functionary, like a zombie, like a robot — you scarcely know anymore who you are. Perhaps you express only dry criticism. You are rusted fast into a pattern, from which you no longer can get out anymore; but, by these symptoms you are shown just how you have dulled yourself.

Break out of this tight armor! No longer push your emotional world away; allow everything to stream freely. Don't be so stiff, not with yourself nor with others. Don't pin yourself down to vapid material business; your life has much more to offer. Change direction, lay down your function and your habits, if necessary, and allow your Heart to show an open structure. Don't build your life on self-limiting laws, but on love and flexibility.

Transformation! Give room to your Total Self!

CHEST WALL PAIN
pain in the chest, caused for instance by muscles, nerves, joints in the chest wall (so there's no question of heart disease)

It's as if a nail stabs you, but it is you yourself who keeps the Mars forces directed inwardly. You hurt yourself; you want to go on in a direction that is not good for you, but life holds you back and calls to you: "Stop!" You now may first STAND STILL AND REFLECT about yourself and wonder why you called up this specific pain. WHY? Possibly you have again and again resisted a thorough investigation, resisted going deeper than the purely superficial, perceptible level. Have you too often passed by a deeper investigation *of life in YOU?* NOW you are being OBLIGED to start looking at the "inside," the deeper layers *of yourself.*

Were you running on too fast, in the meantime cut off from your body, your deeper feelings? Did you run past yourself? Are you afraid of dying? The cause of death for certain people lies in not wanting to see, in not wanting to see farther than their noses, farther than what one can notice on the outside of things (of the body): but you call up a signal that asks you to look, to feel, to go deeper inside yourself... You will/can LIVE, truly and fully live!

Therefore, chest wall pain has to be considered a positive signal, because in time, man calls himself to a halt when he's gone wrong. Then correct yourself right away; look deep inside yourself and feel what is the most powerful and honest way to go on (in all honesty with yourself, doing the things that make you *feel:* "This is what I really have to do now."). Don't forget that, through your body, Consciousness energies are flowing, which you can indeed allow to flow through you in a Conscious or Unconscious way. A call to take your life in your own hands! Get a hold of things in a definite and thorough way! Take the reins in your hands! LIVE! Do something with it. ALLOW THOSE ENERGIES TO FLOW THROUGH!

Now, once you realize "why this pain," don't stay there "thinking." In what area, in which way, do you corner yourself while not realizing that you are doing so? Were you too involved with the outer side of things, with the rational or superficial exterior of things, and in the meantime slid away from yourself, from your body, your feeling, your deeper content? Time to realize that THE FORCES INSIDE YOU, THE POWERFUL CONTENT OF YOUR BEING, ask you to go Onward in a firm and solid way! Now go onward, keeping pace with yourself, closely present in your content, your feeling, your body. For a little while you had to contemplate the facts, the cause of the pain. Now the moment has come, after this deepening of insight into yourself, to go further and to

KNOW: in life nothing "just" happens. Everything has its reasons for being, and this includes occurrences, like illness or pain (or whatever event you encounter on your path). You no longer turn away from the deeper Truth regarding Yourself.

NOW YOU DO OPEN YOURSELF UP TO IT: to (those forces of) truth in yourself! You turn deeply inward, toward the treasure room of gold. Deep inside you lives that true human being with the big heart and the rich consciousness, with his talents and abilities to dig things out, get down to the bottom and go to the depths of existence. THAT is what life now asks of you: GOING DEEPLY INTO THINGS, into yourself, into life, the "why." *And this will liberate you;* the answer will be quite a release. That the life of man can be DIRECTED by man himself, *that healing and elimination of pain are the results of (necessary) changes one brings about* in one's existence, in one's outlook on life, in the steps one takes.

Chin up! Be aware of your worthiness! You now *know* you are not an ostrich that sticks its head in the sand: you look straight ahead of you in the direction of LIFE, in the direction of the HIGHWAY of life, and you no longer deviate from it. You now offer yourself all the opportunities; full speed ahead! Forces are being applied, are coming free for this self-development. You are now proud of your true content, not of an image, but of your true "I." You know what it means: taking your own life in hand and being aware of your worth. Not looking back at anything or anyone beneath the worthiness of true life and . . . going onward!

Allow those life energies to flow; no longer keep fretting, but follow that inner dynamic and answer to this. Now you *know* at least, through that pain, that there are enormous forces inside you that are asking for a free life-current, forces that don't want to be blocked because you didn't recognize them, because you weren't AWARE enough of the fact that there was a huge life-content present in you. Now you know it, now you listen to your Inner Voice and firmly go onward!

Happy to be in your physical body, enjoying being present in yourself, in matter, very close to yourself, very close to your body, to your feeling. From this awareness of your worth, from this knowing that everything is all right — there can be no question of fear, of concern, of nervousness. You always connect yourself with your inner Heart, with your body full of love.

You now cherish your being in a warm, heartfelt way, and this experience of unity in and with yourself does you so much good and offers you the greatest relaxation: YOU EXPERIENCE YOURSELF IN THE HERE AND NOW like a wonderful, clucking chicken, wrapped up in its warm coat of feathers — enjoying life without rushing yourself, no longer finding yourself nervously with your thoughts above or outside your body.

This chest wall pain wanted to bring you deeper and closer within yourself, your body, in order to go onward in full force on the basis of this feeling of worthiness, on the basis of this loving presence in yourself. Rest and powerful dynamics go together in a going-onward, departing from the here-and-now moment . . . and constantly finding yourself very close to your deepest central content, to your blissful, warm earthly body. Being very close to yourself, and — thanks to the fleshy power of your body — you offer a strong passage for all those life forces that wish to flow through you. And when one has satisfied this condition, the pain will disappear like snow in summer. From your own depths, you now continue in a self-assured way, different than before, immediately listening to the signal that calls you back to yourself, very close and deep. Onward on the Path of Life, cheerful, without fear, in healthy pride; you know your worthiness as a powerful, creative Human Being, full of love!

CHILDHOOD ILLNESSES
(Read Children in Part I)

Adenoids; swelling, inflammation

You don't establish yourself truly as an Individual of flesh and blood on earth: you are too absent, too "spiritual," too unreal. Not fully present in your body. You feel dragged along, as it were, by a wave or by the wind. . . . Who *are* you? You experience yourself as an empty pawn, looking for support from a strong shoulder, from paternal authority, from a teacher etc. Unconsciously, you build up a protecting shield. Your feet are soft, you are sensitive — you depend on the protection others offer you. Despondent and lonely; putting yourself under a superpower. Your consciousness doesn't get a true grip on your body; you feel small and rudderless and you hope for the love of a good shepherd, because you are nothing but a sheep? You don't believe in your personal powers, in your "thinking" abilities.

You float too much above your head instead of Consciously making use of your brain. You don't really live in this reality; you fantasize, sometimes living in unreal, blurry Spheres; you dream, not perceiving earthly existence clearly. And when you do stand up for yourself, or get angry, then this is being laughed away or punished.

Become truly Human. Wake up from the unconscious sleep, or the dream of death. Make use of your brain, of your senses: look clearly with your eyes, consciously contemplate your existence. Allow your awareness-powers to crystallize in your body: navigate **yourself,** *don't allow yourself to drift along. Live here-and-now, with your feet solidly on the ground; don't dream, but be attentive and alert!*

Learn to distinguish details; observe nature, the objects around you: feel with all your senses and descend into your earthly existence.

Others treat you like a sheep, as long as you behave that way: take up the responsibility for your life and don't allow yourself to be swallowed up by others.

Free yourself, dare to live, push away all obstacles, go on!
Now allow yourself to be born, let go of everything that is behind you and come into the "flesh".

Trust your nature, come to clarity in your feelings, don't reject the little child in you, but know that Protection lies in your deepest Self.

*Don't **let** yourself grow in an unconscious way, but live Consciously, intensely, going your way. Open the hatch. You are safe in yourself; come completely out of your hiding space!*

Chickenpox

Carried along by the wind, by your mother, by realms — you are easily influenced because you don't yet live autonomously. "Who am I?" Feelings and impressions, sadness and anxieties of the environment: you are open to them because you are still too dependent, and you perceive life like a fish on a hook. It is all too heavy for you; you no longer can carry it this way. You'd like to protect yourself against influences and painful experiences from the outside, but you don't succeed. You feel swallowed up by others: in this way you are "contaminated" psychologically and physically.

Experience the "solid framework" of your home, your "I," in which you are good and safe — even if people in your environment would poison the atmosphere with their anxieties and problems. So, determine your own path by resolutely pointing with your forefinger: dare to stand up for your personal opinion. If need be, in an angry way.

THAT IS WHO I AM! For you are who you are, different from your parents or your friends. Search for yourself, for your personal qualities, and give yourself some time alone; a restful pause for your own "I." Knowing yourself to Become yourself, slowly but surely, in a more autonomous way.

Cradle-cap
**thick , yellow crusts,
sticking on the scalp of the baby**

Anxiety about something or someone bigger than you. You don't trust life very much. Also, afraid of reactions: Did you do something wrong, wet your pants? Afraid to be scolded. Mostly, mother has to deal with her own dark emotions, with *her* anxieties, and the little one reflects this.

A feeling of insecurity, of emotional instability; too little inner rest. The child withdraws, is afraid of new or unfamiliar things. It doesn't trust itself, its own eyes, very well. "A ghost?" Suspicion, mistrust. Afraid of its own powers, of its deep emotions.

Blind anger because of its anxieties, aggression because of its powerlessness, screaming protest against the adults on whom it is dependent.

An inner urge to deal with these anxieties, to realize personal ambitions, however small they might be; sometimes, this leads to stubborn, persistent behavior, as if in this way its own unsureness will disappear. . . .

Feeling safe within a stable structure. Getting a clear view of yourself, of life; dare to take apart an object and study it: matter does not threaten. Rest and love drive anxieties away.

Develop Self-Trust; don't be afraid of feelings, or of punishment. Deep inside you there is no dark hole, but instead a secure, beautiful, divine essence, your individual Self, which lies at the origin of your eternal life. You are the creator of your life; nothing bad happens to you if you have not called it up to begin with. Trust and joy in life! If the parent solves these problems in himself or herself, then the child will feel liberated, then the turtle will dare to show its head.

Croup
acute laryngotracheobronchitis
with subglottic edema

Anxious, without a strong backbone: after all you don't believe in yourself, and you feel targeted by others. You have the impression of being without strength, powerless to stand up for yourself. At first you try for a long time to embrace it all — your anxieties, your sadness, your anger — because you don't dare to express the way you feel.

After all, you look to others for Attention and shelter, also doing so in the form of illness, so that one will give you "flowers." You hide, but finally you feel stuck in such a way, that you can't get out of it anymore. It becomes too heavy for you; you are sad and powerless; you don't care anymore; you let your head hang . . . wanting to get away.

Build up a strong Structure: depend on your own solid basis. Express your feelings! Develop self-confidence and dare to speak up for yourself. Free yourself from this prison, take away that damper from your face, and dare to live in an Active way. Be yourself without hesitation. Be good to yourself first of all and discover your talents, your creative possibilities. Come to action! Trust in that fundamentally strong essence in yourself. (See Anxiety)

Eye disease in children

You feel anxious: because you don't yet see yourself as you really are, because you are afraid of reality. Perhaps you experience much sadness and misery with your parent(s), but because you refuse to see it, you blindfold yourself. But here, too, your parents just hold up a mirror of a deeper sadness INSIDE yourself!

You feel unsafe, would prefer to crawl back into the womb, don't dare to really observe the world around you. Or do you escape into fairy tales? Do you live too much in imaginary realms, so that you confuse reality with your dreams?

If you have a strong, emotional bond with your mother, you no longer see yourself at all, and you take over her "blindness." With small, red, inflamed eyes you translate her sadness and her anger. Even if you don't realize that this sadness, this anger, also lives deep inside you . . . therefore, that "sensitivity" to these emotions in your fellow men.

You don't know very well *which* path to choose; you are being pulled to the left and then to the right, now by father then by mother; both eyes are looking in different directions, anxiously seeking safety and stability.

Balance and clear perspective are beneficial for your eyes; a feeling of peace and relaxation. Your senses being clear and open in the here-and-now; never fleeing from a problem, not the parents, not the children. Honest, clear language. Sadness and anger are being remedied by this. If the parents behave like ostriches, then the child won't be stimulated in the (unconscious) search for a happy solution.

Feverish convulsions
(See also Convulsions, in general)

Powerless, desperate expression of fundamental anxieties. Panic and unsureness: you absolutely feel not safe. Do you feel emotionally dependent on your mother? Then you will have very sensitive antennae which will pick up the emotional problems of your mother. Psychologically, you feel hunted, without a firm hold. In the grip of a dark emotional world, you go to your mama for protection. When she also feels anxious and tense and insecure, then you don't experience her "being" as a safe haven! Still the "cause" lies in the baby itself; the parent is then just a "reflection."

Of course, an extremely tense family situation enhances the feeling of an inner overcharging of emotions, which find an outlet in the form of convulsions. You feel as if you are in the Power of.... You have no defense against it. You seek liberation from an oppressive situation: love, safety, and stability in your surroundings and a solution to the unconscious emotional problems of the parent(s), can help drive away these panicky, mortal fears and enhance restfulness in your soul.

The older the child, the stronger the emphasis should be put on inner wisdom, on its own strong Basis, knowing it is protected in itself. Speak, scream if need be, but don't bottle up suffocating emotions! Fill your lungs with air and breathe out until relaxation is achieved.... Self-manifestation, experiencing your own Power, discussing the family situation and looking at it from a higher level.

You can interact with your environment, but the emotional problem — anxiety — that you'll have to ultimately solve deep inside yourself.

Fifth disease
slapped-cheek disease, erythema infectiosum

Biting, harrowing sorrow. Deep unconscious processes are taking place here: deep-seated emotions require a total purification. A chance for early transformation, also for transformation of the mother, who possibly is stuck with a psychological problem of the same nature. The child is very sensitive to the sadness and the anxieties of its surroundings. It feels lost, afraid of "death" and loneliness. Anxiously clinging to others. Chilliness, emotional tension; having no clear view on life, no perspective on oneself; an absence; being too much of an "unaware

spirit" instead of a Conscious "I." Having nothing to hold on to, no safety, seeing no direction in which to go. In the grip of "Pluto," of the deepest emotions. Feeling overpowered. Painful memories.

The warmth of a mother's womb; secure shelter in oneself. Pride of one's own being; playing joyfully and carefree. A safe home. Knowing that nothing in life happens by accident; knowing that every human being is able at any moment to create his life in a joyful direction, in spite of painful memories from the past.

Fontanel, closing too slowly

Occurs in entities which, in this incarnation, feel "squeezed." One already has certain wisdom in oneself, but often one also has a willfulness: a stubborn refusal to transform. A feeling of power and mastery over others, coupled with a nostalgic memory — perhaps regarding other lives — causes you to revolt against physical life, in which you are now obliged to surrender to others in helpless nakedness. Your body constricts you, and you fight against those who care for you: you'd prefer to have others in your "grip," instead of the other way around. You feel anxious in this state of powerlessness. You were so proud of being a caterpillar, and now you have to transform into a butterfly: you aren't aware of this, but your deepest Self propels you on and on toward an ever-greater worth-fulfillment. Resistance against *having* to listen.

Love drives away every anxiety here; the discovery of a world of possibilities for self-development will be a stimulant to find new paths and to find the power within yourself. Listen and communicate. Be socially directed. Give and take. Don't withdraw into a hole. The heart is your true center in your being: a safe feeling in yourself.

German measles

*(In Dutch language
this disease is called "Red Dog.")*

This illness is like a guide dog for a blind person, steering for the master, who is absent.

Not in the least concentrated in yourself, unaware, rather not being — unable to place the slightest authority in yourself; as a result, the outer world appears threatening to you. Where is your "I"? You *let* yourself "be lived" by, for instance, your mentor, by other children in school — powerless. . . .

The guide dog shows you the way in order to make you descend into your body with your full Awareness! Powerful energies from out of your deepest Self offer themselves in a glowing red way; you no longer can ignore your personal powers.

Now anchor yourself strongly in the earth and become aware of your worth. Build up your own structure and mark off your terrain more distinctly, so that others no longer can penetrate into it, uninvited. Become aware of your Self!

Congenital hip dislocation

He experiences himself to be in chaos; baby lets himself droop, doesn't see any sense in anything, undervalues his worth.

Baby would prefer to shut himself up inside himself: "shut," a refusal to communicate, not truly wanting to be here.

He doesn't believe in himself; he'd prefer to hide behind a mask.

The psychological condition of this baby at birth is one of: "I have to keep the door closed here, because I already have to fight for myself." A little cautious in making contact.

"Because I am "only" this, I will have to hurry to get my share, too!"

The duality: on the one hand, pushing oneself under — finding oneself not good enough, sad self-destruction. On the other

hand, aggressively beginning to fence and standing up for one's own "I." This duality will resolve itself as the years pass. The duality: on the one hand hiding oneself behind a fake posture or a clown mask, and, on the other hand, there is an "I-ego" that strongly stands up for itself. On the one hand, not wanting to be, wanting to be gone, and on the other hand, running as fast as one can, like a chicken that wants to get the biggest kernel of grain. Life seems complicated to this child; he cannot get a perspective, and as a reaction he wants to "pull himself closed."

Feeling of security; life is safe to enter.

Growth of self-awareness; growth toward self-confidence; feeling safe and strong on one's feet. Reconciliation with oneself will lead to cheerful contact with others.

Self-appreciation and trust; an openness to life in the arms of a loving parent. Gradually daring to take up a larger space, without forcing oneself, without having to fall into extremes, be it by withdrawing, be it in exaggerated self-affirmation.

Jaundice, in babies

Confusion, anxiously clinging to a previous situation — to mother. You would actually prefer to quickly run away, preferably back to the situation out of which you just came; but you feel that this is of no use: you experience yourself as a drowning person in the middle of the ocean, anxiously looking for something to hold on to. In powerless anger, because of your own helplessness, you'd like to push your feet against something, but you don't know against what. You don't know what to do with yourself, with your body. You'd like to do more than you now physically can, but this is not possible: you are afraid and impatient. You are in pain, being pricked with needles; your ears are burning; you don't know where it stings, but you know you have to get out of here. You would like to get a firm grip on something, but you don't succeed.

According to how restful, and without anxieties, the mother can become, and according to how safe and assured in herself she can feel — according to how little she "clings" to the infant with an over-concerned grip, and to how well she succeeds in giving love, trust, and shelter to it — then, to this degree will the baby accommodate itself to the new situation and take on her restfulness. Let yourself relax, letting go, trusting in life, allowing feelings to flow freely.

An exaggerated cuddling of the baby will not help; on the contrary, if the mother, joyful and carefree, gives herself over to life then this will have an immediate effect on the tense state of mind of the little one.

Lacrymal canal

Obstruction: Too much in the spirit, too little in the here-and-now, in life on earth.

The baby senses life with the antennae of its consciousness, but is not yet really present with its total Self. That which has a salutary effect here and releases the blockage is, first and foremost, confrontation, contact with a public. Also, sensory exploration in all possible ways: a toy that makes noise, a melody, touching water — "shivering" after a bath — daring to feel cold and warm, etc. Being submerged in the earthly in many ways.

Inflammation: Anxiety and anger because one is fumbled with too much (ears, nose, navel . . .). Fear of pain. "Keep your hands off me!"

He cringes because of fear of being hurt, of being (psychologically) pierced: sadness and anger cause the inflammation.
Let him feel how safe his existence on earth is; put him at ease in joyful, optimistic contact. And, if necessary, work as a parent on the solution of a similar problem in yourself.

Measles

You are like a pearl in a oyster shell: it is time that you become aware of your worth and come out now.

Inner conflict; satisfying the longings of your parents/environment or fighting for yourself?

You don't yet feel totally at home in your body; you feel imprisoned in your own skin; you want to look for space in yourself, but you don't quite know *how.*

This requires unification of spirit and body, consciously taking hold of the rudder of your existence. But for the time being you still feel too dependent on others, and you also feel vulnerable and exposed to the eyes of people around you. On the one hand, you try to hide yourself from this, also in order to protect yourself from pain; on the other hand, you'd like to have wings to free yourself from this oppressive binding.

Still, you cannot yet be without a supporting hand, but your immature attachment irritates you. You cherish ambitions, but you still feel too small. You'd like to test your possibilities, but you feel stuck in a structure that is too oppressive. Your spontaneity is being suppressed by authority. The irritation is directed at your inner insecurity as well as at the resulting communication problems with strangers, and also at the educating authority above you. But above all, this has to do with a feeling of being hopelessly stuck on one's own unsteady ground, and with the longing or urge to liberate yourself from this.

People have power over you; inwardly, you resist, and you long to experience authority in yourself, but you feel like a snail, which cannot tear itself away from its little shell, because it is too dependent on it, because it can hide in that shell! Sometimes you experience life like a tug of war: they or I?

Annoyance disappears when you become fully aware of your specific worth as a human being; when you don't regard as power or pressure the guidance that others give you. Measles ask the parents to give the child sufficient free space so that its own uniqueness is respected, and thus the child is

The Key to Self-Liberation, Christiane Beerlandt © Beerlandt Publications

not made subordinate to formal structures that are no more than facade or tradition.

Spontaneity, self-assuredness, daring to show your naked self without fear that others will hurt you. Daring to freely make contact with others, without constantly withdrawing; daring to speak up for yourself.

When father or mother insufficiently respect themselves — when they would rather place importance on "are we looking good to the outer world?" — then they overlook their valuable content, and deny the individual uniqueness of themselves and their child. Just as they put themselves in a straitjacket, so do they to their child. In this case, measles will break through intensely as a call of the deepest Self for acknowledgment of its worthy content! Does your child have to float along on the stream of the Masses, unaware and without defense?

Every child is different and has its own specific disposition: don't submerge it in a system of laws and structures for the masses, but encourage it to develop its individuality!

Measles are symbolic of inner resistance to anonymity, resistance to being a victim. If one is insufficiently aware of one's divine worth, which means immunity, then measles symbolize "transmission and contamination." A struggle of the child for enhancement of its worth, with the same message to its parents.

Mumps

Self-condemnation, via which comes psychological infertility. An enormous potential of creative powers are being restrained.

A hidden, secretive emotional-world: you are constantly fighting with yourself. You will keep yourself anxiously under control, because creativity and spontaneous self-manifestation are being pulled back — because you have a certain shame with regard to some budding feelings inside you, such as sexuality.

You think you are not to be trusted. Still, you are stuck with a mass of feelings: you

then secretly experience all this inside yourself, perhaps feeling guilty about it.

The cause of this falling-back in yourself, and of the search for some kind of self-gratification, lies in your feeling unable to be yourself, to use your talents: you feel too weak or too bad, too small or too naughty.

Wandering, hesitating, tense, you condemn yourself, see things only in black and white, experience the sexual and aggressive powers in yourself as bad, and to be suppressed. That which one fights becomes stronger. Know, however, that these instincts, these primal-powers in yourself, are good. Know that these powers do their work as positive creative energies when — full of self-confidence — you dare to create in many areas. If you no longer put away — through shame or self-punishment — this inner volcano, this enormous quantity of possibilities and talents, *then,* these healthy energies will no longer form a ball of frustration, neither in sexuality, nor in the mumps. There is nothing wrong with those feelings being there, but you fixate yourself too much on your "inability and your badness," so that active creativity can no longer find a way through. As a consequence, creativity is "beaten down" again into sexuality and into a hidden emotional life full of disappointment.

This oppression of healthy, active powers leads finally to extreme aggression! You would like to box, would like to sound the trumpet, would like to declare your opinion. You get angry with people who play upon your powerlessness; you are angry because you are too pliable, angry because of your so-called weakness; angry because of your sensual longings. But you accumulate this anger. Your longings weigh so heavily on you. You direct at others — perhaps silently — your anger about yourself.

Condemning yourself, you turn your back on yourself and others; communication disturbance.

Raise the Love for yourself; say proudly, "I am here," and then sexuality and other primitive feelings will no longer serve as "compensation" for your feelings of inferi-

ority. Then, in self-respect, you will realize your dreams; then, creativity and sexuality will place themselves in the service of pure Love. Nothing in you is black, but you focus exaggeratedly upon certain feelings within you because of fear of yourself. Allow your powerful energies to circulate freely under your loving eye. When you attribute worth to yourself, then frustrations and anxieties will disappear. Quietly, proud of your Total Self, in the purity of Love for yourself, you will resolutely dare to choose your path; you will say what you have to say and no longer flee from honest, open communication.

Confrontation with your deepest feelings AND acknowledging natural longings to be "good" will lead to spontaneous evolution, by which creativity and fertility will grow at many levels.

Port-wine stain in babies

These are formed because the entity holds on to light energies, to a fairy tale atmosphere which is not from this earthly world.

A symbol of the incarnation of the spirit that reaches into the body. A crossing of various energies which accompany the settling in matter.

But the baby imagines itself to be still "strange" in its body; it dwells with gnomes or Japanese flowers. . . .

It is good for the child to intensely come into contact with its immediate surroundings: earthly, sensory contact with the body of the mother; a solid grounding of the one who is raising the child is beneficial to it; a gentle but intense exploration of the flesh, feeling itself welcome in this new world, leads to earthly "flesh-color." Feeling at home, in trust — in material reality, in its own flesh and blood.

Rickets

You don't live enough for YOURSELF. You live for others, feeling as if you are at the service of other people. You worry about others; you also accumulate their problems inside yourself. You still live too "spiritually," not really descending into earthly, physical existence; you think that earthly life and "happiness" are difficult to combine. Life lies very heavily upon you, like an enormous burden on your back, and you can barely carry it. You don't feel able to cope with life here, although you would like to fight determinedly for an ideal — but you cannot. You are convinced that emotionally you have a weak constitution and that you don't actually belong on earth.

You hold inside you all sadness and worries: it becomes heavier all the time.

Dare to bathe in your own bodily warmth: live for yourself first of all! For once, let go of all burdens and put your feet on the earth. Participate in joy on earth and take care of yourself. Cherish yourself with warm feelings: you are part of physical life, which is a manifestation of the divine Energy of Consciousness, but this incarnation requires a letting-go of a TOO-spiritual state of being — get a grip on earthly existence, in thankfulness. You, too, deserve it. No longer degrade yourself to a condition of slavery. Manifest yourself fully in matter.

Scarlet Fever

You feel unsure and unsafe in a certain structure: you think you have to protect yourself with armor, where no one can find you. Anxiety — especially when you feel physically separated from someone dear to you (at school or nursery) and you don't at all feel at ease in this new structure.

You are so unstable on your little legs, can't get a grip on anything — you look for affection, but sometimes you get so angry because of your Powerlessness. Your heated feelings sometimes boil over with aggression, and your little head burns with negative, poisonous thoughts. A conflict: passively docile — hot-tempered aggression.

You hold in your feelings too long, afraid that something catastrophic might happen. . . .

You are afraid of failure and punishment; you anxiously hold on to your feelings. You keep hidden in order to protect yourself — until with a waving fork you protest against the food mother serves you: the bomb explodes in response to a minor detail. The cause lies deeper: an anxious little soul that doesn't feel truly safe.

The safe, close physical feeling of cuddling does you a lot of good.

When parents reach a state of restful self-assuredness and trust in themselves, the child will experience its influence. Allow the child's spontaneous feelings to flow freely, don't smother the crying out, allow the child to scream at the top of its voice without mother getting angry about it. Not having to hold it in, being allowed to weep and still experiencing shelter. Reconciliation on every level. Allow emotions to go freely before they become too glowing red. Aggression, anxiety, and feelings of insecurity in the mother can intensify scarlet fever in the little one. Come to rest within yourself.

Swelling of the sebaceous glands in babies

Asking for attention.

You still feel so clumsy and dependent; you want a lot, but you don't succeed in everything. You cling to your mother (or to another mentor or person who brings you up) but a crushing authority scares you a bit. You ask for her attention, but still you long to experience yourself in freedom. You push away, you attract toward yourself.

Quietly take time to grow, don't rush, don't go too fast for your own good! Reins not too tight, not too loose. No suffocation.

A feeling of being securely sheltered, gratefully accepting loving care.

Powers and feelings develop inside you — don't put a check on them.

Umbilical hernia in babies

As a baby, you cautiously come and take a look in this world, but you don't very well dare to make the step; you are not very sure yet if you want to stay here. With one foot you are still in the non-earthly world, are only in your original awareness state, with your other foot you are over the border as it were. But you are afraid; you don't really dare to make the step completely; unconsciously you ring the alarm bell: an umbilical hernia.

The awareness state of these children is silent, an endless sphere, being a "spirit," not really living Here; the baby unconsciously blocks itself from moving on, from making the tie with life. Anxiety and unsureness are the cause; the more the mother resolves her anxieties and unsureness, the better the atmosphere will be for the baby.

Something's wrong: "I don't dare to go on in this way." Emotions and tensions are piling up, until the alarm bell sounds. Sometimes, the baby would prefer to withdraw into another existence. As long as the umbilical cord was connected with the mother, there didn't have to be an emphatic "ensoulment" of the Individual, of the new being; after all the body was being nourished spiritually and physically by the mother. By cutting the umbilical cord, the body of the baby will react much more strongly to the impulses of its own deepest Self, although the radiation of the mother also will remain strongly present. An independent existence, a descending into the earthly sphere, requires adaptation, which doesn't always go smoothly.

It is necessary that the being dare to pull a powerful "tube" to its earthly existence, to its body, from its prime source, the living

Self, from the other dimension. Allowing himself to really be born.

This "entering into earthly life" can only begin with a little flame: it's impossible for the baby already to find a solid grip on life here. That's why he looks for support in the mother, in the "mother source," tapping life for the moment in a comforting way; he feels, after all, so insecure in this new form of existing. If the mother feels calm and secure, not in an anxious nervousness, then the little one, while depending on her, will dare to extend the connection, without anxieties, from his Inner Self toward earthly existence.

An umbilical hernia provokes a reaction from those who care about the baby: a fire arrow which doesn't miss its mark; it's about baby's aim to be able to feel more strongly present in life, to bring himself into life via the sensory stimuli of his own body, via contacts with others. Loving, relaxed care gives him a feeling of security and welcome in the new life. No more is necessary; a warm, sheltered feeling that is able to drive away anxieties.

Experiencing joy, the great objective of earthly life, in the warmth of the sun, in the warmth of the mother heart.

Umbilical hernia in adults: the same "essential" causes are to be considered.

Umbilical redness and inflammation in babies

Aggression because of impotence. You feel weak, helpless, dependent, and you would like to do much more already than you are able to. Your care-givers fiddle with your little nose, at your little navel and you resist. You feel stuck, anxious, because of your powerlessness. Because of this you would cling to your mother with your little claws, but actually you long for room to move, for freedom, for your own power of expression. Sometimes someone hurts you, with a needle or a piece of cloth; you get really angry about this.

The baby also collects the mother's feelings: if, for instance, Mama feels powerless then the baby will unconsciously drink in these feelings; this also goes for anxiety and anger.

Give the child as much room as possible, don't put too many clothes on it, don't force it, don't oblige it, but follow the rhythm of its nature!

No matter how small it is, it has its unique characteristics: let it be itself and don't mold it according to your nature: its freedom to be "I"; a separation into two autonomous beings, mother and baby. Love gives and doesn't grab, doesn't claw.

It is beneficial for the child when the mother is aware of her powers and possibilities, when she can stand up for herself and doesn't bottle up any anger! Trust in one's deepest Self, a comforting, calming attitude of the mother, is beneficial to healing.

Whooping cough

Protest. Someone wants to look inside you, or someone hurts you — at least that is how you feel. You feel as if you are suffocating; you close yourself off! Unloading feelings, longing for liberation; anxiety and powerlessness.

Searching, disorientation, having no perspective on yourself, nor on the situation around you. A powerless, anxious protest: you feel like one who is condemned to be hanged, at the mercy of your parents or mentors, imprisoned in a structure; it is as if one can do what one wants with you. . . . You feel as if you are in the spotlight — exposed to the criticism, the orders of others. They make decisions for you; they expect from you a beautiful report card so that they might boast about you to their relations, etc. — that is how it seems to you (no matter whether your impression is based upon reality or not).

You feel as if you are the fool who has to go along with someone, like a dog with its master. You have to play a certain role, but you don't have true contact with your deepest Self; your basic instincts, your psychological survival instinct, and the early sexuality sometimes come too strongly to the fore. This is all because you are not yet able to direct your life yourself in a Self-assured and Aware way.

Transform these inner powers into energetic action and self-realization: don't flee into a shell, but feel protected in your safe, deepest Self. Listen to this inner voice; don't allow your feelings to be looked into if you don't wish it; don't allow yourself to be hurt by others, but don't hide yourself away from your own feelings and potential energies, because this only leads to powerless frustration. Mark off your terrain; no one has to aim spotlights at you; it is you who has to express your opinion, your creativity. No longer bottle it up; dare, in love, to experience yourself to the fullest. Discover the peace in yourself, the unity, by being consistent: live in honest contact with your deepest being, without outwardly playing a role to please others. Transform aggression and suffocation into resolute, constructive Action!

CHILL, COLD SHIVERS

Insufficiently present in your own warmth, in your heart; you are insufficiently aware of your worth. You block the love for yourself; you block life energies.

You cannot truly be yourself because you recoil too much in anxiety and chilliness.

All energies in your body constrict, so to speak: your spiritual attention fixates on *one* point; you bind yourself, you reject, you draw back into yourself. You put a muzzle on yourself; your broad thinking capacity limits itself now; a concentrated energy in your head, chilled spirit, too little earth.

Sharp energies that are driven to a peak are penetrating your brain, your body; you allow yourself to be pulled along in a stream of light energies that are called up out of fear.

Anxiety is the cause of your calling up sharp energies which shut you off emotionally from the outer world so that you no longer really want to think, so that you would rather draw back into yourself. Sometimes it all becomes too much for you.

Wrap yourself with the warmth of your heart: come out of your house instead of locking yourself up. Don't block yourself in; don't be afraid of being yourself. Allow energies to exist freely; express yourself; don't be afraid to be the way you are. Dare to burst open with all your powers and possibilities, feel the earth beneath your feet, bid yourself welcome amongst others, don't tie your nature down. Speak and sing! When you don't acknowledge your warm heart-center, anxiety and coldness will dominate your life. Allow life energies to flow freely. Don't lock yourself up in chilly isolation. Powerful consciousness in a warm body.

THE CHIN

Psychological correspondence

An antenna directed toward earth; carrying your face. Knowing yourself to be safe on your foundation. A strong grounding, being rooted in your deepest Self. The Power of Unity within yourself. A reflection of your self-assuredness, of your strong inner essence, the radiating sun center in yourself. No masks, no lies, no weakness.

Resolutely going on in life, without detours, without hesitations. Leadership in your Self; all authority and support lies in your Self. Feeling warm and welcome with your fellow men without question, without forcing, because you love yourself the way you are. When you are whole, satisfied with yourself, without inner discord, then you will not experience a wall between you and other people, then you don't have to ask pointedly for affirmation.

An harmonious merging of heaven and earth, of your living Self and your earthly body.

Ailments of the chin

Are you insufficiently grounded in yourself? Do you feel unsafe? Do you withdraw from your own roots, from your deepest Self, from the Consciousness that propels your body? Then you only live on the surface, and you feel unsafe, weak, unsure. Your chin will be sharply and aggressively on guard, ready to defend itself or to attack. When you don't place value and Authority inside yourself, you will become dependent on confirmations, on affirmation from the outside world. Your outer Image will become more important than the way you feel inwardly. Insecurity is compensated for by fighting spirit, by glittering outwardly. Do you find nothing to hold on to? Do you feel anxious? Don't look for it outside yourself! Do you only acknowledge the "spirit" and ignore the physical, the enjoying, the physical pleasures?... Do you think that your foundation, your deep feelings and longings, are "bad"? Do you not trust yourself?

Too little grounding leads to unbalance: come with both feet on the ground and put your trust in your total Self, don't put up any stop-signs. Don't lift your chin too high above the earthly: dare to be human amongst humans, feel welcome, don't withdraw.

On the other hand: do you allow yourself to be led by materialism, by the physical, by sexual lust or other compulsions? Bring yourself in contact with your deep Essence and stop fooling yourself by thinking you are not worth anything, that you are but a weakling; these are only convictions. Get a hold of your self and direct your emotional-world

in a self-aware way, without becoming a slave to it.

Become master over yourself, not over others, which would only be a frustrated reaction to the feelings of powerlessness inside yourself. Be proud of your content, not of your masquerade or your act. Experience the unity in yourself and don't place a thick wall between yourself and others. Is your attitude toward yourself so condemning and critical? Then you will also approach others too critically. Self-contentment leads to friendship.

CHOLERA

You consider yourself an anonymous element that ought to show love to something greater and higher above itself, to a super-god. You aren't aware enough of your own divinity, of your Powerful creative center. You surrender to the passion of love and hate; you let yourself be dragged along by emotions, by religions, by the opinion of the masses — you are being absorbed, sucked up by great energies over which, according to your convictions, you have no say. You think your safety doesn't lie inside yourself, but that it depends on something or someone else, on a god, a devil or on Destiny. You allow yourself to "be lived": this leads to even more miserable circumstances — it makes you angry, aggressive, wanting to call out loudly for attention. As a people or race, feeling lost in this condition of unawareness, of powerlessness, of self-deception ("We are but helpless poor souls, unable to change our situation."). You become increasingly more anxious about the grip of evil until the "evil" absolutely strikes. Helpless, you throw your arms in the sky, toward the rest of the world. . . .

Negative expectations about the future, and a fatalistic vision regarding existence, only *perpetuate miserable situations. Every individual may come to holy self-respect, marking the borders around the sanctuary of his being. Self-respect. Insight into the possibilities of programming the world differently: first of all realizing that no one — no god nor commandment — outside ourselves will offer rescue. That we ourselves are responsible for the life that we now lead, **and** that we are able to change this in the future. Not by feelings of aggression and revolt, which only worsen the negativity in the world. But by resolute projection in love and longing toward the future. By the belief in these creative powers of the human being (and mankind), changes will be created in the world which finally will lead to the solution of misery. If, however, you believe in the powerlessness of humanity — in its defenselessness, in its evilness and guilt — then this blindness hinders the healing of the Earth and the recovery from all epidemics which have come into existence as a result of despair and of the belief in the powerlessness of mankind. Faith, Love, and the achieving of Consciousness by the human being (and mankind) means also reaching "immunity" against whatever illness. (See Part I.)*

CHOLESTEROL LEVEL, TOO HIGH

Your natural aggression is being restrained; a holding-on to ideals, to dreams, but without *really* coming to action in your life! Yes, you do a lot, but only "to give a good impression" or to achieve or to win a trophy or a competition, or you play the clown to satisfy others. You project your deeper longings or dreams toward the future, limiting your life, even putting your head in the sand. You don't really build from the here-and-now. "Ah, it will come one day" — good

fortune. Meanwhile, you drift about in a life that is too restricted. You believe in a lucky horseshoe or in a saint, but you don't make use of your own creative possibilities. You retain sadness from the past, virtuously following rules that have been put upon you by systems or religions; you neglect the spontaneous, happy child within you! You are so serious in your heart, while life is *one* joyful stream, but you refuse to feel this joyful heart; with steely sternness you constantly grill yourself (on a metal gridiron, as it were): "What have I done wrong today?" You forget to enjoy. As long as everything looks good and beautiful on the surface. You completely constrict yourself in order to satisfy the judgment of others — you don't really *live;* you are unfaithful to your deep, natural, spontaneous nature. You are plainly afraid to truly experience joy, to surrender to this endless stream of life. Is this perhaps because you think that in the end you will die anyway? Do you prefer a slow departure from this life, with the prospect of death? In this way, you deprive yourself of all joy.

Now, realize your own dreams! Liberation, resurrection! No one dies if he does not wish to. Stir yourself and exploit all your possibilities. Allow joy to free your veins in gratitude for life. Leave the past behind and go on: build your own castle; don't let life pass you by. Complete surrender to yourself; come out of your shell in honest openness instead of playing a social role. Be YOURSELF in all your facets! The child in you is truly King: follow this simple heart, these intuitive, natural powers. Don't hide yourself in sadness or dark thoughts. Become master over your life and play the game of life in a grand way, taking up all your space. . . .

A cholesterol level that is "too high" or "too low" — this is a very relative notion. A level that is perfect for one person might be too high for someone else, or vice versa.

CHROME
Deficiency, insufficient assimilation of

You feel yourself cold and at the mercy of others, unable to guide your life in a well-determined direction. You surrender; you have difficulty seeing a solution; it all doesn't matter anymore. You are angry because you make compromises that betray your own nature and longings, but, after all, you bear the burdens. Possibly, you live or work in "forced servitude," or you are being confronted in a hard way with your own nature, with your feelings, although you would rather have kept them hidden: others now also seem to have their say in it. You are insufficiently grounded in your own roots, so that problems in communication can occur. You'd like to get a grip on others, but they only seem to have power over you. You refuse to look for depth and power in yourself; a refusal to transform, to acknowledge your own powers of consciousness. Out of sheer necessity, you yield to the so-called "authority" of another, because you refuse to acknowledge the authority in yourself. Possibly, painful memories from the past are burdening you; instead of evolving onward in a self-aware way, you try to get a grip on everything and everyone, but you realize soon enough that this is of no use.

Live from out of yourself: stand behind something completely or don't do it. Come to beautiful cooperation with others, to unity in yourself. Don't dredge up problems from the past; no longer carry needless burdens on your shoulders. Be alert and critical in a healthy way: allow Mars powers to break through in active self-realization. Transformation: work on yourself, free yourself, be faithful to your nature. Work, labor, on yourself, toward depth, toward height, toward all regions! Don't reach outside yourself, but discover this fundamental power in your Self. Place inside you all Authority over your life.

CLAUSTROPHOBIA
fear of confined places

You are filled to the brim with energies: with sad emotions, anxieties, as well as with a richness of creativity! But you run away from yourself, especially from the small child in you, who asks to express itself in a free, natural way. This mass of suppressed powers — sadness, anxieties — asks for complete liberation, like an erupting volcano.

You suffocate yourself with anxieties and the feeling of not being safe in yourself. Trust in your own powerful self is lacking!

You yearn for space, space — and you cannot get enough oxygen — but in fact you ignore the space of your "I": you run away from it!

Come into yourself, resolutely and self-aware! Come to fusion with yourself: draw the poor, helpless child close to you instead of abandoning it and taking flight.

Come close to yourself in tenderness and love: on your strong basis. Love for yourself drives away anxiety and panic. Rest and balance will be found when you resolutely and consciously take hold of yourself in order to look at your deeper feelings and powers and to allow them to exist Freely, under your mastery. Free yourself from the grip of power: let your anxieties, your emotions, go free — don't run away! No longer be afraid of your deep essence, your deep feelings.

CLEFT LIP — CLEFT PALATE, CONGENITAL

Here, we're not dealing with an illness. Just look at the reasons why your Self-core gives you this signal at birth. It doesn't have to disappear at all! Truth, goodness, and beauty follow each other naturally.

You are born with a certain conviction regarding yourself: your body translates this conviction. Therefore, negative convictions ask for a psychological growth and transformation into positive thoughts so that inner harmony and joy will be the result.

You have the feeling that others dominate you and that you are not worth very much. You feel yourself to be inferior.

You think that others "force their way into you"; you think they will again rape you psychologically; you hide yourself anxiously; you look for shelter; you look for a hold somewhere. Sometimes, you'd prefer to withdraw, to close yourself up: no one has any say over you after all! You've allowed others to treat you the way they wanted, allowing yourself to be hurt, because you insufficiently believe in yourself. Instead of manifesting yourself resolutely and taking action, you withdraw.

It is very possible that, as a consequence of your negative convictions regarding yourself, you actually have attracted an environment that even intensifies your negative thoughts! Therefore, it's through such a confrontation that you can solve your problems!

Now, be completely open to yourself, to your worth and possibilities; no longer push yourself into the background, and allow yourself to be truly born now, independent of others, in love for yourself. Only then can you really grow from out of your own basis, not from out of that "which a society or others expect from you."

Dare to be yourself; come to true consciousness: come into contact with that which is deepest in yourself, with your intuition, and now determine entirely your life path! Become aware of the value of content and of the relativity of image and outer appearance. Come to the essence of yourself, to the core of life, and be faithful to your unique nature; no one but you can indicate

the direction which is good for you. Determine your limits regarding others, and achieve communication with the people whom you wish to encounter; don't allow anything to be forced upon you.

COBALT
Deficiency, insufficient assimilation of

Crushing anxiety; you feel irretrievably lost; powerless in the face of your overwhelming emotional content. You think you are being manipulated by Destiny, by your those who raise you, by those who would squeeze you, oppress you, hold you — you cannot get a grip on anything. You drop yourself, so to speak. . . .

Determine your life yourself, no longer allowing yourself to be dominated or suffocated by others; feel Protected by the powers of your deepest Self; be fearless, but resolutely take hold of your rudder. Change your false convictions: you are not a weak, powerless creature. Nothing, or no one, has a hold on your life unless you allow it yourself; Destiny does not exist unless you call it into being; create your life according to your longings.

COLDS

You but live behind a chilly "death mask"; you withdraw from life somewhat because you don't connect with your warm, joyful, inner Center.

Your head is ravaged; it is as if your head is empty, but it is full to bursting: filled with all sorts of things, because you constantly are working at something outside yourself instead of existing yourself and living from out of your warm essence.

You chisel a sculpture instead of chiseling yourself. You feel cold, gray, sad, small: you don't place yourself in the warm sun center; you would rather retreat; you hide behind a dark mask. You think you cannot *really* take your life in your own hands; you allow yourself to *"be* lived." You don't place mastery and Authority over your nature, over your life in yourself!

(Moreover, you are convinced that you can be a victim of a psychological as well as a bacterial infection. You don't believe in individual immunity: you are a follower, or you take on certain traditional ideas from the anonymous mass. Because of this, you will of course be infected on all kinds of levels.)

You don't truly *live!* Where is that warmth of life, the joy deep inside yourself? Are you cut off from your warm heart because you don't believe in the power and authority of your deepest Self?

You underestimate the divine abilities of a human being: you can create your life *yourself;* you are not the victim of circumstance; you need to build up your personal ideas, independent of the expectations of others. Don't expect love and warmth from others if you haven't first welcomed yourself warmheartedly, if your body has not first received the radiant power, full of love, from your Self, your Heart. Free yourself from the somber, negative thoughts you have absorbed from the outer world. You are naturally immune (See Infections). You don't need to protect yourself against dim surroundings with a dark mask, because you are naturally protected in your Self. Come forth in life with all your power and warm energies. No one can infect you; enjoy life without anxieties. You are not a sad, poor, minuscule individual! Every human being possesses the ability to build up his life as an Authority, in joy: feel this completeness in yourself and stop degrading yourself, pushing yourself aside.

Dare to inhale the most beautiful fragrances of life, and don't shut yourself off from them! Don't close yourself off from joyful participation in life! Don't pile things up in your head, like a machine, but integrate only that which you wish to take in — that which is in accord with your heart. You are not a wooden doll: allow warm energies, emotions, personal longings, all to circulate freely. Don't belie your nature in social relationships. Don't kill your nature, life in your existence, by exaggerated "thinking and brooding" or by a structure which oppresses you, in which there is no longer room for spontaneous, enjoyable existence. Make it warm and cozy for yourself; bring about changes in an existence that is too cold, too deadly, and too sad. Now, you also close yourself off from the world around you in order to be able first to find rest with yourself, and delightfully spoil yourself. Don't fight against this.

COLD SORE
herpes labialis

You long to stretch yourself, to blossom out of a tightly strung psychological situation; impatience, irritation — because you aren't, or can't, be yourself.

You want to say something, express your feelings and personal opinions, but you are being stopped, held back, and you keep silent. From fear of not being accepted or loved by others, you don't express yourself enough.

You feel squeezed, tied down; then, you often force yourself to get out of it.

With a heavy head, you inwardly direct your irritation or accusations toward those who — so you think — don't let you be who you are; it is you, however, who lives on half your strength, in anxiety and sadness, feeling yourself too small.

Do you allow your life to be too strongly influenced by authorities outside yourself (parents, partner. . .)? This irritates you inwardly, but you bottle up your anger. By not trusting your own basis, you see everything in fragments, pulled apart into details, you can't get a perspective. In this way you sometimes feel anxious because you can't get a grip on yourself and because you are too dependent.

Be faithful to your nature, dare to be yourself; express yourself!

No one can live or speak in your place: in self-confidence, be aware of the uniqueness of your being. The little bird will first have to spit out something before it can sing the way it's meant to: actually, there's insufficient confidence in what it feels, itself. Speak up and say what you feel: in this way you are faithful to yourself and, in dialogue with someone else, you can both grow. Build your life on your own authority.

When the time is ripe, joyfully say goodbye to previous "teachers" or systems that used to make you feel good. Look for the right path for yourself, via your intuition and inner wisdom.

Feel how energies are ready to let you grow; free yourself.

COMA

Nature covers you with a friendly, protecting gesture: now you are safe. You really wanted to be *gone,* to step out of time, unconsciously go toward death, because you long for rest, because you experience yourself to be powerless, unable to solve one or more problems in your life, or "have" life the way you would like it to be.

This is an emotional reaction: you sit there, as it were, in your little hole, in a safe womb where you no longer have to bear any responsibilities, where no one can hurt you.

Possibly, you fled from an obstacle in your life. You would have had to go through it, but you did not dare. You probably knew unconsciously that you were not on your *real* path, on the right path of life, but did not

dare do otherwise. You have now *fled from transformation, from change.* Emotionally it became too much for you; you felt powerless, seized by something of which you could not get a clear perspective. Anxiety.

Possibly, you also have placed "conditions" on life (and have not obtained their fulfillment) instead of *thankfully* and *receptively* throwing yourself in unconditional surrender into the arms of life. "BEING," "LIVING" . . . as "YOU"!?

A person who is in a coma will make the choice to live or to die himself, although this choice will be made while in a rather unconscious state — on the basis of convictions. It is possible to speak to him: the deeper "I" will register the message. The feeling of safety, security, and love will make anxieties disappear. Self-trust is strengthened by the suggestion of Power and Daring, and by being Aware of the enormously strong possibilities present in every person, and so also in this human being. This trust can lead to joy. Joy leads the life energies "away" from death. The suggestion that — if he wishes it so — his life will be a promise, a rebirth, and that he is not alone in it.

Also tell him how Happiness is waiting for him if he lives in "thankfulness," without placing demands or conditions on life.

If he has reason to finally stay "away," then he is entitled to do that. In one way or another, the comatose person registers and "hears" you. Speak to him in a positive way.

COMPUTER MOUSE ARM
repetitive strain injury, RSI
tendon inflammation caused by working too much, too long, with the mouse of a computer

It seems as if a mouse has bitten you. "Ow!" It painfully pulls in your forearm. The moment has come to realize where and why you have filled yourself with things and/or people outside yourself and therefore life now sends you painful signals so that you will become aware of it. The emergency brake is being pulled; stop hurting, forcing yourself so. Why do you push yourself away? Why don't you allow gentle love?

As a result you can feel painfully pushed out, sometimes shut out by others or by those you love. This, indeed, is the result of shutting yourself out, pushing away that which is gentle, as if you don't want to lovingly embrace yourself, as if you demand of yourself to do this or that; you can be painfully hard on yourself, punishing yourself. It makes no sense to go on this way.

Look at the sadness about you that you push away, look at it first and see how it's your body that begs you to love it. As a beautiful piece of nature, no longer push it down or reject it (by, for instance, looking down on it or placing it on a strict diet, or obligating it to do certain work with which it is not at all in harmony at the moment, etc.). Give yourself all chances for rehabilitation. In gentleness, enter into your complete being! Are you angry with yourself? Do you think that you don't answer to this or that "law"? Would you hurt yourself because you think yourself to be nothing or inadequate? Then, it's time to realize now that you are beautiful as a human being, if only you live in "goodness," in love and harmony with yourself and, as a result, also with others. Stop hurting yourself, feeling shut out; it is you who are so hard on yourself! Don't expect anything, don't demand anything of others, especially not if you already treat yourself less worthily than you deserve and hurt yourself.

Don't try to satisfy an ambitious plan, a job because you think you have to (because otherwise you wouldn't think yourself very worthy). Don't escape from yourself in a job — for instance, in a computer job, in the meantime suppressing deeper sadness, not allowing yourself all the space to exist!

Don't place your "work" above your life. A signal to stop for a while and have a good look at yourself, at your inner sense of being hurt, of pain; to see how you have immobilized yourself without much love, how you have not respected yourself in Worthiness — and we are talking here about your true worthiness.

Do you, for instance, attract financial problems? Don't just rush over them, don't just frenetically begin to work, but first look at why you have attracted such a situation. Warm yourself now in a hearty way, give yourself the needed support, and make your heart welcome; allow yourself to "melt" a little, as it were, don't adopt such an icy cold, hard attitude. Don't try to satisfy others, image, achievements or ambition and especially: don't fly from your problems, but look at them. And you will see how you actually long for a deep acknowledgement of your inner world, for a going-under the surface of your being; how you really want to transform a kind of primal sadness into joy. Then become happy about your total being; don't live according to the conviction that you are a "victim" who always will attract painful situations. Don't live according to the conviction that being on earth means hard work and suffering pain — because as a result you will attract circumstances which will be a conformation of this.

Disconnect yourself from this perspective to life, and change things around. CONFRONT yourself with the bottleneck inside you and (as a result) also with the bottleneck in relationship with your surroundings, with certain other people. Speak , express yourself and pull yourself up. Express yourself in an honest way. Bring the deepest pressure points above board, don't hold back, don't suppress. With honest communications you get much further, you come to a solution. You become honest with yourself; step out of your shadow, and others will look at you respectfully, will treat you respectfully, as long as you no longer push yourself painfully away. Don't try to constantly live in a such a way that you think you have to/want to always satisfy something or others outside yourself, but satisfy your own highest feeling of Love. *Give* yourself what you deserve, and come into the world with open eyes; say to others what's on your mind when necessary, express your burdens and in the meantime solve the hard dictatorship inside yourself!

Do you doubt your "belonging"? Do you doubt your worthiness for Life, doubt your ability to remain standing up straight in life, perhaps under the pressure of emotions or under the pressure of a power, an authority, you place above yourself? Know that the essence of the solution to this problem begins by "getting yourself on dry land": allowing yourself to enter into the ark of security and self-protection; showing yourself the way toward warmth and shelter in life, in your total body. Realizing you don't gain anything at all by leaving yourself in the cold — and that this doesn't at all depend on something, an authority, outside yourself, and that only YOU decide what will become of your life. Only you know your limits. You know when, and in what way you DENY your total being, your nature, your body, your broad content! So take good care of yourself, offer yourself warmth, attention, bring yourself in. You no longer have to stand crying outside in the cold waiting for someone to let you in. This letting-in, in a loving way, into your earthly body — that you will have to do yourself. And as a result, you will notice that it's comfortably warm around the inner hearth! And you decide that you are allowed to be, that you are worthy, as a Human Being, that you are allowed to offer yourself that which is beautiful, gentle, and sweet!

Communicate in an open, warm way with others and feel welcome in the warm home of mother earth. The rest will follow by itself. But go onward! in the right way and stop losing yourself in a task, or job or hobby in which you escape from yourself, behind which you "hide." Now, come to the fore in full beauty, in the uniqueness of your being. You now OPEN yourself, become RECEPTIVE to all the beauty you carry inside yourself; you no longer PUSH it AWAY from yourself. In a flexible way, sweetly and gently, listen to the female voice inside you, which asks you not to take a hard, sharp, aggressive, red attitude toward yourself (as if you might stab yourself in the arm with a sharp object), but to allow beautiful things to smoothly flow in you in a blue-hued, open way: all those beautiful consciousness-energies, full of love, which want to fill, to circulate, in your body.

Let go of that to which you so clamped on before, don't be coldly ambitious, don't be hard as a stone toward yourself, let go! Don't direct yourself in a red, intense way to the work that "has" to be finished. Where is there anger hiding, a being-wronged? Regarding who? This is, however, only the result of the fact that you place yourself in the cold and that you keep yourself powerless to do and say what you feel you have to do/say. Bring yourself warmly inside! Don't blame someone else, but ACKNOWLEDGE yourself in your fullness! As a result, others will also listen to you, and begin to communicate with you in an honest way. But *first* you have to bring yourself in.

Anger only pops up as a result of the feeling of powerlessness to be yourself and to acknowledge yourself in totality, separate from your job, separate from the computer for instance! And, now look deep inward to the warm light inside yourself; that is what is essential in Life. The rest follows by itself. First, come home to yourself; let go where necessary and no longer hurt yourself by racing on, wanting to reach, absolutely wanting to push things through. YOU as Human Being come first, as do other human beings. Only then comes the rest: work, ambition, etc. And know you never have to prove yourself, but instead cherish yourself first of all, warmly welcoming yourself in life. By doing so, it will be necessary that you "let go" of certain things for a while in order to direct your EYES clearly toward the inner, deeper soul-world that lies under the surface of a hectic, hard existence full of obligations. Make yourself softer and warmer! As a result, you will no longer make yourself sad and silently angry, throwing yourself furiously into your work, feeling shut out — because YOU have shut yourself out! Life circumstances change when first you look at yourself and welcome yourself in a heartfelt way; when you put Life and Love for yourself in the first place! Don't blame others for what you do to yourself.

Now, turn deeply inward and work in all honesty with yourself without forcing yourself or "pushing out" your nature, your heart, your body. If you keep on "pushing out," then it's better to stop! Nothing stands above Life, nor above the warmth of the heart and complete self-acknowledgment, according to soul and body! Now, arrive at JOY regarding yourself: joy can only exist if you acknowledge yourself in TOTALITY, if you don't shut out any part of yourself (and might as a result expect love and acknowledgment from others). Be THANKFUL for who you are, for the earthly body in which you live; no longer close yourself off from your content, from your feelings, your heart. Listen to your signals and don't live just to prove yourself in your work or to please someone else — all the while pushing yourself away from yourself. Lovingly take yourself in and listen to yourself, to your heart. Speak when it's necessary to speak with others; only you can sense when you are too hard on yourself, when you sting yourself and hurt yourself (and as a result you might feel that others are hurting you, are severe toward you: so, begin with being gentle with yourself). Don't fill yourself with things outside you, but acknowledge now that magnificent fullness of your being!

Other types of RSI are discussed in other chapters: achilles tendon, bursitis, fibromyalgia, PSH, tendinitis, tennis elbow, etc.

CONGENITAL PHYSICAL DEFECTS — BEING BORN IN MISERABLE LIFE CIRCUMSTANCES

Every physical symptom is actually the key to solving inner problems which are at the bottom. Every life situation is a mirror of what dwells in your inner being, a rendering of your deepest convictions about yourself. If you were born blind, this indicates that deep within yourself is the conviction, "I need to suffer first before I can arrive at insight," or "I don't see clearly; I have my eyes too closed to deeper inner values," and so forth.

Many call this "karma." No, it has to do with something completely different: no one's being punished; no one has to feel guilty for "mistakes." We can start again at any moment with a clean slate. No one has to be born blind or to be born in miserable circumstances.

On the one hand, one has the irresistible urge to Be; and on the other hand, one is stuck emotionally at certain points. Being ever again on the way to fulfillment — to enrichment of itself — the Self will automatically lead every inner problem to a solution. So, through specific defects, we are confronted with the negative convictions we have about ourselves: "I'm bad and guilty, so . . ." or "I'm tiny and powerless, so. . . ." Unconscious opinions about yourself are brought to light via a physical defect — in order to destroy them! Nobody is tiny, small, powerless or bad, even though certain religions or philosophies would like us to believe so.

If you have been born among a pursued, discriminated-against race that is almost extinct because of hunger and thirst, then this is a consequence of your deeper unconscious conviction patterns: "As a human being, I'm a powerless victim of situations which are there simply as fate or as a consequence of a punishing god or devil. I always will be persecuted. I must simply be bad, or at least don't have the right to live happily." Lies, of course, which you convince yourself of consciously or unconsciously. Therefore . . . the sooner we human beings, young and old, become AWARE that we ourselves create our lives on the basis of expectations — the outlook on Life — which we carry inside us, then the better it will be. The sooner we become AWARE of the fact that we are able to change our convictions, guide our energies in a new direction . . . the better it will be! Circumstances will change for the better when first of all we change our convictions according to the knowledge that WE have our happiness in our own hands. (Read Part I)

Genetic determination . . . or not?

Genetic PREDISPOSITION . . . yes! But HOW that predisposition unfolds in evolution — that depends on you!

The physical genetic structure is determined mainly by your ancestors. It's your psyche, however, your inner convictions, which determine whether or not genetic instructions come through! If you acknowledge the mastery of your conscious "I," *if, where necessary, you bring about changes in your thoughts and convictions, then the genetic pattern will automatically also change!*
We have not "accidentally" been born here or there; neither has it been a real "conscious" choice, such as choosing between an apple or a pear. We have been born in this family because this frame-work corresponds best with our deepest convictions regarding a new life. It has to do with a constant flow of spontaneous growth of Life itself: *your Self, for growth and self-realization, will be born where — for you — lies the Confrontation with your unconscious convictions.* Were you stuck with feelings of

inferiority? Being born as a child of a father who, for instance, belittles you again and again, will ultimately make you jump up and evolve.

No blaming, no self-blame. Becoming conscious, once and for all. Become conscious that no one or nothing but you, yourself, leads or "suffers" your life. Take up this responsibility out of love for yourself and for mankind.

You can do much more than you "think." The genetic system is a DYNAMIC data base that is constantly in motion and susceptible to influences of the positive — as well as negative — convictions, feelings, and thoughts of the human being.

CONGESTION
rush of blood to the head

Suppressed feelings, emotions, bring you into a constant state of stress. You don't dare fully experience your emotional world. You keep yourself tense, like a mouse in a trap. You consider yourself to be not "good" enough; you don't dare show the way you feel. Energies leading toward self-liberation are pressing forward! You think you are navigating on an unsafe, dirty ocean; you don't trust your deep, unconscious content. You arm yourself against this situation. You feel uneasy because you fear that sooner or later something "bad" will rise up out of you. You anxiously keep yourself from living in a natural and free way.

By playing an important "angel" role, or by taking on a showy attitude, you already feel safer. Instead of building your life on a self-assured basis, you depend upon a false backbone. A discharge of your most natural, suppressed feelings and talents is now taking place; they want acknowledgment, they want to be experienced from out of yourself without your asking any longer, "What will others say?" You live too deeply in the world of thought, too little on Earth. Do you exaggerate the importance of the "spiritual"? Do you ignore the worth of the "earthly"?

Now integrate all your feelings, enjoy the physical also; feel yourself taken up in the fire of the earth with your feet on the ground. Don't float away with your thoughts, with your spirituality: keep yourself here-and-now, experience your intuition. Balance between body and spirit is necessary! We are people of flesh and blood; don't exaggerate the spiritual or mental aspect. Our soul essence will flood through the body with powerful, joyful energies: try not to oppress this, neither in purely thinking nor in spiritual one-sidedness. Via your senses you taste the Earth, the beauty of Nature. Allow your nature to grow freely; don't block this exchange between the body and the soul-essence. Feel relaxed and free in yourself.

CONVULSIONS

An inner contradiction: on the one hand one feels anxious, in the grip of Authority (parents, mentors, Leaders, religions, philosophy . . .), one experiences oneself as powerless and suppressed; one allows oneself to be led through the life or the thoughts of someone with whom one identifies oneself, or in whose power one finds oneself; one experiences oneself as fragile and unprotected, bent under a heavy load, because one's own identity cannot or may not powerfully exist. A tense, restless nervousness results from this. On the other hand, this frustrating suppression leads to anger, to (mostly) unconscious aggression; one is ready to burst, to break loose. This inner dilemma between docility or being one's own master derives from mistrust of one's own intuition, mistrust

of the deeper inner divine Self, mistrust of one's own creative Ability. Higher, intuitive energies are being blocked. One tries to save oneself with sheer one-sided rationality, with confused searching in thoughts. Until this situation becomes unbearable: a one-sided overburdening of certain parts of the brain, a convulsion.

This is a Request for straightening things out, coming from the Living Self: "No longer deny your deepest Source; allow your feelings, your intuition, your personal powers, to circulate freely now; acknowledge your higher awareness; now tune in to your own creative, Living self, which guarantees autonomy and mastery over yourself."

Pull that plug: allow all possibilities to come through. No longer dam up your being human. Don't overburden yourself with thinking and fretting, nor with book-knowledge or with obtrusive pedantry from sources outside yourself (TV, teachers . . .). Come to rest in your total self: a balance in yourself. Acknowledge the physical and your nature, don't only live in your head. As an Earthly human being you are allowed to enjoy with all your senses; don't neglect this. Don't try to achieve, but try to inwardly realize yourself. Complete wisdom will unfold within you. Experience all these mental and physical powers inside yourself and no longer suppress these creative qualities. Stop fretting and becoming excited because of insecurity: as a human being you are unique, not subordinate to anyone. Quietly turn yourself inward, feel yourself safe, sheltered in your Nature. Then come to true, energetic action, externalize, from out of your natural longings — no longer because you "have to." Dare to feel "good" about yourself!

If a child suffers from convulsions, the above-mentioned causes are often also present in the psychological condition of the mother (or of the person with whom the emotional tie is strongest). Both can learn from each other and help each other in the process of healing and transformation.

Convulsions in "contractions": hands tightly closed, eyes turned downward and showing white above, feet usually warm

Psychological causes: pent-up energies, emotions are looking for their outlet.

Full of sensitivity, of softness, and too flexible towards others. You feel as if you were hollowed out; you insufficiently stand on your own legs; as a result, you very strongly undergo the influence of your "home," of your mentors or another "haven"; emotional dependence; too weak a grip, you can no longer handle it; insufficient faith in your own Power; this way you cannot handle life, you surrender completely, without resistance; emotionally you try to embrace *very* much, but it overflows; powerless, unsure of yourself, withdrawing yourself; your deepest Self tightens itself as it were, to show you your powers. You doubt your worth! The female, soft, weak aspect achieves the upper hand; you are no longer aware of your strong "I". You flee away. The convulsions protect your life: *allow* energies and emotions to turn outward!

Psychological lesson to be learned from this: here and now, come to a Self-aware, powerful trust in your "I." Don't allow emotions to have the upper hand: become master over yourself. Allow energies to circulate freely; no longer bottle things up, and know yourself to be safe and strong on your solid Basis, your Living Self. Build beautiful, clear structures for yourself. Don't allow anyone to "worm their way in," and take good care of yourself.

Feel the masculine force inside yourself and experience the power in your legs, in your feet: experience your total BEING. Know you are protected in yourself; experience your primitive powers and allow them to come through! Use these energies in creativity, in emotional experiences by which the sensory will not be overlooked.

Smell, taste, feel, breathe, see — and enjoy the beauty of the earthly: a focused presence in nature, in your nature. Self-assured

participation in life. Acknowledge your worth as being distinct from others; don't LET yourself "be lived." Put all power over your life in yourself. "I AM." Don't let yourself glide away, but establish yourself firmly on your feet!

Convulsions in which the hands are open, feet cold, and the eyes are directed upward, with white showing below the pupils

Psychological causes: aggression; you try to get a "grip" on others, on your surroundings, sometimes clawing, but you feel lost, anxious, hurt, and insecure, for all that you are trying to get a grip; you would like to achieve and climb up ever further. "See how good I am." A high concentration of spirit, a strong fixation upon certain points, for instance upon study or career; in an authoritarian way, you'd like to compel others to give you attention. Possibly, you attach a lot of significance to your "exterior" in order to get others in your grip; you leave yourself standing, lonely, out in the cold. You feel painfully hurt, sometimes in panicky anxiety, but you resist this, taking it out on the outer world in anger, aggression — sometimes in resentment — as if the outer world is the cause of your not liking yourself!

You want more, more, more — further and higher — but you don't realize that you never will find a firm handhold in the outer world, that the world will never give you what you don't *give* to yourself. Your anxieties manifest themselves in aggression, revolt, and the urge to achieve, compulsively going on without end in order to "find" yourself; but you run away, further and further from the most beautiful aspects inside yourself.

Live from within now, NOT directed toward the outer world. Discover your sensitivity, your intuition: free yourself from this prison of HAVING TO, of stress, and of bustling in order to find yourself good, to feel powerful, and to confirm your value.

Now give yourself all the space and open your lungs wide. Enjoy the softness, the love in yourself; no longer reject yourself, and no longer try to satisfy the expectations of your "masculine ego" while at the same time destroying the "feminine aspect." You don't have to be angry with yourself: you are good just the way you are. Descend into your deepest Self and trust that warm soul inside yourself! Don't allow your life to be determined only by rational understanding and outer manifestation: acknowledge these talents, the gentle feelings in you; listen to music and let your heart thaw out; dare to enjoy — relax.

COPPER
Deficiency, insufficient assimilation of

Sensitive, fragile, helpless, flexible, small — but you resist all this! You clash, you are angry, you fight *against* people who want to help you in your "weakness"; you try hard to appear stronger than you inwardly feel, but this gets out of hand. You'd like to turn your back on your emotional world, but you are all the more strongly being confronted with it. You would like to take charge of your life *yourself*, but you don't succeed very well. . . . You look to someone else for help, but in fact you cannot at all tolerate this attachment! You feel stuck, and for the moment see no way out.

A clear view on yourself is beneficial; quietly get a perspective upon your situation via a balanced cooperation of intuition and reason. Experience very deeply your personal roots and plant your present existence in them; be aware of the true worth of your "I," don't remain stuck on outer show. Allow these powerful, creative energies to come through freely. Don't fight against, but build

your own Structure from the basis to the higher awareness. Establish yourself solidly upon your Basis.

CREUTZFELDT-JAKOB DISEASE

You aren't truly aware of your worth and possibilities AS A HUMAN BEING; possibly you perform your tasks because "that is the way it's supposed to be," or you perform it like a robot. But you don't ask yourself many questions about this. You remain stuck too much to the superficial, material reality, without making contact with your deepest essence. Do you live like a functionary, hooked up in a system? Then you will fulfill your role properly, but you seem not to truly LIVE. The look in your eyes shows us your Absence: Where are you, then? It seems as if you are cut off from your feelings, as if you only function via habits, routine or instinctive actions. Your friends can even get the impression that you don't really like to live, that you don't really take pleasure in life.

You let your level of consciousness drop to the primitive, to life's essentials, like that of an animal: because you don't at all believe in the lofty possibilities of yourself as a Human Being. A rich potential is not being used in creativity: you obstruct the genesis of your true "I"! You numb yourself, so to speak, so that you might appear apathetic, indifferent, or like a zombie. You don't really believe in yourself. . . . . You aren't really thankful for Life in yourself; you don't experience any joy in it. Is this possibly because you think that death is always lurking around the corner? You remain on the surface, on the outside of yourself, as it were. It seems as if you have no clue about true FEELING: feeling yourself in Life.

This is a matter of REJECTION; you close the doors. You withdraw to another, lower level, where you are left in peace, where you don't really have to live, where you no longer have to take responsibility for yourself. You are tired, and you close the curtains. By doing this you easily flee from life — this, however, will not bring you any further at all. You take away from yourself all chance for a (happy) existence! "I quit!" you say, doing great injustice to yourself in this way! You have never truly known life; you don't believe in true joy and happiness. Now you need to turn the Tide: if you give yourself every chance for a true existence and come to truly LIVING, then you will be surprised by the enormous possibilities that are present in you, by the pleasant experiences which will present themselves upon your path. But as long as you don't believe in yourself and ignore or degrade your own Worth, it is impossible of course for you to experience this.

You actually live behind a screen, behind a door, behind a newspaper, behind a book, behind a system, behind a job, behind a tasks, etc.; you don't come forward as "I," THE HUMAN BEING! You mistrust life and you hide your deeper Content — hiding it from yourself as well as from others. You keep yourself occupied with primary needs, but you refuse to engage yourself totally in life. You peer at life from behind a wall. You consider yourself to be well and safely protected behind this wall, but by doing this you take away from yourself all chance for a true life. You hide yourself; you are not honest with yourself. Instinctive mechanisms for safeguarding your earthly being can put such a damper on your life that there is nothing left but this "ducking away" from life. And you don't WANT to go deeper; you wish only to forget, wanting to not think things through, not truly coming out with your "I"; you would rather keep hidden, living in self-castration.

You don't truly come into contact with Life, nor with other people. You would even avoid contacts or flee, because people might hold a mirror up to you. You don't really trust things, and moreover you are afraid of being hurt: you therefore keep yourself safely "inside"; you keep others at a distance, especially when a "closer" contact presents itself. A problem of COMMUNICATION needs to be solved by this illness: if you — in trust, in Love —learn to communicate with yourself, with your "I," and no longer shut out a part of your being, then the anxieties will disappear and you will be able to establish true communication with others, and to experience pleasure from this.

As if your Skin and the Roots of your hair ache (Read the related subject, Skin; symbolism and Ailments, in general) as soon as you come in contact with the wind of Life; you try to escape. . . . On this route of escape your spiritual essence pulls back slowly out of your body until you are no longer here-and-now at all. At this point, you urgently need to call out "Halt!" and make a U-turn; return with your soul powers into your body and allow yourself to come to life! Life is a painful happening only for those who stubbornly hold on to the conviction that life is just a painful, worthless affair: so change this conviction in yourself. When you decide to lead a life in joy, without pain, when you are convinced that you, YOURSELF, are worthy to blossom, then Life will help you; then your Self will thankfully make use of all your brain-cells in order to make you sense the most beautiful experiences. Then your Brain will Blossom, according to human dignity! You know now that you are a Human-Being in Growth and that your spiritual essence directs your body, that your brain will RE-GENERATE until it can optimally fulfill its task and do so in a wholesome way. If, however, you degrade yourself to an animal or to an object, to a mechanically working-being, to a worthless object, then your brain sees no more reason to exist further or to function. You no longer give it any order, except that which says: "It has no use, let it be." You, yourself, put it to silence.

(Read "The Brain")

You now have to make a choice: you either let yourself be ABSORBED into something, into someone, into a system, a group, a religious society, a deity, a mass, a Task, an Energy — by which your own "I" DISAPPEARS in the mist (This means FLEEING from yourself, away from the earth). Or you choose to quit these fleeing-mechanisms and start a new Life: a voyage of discovery gradually leading to your SELF, in trust, whereby your spiritual energies again CONCENTRATE themselves more and more in your BODY, in your brain, so that you can feel better and better and will have ever more possibilities at your disposal. It is this Path which leads to Joy. If you no longer run away from yourself, then you will gradually find that you, YOURSELF, can guide your life in the direction you choose, without pain. As long as you maintain the conviction that a human being is doomed to live in pain and anxiety, then it is totally normal that you don't see the sense of it all and would rather sound the retreat. Still, life is put together totally differently than you think: YOU, as a CREATIVE HUMAN BEING, determine whether your life will be joyful or painful! Seize that opportunity! Come INTO YOURSELF again with ALL YOUR LIFE-FORCES. Stop DEGRADING yourself. Come into yourself, step into Life! No longer flee from that wonderful Content in yourself, but realize yourself as "I" — the CONSCIOUSLY LIVING HUMAN BEING. (Read Part I)

Probably you have rather considered the HUMAN BEING as something ugly, perhaps even as a Monster: break with this Lie and discover now that Divine Power, that which is most beautiful in you, in the Human Being. If you consider yourself a Good and Beautiful Human Being, then you will ultimately radiate this goodness and beauty. If, however, you experience yourself (and mankind in general) as something awful, as limited or animalistic, as a miserable soul, then you will begin to live according to this. The human being lives again and again according to this Self-image: so make something beautiful of it!

Raise yourself up to a higher level and take full responsibility for your existence as a true Human Being.

No longer keep yourself "ignorant"; no longer keep yourself tied to an instinctive pattern which limits you, in the lower-consciousness way of life, like an animal, like a programmed robot. . . . Discover your ORIGINALITY as a human being, your highly unique "I," and no longer follow the habitual patterns from the past! Now, shake yourself awake and put your brain to work: give it the Task to recover, to bring about regeneration in the tissue. Now, become aware of your masterful possibilities! Stop keeping yourself in a "state of sleep," and follow a totally New Course now: you will hereby come closer and closer to yourself and will place your powers in the service of love and goodness. Now, you give yourself, your brain, the chance to richly blossom. You fearlessly face life because you know that you, yourself, can create your life, your health, your happiness — as a WORTHY HUMAN BEING. You are now happy TO BE "I"; you no longer want to flee out of yourself. You come out of your hiding place and dare to take a good LOOK at yourself, at mankind, at life. You now look at life with new eyes; you now dare to take initiative and to bring about complete changes if necessary. You don't flee from problems, but you solve them through confrontation. You learn from this, you grow, on the way to more Humanity and inner warmth. You now live, motivated, having become Aware of your Worth and the Worth of Life. More and more, you feel your HEART: you now discover Self-love, and with this you offer Life to yourself.

CRUSHING OF A BODY PART

**(See also the category
for the body part concerned)**

You constantly flee, as it were, from yourself. You don't acknowledge the solid, inner "I"-force, nor the gentle, sensitive little one inside you. You hesitate, you experience your basis as unstable and unsafe; you'd prefer to launch yourself on a rocket, as if on a flight to greater heights. A nervousness, an unbelievable aggressive agitation inside you — but you keep running in place after all; energies bottle up. You'd like to get out of the situation you are in now; you don't want to "give" yourself, you offer resistance to evolution. Rather fleeing than changing.

In the outer world you strive, you work, you possibly make a super flight, but you run away from yourself. You overburden yourself with emotions, with doubts. Deep anxieties lie at the basis of this escape. You think you have to "protect" yourself, because you don't believe in the protective power of faith in your Self. You are afraid of the "weak," sensitive side of yourself; you'd prefer to identify yourself with Superman, but you don't even trust the chair you are sitting on.

Acknowledge the tough "I" force in yourself; surrender trustfully to your deepest, immortal Self. Anxieties are unnecessary; you yourself can create your life! Feel safe and protected; nothing "just" happens to you. Now, come very close to yourself and acknowledge that gentle, sensitive child inside you. Don't run away from it: your gentle side is no threat to you. Instead of running away from it, give in to that aspect in yourself which begs for attention and love. This can only happen when you become aware of a solid structure in yourself. Determine your borders in a self-aware way and push way

from you that which doesn't really belong to you. No flight, but a fearless "I"-manifestation, going onward self-assuredly, without hesitation. Determining, yourself, where your path lies. Being open to your deepest feelings. A homecoming, in peace, to yourself.

Also read, if necessary, "Crushed Finger," or "Crushed Toe."

EXAGGERATED TENDENCY TO CURSE

You are a barrel full of compressed energy, and you unconsciously seek release so the barrel will not burst. You feel stuck, and you feel an urge to let go of yourself without restraint, flying out of the cage in complete freedom.

You are looking for all possible ways to get out and express yourself, so much feeling as if you are locked up and powerless in yourself!

Your powerlessness and your distrust regarding yourself and your energies are the foundation of this. You are afraid of not having control over yourself, afraid that everything might overwhelm you — so you hold back, again and again withdrawing a little, not letting yourself *truly* come through, until at last the barrel bursts.

Most of all, you'd like to curse and throw yourself and also your concentrated, repressed powers away: and so you do, with a curse.

Dare to be yourself, in full activity: seek out your channels and don't hold back!

In an alchemical sense, transform primitive instincts and emotions into "awareness." Become aware of your emotions, of your self-deprecating thoughts, and of all convictions regarding yourself. Healthy aggression is not bad. It is even the motor for evolution;

your emotions are not a threat. Look at them and deal with them. Transformation of the primitive into channeled beams of energy, into true creativity on the basis of Self-trust. This also indicates the prime requirement: first, set your foundations very deeply into the Earth, feel your powerful Basis, no longer doubt the Security within your Self. Only then can these healthy, exuberant energies be fruitful.

life. You can lean on yourself in confidence and feel joyful about your existence. A beautiful future can only be created from an intense awareness of the here-and-now. Thus, live very strongly in the present; be master of yourself. Don't shut yourself off anymore! Transform powerless fury into creative, energetic action. Stop being angry any longer with your own powerlessness; soften yourself, appreciate yourself in love.

CUSHING'S SYNDROME
caused by overproduction of, or an exaggerated intake of, corticosteroids

You project many dreams, ideal expectations — outside yourself. You expect so much that your head is full to bursting with longing, with creative dreams. . . .

But you suffocate yourself in powerless fury! One disappointment follows another. You blame it on others; you don't see that your own feelings of insecurity, your lack of belief in yourself, make it impossible for you to realize even the slightest part of your dreams. You "expect" things from the future, from others, without realizing that your destructive, hard, negative convictions about yourself — the fact that you restrict your self-fulfillment — hinder beautiful things from coming to you. You become more and more displeased and angry over disappointments, about which you claim you can do nothing. A mass of radioactivity discharges itself in order to be managed by you and transformed into magnificent realizations. But you neglect these beautiful powers in yourself. This leads to self-destruction. You are so hard on yourself! You no longer know where your soft, gentle feelings are because, deep inside, you are angry with yourself, even though you don't realize it. Love for yourself is far gone.

Feel the solidity in yourself: allow all these powers to flow outward and construct your

CUTS
being struck by sharp objects

Anxious, nervous tension, self-destruction, frustration, anger: "I cannot be myself." You undermine yourself. Perhaps, with great conviction, you strive after ideals or ambitions; perhaps you stand up for your opinion, your career, in a pugnacious or fanatic way — too nervous, because you feel anxious and not safe, because you don't really live from out of your true feelings. You revolt in resistance to the feeling "I'm stuck, I cannot really be myself; my emotions, my powers, are suppressed; I'm dependent on others, on society —" You want to be free; you resist this feeling of "self-limitation." Unconsciously, the longing wells up to open the door of the cage and give the bird its freedom.

Still, you don't really go on; you doubt, not really feeling protected in yourself because you feel cut off from your deepest Essence. You look for a grip outside yourself instead of turning in upon yourself and achieving a thorough self-evaluation. It is not the outer world that counts, not the norms of others, but that which you feel!

You hurt yourself, or you call up situations in your life wherein others "thrust at you with daggers." This is because you unconsciously refuse to surrender to your true nature. You imprison yourself in a situation; you refuse to go on at full force, to live in harmony with your own nature. You limit yourself because you don't believe in the Power of your inner Self.

Anxieties, emotions, oppress you, and require you to break through. Healthy, aggressive powers are not really put to work to benefit the building-up of your life in a fruitful and multifaceted way. You are hard and sharp with yourself. You are frustrated because you cannot truly be yourself — this suppression of your "I" will give cause for collisions with others! You are convinced that others can hurt you; you are convinced that you cannot trust others, and thus you live anxiously and on guard. You mistrust because you don't really trust in your deepest Self! Perhaps you are angry with others, but in fact this is about your own powerlessness.

You are not a victim: become Master over your life! Dare to let your feelings and your powers circulate freely from your heart. Come to honest communication with your inner SELF and with others. Know yourself to be protected within yourself, and free yourself from this self-limitation: live in joy, in harmony with your emotional world, steadily going on and not allowing yourself to be pulled down by anxiety or by negative convictions regarding yourself. That lack of power to be yourself is a lie: free yourself and direct your being with certainty on the path you have chosen — a path which links with your true inner nature. Don't fight against things or people, but build up! Don't be angry with others: they are not the cause of your feeling so oppressed. Resolve that emotional tension within yourself by believing in your possibilities, by realizing yourself, without frustration. Don't try to "achieve"; don't strive after an ideal "outside" yourself; don't fight for a tinsel trophy. Discover that splendid diamond in your heart and live in love for yourself. Give yourself all the space — gentling, trusting, going on (Mars); inner peace.

CYSTS

Your thoughts remain fixated on certain experiences. Not only problems of Now, but sad remembrances of the past keep you in their grip.

You cling to certain experiences that can be permeated with feelings of pain, vengeance, regret or hate, so that they begin, as it were, to dominate your life: they stick to you as a ball, a cyst, full of negativity. The true cause of this holding-on lies in your feelings of powerlessness, anxiety, self-doubt, the ignoring of your own solid Basic structure. You have made your life too dependent on others. You are not truly evolving from out of yourself! Because you have allowed yourself to be "drained" too much, instead of building up your life in a very personal, active way; because you have lived like a "victim" without building up your existence in a creative way; because you have put the Power over your life in the hands of others or of the outer world: therefore, by this negative, empty attitude to life, you have attracted situations in which you were hurt, as a victim, by which one "invaded" you psychologically, in a painful way. You were hurt in your most intimate feelings, and you considered yourself the victim of circumstances, not able to do anything about it. Unable. This feeling of inability has attracted sad circumstances toward you. "No one has any say over me," is how you sometimes close yourself off, as a reaction.

Your energies, your feelings — turn themselves inward; you draw in instead of radiating outward. You bottle up, you cannot let go or forget.

Dare to express yourself now, dare to cry, dare to say what you have to say; no longer live the Hard way, bottled up.

Let go of everything, leave the past behind, turn your mind to the here-and-now.

Let go of all feelings, like a balloon that loses its gas; in this way your cyst can disappear: sadness, aggression, pain, etc. — let go of everything. Come to Insight: know that no matter what has happened to you in life or how painful it might have been, this was called up unconsciously by you yourself.

Go ONWARD now like a locomotive; use these bottled-up energies in actively building up your life, in positive creativity. Allow all the sad thoughts to slide from you, and turn toward the wisdom in yourself. Be your own Leader in an autonomous way and dare to live from out of your specific longings, in Love.

Discover that solid Essence in yourself, know yourself to be safe and protected herein; come to rest and balance, and allow yourself to enjoy. When you acknowledge love and power in yourself, when you put trust in your deepest Self, then you can calmly let go of everything and everyone. . . . (Also read Anxiety and Part I.)

CYSTIC FIBROSIS

Aggression, callousness, as an inner resistance against one's own feelings of powerlessness.

You see everything as being dark, senseless — you have no real goals.

You sit and wait; you might even fall asleep, bored and Absent.

"Where are you?" You feel like a victim, a poor soul — you don't at all experience your Worth. What is mainly missing in you is the solid Structure, a strong Basis in yourself. You don't experience yourself as a unified being; you let yourself droop, with the feeling that you are inferior to others, that you are only there to sacrifice yourself or to do an unpleasant task. . . .

In this way, you do everything except depend upon your deepest Self, your basic structure.

You feel estranged and cut off from your nature: at a distance from yourself. In this way, you can't experience any Joy, since every joy begins with self-contentment and experiencing happiness with Life itself.

But you feel so oppressed, so imprisoned, because your nature isn't allowed to exist, because you experience life as sad, because you suppress emotions and powerful energies! These energies of emotion and creativity suffocate you. You load up your wheelbarrow without ever unloading it. Because it all has no purpose anyway — or so you think, because you don't make any contact with your heart, with your gentle, deep core.

There seem to be thick walls between you and your own physical nature, between you and your own natural feelings. And because you live in this inner rift, you can't really come in contact with the gentle core of others either. This leads to feelings of powerless anger, to hard phlegm.

Inner collision, an inner battle in thoughts and emotions; you want to go here, and then there — you don't know. Powerlessness, and because of this, unused energies pile up, and there's no question of true evolution or progress. These pent-up potential powers suffocate you. A standing still.

You'd rather wait passively than believe in an active process. Anxiety about going on? You feel pain, deep sadness, powerlessness, anxiety — you can't see through it; it all seems desperately black to you. You don't realize how precisely these negative expectations of life are the true cause of your ailment.

Your solution lies in liberation through deepening and softening.

Deepening: turn into your deepest Self, your fundamentally strong Basis. Make contact with your worthy inner core, discover yourself, and very strongly build your own structure. Don't depend on the philo-

sophical frameworks of others; discover your inner Wisdom, your intuition, your rich emotional life. Your life won't offer you any satisfaction or joy as long as you don't dare to live from out of your longings, from out of your spontaneous wishes or impulsive inspirations — look deeper at life and stretch it open into a very large space.

Be gentle and sweet, very close to yourself. Acknowledge those gentle, female feelings very deep inside you. No longer suffocate yourself with anxieties and anger, with revolt and battle. Arrive at unity, at peace in yourself; stop this fighting and surrender to the gentleness in your heart.

If you have positive expectations regarding your life, then you will attract beautiful experiences. If you doom yourself with pessimistic expectations, then you will attract a suffocating illness.

You're not pitiable; you're not a poor soul — but you are a worthy human being with many potentialities! Do you allow these life energies to flow freely? Then you free yourself. Do you acknowledge your rich emotional content? Do you love your body? Do you enjoy with your senses? Do you breathe life in with grateful breaths? And do you now OPEN yourself to a total change, to healing, to your liberation? Then, every cell in your body will react to this positive openness and will allow healing energies to go through. Healing energies that will get rid of superfluity, energies that will hinder new, exaggerated production of mucus — powerful magnetic streams which will be directed very simply by your Consciousness. Open yourself up to YOURSELF, in loving gentleness; offer trust to your deepest Self. This illness has served its purpose: it has opened your eyes and given you the chance to go in another, happy, meaningful direction.

D

VITAMIN D
Deficiency, insufficient assimilation of

Fear of truly living. The feeling that you cannot *really* come through; you experience pressure from others, from a structure which has been put upon you. Unconsciously, you are afraid they will beat you down again if you would begin to live for yourself. Therefore, you don't dare open your mouth to voice your true opinion. You feel small and naked, at the mercy of evil in general and of the negativity of others.

Break through; manifest yourself, conquer all obstacles, clear a path for yourself! Believe in the good; no longer pay any attention to the negative. You don't have to fight; simply allow all your powers to come through. Be convinced of the natural production of healthy building materials in your body, if you simply allow this growth.... Don't hinder the working of these powers by underestimating yourself or by anxieties.

DEATH
(Also read Part I)

Apparent death

Inner conflict: shall I keep on living? Yes or no? You don't see a way out any more; deep anxieties prevent your continuation in life.

You feel stuck, with a padlock on your mouth, as if you have no say over your life. Your head has for quite a while been "muddled," full of thoughts and considerations. On the one hand emotional suppression, on the other hand clutching onto structures and "thinking," in an exaggerated way. With squealing brakes you have come to a halt on your life-course, anxious and shocked; you did not see any sense in it any more.

Also, fear of pain; you cling to a false posture; you don't really want to die, but underneath you the swirling river of life threatens and you don't really dare to go back.

You have escaped into exaggerated "spiritual" brain-activity: the spiritual no longer concentrates in the body, although your deepest Self keeps directing your body.

Body and "spirit" are not truly united. You were filled to the brim with negative thoughts; instead of really confirming your "I" and going ahead on your path, you flee into another dimension; you cannot or dare not manifest yourself as a Human-Being. You live too rigidly within a structure: there was no room for your feelings, your intuition; you are afraid of them! Insufficient awareness of your deep Worthiness; not feeling safe, cut off from your inner Self. An escape out of the body, into the spirit.

No matter what circumstance has brought you into this situation, you unconsciously (or consciously) called this up in order to make yourself contemplate death and life. What is Life? Time for transformation: discover your warm Heart, feel safe in your deepest Self; death is the going into another dimension, but your Self keeps on existing and growing forever. Did you perhaps pay too little attention to your intuition, because of fear of death? Then you now may enlarge your space. Discover the possibilities, the creative powers of your Self in earthly life. If you wish to live, you will live; if you wish to die, you will die. How you wish to live — this you determine yourself! Know that you have your destiny in hand, that no one else decides this. Negative expectations about the future lead to negative experiences: become aware of this and adjust these expectations! You are far mightier than you think: take your life in hand and don't lock yourself up in a suffocating structure — open yourself up to beautiful feelings and trust your intuition. Don't limit yourself to the rational, nor to the material nor to the "spirit." Discover earthly joy!

The foregoing is also useful for the close relations of the patient: changes of consciousness in the relations are unconsciously perceived by the patient, so that it is possible to influence the patient in this way. A strong life-concentration of Consciousness in the body, a strong awareness of worthiness, a feeling of safety, standing solidly with both feet on the ground, an harmonious cooperation of feeling and reason, a loving expulsion of all anxieties: these are conditions for being able to appreciate the new life. . . .

Build your Paradise here on Earth, not in vague spiritual spheres.

Don't flee from the Truth, from Actual Life.

Crib death

Mother has (unconscious) feelings of guilt, self-condemnation, and unconsciously she wants to punish herself. Possibly, she was burdened by a feeling of inferiority, again and again having to live according to norms that others preached, sometimes under a dominant authority — still, she doesn't give herself room to exist. Nervous aggression

and dissatisfaction with oneself. Anger toward oneself.

"I'm not good enough."

She kicks herself, as it were, kicks her own "I": self-destruction or killing oneself. She constantly pierces her own heart with a dagger, calling up, as a result, even more heartache with the death of the baby.

The baby experiences life as a burdensome pressure and chooses instead to break the umbilical cord with the mother in order to return later, if desired, to physical life.

Mothers, be aware of your self-worth, achieve an unfolding of yourself and dig for your aggression: pull that nail out and look well from whence it comes. First of all, give yourself the love you deserve and stop breaking yourself down.

Death, as such, does not exist: don't mourn, but understand this message in the right way. You are actually allowed at last to live for yourself in complete self-acceptance. It is now time for you to completely acknowledge yourself; don't first of all expect this of others. Don't look to the past, which was a reflection of your inner convictions about yourself. Be convinced, now, that you are good, and that you can be there one hundred percent because of *yourself*. No feelings of guilt! Every being chooses (unconsciously) his moment of departure. But "why" you unconsciously attract such a happening — that's important to consider, in order for you to make a big step forward in life.

For you, this happening was a result of an unconscious life of self-negation: no guilt, but the consequence of causes, in the mother as well as in the child, of which you were not conscious. Time for psychological transformation — become aware of your unique, worthy "I"!

Near-death experiences
(See also Coma)

On the one hand, one refuses to transform, one offers resistance to true life-evolution (which means that one lets go of things or people which are no longer really good in one's life, and that one no longer offers opposition to a new direction which must be taken for one's own good).

Rather die than change or let go.

Life is experienced as a pressure that is too great or as too great a task; one chooses self-destruction. One is in an emotional knot; one can no longer keep things in perspective. On the other hand, one still wants to stay here. One does not really want to die.

Still, there is a questioning: "Will I stay or not?" Via all sorts of experiences that are called up, and after this pondering and weighing, one wishes to come to an answer; finally, one chooses death or life.

The unconscious longing for taking a look across the border of life; the fear of death; a firm belief, as it were, in the Fates, which weave your life and Destiny into a network, and you cannot change anything about it. . . . But emotionally you are still being drawn to life.

After such an experience, one will often begin to take up the space which one previously did not realize one needed: beginning to fly with one's own wings, and standing on the Earth in a more conscious way and in greater wisdom.

Stillborn child, full-grown

Here, feelings of guilt are totally superfluous: it is a choice of the child and an unconscious evocation of the mother. At this moment, it is the best solution for both.

Mother hasn't yet found herself. She still lives encapsulated, her feelings are being restrained, held back; pain and sadness are being pushed away. She does not really know what she means to herself; she is anxious, fleeing from herself. First, it is necessary she find herself, in all trust, and then there will be space for a child. She experiences an emptiness in herself; she draws in everything from her surroundings to fill up her emptiness. There is no solid direction, but rather

blindly pushing through in life, no well-determined goal for the mother, herself.

An empty little heart that wants to fill itself up with a baby — this of course is not possible.

First, mother will have to learn to discover her own self-aware sun-center and learn to unfold the love for herself, discovering the large range of possibilities in herself, no longer closing ears and eyes to her own deep emotions, no longer fleeing, but Confronting herself with herself! First of all, resolve all anxieties.

The child has its own reasons for going back for a while to the other dimension before incarnating; mostly, it feels smothered in the "custom-made" design in which it has to live here, like a captive in a net, and it chooses to take flight.

DEHYDRATION OF THE BODY

You are slowly taking life away from yourself, because it can't go on like this.

You allow yourself to be dragged along into the depths, into death. You have so many emotional pains.

You withdraw from life. You, yourself, are barely living; you place all authority outside yourself. You see no way out; you feel weak and limp; you don't succeed in standing at the rudder of your ship; you let yourself droop, you let go of all hold on yourself; energies flow away without a goal. Pain, the feeling of being hopelessly stuck. Dematerialization, spiritualization. No more faith in your own creative power. You place yourself next to the earth, at a distance.

Self-awareness! Active participation in life! Creativity of the spirit. Your expectations from life determine reality — the circumstances which will appear in your life — even if this seems impossible to you now. Allow life-energies to come in; let your Conscious spirit feed your body.

Don't reject your feelings, don't extinguish your life-fire, because you need both (water and fire) to be able to live towards a new perspective.

When a whole population suffers from massive dehydration, it is necessary that it achieve awareness-growth as a group, on a world-wide scale. (Read Part I.)

DEMENTIA — ALZHEIMER'S DISEASE

One runs away from Life; in this way, one no longer has to take responsibilities anymore; in this way, one can throw off certain burdens without the need for death. Yes, often it's the fear of death that also calls up this in-between stage.

An escape from reality; the anchor is being thrown into another world: demented persons no longer wish to experience themselves in totality, here and now, on earth. For the most part they already live in a world that has gone beyond the borders of our three-dimensional existence.

Out of anxious self-protection, they close themselves off behind an impenetrable fog; they fear that if they would come out of their box then the lid might fall on their heads — so they stay where they are. These are unconscious processes.

They no longer wish to participate — they no longer feel at home here — possibly, they consider the physical and the earthly to be just a useless burden, inferior to the "heaven above." Anxieties. All these are possible inner motives. Anxiety, fleeing from a confrontation with one's own deepest source of feelings.

One has tried desperately in one's life to find the might and the power in oneself, but one has found this only outside oneself; one has not succeeded in coming into contact with one's deepest, divine essence, nor has one discovered the value of the creative possibilities of Self-awareness. One has lived unconsciously rather than consciously, resulting of course in anxieties raising their heads: dementia is only one step further on.

As a reaction against one's own powerlessness, one has possibly tried to dominate others or to dictate to them, possibly putting up a tough outer appearance, a camouflage. An intense effort to get a "grip" on something: "I know! I don't listen to anyone — I will say it, and if that is not possible then I will close myself off!" Dementia. In this way, one still gets attention and the care of others without being confronted any longer with one's own powerlessness. It is the only possible way to still be able to "manipulate" the situation around you. Sudden aggressive discharges can occur as a consequence of this passive self-suppression: feelings of powerlessness.

The cheerful, childlike aspect that is always present in every human being is often suppressed behind a mask that is too stiff, too hard: thinking too narrowly. An unconscious longing to experience this candid cheerfulness again calls up dementia, second childhood. (See also Senility)

A primarily preventive approach is necessary. Don't close yourself off from life, from society, or from Nature. Feel at home and know yourself to be safely integrated into the life process: life does not "just happen to you": you are the master, and you need to resolutely take the rudder in hand and steer in the direction you wish. Dare to acknowledge the earthly, tenderness, the body, and to share love. Don't withdraw into barren isolation, but participate in activities, in the joy of life itself. Take up your task! Lead your energies to productivity! Don't force things, but quietly come into yourself; acknowledge your feelings in a balanced relationship with your rational abilities. Don't push away the child in yourself, but integrate these simple, beautiful feelings in your life. Experience yourself creatively, in spontaneous joy. This intensely being present in life is completely opposite to the escape that dementia is.

GENERAL DEMINERALIZATION
(See also Deficiency of fluoride, calcium, etc.)

Anxiety paralyzes energetic production.

Being emotionally stuck; your emotions direct your life. You don't know how to get a grip on your emotional world, on your life. You are afraid that at any moment something bad can happen to you. You feel seized by the throat, as it were.

Afraid of death.

Negative thoughts and gloomy convictions drain you dry; your powers flow away. Suppression of a normal, healthy stream of joy and of your creativity leads to ever-greater anxieties and insecurity: at any moment this time bomb, this tangible self-negation, can explode. In the worst case, it at last becomes extreme fear of yourself! Cramped tension; at the ready in a defensive posture — stress, mistrust, cold.

Light the flame of life: come to love inside yourself. Warmth.

No longer ignore that which is beautiful in yourself, in life. You mistrust erroneously.

Don't feel so threatened: no one can harm you if you don't call it down upon yourself. Quietly open yourself to the outside; relax. . . .

Labor, healthy activity, fire, fruitfulness, creativity! Acknowledge your productivity: once the vicious circle begins to turn in the opposite direction because of your belief in your own powers, then your batteries automatically will charge themselves because of the energetic, joyful stream of life.

No longer keep yourself stressfully tense; flexibly bend, work out your emotions without anxieties. Opt for life: give your trust, and life will reward you. If you allow yourself to be led by anxieties, then you will attract negative experiences. Take up your royal scepter and become master of your Life.

DEPRESSION

Anxiety and depression are indications that you have to bring about a change in *your* life: you pull and drag in order to get something into motion; you desperately try to realize a certain something, to make a certain path or ambition come true or to push through a certain change in others — your partner or someone at work. And again and again you don't succeed.

It is of no avail; it's not working. In this way, you hurt yourself: you constantly try to force something — doing so against the natural flow — because you WANT it to be just so. But you are in fact blind! That which you so absolutely want is perhaps not at all good for you: your deepest convictions hinder everything from going along smoothly. Your path probably lies somewhere else completely; time to let go and broaden your philosophy of life! (Read about this in Part I.)

This period is meant to bring you in contact with your deepest Self in order to deal with anxieties and death, to surrender to your Living Self, and to learn how to interpret signals that come to you from your surroundings. Nothing "just" happens; life is put together so beautifully; find trust in yourself, come to action in the direction which your deepest Self shows you by sending you signals along your path.

Everything in the past has had its meaning; regret, guilt, and anger will resolve themselves when you come to a broad understanding of life itself.

Life is not a fatalistic fact, but it also is not a matter of forcing things. Let go of everything and call up the solution in yourself: it will present itself as an answer to the question that has been posed. Trust; no longer stubbornly resist the true direction of life. Open yourself up: that which is good for you (and which will at last bring you to happiness) is difficult to evaluate in a rational way beforehand. Therefore, follow the signals of your body, of your environment, but especially follow the signals which your deepest Self constantly sends you. Then follow, in a self-aware way, your path.

Do you feel so empty and lonely in the midst of the masses? Does life bore you, and are you thinking of suicide? Do you not achieve true communication with others? It is you who doesn't seek contact with your deepest Self, but who flees out of yourself while the solution lies in you. Turn deeply inward and seek that immortal Essence. Give up your resistance to Life, and then you will be able to experience joy in the simple circulation of it. If you come into closer contact with this Living Self, then joyful contacts with others will result from it.

perience your Fullness; you feel empty, lonely, incomplete "In Yourself". Possibly, you are even unconsciously angry with the baby because he or she doesn't solve your problem. You refuse to take your life in your own hands in a self-aware way because you don't really believe in yourself. It seems as if you have no perspective, because you don't live from out of the awareness of your valuable, creative power-source. You are not yet master over your life: your thoughts are self-destructive because you don't open yourself up to your deepest, divine Self, to your intuitive channels. Possibly, you are still following limitative thinking patterns and ancient prejudices. In this way your "head" is being kept in a tight grip, and as a result hormonal reactions appear in your body, urging you to choose a new path: after all, anxieties and depression indicate that you are following a direction and a thinking pattern which are contradictory to Life and to your well-being. Does it all tend to crush you? Are you afraid to be walked all over? Find the path to yourself, free yourself, *allow your Self to be born;* life is much lighter than you see it now. Discover the Joy FOR YOURSELF: go and search for it!

See also the categories Depression and Anxieties, and Part I.

DEPRESSION, POSTNATAL

The baby in your belly has temporarily filled up your "psychological emptiness"; at birth you need to say good bye to that which partly had become "you". You thought possibly this little one was going to fill up your emptiness, but of course this is not possible. Now, again, you are totally confronted with yourself and with your fundamental problem with which you had already struggled before your pregnancy. You did not and don't ex-

DIABETES
problems with the blood sugar level

Diabetes, in general
hyperglycemia;
blood sugar level is too high
(See also Hypoglycemia)

Your sadness is getting out of hand; you cannot "grasp" hold of happiness. An inner pining for warmth, love. You might "grab" for it.

Experiencing oneself as being too small and powerless, and wanting to reverse this by being taken up in the "sweetness" outside oneself, in an energy-stream of warmth from others. But of course this need can never be satisfied if one considers oneself worthless and denies oneself love, denies oneself "sweetness."

You are lacking in courage; experiencing yourself as helpless: this tends toward irritability and aggression because others don't give you what you need. With an inner, fearful, aggressive feeling, you try to grasp everything, to arrange, to organize. The convictions upon which you have built your life give you the feeling that life is a pool of sorrow and that nothing beautiful is reserved for you, and that if you don't really grasp it or draw it toward you, then life will offer you nothing at all.... Thus, you have absolutely no faith in life. You don't realize that all sadness and sorrowful situations in your life have been caused — yes, called up — by your negative convictions. To be sure of "having" a little love, you clutch — to a partner, for instance — and often hurt yourself by sacrificing yourself in exchange for having a little hand-hold in life. In this way, your life becomes a prison.

You are making your happiness dependent on a partner, on others — not on your Self. This is exactly where you make your mistake: happiness *can only* begin with *you*; arrive at love in harmony with yourself, and only *then* will a delightful relationship follow.

You don't live upon your own foundations. There might be a land mine underneath.... Distrust of yourself.

In love, come to yourself. Let go of everything and everyone, and trustfully allow everything to quietly follow its course: stop anxiously wanting to organize everything and trying to get everything in your grip. This simply indicates your fear of creating your life yourself: building a beautiful future

*presided over by your Conscious "I". Life is beautifully put together; love will flow toward you when you let go of everything and place your faith in your deepest Self. Don't, as you have in the past, "let yourself be lived"; don't clutch: it will only bring you more sorrow. Don't allow your life to be directed by emotions and disbelief, because in this way you call up misery. Be convinced of a new beginning, of a joyful future, and of the fact that you deserve it — you, as a worthy, autonomous individual! Only in this way will you see that life **is** worth living. Now allow yourself to enjoy all that which is delightful in life! Sadness disappears when you acknowledge **yourself**, love **yourself**.*
(See further, Part I)

Hypoglycemia
blood sugar level is too low

You refuse (still) to live from out of your powerful self-conscious "I": you allow yourself to drift away with the stream of your emotions, presenting yourself like a small child: you ignore your inner wisdom; your own WILL disappears. You give the impression that you are weaker than you are in order to be able to wallow in misery like a victim — sometimes like a "zombie" or an "underdog" at the feet of a Powerful person, who has command over you: this is a possibly unconscious but dishonest game. But anything is better than having to handle your own strong powers with mastery, because you are afraid of that. You mistrust your own nature. Outwardly exhibiting yourself in an almost untruthful way leads to a sense of guilt and to the feeling that somewhere you are "bad." Nor do you want to you trust others any more. You allow yourself to remain in the grip of others — pent-up aggression makes you nervous. At last you feel totally constricted; you want loose! Peering out from your hiding place, you don't dare, however, to take charge yourself; you look upon life in a one-sided, emotional manner, and you submerge yourself in a pool of black ink, as it were, not allowing your self-Awareness to be.

Difficult as it might seem, escape from this trap, which you have laid for yourself! Come out from under others and, in all honesty, dart ahead! Make people understand that from now on you will live for yourself and not as a servant for them. Be productive! Learn how to laugh again instead of cherishing tears. Work, constant activity, creativity, will do you good. Don't consider yourself a poor lamb, because your body will react to this: if you do, you deny and cast away your powers as a human being. Let your song of life resound in a key of self-awareness, in trumpet sounds that shake you awake out a false sleep. Change your detrimental convictions, which have pulled the wool over your eyes.

Infant, children's diabetes

Fear of your own self-development, fear of BEING. Almost preferring not to be. On the one hand, you brace yourself in order to be able to manage life; on the other hand, you would like to withdraw. An extremely fine sensitivity, which is open for the slightest impulse from the outside world. This world is being experienced as too oppressive; you arrive in an environment wherein many things are pushing themselves upon you. You find yourself unable to handle it. You cannot get the least grip on it. . . .

Vague fears of "devils," as it were, that are getting a hold of you: a result of your own feeling of darkness, insecurity. You don't solve this by clinging to things or people.

The psychological interaction between baby and parents is mostly very strong: it would be good for the parents to read the text under the heading Diabetes (adults).

Sometimes, one of the parents assumes the role of substitute for the "I" of the child: ease children gradually, securely, onto their own small feet and make them aware of how

strong and trustworthy is this "I"! Autonomous power and self-appreciation, love for oneself.

Teach them to trust nature: in a playful way allow them to become acquainted with the physical, the body (with a small dog?). Trust that radiates from the people who raise the child counts as a good medicine!

Love, affection, awareness of self-worth. There is no "devil"; it is only the projection of their anxieties. The well of sadness in which one finds oneself is no well! Land with both feet on the earth and live in the here-and-now, not in the imagination and thoughts. Spontaneous play, joyfulness. . . . Life is "sweet" and "safe." Love chases away fear. Believe in your fundamentally strong basis, your inner Essence, the angel deep inside you; let go . . . and create your life yourself. Allow your heart to radiate!

Diabetes of pregnancy
(See also Diabetes, in general, and Pancreas)

You are really still pregnant with yourself and there's the little one already. You feel still dependent and small, rather inferior and withdrawn, perhaps shy. Possibly you put on a big front, with a strong feeling of responsibility, and you do try to embrace it all; but inwardly you feel anxious, also about that what has yet to come. It seems sometimes as if that little one threatens you, as if he'd climb on you and take your place. You feel threatened, because you don't yet dare to completely take up your worthy space Now. You don't really dare to allow your consciousness powers to flow through: you slow yourself down. You feel like a dolt, clumsy; you don't really dare to show your true nature, your feelings. Possibly you were already ashamed about your stoutness (See Part I, Cult of External Appearance) and now you get more weight added onto it; now you don't feel at all accepted by the outer world anymore, because you make yourself subordinate to others. You, yourself, are still somewhat a baby; you don't live on your own firm foundations. On the contrary: you doubt your Self. You feel languid, slow or lazy; you constantly run yourself down. Sometimes you are so sad about yourself.

Sometimes you just feel like a silly donkey. Your natural spontaneity and your feelings aren't "unfolded" enough outwardly. You long for love and approval from the outside instead of offering love to yourself. Anxiety about it all becoming too much for you.

Allow the flower you are to blossom and discover your own beauty.

Independence, autonomy, pride, humor about your possible temporary clumsiness or listlessness; trust in your powers. You are good the way you are at any moment in your life, stout or thin, also when you are not pregnant. Don't pull yourself down; you will only feel threatened by someone new, as long as you refuse to take your life in hands in a Self-Aware way, as long as you don't trust in that immortal Basis in yourself. It is time you offer yourself the love you need; don't expect from someone else that which you don't give yourself. Anxieties are unnecessary; trust in yourself leads to a positive life-course.

Nothing just happens by accident; now take the reins yourself, no longer hiding yourself. You are allowed to be who you are, without even for a moment caring for what others say about you. Become aware of your unique being, of your specific possibilities, of your worth as a human being, of the possibility to create your life yourself.

DIPHTHERIA

You feel so small and insignificant; you experience mortal fears — you are afraid of totally disappearing, of drowning in your sadness, in your deep, dark feelings.

You experience yourself as ridiculous, ludicrous: "look at him there in the mirror"; self-destruction; you don't give yourself a chance in life! Were you perhaps treated like this by certain people? Then it was simply a reflection of your own deepest convictions regarding yourself.

It can also have to do with discontentment with your outer appearance: you vomit because of yourself and you would like to run away from your own body. In the deepest sense, it has to do with not loving yourself, with not accepting yourself the way you are.

Inner division; powerless to seize the wheel, you allow yourself to "be lived," to be ruled by others, not daring to be straightforward and say what it's all about or in what way someone treats you unjustly, according to you.

In a paranoid way, you constantly feel threatened by others, by death.

You are constantly fleeing from life itself, full of inner anxieties.

This leads to self-suffocation.

Be aware of your own majesty as a Human-Being. Straighten yourself up and resolutely dare to live, to speak, to act. Don't hesitate; become master over your Life: in all creativity build it up according to your longings. It is just waiting for your acknowledgment. In love, call up your self-healing energies so that all anxieties disappear.

FEAR OF DIRT

Obsessive ideas of contamination (e.g. becoming infected by shaking hands, by patting a dog, etc.), followed by, e.g., washing one's hands incessantly

Anxiety; you can't comprehend life. You mistrust your nature, yourself, your body.

You don't live on earth as it were, but far above it. You take distance from that which is earthly. This obsession often occurs with people who have a dislike — who are too critical — regarding their body and the sensual. Women with this problem often don't like to experience themselves in a "earthly female" body: a projection of the fact that they turn away from the "female" aspect in themselves, from their emotions, from what they feel, from receptivity. In this case, they experience themselves as "being powerless to be a woman"; inner aggressive powers are being suppressed. One doesn't believe in the good, in the light, in the joy of the inner self; one considers oneself and one's body as a "dirty" earthworm.

You should allow your "I" powerful self-development, but you say "No" to that which is most beautiful in yourself; you don't believe in the beauty of nature. You don't build your life on inner wisdom because you don't trust in your inner self, in your intuition. Because of this, you quickly feel anxious and threatened. You make a mountain out of a molehill; you see a devil in your nature. You are afraid of "contamination" outside yourself because you consider yourself and human nature as devilish and "contaminated." You'd sooner experience yourself as devilish than as divine. You are on the alert; you are on guard, ready to take flight, as if the Earth is a taint by itself. Your nature lies asleep, almost dead, because you don't really *live* from out of yourself, from out of your nature. You direct your attention and your prayers to something or someone outside yourself, to bookish knowledge or a religious system — because you undervalue your Self and your wisdom. You are afraid of being in the grip of your own emotions. You run away from yourself. You compensate for this by "grasping" at others.

In the meantime, you are stuck in piled-up emotions from the past, too afraid to really work them out. You stab yourself with a dagger; you frightenedly suppress your feelings. You don't dare to really live. You think you have to wash out the evil inside you. You lie with bound feet; you can't evolve because you are so desperately convinced of your powerlessness, of your inability to manifest your "I" in a powerful and self-assured way without having to be afraid of your inner powers, of your nature, of your feelings, of evil.

You live too much in your head, at a loveless distance from your earthly being; you allow your life to be led by false gods or idols because you refuse to take in hand mastery over your life in a Self-aware way. You mistrust your surroundings, life; you try to hide behind something or someone else.

You don't dare to risk an open confrontation, not with yourself nor your surroundings.

Merging of the "male" and the "female" aspects in yourself (See also Left and Right Body Halves). Self-assuredly work your way through nature; joy and trust in your natural earthly being. Sex is allowed, but isn't needed; no reason, however, to condemn your body or earthly enjoyment. Allow yourself to enjoy, to experience joy, to let your feelings flow freely, to use your inner powers in spontaneous creativity. Don't block up your emotions; no longer frustrate yourself. Become your own master and don't hide under an Authority or behind a book or a job. Trustfully surrender to your nature. No imaginings, no paranoia, but be realistic, with your feet on the earth. Dare to experience your body; feel those strong, concentrated, awareness-energies in your body. You are safe in your Self; natural powers don't form a threat. You are naturally immune (See also Part I).

Build your life on that fundamentally strong basis of your living Self. Listen to intuition, to inner wisdom. Be faithful to your nature, to your feelings; don't hide your powers and your feelings; self-manifestation and self-liberation!

DOWN'S SYNDROME
(See also Congenital physical defects)

Why is one born a "Mongoloid"? In this way, you can exist spontaneously, uninhibitedly, cheerfully, unhindered by formal but oppressive human norms, with a free passage for emotions that well up. Those who unconsciously build such an existence are mostly born into an environment with precisely *those* parents who (unconsciously) are convinced that they would better completely open themselves up in this life to things they possibly have neglected or underestimated too much: their *spontaneous,* natural emotions.

In order to become a "complete" human being there are many people who could take an example from a mongoloid. The genuine, loving, sensitivity; the spontaneously natural; the untroubled cheerfulness; the free sense of humor. All life-essential characteristics which are being murdered in our society.

The Consciousness directs the genes: the birth of a mongoloid is not by chance. In addition to this unconscious longing to experience the world as a true child, to learn how to deal with "emotions" — and this counts for the child as well as for the parents — there are yet other reasons why this genetic code is (unconsciously) chosen.

Another unconscious reason is Anxiety: as a mongoloid, one lives "hidden" and happy. One is afraid of living "completely" consciously here on earth, for consciousness means also "daring to take responsibility oneself, daring to consciously build up a life and to lean on your Self." Anxiety and unsureness — you'd like to, but you don't dare to — can attract a situation in which one is allowed to simply enjoy oneself without having any anxiety: being a clown, rather unconsciously. In this way, someone else "takes care" of them and thinks for them. Possibly, one then prefers to "stick" to others, in attachment, rather than growing toward autonomy.

It's therefore of utmost importance that they can safely experience the love, the feelings, and the affection they long for. In this way their unconscious, anxious, negative convictions regarding life on earth can be changed via comforting contact with earthly experi-ences! Thus, they won't have to return in *this* way. Evolution is possible for these people by the (unconscious) altering of convictions. They will also have to learn, via experiences, that "being nice" doesn't mean "Love."

Powerlessness grows because of the fear of truly "coming through," or of "being" in this world. The conviction that "one is not able" to climb to a higher Consciousness; one would actually like to come out of the little hole but doesn't dare. . . . Nevertheless, there are many powerful energies that urge and ask for evolution. But one can't get hold of them. On the other hand, other than feelings of mindless joy, this feeling of "powerlessness" can raise its head in the form of aggression.

In order to alter these negative convictions, it is very good that one allow the child to discover Love of self and its Worth in contact with ordinary, sensorial, earthly things: their playful and original attributes will help them with this. Enjoying the earthly, a strong "awareness of the body," the integration of this body into the total self, pleasant communication with others in true friendship — these are of great importance. A feeling of security, of joy, of light relaxed atmospheres, an intense life, here-and-now. Spontaneously supplementing that which in our world is being so strongly suppressed.

DWARFISM
(See also Growth hormone, insufficient production)

You have been born into this life with a built-in mistrust, a fear of the world and humanity. You don't know what people mean to you, nor what you mean to yourself: you don't dare to let your feelings, your emotions, flow freely. In order to get somewhat of a grip on yourself, you psychologically lock yourself up in a structure that is too tight; you are too tense; you confine your total personality within repressive walls. Because of doubts with regard to yourself, your sun cannot freely radiate. Too tightly wound, too structured, too controlled. . . .

Your body tells you that the above-mentioned oppressiveness certainly should disappear; it is not form, but what you truly feel that is of importance! So, now open up in flexibility; dare to completely surrender to yourself, to your emotional world; no longer restrict yourself, and live in joy, in harmony with yourself. Structure and (self-)control may be there, but then only in service to your worthy content and rich emotional life. Of essential importance is not what others tell you, but what you inwardly know, feel, and build up! Release the grip on yourself, on others, and relax; achieve self-trust; live your life to the fullest, expressing yourself the way you feel, not living for the eye of others. What really counts is not the outer image, but inner joy and development.

You find that happiness only in your Self. Once you have found this, you will no longer punish yourself with a structure that is too limiting and that presses you down. Open up, radiate your being the way you are, now give yourself all the space to live, to enjoy!

DYSENTERY
a kind of intestinal infection

You are derailed — nothing can avail you anymore; you've had it. . . . Desperate: because of the duality in yourself, because of the distance toward yourself (and as a consequence toward others); not being able to feel real contact with your deepest "I." This powerlessness leads to feelings of strong dissatisfaction and rage, largely because of your dependence on others without being able to achieve real feelings of love and unity. The solution here lies in very strong self-contemplation, getting a powerful grip on yourself from out of your central "I," without others being able to influence you.

You blame it on others, but your problem lies deep within yourself.

Amebic dysentery

You believe that you have a very bad, devilish side in you, and you become afraid of this; fear of the devilish in general.

You feel bound like a great martyr; you have been friendly and generous toward everyone, but now it is simply not possible anymore! Now you spit and blow it all out; you are nauseated; you become furious. . . .

You have suppressed your normal aggressive energies for too long: your surroundings have reacted to this electrically charged field and have given you a whack on the head, as it were, after which you began even more to feel in pain — like a victim, more powerless. Now you are furious with others! But with your angry mouth you stay stuck in spite of everything, and you continue to spit out your gall without actually evolving.

It is your enormous energies and feelings which beg for acknowledgment and to be able to exist freely: but you are afraid to experience yourself. So you play the underdog or the victim.

Still, you are being confronted with the duality in yourself: on the one hand you want to do good to others, but on the other hand you would aggressively attack. There is a feeling of powerlessness to become master over yourself; mistrust, anxieties.

Call yourself into line: you are a human-being, a frustrated human-being, who doesn't dare to experience himself as he truly feels. Stop suppressing your feelings and longings, but be completely aware of your human worth! If a boat would sink because it has a hole in it, then stop endlessly bailing out the water, take it to shore, and fix the leak! So, also, with yourself: come solidly with your feet on Earth, don't allow fear and unsureness to suck you dry, fill yourself with self-respect, and energetically bring yourself to realization. Integrate all your feelings into a self-aware existence; deal with that which has become unbearable to you. When your emotional world and your active deeds are in harmony with each other, then this means the end of your inner conflict. You are good, but suppressed powers and emotions can lead to eruptions.

Anxiety and aggression go hand in hand: only trust in your Living Self (See Part I), and a loving acceptance of your total personality, without compromise with the outer world, will drive away these negative feelings.

Bacillary dysentery

Furious revolt; the barriers are being thrown down, so that a true emotional flood drags you to the bottom. You built your life too much upon putting up a brave, bold face toward the outside, the aggressive, the masculine — with powerful energy you fly onward like a superman: you are angry, your pride is hurt, you will show for once who is the strongest! You allow yourself to be dragged along by your feelings in such a way that you no longer have control over them. . . .

You would like to perform stunts and with resolute power reach farther than you can, forcing yourself (all of this in reality or in thoughts). In fact you are weeping, but you roughly wipe away your tears.

It is about reacting in powerlessness, anxiety, and sadness; you become so hard because of this — in the first place hard with yourself!

Feelings that have been bottled up too long; you even have been angry with your feelings. You demand of yourself that you become master over yourself in a tough and strong way, but instead of believing in your inner mastery and in the strong Basis in yourself, instead of truly realizing yourself, you fixate too much on a part of life, on basic instincts like sexuality, on emotional pas-

sions — powerlessness to experience your total human existence.

An unconscious longing to achieve Power over yourself. Now, out of desperate protest because of your Powerlessness, you shake loose everything that is in you, you throw off everything; a cry to your deepest Self so that at last it will become Master. You are furious, and you feel pain; there are no more borders. Anxiously searching for yourself. . . .

Sit proud and comfortable on your throne: no longer inflate yourself, but become aware of your true worth. Acknowledge your total personality and be good to yourself; allow your heart to relax and soften. Turn IN-WARD, come very close to your feelings and allow emotional burdens to flow out of you. Anxieties are needless when you achieve an overview: quietly become master over yourself, feel your inner Power which will drive away feelings of powerlessness. A steady progress, an even development of your longings, of your possibilities, your ambitions, pushing yourself through with your feet solidly on the ground in a balanced way, a constant, quiet streaming of your energies — instead of going wild. Don't become a caricature of yourself, but confirm your true worth in self-respect; don't shut out a part of yourself, acknowledge especially those soft, gentle, beautiful feelings deep inside you. Get a grip on yourself and allow primitive instincts to be transformed into Self-awareness! Peace. . . .

DYSLEXIA

Dyslexia is not an illness, but instead has to do with a twisting path which the brain sometimes takes as a consequence of a certain personality, a certain (albeit unconscious) disposition.

This has to do with an urge of the human being for inner liberation, with an urge to be or to become totally faithful to one's highly unique, original Nature — without compromise!

This human being knows THE LANGUAGE very well, but does not want to live, speak, or communicate in "words or little words," wants to do so in HIS OWN LANGUAGE. If he keeps himself to this, then he knows in his deepest Self that those who are on his wavelength will understand him very well! The brain of a "dyslexic" is definitely tuned in to the usage of language, but not to the word-language the way our society has presented it as a "must" for everyone. Unconsciously, this person wishes only to see the ESSENCE of things and to communicate essentially. It is sad enough that society pushes THIS use of language onto every individual from childhood without taking into account other possibilities of communication, and as a result much of the originality of the child gets lost.

When, with such human beings, one finds an "organic" so-called "abnormality" of certain parts of the brain, then this "abnormality" is not the CAUSE, but the CONSEQUENCE of the dyslexic spiritual attunement of such people, who direct their brains in such a way that their appearance will be different from those of non-dyslexic persons. This is not an abnormality, nor an illness, but a certain construction which is the consequence of the "special" nature of the individual.

We are often dealing here with headstrong or self-willed people who want to follow THEIR ORIGINAL path. And this is good with regard to the development of one's own Nature in all its possibilities: creativity, originality, and talents. . . .

These people are not, however, allowed to push their language and their will on others. For dyslexia sometimes also means being unwilling to — or not wishing to — hear what others have to say or what written words have to say in their own way. This person would rather impose HIS version in his OWN way, or at least give it preference over the versions of the external world. Not always, but often, it then happens that one is being "forced" to read something the way it is written — a battle of wills can develop, a resistance to the "compulsory" reading lesson, a refusal to read things the way they are written. (Of course, we are dealing here with an unconscious process.)

This occurs with people who, in fact, want to build completely upon their own Authority (and taken by itself, this is very good), but in extreme cases what goes along with this sometimes, and which is not so good, is that those people no longer wish to hear anything or listen to others — yes, sometimes would prefer to boss others. They might even impose their wills on nature, so that they see only what they want to see and can no longer take notice of "objective" truth or facts. It shall be made clear to them that it is all right for them to live their original dreams in creativity — but that they must be considerate of other people and the nature of things as they are. They unconsciously call up situations in which it is made clear to them that in life it is not at all about being the first or being the best, or standing out or projecting a proud image to the outer world. . . . For this process to be completed in themselves, they might attract situations in which they feel shame or powerlessness, or in which they are ridiculed because of their dyslexia. The point is to develop a realization of worthiness, pride in their authentic Beings, and not to assert their image, their power, or their desires, which are only oriented toward outer achievement.

It is marvelous in these people that deep within themselves they really wish to evolve in a highly unique way and that they are able to come to original findings, yes even to achieve original discoveries without being hindered by that which others want to force upon them. Their self-essence directs the working of the brain in such a way that dyslexia appears. This is because these people really wish to come to the ESSENCE of things — to essential understanding, to essential communication — and to do so without having to listen to what someone or something from outside themselves has to say. Inspiration and creativity seek their courses in very individualized ways, as a result of which aspects of genius sometimes can be developed via intuitive and rational twists and turns.

In dyslexia, one often finds an (unconscious) hidden resistance to the rules and regulations of "society," to parents or mentors — "one shall find out for *oneself.*" On the other hand, hidden here is a feeling of inadequacy which is a consequence of: "I no longer want to" understand the others nor to read the way the others want me to.

The self-willed way of wanting to develop oneself is not good if it goes together with Self-righteousness and Vanity, with "I am in charge" and "I know everything better." When dyslexia goes together with these characteristics — and this is sometimes the case — then the deepest Self of this human being can call up situations in life by which the child is humiliated or ridiculed so that it immediately will be confronted with its less appealing characteristics: the vain person ought to now come down a peg or two. (Because he cannot, for example, boast "I am the first in the class at reading!") He must learn the lesson to find the worthiness IN himself and to diminish the Image that is shown toward the external world.

Often, we trace a striving-impulse in a child with dyslexia as well as a fear of failure; both go together, both may be alleviated. . . . The most beautiful lesson one can give a child is that it is allowed to BE itself without having to desire, without having to possess or to achieve — these last lead only to discontentment in life.

A healthy BALANCE needs to be found: a healthy communication with other people is necessary; this person may not live isolated in his "dream castle." First, he will learn to understand HIMSELF and to have honest communication with himself; then he will learn how to establish healthy communication with others. He will have to learn the lesson of understanding others in THEIR language without betraying himself and his true nature: he need not at all begin to read and write like others do; he will learn to come to TRUE communication with his deepest SELF, with others — communicating with others in, perhaps, a personal way of his own! He is, therefore, no more or less worthy than others. It is necessary for this human being that he stand solidly with his feet on the ground, in concrete reality, without having to give up his imaginative power and originality! A human being never has to go along with an unhealthy society; it is high time that school systems make space for forms of communication other than the officially standardized and accepted forms. By itself, it is not a healthy situation that everyone in a society MUST know how to read and write in the way THE norm (in this or that culture) dictates. The human being with dyslexia has no handicap at all and is not sick, but it is our western society that suffers from narrow-mindedness and anemia. It is self-evident that difficulties can develop in the child's upbringing when one does not strive after a healthy balance but instead begins to go to extremes — whether it be unbalanced in one way (forcing the child) or in another (allowing the child to have its own way in everything without considering others, without considering reality, without for once truly "listening"). By themselves, however, such difficulties have nothing to do with "dyslexia" in itself.

E

VITAMIN E

Deficiency, insufficient assimilation of

Confusion, insecurity, a feeling of help-lessness, of dependence in your relation-ship with others. You don't really stand on your own legs; you're indecisive, you let yourself droop, and you can't make any autonomous decisions. In doubt re-garding yourself, you carry needless bur-dens; you don't see clearly how to deal with the needless burden of emotions, un-fulfilled longings, feelings of inability; you don't see clearly : "Where am I go-ing? What direction shall I take?" Inde-cisiveness.

Solidly stand in your own shoes, build up your life with resolute power, based on your inner wisdom. Allow that endless stream of energy to come through; no longer block it by disbelief in your Self! Feel good in your skin, in the Now; dare to freely breathe, quietly and deep; take up all your space — be aware of that enormous range you have as a human-being, of those powerful original energies in yourself. Love and peace in yourself, fruitful creativity, active participation in life, self-confidence, radiating from your sun-center toward others: in this way you charge yourself constantly with new en-ergy.

EARS — HEARING

Psychological correspondence

Symbolic of listening to your deepest Self, being open to your inner wisdom. Experi-encing the depths in yourself, feeling safe and at ease in your Self and knowing your deepest awareness-channels, which come toward your physical, earthly existence from underlying dimensions.

Anxieties disappear when you lovingly open yourself up to your deep emotional world, toward your intuitive core, toward the light in yourself — which you might call dark and unknown, but in fact is an eternal living Self, the true center of your individuality.

Thus, symbolic of the intuitive channels through which we gain access to our core, to our inner knowing. Listening to inner signals which we receive as a reaction to impressions from the outer world: don't neglect your inner voice, listen to your intui-tion, the guardian angel is IN you.

Symbolic of controlling energies which come in and go out.

Are we flexibly open to new impres-sions, or do we close ourselves off to the outer world? Symbolic also of generosity: lovingly being open to others.

The auditory organ reflects how much we allow ourselves to flow along supply with our deep emotions, without anxiety, but still under the control of our "I": are we retaining deep emotional experiences too long instead of dealing with them in a flexible way? Or do emotions flood you, so that you no longer have any grip at all on things?

Being open to our deepest emotions; listening also to joy, to sadness, to messages from your environment, and comparing all this to the already present content.

The outlet, letting go of needless emotional burdens — purification.

Pushing powerful energies — coming from your deepest Self, from your emotional core — to the outside. Turning outward anxieties and remnants from the past; freeing yourself.

Calmly dealing with new impressions, with new announcements.

Trusting the intuitive spontaneous working of your nature: you, as master over yourself, as a wise one, listening to your depths.

Ailments of the ear, in general

Anxiety. No contact with your deepest Self; insufficient trust in your intuition. You don't at all listen to your inner wisdom, but you do listen to many channels in your environment. Because of this, do you become alienated from yourself and at last no longer know what is true or not? Do you catch several versions or opinions and become confused? As a child: do your mother and father each declare their opinions, and do you stand between two fires? Then, you might stop up your ears. Or are you tired of always hearing the same thing? Do you feel guilty? Do you want to hide something? Do you think you are bad and have to hide yourself? Are you angry with yourself?

Can't you become master over your feelings? Do certain impressions overwhelm you, and do you close your ears out of self-protection? Do you crawl into a hole where no one can find you? Do you feel weak, closing yourself off from your intuition? Do you become aggressive, wanting to reach out as a result of this weakness? Do you become angry, in powerless anxiety? Children with

ear problems often reflect the problem of the parent(s): refusing to listen to the inner signals, and still going forward on a path that lies far away from joy or authenticity!

Do you no longer wish to have contact with others or do you open yourself up in love? An inner conflict; you don't very well see what to choose because you don't give ear to yourself; you don't very well know who you are. You have insufficient control over your life, your body, your feelings.

Do you save up your negative memories from the past?

Deal with them! Purify everything in your emotional life, which is now in the way of your self-development. Purification, becoming master over yourself and being open, listening to your intuition, to inner knowing or feeling.

Calmly turn inward and contemplate: anxieties are being replaced by a loving openness toward yourself, toward others.

Trust in your deepest, divine Self.

Deafness, being hard of hearing

You drift down to the depths instead of going onward in a self-aware way! You close yourself off, often stubbornly: "I will help myself; I will solve my sadness, my problems, myself."

A damper is being put on your aggression, on your spontaneous energies, which are being turned inward; with dark thoughts, you demolish yourself. Light, joyful energies which wish to exist are being immediately obscured by pessimistic or worrisome thoughts. You feel stuck, unable to go one way or the other. You feel hurt in your deepest "I"; you make yourself inwardly angry, but you don't dare to express your thoughts, your longings, or your feelings. You lock yourself up. Your life is not built on intuition, on your deepest Self: you refuse to listen to your inner wisdom. In the same way, you will close yourself off from others:

"Leave me alone, I know what I'm doing." In the meantime, you blindly go on.

You refuse to listen to a voice inside you which asks for a change in your life! Your deepest powers can't come through. You fixate too much on the negative, on that which constitutes a limitation. You are stuck in an iron suit of armor that you've created yourself. Cut off from your deepest "I," you don't very well see which path would be best to take. Confused, you search in all directions; you don't know what direction to choose. You hear many bells ringing, and — dependent as you make yourself upon others — this has a strong influence on you: one time you're inclined to go here, then another time take that path, until you don't know at all anymore, and you shut your ears in order to no longer hear anything anymore! You feel lonely, alone, isolated, sometimes anxious, because you isolate yourself from your intuitive fundamental being. You feel too unsure to come out of your cocoon, to transform from caterpillar into butterfly, especially as long as the environment appear to you to be unsafe or ambiguous (this particularly occurs in children).

Unsure — you feel there are beautiful energies ready to break free, but you don't very well know how to realize yourself.

You have anxiety about death. You crawl into your shell; you feel unsafe.

Put yourself under the authority of your inner Lamp, your deepest "I," your center: one-pointedly direct yourself to this, so that you no longer swing from left to right. The truth lies within you. Now, open yourself up completely for signals from your deepest Self.

Become aware of your Worth, of your possibilities, and come to peace in yourself. Nothing or no one can threaten you: build up your existence in a self-assured way, daring to be open for the beautiful. Enjoy the small things in life; don't constantly worry. Stop your gloomy brooding. Ask your spontane-

ous intuition for the answer to your problems. Dare to change direction! Listen to the voice of your heart: don't lay a prohibition on yourself; allow your feelings to flow freely. Don't live like a dead person.

You don't die if your deepest "I" doesn't long for it: give yourself over to lighter thoughts, to lighter feelings in yourself. Now, come completely out of your dark tunnel and listen to your wishes: allow yourself to live the way you really would like to live, in harmony with your deepest nature. Enjoy a sunbeam; start from Pluto and come to life.

Earache

You curl, as it were, into yourself; you don't dare to experience fully your deepest feelings, to allow your true "I" to come through, for you are afraid.

Restless thoughts, feeling unsafe; you demolish yourself with gloomy fretting. You don't see clearly into your unconscious foundation; you experience it as an unpleasant cellar; you don't really trust your deepest core.

Frightening fantasies, unrealistic anxieties, fearful expectations of the future, a holding-on to dark memories of the past. Locked up in yourself. You accumulate a lot of emotions, sometimes feeling uneasy and bloated because of the black thoughts in your head. Don't you consider yourself good enough? What gnaws at you? Feelings of guilt? Don't you consider yourself worthy enough to bloom? You are angry with yourself. Beautiful energies are being kept prisoner: you are hurting yourself. Or are others the ones who are hurting you? Then this is only a consequence of your convictions!

Come entirely into daylight with your creative possibilities and secure your thoughts. Do, produce, dare to be yourself without holding back; don't be ashamed of yourself. You are good the way you are. Take up all your space and allow yourself to blossom in

all joy. Build up your life with all your powers; don't allow anxieties to stop you. Fear
is unfounded: fully trust in your deepest divine Self, which lies at the basis of your immortal existence.

Come to powerful self-manifestation and
be proud of yourself. Death doesn't exist in
your life if you don't permit it. Trust your
intuition and live spontaneously from out of
your deepest Self. Don't be afraid of your
emotions: observe them, deal with them,
come to clear insight, and go on. Transform
aggression into action. Loudly question
those who "hurt" you. Create clarity in
chaos. Find peace in yourself. If certain
family circumstances enhance a child's feel-
ing of being unsafe, then the parents need to
look for a solution. Do they, too, deny their
worthiness and refuse to listen to their deep-
est inner Self? Fundamental anxieties in the
parent(s) ask for a growth in Trust in the
whole family. This promotes healing.

Mastoiditis
inflammation of the bone just behind the ear

No longer wanting to see or hear; an aggressive refusal, "Now it's enough!"

Deep anxieties. You feel as if you are in
the iron grip of something ("or someone")
big and threatening. You barely dare to
glimpse at that which you fear you'll see.
Your imagination can go wild under the influence of your anxieties. Frustration, pent-
up aggression, feelings of utter limitation.

For the moment, you fearfully draw back,
but you have a great inner longing to strike
back in anger.

Feel safe and strong in your deepest Self.
Know yourself to be protected and supported
by that powerful Basis in you. Allow new ex-
periences to come in, and don't judge them
according to painful memories of the past.
Let the parents of such children achieve in-
trospection and strive after peace in their
household. Anxiety disappears when it dis-
cerns the mantle of love.

Otitis media
inflammation of the middle ear

An anxious flight away from the hard world.

A feeling of being psychologically strangled, of limitation and frustration, of powerlessness and anger.

One experiences an enormous pressure on
the head; one feels curtailed; children feel restricted or anxious (sometimes also under the
influence of mentors who themselves are
wrestling with anxieties and who put restrictions on themselves).

Inwardly, one feels small, fragile, and
soft, but one receives darkness instead of
light — from memories of one's own past
(from this or another life) as well as from
one's immediate surroundings — and poisonous thoughts instead of joy, thoughts of
death instead of life, anxious clinging instead
of love, coolness instead of warmth. The
small and gentle is being poisoned by angry
and dark thoughts.

One often withdraws into one's own
dream world, where everything is fairytale-
beautiful, where time doesn't exist, where
there are no more limitations. An absence, a
floating, in order to escape problems and
anxieties; one withdraws into an isolated
sanctuary. The lightest, most beautiful philosophies in a high-consciousness level —
which are mostly not understood by others —
alternate with dark, dead atmospheres.

A child often is being confronted with
other people in its surroundings
who are themselves cut off from their divine
Living Self, and because of this anxiety and
thoughts of death appear. The child experiences a soft light deep in itself, but, on the
other hand, is being confronted with dark
spheres from the outside and will close itself
off. Fearful thoughts will chase around its
little head; higher energies are being bottled
up and not allowed to exist freely.

People who raise the child would do well
by strengthening the Trust in their own nature, and the child will receive the positive
influence of this. Also, deeply rooted, un-

pleasant memories from the remote past can again arise in confrontation with oppressive present situations.

One can drag oneself along in streams of thought without end; one desperately seeks answers to life-questions; one allows oneself to flow along unconsciously in endless dreams or philosophies, but one separates oneself too much from the earthly here-and-now. One doesn't stand solidly with both feet on the ground.

Inner anger, powerlessness, because one doesn't dare to fully experience oneself, because one restrains one's own energies — often unconsciously — because the surroundings can't be a sounding board, or because one fears one is not good enough the way one IS.

Paint out the past and start again: believe in Love at the highest level. Determinedly take hold of your life yourself and don't let go anymore: be proud of your earthly existence, be aware of your Worth as a unique human being. Don't hold back your spontaneous nature, your feelings, your beautiful energies. Parents have to become aware that children might be carrying a message, a wisdom: don't curtail the uniqueness and greatness of a child and its inner wisdom. Don't force your anxiety and unsureness upon it. Allow the light of Consciousness to come through into incarnation. Produce, create a life full of joy and love. Allow happy thoughts to purify the dark head. Feel safe in your earthly existence, on the basis of your deepest Self. Don't flee into a confused thought-world, but draw to your body all powers of consciousness, all your deep feelings, and allow those happy spheres to permeate your body from out of your spontaneous, living, playful Self; push that lie of anxiety out of your ear, open up outwardly, and loudly proclaim the true message to your surroundings: that anxiety, death, and sorrow are a regrettable remembrance of the unconscious existence of humanity; that every human being is able to Consciously create his or her own life, eternally, and in joy! Open your ears and take up your responsibility to lift the world to a higher level.

Earwax plug — too much wax

You have pain; you try to defend yourself. Enormous anxieties; afraid of sharp contacts, of stinging words from people to whom you are attached. You feel too small, too absent; you are too much "spirit," too little here in your body. You don't get a grip on the new, and you should let go of the old. You don't see clearly; you too much allow yourself to "be lived." In your imagination you'd courageously go into battle, building upon your own authority, but you refuse to acknowledge your authority, just as you angrily call out NO to authority that is above you.

Shutting off, being stuck, resisting the outer world. You hold on to a lot with your feelings, your desires, your thoughts. You want to seize and embrace too much; an angry urge for power, but you feel powerless! On the one hand you cling to others, in confusion, and on the other hand you want to fight free of this dependence; you allow yourself to be ruled by others, and then you feel manipulated. You draw another toward you, but then again you'd indignantly and angrily push him away. Aggressive feelings are looking for a way out. You feel forced, imprisoned, stuck, and you develop enormous energies of resistance against this.

Powerful creative energies are left unused, with the consequence being frustration.

Unconscious, primitive powers are asking for a breakthrough, for a transformation into action and creativity, but you don't go on in a self-aware way. You bottle up these powers. You don't really live fully.

You feel misunderstood — as a child, by your mother; as a partner, by your equal — and you close your ears to fights or arguments. You don't agree with what is happening around you. You become angry with your relations who, according to you, are the cause of the Tower of Babel. Self-destruction, closing up in anger, stubborn resistance, revolt against a situation that for you is unbearable. "I don't want to go on this way." Feeling wronged. An inner urge for self-liberation.

Allow negative feelings and thoughts to escape! Direct your attention to your worthy content. No longer hold back your creative energies; produce, be fruitful, and let go of the darkness in you. Seize all power in yourself, grow in self-awareness, but let go of others. Go on without hesitation, position yourself independently, and listen to your inner voice: unfold your particular possibilities, direct your glance at your content, and don't grasp for that which lies outside yourself. Open yourself in love toward your content, transform primitive powers into creativity. Peace and harmony are found deep inside yourself! Transform aggressive powers into active self-realization. Don't isolate yourself from others, but speak openly with them, and express your feelings. Accept your process of growth and don't force anything. Acknowledge your worth as a human being and feel welcome.

Ringing or buzzing in the ears

Locked up in your own negative thoughts. False pride; you push others away from you. Resistance, stubbornness, fear of listening to your deepest Self, of listening to wise and beautiful truth-loving messages. You'd rather fixate on the darkness of the world, on the "sins" of others, on gossip in tabloids, on strange things which are far-removed from you, so you think — in fact these are reflections of your own pessimistic view of life, of your dark emptiness, of anxieties. You cling to the darkness, to that which is lower.

You don't really live in reality, here-and-now: you live in a very subjective thought-circle — "I know better anyway" — you imprison yourself in your prejudicial, imaginary world. Maybe you'll meet comrades, members of sects or gossip groups, whereby all small-minded, dark things are put on the table.

You collide with others; you are not completely honest with your deepest Self.

You leer at the devilish; you forge secretive plans in your head; you fight against your own delusions; you think you have to be ready for evil.

You glare, with a certain hardness in your thoughts, at that which smells unfresh; you fill up your own emptiness with dark delusions. You fly with your thoughts from here to there, but emotionally you are angular and cold; you warm yourself with the fire of "strange things."

You bite into the otherness, into that which is dark; you hinder yourself from living flexibly and happily from out of your heart. You don't believe in joy, in the sun, in happiness. Often, we are dealing here with very dark UNCONSCIOUS spheres and expectations. . . .

Upbringing and indoctrination, religious small-mindedness and prejudices: do you build your life upon this false Authority? Now, turn in all honesty toward the divine authority deep in yourself, and listen to your inner wisdom. No longer allow yourself to be manipulated unconsciously by small-minded life philosophies that don't have any respect for the individual and that divide humanity into categories, white and black.

Look at yourself, stand here-and-now with both feet on the ground and become sober: curb your fantasies. Stay present in reality and discover now the beautiful in yourself, in life. The evil in the world is but the consequence of a lack of insight. When you turn your mind toward darkness — or that which you condemn as darkness — then this indicates that you don't really believe in that power of goodness in yourself. Has someone made you believe that the human being is "bad," and that you have to watch out for this? Then you will be lurking, then you will strengthen the evil in the world, because you concentrate on it.

If you'd dare, however, to allow love into your life and true joy of life — lighter expectations, instead of anxieties — then you'd be doing your part in the building up of a new earth. Allow light and joy into your life!

Let go of that resistance to your inner Self; don't build your life on dark prejudices; acknowledge that which is beautiful in yourself and others; surrender yourself; for once, bend flexibly instead of thinking, in an obstinate and narrow-minded way, that you know it all, for your judgment is not built on a true basis. No longer listen to destructive influences from your upbringing, but open yourself up to the diversity of people; everyone has his or her story. No authority, no system, no law outside yourself, has a lease on the truth. Listen to your heart, and look at that which is the most beautiful in life.

Break that stubborn obstinacy; become flexible and softer; direct yourself inwardly and don't play the judge.

EDEMA
dropsy, swelling caused by accumulation of fluid in the body

You live according to a certain pattern, within a certain structure, too tightly, because you insufficiently trust your nature, your spontaneous feelings.

You hold on to others, to certain things, because of fear and powerlessness.

You FLEE from yourself; you go beyond your own borders and even try constantly to crawl into someone else's skin, like a chameleon, so as not to have to face yourself. For you want to please others, because you believe insufficiently in yourself. You feel unsure, vulnerable, at the mercy of others, afraid; you roll yourself up in a ball, as it were, like a porcupine, to protect yourself; you conceal yourself; your feelings and your creative energies are being rolled up, not allowed to exist or to "be lived." You feel like a doll, or like a person who isn't able to just be himself. You are so afraid of your own feelings that you hide behind a pose, a structure, or behind someone else. You will assume various poses depending on the person you are facing, in order to please him or her; you live too much for others, so that you play many roles, but never can really be spontaneously yourself.

Your personal feelings, anxieties, and suppressed aggression ask for liberation.

Fixated thoughts suffocate intuition and impulses.

Allow yourself to be carried along on the waves of *your* nature; don't allow yourself to "be lived" by others. Follow your own path in a Self-aware way. At all times, be honest with yourself; don't bend so deeply, don't be too compliant, intending to please others. Follow your Nature, your intuition, one hundred percent: self-contentment will result when you are in harmony with yourself and do only that which is inspired by your heart, by your inner Self. If you don't first of all let go of everything and everyone and come very close to yourself — if you don't first of all offer yourself the necessary attention and love — then how can you experience happiness? Take the rudder in your own hands, resolutely determine your course, come to self-respect so that you also will get respect from others.

Feel the joy in yourself and radiate it to others; know yourself to be safe and protected in your Self; allow your emotions to flow freely, deal with them, and build up a new life in the Now, separate from the past.

No longer hold on with your thoughts; trust those impulsive inspirations.

Action in self-confidence, going on without hesitation!

EHLERS-DANLOS SYNDROME

**congenital disorder of connective tissue with
hyperextensible skin, loose joints, and easy bruising**

You'd prefer to withdraw completely into yourself, anxious and unsure. You are afraid to be seen — possibly ashamed — because you don't find yourself good enough, because you doubt your worth. You constantly ask yourself whether you are on the right path; you hold yourself in, pull the reins tight, because you have no faith in your nature, in your feelings. You leer at others, sometimes, angry and hidden, because you mistrust yourself *and* others; you are afraid of being hurt; moreover, you feel bad, possibly experiencing certain feelings in yourself as devilish (such as sexual feelings), or you are ashamed. Despite the fact that you conceal yourself and your emotions, there lies in you the ambitious inner urge to stick out your chest, to behave as if nothing is the matter, outwardly trying to achieve, although you feel emotionally so clumsy and awkward that most of the time you don't get very far in this outward manifestation — but you'd like to, because you are very sensitive to appreciative, admiring, loving words or glances from others. These are needed to compensate for your own feelings of self-negation and emptiness. You put your nature into armor. You don't allow yourself to Become. Sometimes you think you have to act like a thief in the night; you think you have to secretly hide your emotions and longings because it would be bad or wrong! It seems as if you feel guilty about your feelings, about that which you emotionally take in from the outer world. You refuse to acknowledge yourself the way you are; you make yourself powerless; this can lead to thoughts that are angry and aggressive or even vengeful because of your own powerlessness.

It seems as if your body "hangs" on you: you unconsciously refuse to become master over your own body, because you don't at all approve of yourself! Instead of seizing power over yourself, you feel threatened by those powers inside yourself, by the powers outside yourself. Afraid of the power that the Eye of the outer world has on you: because you refuse to acknowledge in yourself this power over your life.

Because you experience yourself as soft ice cream, you'll sometimes cloak yourself in a stubborn silence of false pride: so that others won't be able to intrude — because you feel too vulnerable. Your surroundings, therefore, quickly appear threatening and obtrusive; sometimes, it seems to you as if someone wants to push something down the throat of the bird in a brutal way. You don't really dare to surface, to be yourself, despite the fact that your head is full of productive ideas; but they are being smothered in emotions of anxiety. You are afraid of punishment; you think you have to protect yourself; you are in inner emotional conflict because you constantly resist your spontaneous feelings. On the one hand, you experience yourself as a "trash can," and on the other hand, you want others to no longer treat you like a trash can: and, of course, this is not possible. Perhaps you force certain things: let go, and open yourself up without forcing it.

A self-assured fundamental structure, building up trust in yourself, knowing that you, as a human being, are good and unique in your own way. Come to a cheerful openness; trust your spontaneous feelings, your nature, no longer questioning what others say about you. Knowing yourself to be protected in your inner Authority: you are master over your life, over your body. Know yourself to be safe and protected in yourself. Feel yourself as being loose and free in your nature; allow these emotions to flow freely: you may be yourself, one hundred per cent. Your worth and your goodness are not dependent on the norms or the approval of a society.

*You are who you are: reveal yourself in the sunlight of yourself; don't force your nature. No longer hold in your creative energies, and create your life yourself. Build up the solid foundations of your existence just by believing in your Self. Transform suppressed aggression into active self-realization. Hesitate no longer: allow negative thoughts to escape from your head. That which you suppress in yourself can accumulate in such a way that you experience it as being devilish; laugh about it. The only problem is Self-suppression! Be nice and flexible to yourself; there is nothing you **MUST** do, but you have the right to completely be yourself; don't hide yourself. Only look for those contacts with whom you feel emotionally good right Now; simply "open" yourself up, and don't force it. In this way, you will attract people who are good for you.*

ELBOWS
(See also Enthesitis, Tennis elbow)

Psychological correspondence

The elbows represent an "electric alertness," a receiving of new impressions, an openness to inner wisdom, a readiness to allow new higher energies to come in — a complete openness for signals which you, yourself, have called up (perhaps unconsciously); don't resist these signals, but receive them in a relaxed way. Don't fight against yourself: follow the right direction. . . .

Dare to go and explore in freedom, like a true "Sagittarius," being open to every new life adventure, without limiting yourself.

The elbows are in solid contact with the lower part of your spine: a cooperative unity which symbolizes safety, certainty in yourself, grounding, self-protection. From this secure feeling in yourself you can open your hands in receptivity.

They are also a symbol of productive and flexible functioning and a symbol of labor, for yourself and for others — in your feeling of security, taking up certain responsibilities for yourself and for others and carrying out a task with ease and in a relaxed way for those who are less able than you are in a certain area.

Fearlessly going through everything! Making yourself a path and allowing energies to pass through freely.

Ailments, in general

Do you remain turned inward too much, like a fetus, afraid of new experiences, in a defensive and mistrustful attitude toward the outer world? You can't get out, you are stuck, you keep running in place, without truly going on in life; you hinder evolution; maybe you want too much or want that which is not at all good for you — let go, no longer fight, but follow the signals! Why any longer resist changes that are necessary? Or do you prefer to wait apathetically until you rust?

Or are you extremely strained in your nerves, unsure in yourself and fighting against others: do you think you have to prove yourself in one direction or another instead of accepting and finding yourself good one hundred percent, without having to find affirmation from others? Do you consider the world an enemy, and do you live "on guard," ready to shoot or to crawl back into your shell?

You hold on to certain ideas, traditional theories or philosophies, and you refuse to distance yourself from them, even if certain signals clearly show you it is high time to revise certain things! But because your life is too little built on your own secure basis, you don't even dare deviate from an ancient path. This becomes a stubborn battle with pain in the elbow!

With openness, you will be able to get further.

Don't attach yourself to, or worship, anything outside yourself! Allow that which is deepest in yourself to come to the surface, to come out, and send out your powerful energies.

Acknowledge your pure, primitive nature-powers, but don't force anything. Act and live from out of your Self, not according to "habits," not according to the eyes or norms of others. Allow the flower to grow up out of its seed, which perhaps has been held hidden for too long under what "had to be"; allow your feelings, your longings, your nature, to exist freely, and no longer offer resistance to necessary adaptations, nor to your Self, which asks for acknowledgement of its inner worth! All authority over yourself lies in you: acknowledge this and don't fight against yourself.

Every human being is unique, has his or her own nature: acknowledge this also and don't fight *against* yourself, nor against others.

Enthesitis
**painful inflammation where
the tendon attaches to the bone,
e.g. Tennis elbow (See also Elbow)**

Because you don't build your life on your Inner richness, you force yourself to satisfy certain expectations which you or the outer world place upon you.

You pull back under the wing, under the protection of a philosophy, a way of thinking, an organization, a social trend, a system, without wanting to acknowledge or explore your own inner reality! You force yourself because you don't listen to your nature, to your Self.

You hide behind a facade, an image, preferably with headphones, blind to your deeper values or to the inner values of others.

You are closed off from your inner Source. You have no true contact with it: your inner soul light, your core, is caught in an iron grip.

What else is behind this but anxiety! The Mole is afraid to come above ground and be struck on its head; fear of being yourself, of

experiencing yourself. You don't trust your deepest "I"; you only allow your outer Ego to radiate! So be aware of your inner grandeur and experience yourself to the deepest regions; become aware of all your powers, your possibilities, and don't hide them. Discover this rich world and the world of others *beneath* the surface! Go into your own depths; don't resist, take full responsibility for your total life — not only for part of it or for just the material, outer aspect. Dare to make contact with new people, who also are open to their inner wisdom, and don't get stuck on false values. Your life is not "empty." . . .

Be more flexible with yourself and listen to your deepest Self, to your nature; you don't have to prove yourself when you acknowledge your inner worth.

Don't let your body function purely as a "body," but let it be animated by Self-awareness that is conscious of its unique being, which reaches beyond anonymity.

EMOTIONAL PROBLEMS, IN GENERAL
(Also read Part I)

Inwardly, there will be an enormous urge to emerge, to evolve: your emotions impel you and make you sense whenever you put the brakes to the evolutionary process that is best for you. One will reconcile conflicting feelings in order to achieve a step further.

If, however, you suppress your feelings, suppress this natural stream of longings, of energies, then at last this build-up will lead to frustration and to powder kegs that sooner or later will explode, or which ultimately will cause physical illness. Suppression of self-realization, and refusing to develop your powers, will then result in uncontrollable aggression, in violence, in anger or jealousy directed at others.

Feelings come to the surface out of your deepest soul and make something clear to you. Are you so afraid? If so, then something is not right with your self-trust and with your convictions regarding life and death. Don't push this emotion away, but resolve it.

A heavy emotion, however unpleasant it might be, requires the solving of the problem that underlies it: observe your emotion, look at it, and deal with it. Don't be afraid of your gloomy feelings, but allow them to flow freely. In this way, one emotion will flow into the other, and you will ultimately come to a solution. This can lead to depression and hopelessness if, from the beginning on, you avoid and suppress your emotions.

Your inner convictions direct your emotions: if you are convinced that you are a nothing, a poor mortal being without your own power, then this will call up emotions in you which will point out to you this conviction you have regarding yourself. This conviction of "inferiority" and "sadness" will attract in its turn situations which again will cause sadness and feelings of humiliation. The cause doesn't lie in the Situations, in the happenings. Resolve these convictions!

By observing emotions, you can arrive at the cause of the true problem in your life. Then change these convictions, and the change in your emotional world will indicate whether or not you are on the right path: if these newly formed convictions lead you to joy, then you are on the right path!

It is, therefore, very important to dare to totally observe your emotions in order to come to a clear feeling regarding the original reasons for your present problems and sorrow: often, this leads to "powerlessness and self-undervaluation."

Feel safely and warmly taken up in the earthly magnetic stream, in earthly energies, and, especially, don't float away. Put both feet on the ground and accept your emotions. Higher energies of consciousness and clear insight can free you from an exaggerated in-flux of sad emotions. When you allow all energies and feelings to come through freely, and no longer block them, then the transformation process in you can begin: a volcano that frees itself transforms all primitive emotions into consciousness. It is much better not to bottle up your natural stream of anger or aggression: express yourself and speak to the person concerned. Thus, in confrontation with others, you will ultimately be confronted with your deepest Self. Bottling-up and frustration lead to illness, violence, crime, perversities, and injuries; when, however, you let yourself go free without inhibitions — daring to let your emotions come through, expressing your anger — then you and your surroundings are no longer being contaminated by a tense, poisoned energy field full of hate or aggression. Via the letting-go, the expressing, one deals with things, and feelings will no longer get out of hand, nor will they cause insane situations (fights, war, etc.). Trust in this spontaneous, healthy pattern; follow your feelings into your deepest core, and know how to bring about the needed corrections in your convictions so that you will become a liberated, happy human being, purified, and filled to the brim with positive energies.

One doesn't need to go back to childhood via rebirth or psychoanalysis; one doesn't have to root about in the "subconsciousness": dare to experience powerfully the Now, with all your emotions, and in this way achieve the resolution of your problems.

See where these emotions lead you, and bring about transformation in the way described above. After all, situations from the past were reflections of your deepest convictions, with which you came into the world: the events from the past are not, therefore, the true cause of your problems, the trauma, or the sadness which you have encountered in the course of your life; nor does the cause lie in "other" lives. . . . Happenings are only "occasions" by which deeper emotion surfaces: the "cause" lies in yourself, in your convictions regarding yourself and life. Therefore, resolve it "here." Happenings are a "result" of a vibration already dwelling in you.

Look at your fundamental convictions, which are the true cause of all your sadness, and change them NOW.

For example: do you now feel anger, aggression? . . . Accept it and come to communication, to action. In a subsequent phase, you will notice how hatred possibly lies hidden under your anger. Pain and sadness will clearly make you feel that something lies deep beneath your aggression: self-negation, insufficient self-love (because of which you've attracted even more loveless situations in your life), powerlessness. You are convinced that you, as a human being, have no power over yourself, your life, or your feelings: this feeling of powerlessness causes you anxieties! Instead of suppressing aggressive anger — which ultimately can be a consequence of all this and can result in violence or illness — it would be much better if, from the beginning, you allowed yourself to experience your feelings and dealt with them.

Become aware that your "I" is not powerless in relation to your emotions, nor in relation to happenings from the outside. It's of no harm to have aggressive feelings; don't deny them; don't think yourself bad or feel guilty because of them: under the supervision of your Conscious "I" they will come through, and you will deal with them. Under your Mastery, feelings are allowed to flow freely: put all power in your Self, don't LET yourself "be lived," but — in an active way — create life the way you wish it to be. No longer deny these possibilities.

There's no need for the "re-experiencing" of certain negative experiences from the past; they were already the consequence of a deeper-rooted conviction.

Now, give expression to emotions if needed, but this is not always necessary; transformation of primitive impulses and

feelings into Understanding and Consciousness makes it possible that pent-up sadness doesn't have to be worked out in an emotional way! For certain people, however, it can mean faster relief to bring out certain emotions completely; with the right understanding and insight into the "why" this release will by itself come to a quicker end.

Insight and understanding into "Why did I attract these things into my life? Which conviction lies at the foundation here? How will I change my life?" Self-awareness and clear insight drive away powerlessness and sadness. (Read Part I.)

EPILEPSY

Grand mal
generalized tonic-clonic seizures

Unstable. Seeking outside yourself, sometimes maniacally.

Epilepsy breaks through as a result of a combination of various causes.

On the one hand, you suppress your true, deep feelings, your sadness, your anger, your anxieties; you hinder yourself from freely living, using only a few antennae in your head; your thoughts nervously roll back and forth because of a feeling of uncertainty and powerlessness. Sometimes you become furious because of this powerlessness, and you try to seize power over others. Possibly, you've felt yourself all along to be under the power of others; you felt rejected by those who limited you or allegedly brought about an inferiority complex in you, and by those who did not want to give you love or appreciation. But, in fact, it was you who condemned yourself and withheld appreciation from yourself! Your environment only responded to those inner negative convictions regarding yourself! Because of this, you've accumulated energies, feelings, confused thoughts, in a powerlessness or a refusal to let yourself go, to let yourself live — until ultimately all resistance collapses, and your deepest Self calls for an outlet, epilepsy, to break out of your prison, your self-oppression. Your natural being pushes away all the constricting armor; your body now makes you feel "I am allowed to be here, too; don't only live in your head." Your deep feelings and impulses protest against the exclusive right of the thinking, of the superficial sensory, or of bottled-up tensions.

This, then, is a second important factor. Because of these feelings of powerlessness, rejection, and lack of self-worth, one will flee into, — or throw oneself maniacally into — a focused occupation in this life, wherein one has the feeling of still having a "grip," or "power," on something, still possessing worth and power in, for instance, achievement in an intellectual or practical level. But you limit yourself; it remains a rejection of the TOTAL WORTH of yourself.

You run ahead of yourself; you think and think — you flee as if pursued, without truly finding enjoyment in yourself, in the earthly. You obligate yourself; you MUST; it even becomes a compulsion in certain cases: why punish yourself so? You don't live in the joyful NOW-moment; you are hard on yourself. In a labyrinth of thinking, you try to get a grip on yourself in an agitated, sometimes aggressive, impatient way. Extremely demanding, anxious, mistrustful, sometimes paranoid. You don't give yourself any open chances! Bid yourself welcome and don't observe yourself through the eyes of others, or through "severe" eyes: don't follow "norms," like a slave, for then you can never be yourself. Build up a new life, with new, free, flexible rules; achieve relaxation and take your freedom — in yourself.

Energies accumulate in your head in a nervous swarm because of your restless and confused seeking. You live in your head in such a way that you might lose all grounding. You feel insufficiently safe in yourself, don't trust your deepest Core, and do everything except call upon your intuitive higher awareness. On the contrary, because of denying your own trustworthy basis, denying your own inner wisdom, your powers, you completely cling to what you can seize with your external senses or with the purely rational.

Because you don't allow yourself to flow along with your intuitive emotional stream, everything seems to slip away from you — you think you always have to get a grip, or power, over certain situations. Actually, it's all about a search for yourself! Of course, this search isn't possible via confused thinking or via fixating your senses on the outer world (or an image); it's only possible via calmly turning inward.

It doesn't do any good to run away nervously from yourself. But inwardly you are desperately looking for Love, because you don't offer this love to yourself. You'd desperately *"shake"* others, as it were, to force love from them, but your deepest Self knows that it is you who should be shaken awake from self-rejection! You feel yourself to be a victim, suffering: at the same time, you are angry — "Now, look at me!" — but in spite of this you feel you can't force love from others. Ultimately, you release every *power-grip* on others . . . and you *flee*.

Let go; don't expect anything from others, but depend first of all on yourself: it's not the others who push you away, but you waste your time. An enormous amount of accumulated energy wishes to come through, but you allow it to exist only in an iron framework; you constantly collide with yourself, energy becomes fireworks, you fight with yourself and don't really allow yourself to freely live!

Filled to the brim with energies, but they are retained in your head: you live too much like an island in the air, seeking, thinking, dreaming, restlessly fighting with yourself.

Let go of this grip — trust the life system, let go of everything. No longer try to "hold on to or control" everything with your mind or senses. Give yourself over to yourself and let go of everything — know yourself to be safe and at peace in yourself, give yourself the life you deserve; you have the right to happiness, not to suffering!

No longer go against the stream, but follow your feelings and come with your feet *on the Ground:* enjoy your physical body, your skin, the sun, food. . . . Your head is too isolated from the earth, your spirit floating too much and away from your body. You FLEE. . . .

Now become aware of your own worth and stop your self-rejection: live here-and-now. Life is everything but "theory." Keep your feet on the ground and no longer run away with your thoughts. Breathe, see, taste, feel — and relax. Anxieties and nervousness disappear only when you acknowledge your own strong autonomy and know that you have the power to create your world, and that your rest and joy are not dependent on others, nor on the measure in which you acquire a greater "grip" on things. Let go of everything — put all power into your intuitive Self and no longer want to suffer: in self-respect, climb onto your throne. No one can pursue you; stop needling yourself. Dare to Live to the fullest! See clearly; nothing and no one threatens you. Allow yourself to exist freely. Be master over yourself through self-surrender.

*   *   *

Somewhere there's a small voice inside you that says: "No I don't want to!" As a result, you obstinately concentrate on things that have nothing to do with the "essence" of Life. You bottle up your anger and stubbornness and at the same time are irritated with yourself about remaining stuck in the old phase. Possibly, you get angry with people in your surroundings, but actually they have nothing to do with it; it all begins in yourself, circumstances are only a result!

You'd like, as it were, to sweep the floor on which you stand with such intensity, force and power, so that everything "old" — yes,

everything that still sticks to the present and which irritates you — would be gone! But you concentrate too much on the upper side, the outside of things, instead of blossoming from within. Frantically, you fixate on a task, a work, possibly with somewhat aggressive thoughts, repressed anger and powerlessness. If things don't immediately go the way you want, you mostly suppress this silently, inwardly, and as a reaction throw yourself more intensely into your task or whatever. But actually you are unconsciously irritated by the fact that you remain stuck to certain habits, certain things or people: you want it to be "gone"! Out of your existence. Forcefully, with all your might . . . you scrub the hard surface of the floor, instead of directing yourself from your roots upward, from out of your inner heart, from your gentle feelings, toward your own further growth, and looking ahead, opening yourself up and *"letting go" of that "outside" yourself upon which you remain so "fixated."* Forces, bottled-up emotions, suppressed anger, energies, thoughts, are frustrated looking for their way out . . . but your head directs itself too much downwards instead of realizing that life inside you asks to now grow *"to a higher level." Asks also to break with being frustrated, angry and with keeping yourself locked up or suppressing everything inwardly. Not just to remain in your old patterns and thinking mechanisms, or in the material aspect, in forever the same thing.*

The head covering — that behind or underneath which, you kept "hidden" in order not to become yourself, to expose yourself — is now suddenly lifted from your head, as it were, and you experience now that the Light in yourself, in your brain, in your head, asks for all the attention.

No longer imprison that mass of "Uranian light forces," those energies in your being. This means the clear, bright light in your head asks for all the attention: in order to arrive at new insight, a renewed vision regarding life, itself. Don't hold on to things in powerless anger, nor in a narrow-minded, rational way. Bring about changes where needed; don't frenetically cling to the old things, because they will never come back, and thinking of it will only stagnate your growth. Time to revise certain convictions, prejudiced thoughts, philosophies concerning life. (Read about this in Part I). Time to listen to the voice inside you, which asks you to give yourself the "inner enlightenment" you need, which asks for *expansion of your awareness, for HONEST openness, for your own being to honestly flow through.* In order to literally "raise" yourself from the *Essence* of your own being (no longer remaining stuck, full of desire, in purely rational thinking or in the material things, on the surface or the periphery of life), which doesn't mean floating with your head in the clouds! Coming to inner wisdom via new insights. Thus, to make a step upward, going *onward* and leaving certain old things completely *behind.* You have nothing to expect from others, nothing to *"desire"* from life, with power; only you can offer yourself happiness and thankfulness . . . *raise yourself, let go of everything and everyone and allow those fruitful energies in yourself to freely create and flow!* No longer turn your mind in a *grim,* sometimes discontented, angry way to the unimportant things in life; don't get angry inside, but bring yourself to realization! Don't *"escape"* into certain enterprises, tasks, hobbies, exaggerated spiritual meditations — or in worldly superficialities — not in TV, computer games, etc. . . . but enter into yourself. OPEN your being toward inner contentment regarding yourself, toward further growth and development, toward an honest flow of feelings, energies. Enter into deep communication with your "warm heart" instead of wanting certain things or people outside yourself to be different; change yourself, go onward! Don't get stuck — in a fierce, sometimes demanding, way — to "thoughts, emotions" which don't really serve life in you. *Let go, and make a step forward, from out of your Essence!*

You might have the feeling that your brain is overexposed to light; it's important then that you keep your *feet on the ground,* that you keep *very close to yourself, to your body* . . . that you don't allow yourself to slip away, that you become "master" OVER YOURSELF, that you tell yourself: "I don't resist 'renewal,' a letting-go of the old; I open myself up to transformation and now enter very strongly and solidly into my body; I lovingly become master over MY life, over myself, *without FORCING myself in a hard or ambitious way, having to do this or that (nor demanding such things of others).* I *Stay with myself,* and nothing or no one outside myself, no single light, can blind me. Because I now listen very closely to my inner source, to my inner light-force, which lies very close to my heart. I no longer put on *blinders;* I no longer hide my head behind all kinds of systems and thoughts; *I radiate my being outward, instead of keeping everything inside me, in my head.* Yes, I want to and will *LOOK* at the new, at the elevated, at the broader view . . . *I no longer hide.*"

It's only when you yourself refuse to go on, to move toward further evolution, that life inside you takes away, as it were, your head covering so that it suddenly looks as if you have lost all mastery over yourself. You are thrown from your horse: it's about a "Uranian" atmosphere that calls for recognition of Life, of true Love, in and toward yourself — of a setting-free of energies that for too long and too restrictedly were suppressed and held back, so that no growth was allowed; a demand for opening yourself up completely to changes, to renewal and awareness, to looking "further" than again and again doing the same tasks, repeating the same thoughts, often with anger and discontentment — like a dissatisfied Cinderella. You, as the wicked stepmother toward yourself, because unconsciously you do feel: "I have to go onward, this is not the/my life!"

You want to get out! Out of this feeling of imprisonment . . . but, initially, instead of "becoming" yourself, you sometimes fixate with devilish thoughts, sometimes with feelings of power and vengeance and hatred, on something or on a certain person allegedly standing in your way — on that which cannot "be," in desire; but know then that every outer circumstance is just a result of your inner situation.

So, desire nothing, and liberate yourself and allow yourself to exist in thankfulness!

You now have to go "higher up"! *No longer lock up your energies.* Open yourself up to *broadening* your field and go along with that giant nuclear power-center in yourself which sends you fire and light; so that, in a highly personal way, you liberate yourself, YOUR REAL "I," bringing it out, showing it the way it is. Be master over your energies, no longer living as a thinking automatic machine, as a working robot, or angrily turned off to life in general, living on a too superficial, closed, narrow-minded level. *Therefore, open up all space in yourself. No longer flee from this evolution in yourself . . .* no longer hide. *Break open,* so that you don't have to be "forced" by your living self via an epileptic attack. Let go of the old, no longer fixate on certain things outside yourself, in a frustrated and discontented way, but open up your hands to Life in yourself which asks for a powerful, free passage. Go onward, honestly and decisively. In this way, you no longer will move through life in frustration. Open up the flood gates and raise yourself up as a Human Being! In your hands lies all power over your life, over allowing your honest "being," your energies, to flow freely and originally: do something with it. Inner liberation!

Absence seizures, petit mal

You'd like to be gone, to flee. The burden weighs heavily.

Anxious thoughts with regard to your past, frightful projections to the future. You don't get any perspective on your chaotic emotional situation; you can't comprehend it, especially because you lean too much on the thinking, the rational: with this one-sidedness you cut yourself off from that in you which you can always calmly trust — your basic intuition, your deep Inner self, knowing without having to rationalize, feelings of warmth and love.

Impatient, nervous, irritated, a great agitation in your head. You'd run from here to there, wanting to do everything at the same time.

Actually, you are irritated about yourself, even though you might project it on others. Powerless to get a grip on your feelings, doubting yourself, cut off from your gentle, sensitive side.

Your feelings are stuck, so to speak, and with your rational ego you stagnate your intuition: communication disturbance in yourself, also toward the outer world.

Nevertheless: your deep emotional roots are strongly present, but the emotional flow is being held back. You have a lack of self-appreciation; you feel you are bad; you condemn yourself and then withdraw within yourself, like a snail into its shell, so that you don't have to show yourself here, and they also can't hurt you or point out your weaknesses, for which you've already punished yourself for such a long time.

Perhaps you find your outer appearance ugly. Are you afraid of communication because of your feeling of inferiority? In this way you direct your energy — which is supposed to go outward — to flow inward. Do you reject your body, nature? Do you limit life to the "spiritual"?

Connect the head with your heart! Love for yourself!

Self-confidence: stop that self-condemnation! Did you not satisfy the expectations of your mentors, and therefore do you think you haven't succeeded? In fact, it's you who makes conditions/demands on yourself. Don't build your life upon "rules and norms." You are unique, with different possibilities than, for instance, your mentors.

Don't compare yourself with others: be happy with yourself, with your own nature! Your motor is the warm heart: from here, power flows throughout your entire body. With a lack of self-love, you block this supple flow. Give love and let go! You don't have to get a grip, not on others nor on yourself.

Don't constantly sit there anxiously thinking or fretting: trust your intuition. Co-operating energies: left and right brain-halves, mind and feelings, intuition.

Trust in your deep Inner self; you don't have to dominate everything with your mind, your thoughts: leave this to your awareness, which finds its solid pillars in your total self.

You are no spirit; the body exists, too: cherish the world, the earthly, with your senses. Relax, enjoy! Press nature to you.

*Via a good Grounding, you get rid of an excess of electricity. Dare to experience **yourself**, your own being, in the here-and-now; you are good the way you are. Don't flee.*

Partial seizures
occurring within
discrete regions of the brain

You have the feeling you have to go through a gate — the gate of life — but it seems as if you are standing on a rotating metal tube, and in an anxious way *trying to stabilize a shaky balance.* You might perspire from it: you live according to the conviction that life really is a matter that's difficult to keep in balance, that you constantly have to be on guard, that you —constantly alert, in a state of nervous tension — have to try to keep your life in balance, and that this is a delicate situation. The conviction that your life is built upon an unstable Basis. (Time to start looking for that solid Basis inside yourself!) Inner restlessness and insecurity are being compensated for by wanting to make a "good" impression in the eye of the public. This only makes you more nervous. In this way you not only place "power" and "pressure" tensely on yourself, but you also

want to get a certain grip on the perspective of others (regarding you): "Will they acknowledge me, approve of me, think me beautiful or proper or intelligent? etc." You put the demands of a perfectionist on yourself sometimes, especially regarding the superficial aspect of life. The head, the thinking, looking around, anxiously wanting to keep an eye on everything — from out of your head, the "spirit."

Trust, coming from your inner heart: that will do you good! Knowing that you don't have to look at your life from an anxious, unstable point of view, that you may "let go" instead of constantly concentrating yourself and trying to keep your balance. This balance will be there BY ITSELF when you stop thinking that there's no other way to live than by experiencing it in this anxiety. Nothing is less true. Let go! Squeeze yourself no longer within structures, laws of appearances and exteriors, within Saturnal, compulsory rules. Make it easy on yourself, quietly sit down, don't rush yourself constantly — "oh this and oh that . . . I must see that I do this and then that, because otherwise my boat will capsize!" You will have to learn to "let go" and begin to search for your inner, solid basis in such a way that you no longer have to keep yourself nervously fixated on things.

Inner insecurity gnaws; the doubt: "What shall I do? Shall I come out with it — with myself, my words, my *true* I — or not? Am I really allowed to be myself? But, no: I will first see if my suit or my dress fits 'properly.'" This staying at the surface, or outside, of life — at the superficial thinking side, or too strongly and purely and alone in the spirit — makes you feel anxious: go searching for your heart, for your deep foundation, and live from within, very pure and simple and more natural, more impulsive!

Not being spontaneously yourself, not trusting in the natural flow of energies in yourself. This fixating yourself in "thought" on certain points inside you, is reflected in your attitude regarding the "outer world." "Shall I keep myself hidden in my room, in my head, or shall I step out, self-assuredly and "sensible," with a "reasonable" attitude of life? How will I explain it to THEM?" (Instead of just being yourself!) A kind of fear — stage fright, perhaps — of confrontation with others. Wanting to step outward with an attitude that is too tight, too stiff; you already clear your throat, hyper-nervously. Afraid that the unstable balance in you, the "peace," might be disturbed, that others might not understand you or approve of you, that you might start feeling very uncomfortable when you speak and behave the way you feel: you take others, the reaction of society, too much into account.

"Do I do right? What shall I do?" You'd almost chew down your nails; nervousness goes to your head, affects your total nervous system. Considering things back and forth till you can't anymore. It makes us think somewhat of the "Libra"-element. Anxiety: "What will they say? What will they do?" And as a result you behave accordingly. Tension, too much taking into account the following: "How are they going to react, or are they going to accuse me, question me — will I be able to deal with this?" Certain people will accommodate their entire behavior and lifestyle to their environment, whereby they deviate further and further from their "inner feeling," from their own inner nature! The throat calls for self-acknowledgment, for inner dignity, for a complete descent into your body. Perhaps a situation just has occurred in your life, or you had to do something about which you feel guilty and think you at least have to explain/account for it to others. This is not true! Don't make your security and happiness dependent on something that lies outside your inner basic "I." Come close to yourself! Deep inside, you feel guilty because you don't answer enough to Life in yourself, don't turn yourself enough inward. All the rest is a result of this.

Dare to express yourself the way you *are*, the way you feel about it very deeply inside yourself. Just BE YOURSELF, without caring what others will say about it. You don't owe anyone an explanation, not even for something that has "happened," or for a decision you make — not for your "appearance," not for the way you act. Only you make decisions about your life, and others have nothing to do with it: it's of course the object of Life that you live from out of your Heart, in self-assuredness and trust. First, establish that solid, Secure Basis in yourself. Know that you don't have to be ashamed of anything or nervous about anything — as long as you live according to "the truth" and are yourself in all honesty.

Therefore, don't force yourself in anything. Just be yourself. First, turn deeply inward and don't "think" too much on a low, nervous level. Open yourself up to that which is highest in you, allowing those energies that are too red to escape from your head. Step outward, amongst the people, from out of the highest feelings inside you. You never have to "prepare" something; you never have to "take into account." You don't have to have any fear of others — not to accommodate or please them (let go of this power too): as long as you live honestly from out of yourself; as long as you know that you have only one fundamental responsibility: Love toward yourself and be yourself in truth. Not ARTIFICIALLY and calculated, but NATURAL, honest, and spontaneous!

No one can floor you; only you can pull yourself down. Don't pay any attention at all to what society has to say about you. Dare to dismiss the "official, artificial" nonsense and at all times be yourself.

MANIFEST YOURSELF WITH YOUR TRUE "I" AND ALLOW THOSE emotional ENERGIES TO FLOW. Don't only live from out of your head, thoughts, spirit; don't escape from your total incarnation! Dare to say the Truth that comes from within you, and don't bother about: "What will they say?" "How do I have to proceed?" "Oh, they are going to bomb me, taunt or attack me." Don't hide. Show yourself in all simplicity, in true form. No longer try to "keep yourself in balance" like this, like a circus performer on a "rotating tube," as if you can fall off at any moment — but come outward in an assertive way, proud of your goodness, your living force, in self-assuredness, from the fundamentally strong basis that is inside you. You now fearlessly manifest yourself and don't care at all what others will say about it: you are you — you live from within, without anxiously fretting. You now acknowledge your full Worthiness, standing solidly on your feet, taking responsibility for yourself, your words, your deeds. And because you do everything with heart, nothing or no one will frighten you anymore; you won't fear confusion, rejection, or battles outside yourself. Because you now have made a peaceful alliance with yourself, have unified yourself with yourself; because you now experience yourself as STRONG, straightforward, on a fundamentally strong basis. Feet on the earth, chest out, head high, energies flowing from the warmly radiating heart. All the rest is of minor importance. You raise yourself in all pride, not according to false norms or "what one expects of you" or according to "that which you think you MUST do because one expects it that way from you." You are NOT ACCOUNTABLE TO ANYONE; you don't at all have to behave this way or that way: be yourself, like a divine human being, acknowledging himself, powerful, unbeatable, solid and steadfast in the Faith of YOUR wonderful "I" Basis Center.

No single stiff, tense attitude, strictly tied within structural lines, exists anymore. You are now FREE, yourself, and allow your honest energies to flow freely, because you have let go of everything and everyone around you, and from now on live out of a fundamentally strong faith that everything in life will happen the way it is best for you. You let go, and come to inner peace; you no

longer force yourself for the sake of the outer world; you now live from out of your deepest emotional nature, very deep and warm, from your heartfelt basis of life, relaxed and self-assured. The "controlling aspect" has disappeared; you allow yourself to "be," fully, from within.

EPIPHYSIS
pineal gland

Psychological correspondence

Just as a vase can hold flowers, so does the epiphysis stand open for the filling of its content: it's an important link, a contact point, for both sensory impressions from the outer world and for experiences from our inner Self. Images we observe from the outer world can take concrete form in our inner eye and be transmitted to the entire body. Also via the epiphysis, we are able to grasp the total existence of our present being, the here-and-now of our self. The Lion roars in its complete power of life-awareness; the cock crows out the glory and joy of the present moment.

Nothing ethereal is sought after by the functioning of the epiphysis; one should not too much consider this organ as being essentially "spiritual." Also because of the working of the epiphysis, we, as human beings, strongly comprehend our power, our "being," from head to foot in earthly life. Just as strongly, we experience our divinity, our deep inner knowing, our intuition; a meeting point between heaven and earth, between matter and psyche, between external and internal. This gland is like a central tower in a network of high-voltage wires; it's the receiving pool for earthly observations; it impels us toward the earth; intense contact with the world around us immediately resonates with our inner emotional world, with the memory in our brain, the past, our total content. The epiphysis functions here like a funnel and is in direct contact with the hypophysis and the other glands of our body.

I Am: also via a physical organ, the gland (epiphysis), we become strongly aware of "being on earth" with our feet on the ground. This is possible because of the fact that the epiphysis stands open to our total soul content, to our inner Self, and allows this non-material being of ourselves to have a look, making contact with the material, the earthly. A balance is being sought between the earthly and the psychological or the content of a human being or an animal.

One can't consider the epiphysis separately from the brain, nor from the other glands: there is constant cooperation. Also, the epiphysis is susceptible to — yes, immediately under the influence of — changes in the human psyche: the glands are a translation of the inner Self. The epiphysis gives a reflection of the inner light and is also able to receive the Light of the outer world. Insofar as we evolve regarding "reception of the inner light," the epiphysis will react to this and possibly change its form and discharge certain hormones to a lesser or greater extent. The same goes for the influences from the outside.

The following is important: the epiphysis will be healthy insofar as we don't close ourselves off from the feeling that gives us light — "the joy of living" — and from the consciousness of living in a light, happy environment: if only we maintain the balance between soul and body, the epiphysis, like a yellow Easter daffodil, is able to totally fill our head and psychological field with an enormous blossoming, joyful, radiating flower-chalice. Consciously happy to be on earth.

Yet, there's *more* than head, epiphysis, or sphere-experiences in the brain.

What does it avail if you have a head but no heart, a psyche without love? This "light yellow" joy for life requires a "warm, red"

presence in our heart, with both feet on the magnetic earth. The epiphysis is only a link. It is self-evident that this true "joy of life" arrives at a new dimension when the spontaneous, the lively, the happiness for existence itself — the way animals also experience it — are nourished by a feeling of love, of warmth, of being able to choose a higher feeling of peace, "a self-aware human existence in Love": truly becoming aware is therefore only possible via an inner propelling force, via the longing of our deepest Self for growth. This inner engine, our eternal Living Self, finds its channels in our total body, not only in the epiphysis. The heart and the thymus gland are symbolic of the warm, loving, peaceful autonomy of a human being: these are in direct contact with the epiphysis.

One can't be unlinked from the other.

Ailments, in general

By becoming more aware in daily life, by development of personal Love toward ourselves and others, by wisdom and evolution, one will automatically come to a new state of consciousness without having to especially stimulate the epiphysis and other glands!

Forcing the epiphysis via certain drugs, certain yoga exercises, or other tricks, by which you force yourself, is harmful for your health. Through artificially stimulating the epiphysis, one achieves an artificially light state of consciousness and internal and external senses are being extremely stimulated. The sending out of impulses by the epiphysis via hormones, among other things, influences the body in its totality, and also the brain; one arrives at super-sensitive psychological state of being, but in an unnatural way. Here, one sins against the necessary balance, against the natural spontaneous growth of the human being. The harmony between psyche and earth has been broken; the epiphysis can function in a healthy way only via a gradual discovery of the earthly life and an equally steady discovery of the inner self. This can only happen in Life, itself, step-by-step, under the supervision of the heart. A change in the epiphysis, in the state of consciousness of a human being, is negative and harmful if it doesn't happen SPONTANEOUSLY and if it doesn't come FROM THE HEART and IN-SIGHT!!!

Epiphysis, overactivity, overproduction

Out of anxiety and because of insufficient trust in your own strong earthly Basis, you might start looking for security in the great "Universal Mother," or in a "paranormal" sphere, in which you might call up all kinds of spirit things. But because you are afraid of your self, you might also attract unpleasant images.

Your emotional side is going wild because you have too little contact with the earth, with your body: you withdraw into the spiritual. You are afraid of certain things; you see certain things, which for others are not really there, because your anxiety has created them.

You believe too little in your own Power over yourself, and then you are afraid of the "Power," death, the negativity surrounding you — you are not aware that this is pure self-projection, caused by your anxieties.

Your awareness is there, but cut off from the rest of your body and petrified, without being nourished by the warm heart, the love. Therefore, also, it is dangerous to do certain spiritual exercises without first having, in love, discovered yourself: the epiphysis that functions too intensely, without your having kept sufficient contact with your total Self — your warm body and your warm heart — can have insane consequences; this leads to chilliness, not to life. Life requires being completely present; we won't be a "ghost, spirit entity, or dead"! Your basis is too weak; you feel unsafe in yourself; you cut yourself off from the earthly and might flee into the spiritual, into spiritism or channeling: wrong! You find true wisdom in yourself: therefore, descend totally into life, in your body.

Experience that gentle peace from out of your warm heart: *feel* life flow through your veins. Turn yourself one hundred percent toward the earth and place the basis in your strong Self. No one has more mastery and power over you than do you! Feel the heart beating in Nature.

Epiphysis, diminished or insufficient activity or production

You are afraid of your intuition; you don't really dare explore your inner richness.

You strongly limit the experiencing of reality: you put up borders; you put limitations on yourself; there are taboos for you. You might be busy with material things, with "the buying of food"; you live rather impersonally and mechanically, or totally indoctrinated, you live superficially. You dwell inside yourself and fulfill certain actions or tasks, but there is no question of *true* awareness. You've tied yourself down; you are not at all connected with your inner Source; you live in a vacuum. . . . You barely stand on your own feet, and are a little like a robot or a zombie. . . . This is all because of the lack of belief in yourself: you stand on unsteady ground, and to build a life on your loose basis wouldn't be possible, so you remain on the surface, in the footsteps of others, of the masses, of your mother.

Achieve strong trust in yourself and for once feel deeper, higher: feel there is more than matter or superficiality. Dare to go on, to break through; dare to question certain matters of life; research and turn deeply inward. Feel safe and secure in your nest; know that inside you there burns a powerful lamp, your personal Awareness, your immortal "I," which you can always count on. Build up your life, no longer cut off from this rich source; don't limit yourself to pure rationality, nor to superficial materialism, but open yourself up to your inner senses, through which true wisdom can reveal itself. Bore through: inward and outward. Discover Life to the fullest.

DISTURBANCES OF EQUILIBRIUM

You lose yourself too much in secondary things, details; you feel overwhelmed by a lot of trivialities. Perhaps you spend too much time on your outer image, your appearance, or on superficial things.

You don't only hold on too much to details, but above all you hold on to a lot of feelings: there is a refusal to allow your feelings, your heart energies, to stream through smoothly. You force yourself. You've been given a lot to swallow, but you bottle up all your sadness. You don't see things clearly anymore.

You grasp onto a lot, things and people, because of doubts regarding yourself: you look for the answers outside yourself. On the other hand, you let yourself be seized, let yourself be drawn down to the bottom, because you're too much absent in yourself!

There is a resistance to truly going on, to evolving; you are not steady on your feet, not sure about your content: you might fall. . . .

It might be that you've "thrown" yourself into something with full force — perhaps a direction, an engagement, a job, a study — and you can't stop yourself anymore. It was too early. Or it's too much for you. You feel powerless to get a grip on it. Anxious, unsure — what now?

Even if you bear heavy loads, mountains of feelings: go on upon your own feet, don't hold yourself back, but arrive at Awareness of your Mastery. Say resolutely, "I will do it MYSELF, will allow all energies to come through, and now will let go of everything." Illuminate everything from above; in self-assuredness, feel your Center; no one can determine your life. Dare to wade through all your feelings and enjoy in love, in joy. Don't pay attention to affirmation from others, for details, but be aware of your unique worth and no longer doubt your possibilities. Clearly and precisely, determine the important things in your life yourself; don't let yourself be put off stride by others. Open your heart and your lungs so that you don't put yourself in the position of being without air or love.

ESOPHAGUS

Psychological correspondence

Granting yourself a substantial passage: gliding through beautifully in life. The road from caterpillar to butterfly starts here in the esophagus: through openness, through dealing with experiences you transform into a further stage of your development. In a relaxed but proud, self-aware way, you allow yourself to climb up.

Your "I," the central inner Authority, knows how to keep a balance in your emotional world and your thought world; you don't keep "holding on," you trust in yourself; you feel safe in your deepest Self. You are on the right track, ON A STRAIGHT COURSE, which keeps the balance between heaven and Earth, between spirit and body. In reverence for your divine worth as a human being, you fight for beautiful ideals: you don't let yourself sink into inconsequential things, into emotions, into the past. You feel "fixed," concentrated, consciously present in yourself. You surrender to that which is the most beautiful, the most "sacred," in yourself.

Ailments, in general

You don't allow yourself to go on, to evolve. You don't trust in the inner Authority; you lean on others. You don't really follow your own Path; you deviate from it by not truly living from out of your heart, your longings;

you hide yourself — behind your parents or those who are close to you, behind laws, systems, programming from the past, behind the material, behind the outer screen. . . . Do you hold on to superficial, material, structural or external values? Do you refuse to explore your own depths? Do you want to gobble up too much at once because of a strong desire-urge in earthly life, without giving attention to the energies of consciousness in yourself? You can't go on because you don't acknowledge that which is most beautiful, most powerful in yourself. You don't *truly* live! You don't really look at life; possibly, you want to reach too *far,* but you want too much and so you fall. Allow yourself to grow peacefully, from the here-and-now! No longer hold on emotionally to the past, to inconsequential things; go on in a self-aware way! Accept new impressions, open yourself up, deal flexibly with your emotions and be proud of your divine essence. Follow that honest, straight path of LIFE; live truthfully with yourself. Speak truth.

Cramps, spasms of the esophagus

You don't dare to really come through; you withdraw. You deny your true Self. Inner emotional tensions; you bottle up too much; you refuse to bring your "I" outward or to push through in *that* direction which you sense is in line with your true nature. Too much flexibility; you bend in such a way that you are no longer faithful to yourself, perhaps in order to keep peace or friendship with others. Possibly, you carry great responsibilities, also for others, and you go beyond your own boundaries; you live too little from out of yourself, too much from out of, or in conformity with, others. You suppress your feelings with rules and rationalities; you destroy your "I." You subordinate yourself to structures or people. Anxious suppression of natural powers, which come from the

depth of your being. You don't resolutely, in love for yourself, determine your path — based on your longings; you doubt yourself, your worth, too much. You make your existence dependent on something or someone outside yourself; you keep yourself tensely closed, or you twist into all sorts of bends.

Don't neglect your core; express your feelings. Say what you have to say. Mark off your terrain and live in reverence for yourself! Acknowledge your worth and your possibilities; don't, first of all, live in conformity with others, with social norms, but live from out of your spontaneous nature. No longer hide, don't hold back: GIVE, offer warmth and feeling to yourself and to your fellow man. FEEL that warm, giving Source in you.

Don't be afraid. Trust in your deepest Self. Don't do anything that conflicts with yourself. Open your "I" in social contacts and dare to show yourself the way you are, the way you inwardly feel; be honest, and also express your aggressive powers, so that you don't block yourself. Action, creativity, expression, an open exchange of feelings. I AM.

Esophageal obstruction

A signal from your Living Self: you can't keep living in this way. Stop! You feel like a powerless child, in the grip of something or someone, because of which you sweat mortal fear. You are not your own boss; you don't really live from out of your feelings, your longings, your heart; you "do" things you think you *must* do according to the norms of others or according to your personal thoughts and convictions. With your thoughts you fixate yourself, you completely get "stuck": You don't allow yourself to flexibly evolve. You are so afraid of being who you are because you don't trust your nature! "Who am I really??" Anxieties.

You feel unprotected in yourself.

You can't go back in a situation; you have to go on, but you don't dare. Intense aggressive powers suppressed for too long suddenly put up a barricade. Your emotions paralyze you into immobility. Possibly, you feel threatened by a crushing authority from your father, an organization, a phobia or an obsession. . . . It holds you fast, it doesn't let go of you anymore. You don't see a clear way out because you don't believe in your intuition or in your feelings. You don't let yourself go. You anxiously block all natural energies; you are afraid of your own deepest content. It all becomes too much for you; you can't swallow it anymore. You don't go onward.

Nothing can seize you, if only you put trust in your Living Self. Become master over your emotions, your anxieties. Seize your energies yourself and create your life in a self-aware way. Authority lies in you, don't place it outside yourself. Choose a radical solution: liberate yourself, your feelings, your longings; listen to this and direct these powers in you!

Don't allow yourself to be stuck fast, don't be afraid of those beautiful depths in yourself. Dare to realize yourself without hesitation! Don't fixate on the negative; LIVE from your heart, from your true nature, not purely from "thoughts" or from superficial, illusory motives. No longer let anxieties dominate your life! Take up your scepter and become aware of your possibilities: go onward!

Gastro-esophageal reflux
in babies and adults
abnormal flow-back of stomach content toward esophagus (and further to the mouth perhaps); in state of wakefulness or during sleep; causes heartburn

Swept along from here to there, full of foaming energies, full of primal female creative forces, but overpowered by them. These creative forces can manifest themselves in the urge to "do" something, to create, to come to creativity. A kind of being over

powered by a mass of energies, where it's best to "do" something with them as soon as possible: *not in desiring, wanting to grasp, wanting to "fill" oneself with all kinds of things or people, but in an active, creative self-development.* An urge for pleasure, strong desire, is the result when a human being cannot yet completely experience and realize his Fullness. Being overwhelmed by these energies, by this current of water, can only happen as long as the human being can't go forward in life as master and be his own leader: *doing what he feels he has to do under the guidance of the Heart, not under pressure from instinctive or desiring urges.*

For Young and Old, therefore, it's of the utmost importance to do something creative with the churning forces in one's own being — directing oneself in goodness; transforming instincts and desires into creativeness and love. *Not grasping and drawing in . . . but GIVING and DOING.* A lesson that a baby has to learn at a very young age; a lesson that mentors or adults should master. Don't let yourself become whipped up by desires and the urge for pleasure, but enjoy life while creating, in self-realization, staying in the here-and-now. *Don't run ahead of things, but intensely stay with yourself and allow to be that which wants to be in you.* Don't fill yourself, but *allow your talents to blossom . . . without desire, without forcing anything.* Give guidance to your healthy, primal female creative energies, which are burning to be allowed to create, to give. Don't long to posses, draw in, attract, submerge in pleasure, but do what Life in you asks from you, and enjoy fully the Being — the Becoming — who you *are*, step by step, without impatience. ***DON'T LONG TO "HAVE" OR "DO" TOO MUCH AT ONCE, NEITHER IN YOUR FEELINGS NOR WITH YOUR THINKING, WHICH MIGHT FIXATE ITSELF ON CERTAIN GOALS . . .*** *but turn the energies inside out, as it were: bring yourself to realization in a*

*constructive way; the animal aspect con-
quered, the human aspect takes shape.*

*   *   *

Are you ashamed of the energies that are inside you? Do you feel longing energies in
your lower abdomen? Are the female creative forces foaming in your abdomen and do
you not know what to do with them? You
experience this as if you are being stirred up
in the surf, as if you are being thrown here
and there by the swirling water, like someone
insignificant. You don't really know if it is
good what you feel, whether this is about
normal, foaming energies and feelings, or
about sexual longings. Know, then, that it's
your body that asks for a kind of (re)birth,
and at the same time for a complete application of all the *primal forces* that are inside
you.

Don't be ashamed of those fiery creative
forces that are manifesting themselves, but
handle them in the right way. Experience the
enjoyment in and about yourself as something sound and good. This can only happen
if, at the same time, you open yourself in
Love toward your total Self, when you live in
goodness toward others. On top of that, your
body, your total being, asks you *to become
yourself in an active, vigorous, creative way*.
Don't fill yourself with things, with others;
don't withdraw into a hiding place, nor abandon yourself to greedy "filling." You can
make yourself happy by using those creative
forces in a constructive way: in the construction of your own being.

Don't fixate on the lower regions, on the
forces from the lower abdomen, but get them
involved in the Total Life-experience, in the
creativity as well as in the experience of love
with a possible partner.

You attract this kind of a signal so that
you will LOOK at the Female Primal Energies that dwell inside you in order to lift
them up to a Higher Level, to a level of true
Love. Sexuality, for instance, is only beneficial where it exists in the function of Love

and Creation. If, however, it only exists
purely on the animalistic level of self-
gratification, not under the mantle of love for
oneself and in service of self-development,
then it will have a burning effect on your
body. Therefore: surrender to that which is
HIGHEST in yourself; break with the lower
animalistic remnants in yourself. Dare to experience your body in the name of Love, and
don't be ashamed of it. Shame is the result
of not being really convinced that you live
and exist and act IN LOVE, but are still on a
level of desire, of an animal, of drawing-in
and being drawn in.

*Therefore, solve the deepest problem by
tuning in to Higher, Generous Love, and
THEN you will feel happy in allowing the
creative forces to flow freely.* Then you can
truly bear beautiful fruits: then you become
the creative person you actually already are.
*The potential of primal creative forces inside
you is very great, but you don't stand enough
at the RUDDER of the ship, so that you are
being thrown back and forth by that mass of
primal female energies — possibly at the
mercy of pleasure, emotions, ambitious desires, urging thoughts or instincts (compare
here the symbolism of the number 5). Now
stand at the Head of your life and be conscious of the fact that you are Master over
your energies, that you have the right to
guide and direct these forces to a higher,
lovingly giving level. Live in the PRESENT
moment; don't live in thoughts about the future.*

In babies this also indicates that there's *a
mass of fundamental female creative energies that can't immediately manifest themselves in action and creativity; an instinctive
desiring urge sometimes to give itself
"pleasure." Also wanting to "grasp" with
its little head; in their feelings/thoughts, it's
all not happening fast enough.* Regarding
the parents, it's good that they read the text
above because there are always reasons
whenever one attracts a baby, like a mirror
— this mirror wants to make something

clear. Allow the child to enjoy itself; when it's hungry, make sure it gets enough good food (also solid food), so that already on this level a kind of healthy psychological "balance" is being achieved! Don't put it on a "diet." Moreover, everything will go much better once the child becomes active, can walk, can actively interact with things, build houses with blocks, sing, make music, etc.. When it begins to realize it should not "grasp" for things, should not "fill" itself with things in animalistic desire, but can grow up in love while truly creating.

It is good from the start to give the child, the growing baby, the nourishment it needs and not deny it anything on the basis of so-called rational health rules.[1] The child may quickly become aware that it may tune in to its heart, to its Being, to the actively being-itself, that it shouldn't turn to the lower animal level, nor has to hold itself in regarding creative safety valves! It will ultimately feel that it can apply its energies in a masterful way, without having to "be lived" by them.

It then is no longer being STIRRED UP by wanting to have/achieve, by (be it unconsciously flowing) thoughts, by whirling instincts, energies: it is at the rudder of its ship, actively stepping outward, creative, expressive, and doesn't store anything up inside itself — so that energy can flow freely while still being directed, and can contribute in this way to a fruitful, creative existence. Desires make way for an active, dynamic existence, full of love. And this of course also goes for the mentors, the adults, who are an Example for the child in this. Becoming a Human Being in the fullest sense of the word asks for masterful guidance of Energy, for a transformation of instinct into consciousness, of desire into love power. Only in this way will the human being no longer fill himself or "draw in" in an urge for pleasure; he breaks through this phase of dependence on the primal womb, no longer clamps on to it with lust, but begins to search for true Happiness,

which has nothing to do with the original, instinctive urge for pleasure. He now feeds himself in love and eats what he likes; he becomes himself, strongly and Consciously; he GIVES, and no longer desires. He fully enjoys his Life in a new way. The animal is gone; the Human Being is born. Powerfully creating, producing, proud of his "I," no longer "curled up" in self-gratification, chained to the primal womb, but OPENLY RADIATING like a magnificent Sunflower. He truly radiates outward. He feels wonderful in this abundantly giving, in this creating outward, no longer "locked up" in the tunnel of his pleasure-intoxicated animal behavior. He is actively creating and happy about his radiating "I"-POWER! He goes onward; nothing overwhelms him anymore; he has both reins of his life in hand and leads his Life in Love, with resolution and awareness!

EYES — EYESIGHT

Psychological symbolism and Ailments, in general

Like two brilliant suns, they radiate the content of your being.

The eyes symbolize being open to your inner Self, to the divine, peaceful light within you, the receiving with open hands of beautiful consciousness energies, of impulses from the depths of your Self. They reflect the warmth of your soul's heart and also your inner wisdom.

They represent the measure in which you as an outer ego have a sound and harmonious contact with your inner Self: being *yourself* in powerful unity.

Your eyes serve as a passageway from outside to inside: To what degree do you close yourself off, build up a defensive shield, not allow any new impressions to come in? Or, are you open, full of self-

---

[1] Read more about this in *The Horn of Plenty.*

confidence and aspiration, to that which is new? Seeing clearly into yourself and being able to "comprehend" or understand clearly the situation you are in.

Fear, anxieties — because one doesn't "see" clearly; insufficient trust.

The eyes reflect to what degree you acknowledge or deny your inner Self, your sun-center. Are you only directed toward the outer world, toward appearance, toward glitter and matter, or do you see everything as it *actually* is, and do you look deeper, under the surface?

Do you, full of anxiety or anger, look too much at details or at problems? Your eyes will reflect joy as well as sadness, your depth or superficiality. Symbol of communicative transferal: do you close the "door" to others? Do you look at them aggressively or critically? Are you the same way toward yourself? To what degree do you radiate toward others your self-contentment, your sun-warmth?

Or, with regard to others, do you use or misuse your eyes as an instrument — power, domination, temptation, compulsion? Do you manipulate yourself or others?

Does Anxiety hinder you from looking deep inside yourself, from acknowledging your feelings and sharing them with others? Do you shield yourself from your own deep emotions? Do you flee? Or inversely do you drown in your emotions and can't look further than the mire in which you find yourself now? Then, this means only that you have insufficient trust in your deepest Self: that you have to look deeper to find that unshakable, joyful core of yourself.

An optimistic look at the future is only possible when you are in deep contact with your creative Self, when you are aware of the possibilities of building your life *yourself,* when you no longer SEE things that are not there, such as Destiny, the devil, an idol, guilt or penance, etc.

Truly seeing clearly means peace, joy, warmth; receiving this atmosphere from your

deepest Self and radiating it outward via the Eyes.

Symbol of *self-LIBERATION, a clear, open look through inner freedom: don't imprison yourself in emotions, in dark brooding, in self-destructive aggression. . . . The freedom to be yourself, faithful to your true nature; allowing your feelings to flow freely; the freedom to turn your eyes in the direction which will bring the most joy for you; no longer fixating yourself on the past, on those things which are best to be let go of.*

When you direct your glance inwardly at that which is most beautiful in yourself, then your eyes will also see outer circumstances that mirror this. Do you consider yourself bad? Then unconsciously you look for confirmation of this in the outer world. If you are aware of the goodness in the core of yourself, then you will notice the goodness around you.

Honest Insight into yourself and others; *don't fool yourself;* dare to evolve. Your eyes will tell it.

LEFT EYE

Ailments, in general;
tearing, possibly discharging pus

Emotionally, you are "stuck" on something: emotions push through and require clear sight, a solution. In a frustrated way, you hold on to certain things (as if you are cultivating warts on your palms: read the subject Warts); you look at yourself, your emotions with amazement. Possibly, you don't have a very nice idea about your content, your feelings. Don't you trust your feelings? Possibly, you then start to "cling" emotionally to your partner, to your relations. Mostly, it has to do with looking for security in the "female" outside yourself because you don't have a clear picture of the "female" inside yourself. Possibly, it has to do with mistrust, anxiety, regarding your own unconscious Content, regarding your inner world. You might be afraid of your own ground; you then look at yourself with misty vision, with a weak feeling.

You still live too much in the "spiritual lap" of the mother. And actually you'd rather stay hidden, sitting quietly in the Egg: you don't allow yourself to Freely be born. The eye, however, calls for emotional liberation! To be able to stand free and happy on your own feet, not bound to another, not bound in emotional dependence to another (which has nothing to do with Love). Yes, also the other, that partner or that mother with whom you have a "tie," only reacts to your trait of wanting to be bound to a sort of lap, from which you don't want to get up.

You don't really trust your emotions: possibly, because of this, you keep yourself "closed." But these feelings, these spontaneous life powers, require a free and open existence: that you no longer might be so much on guard, in watchful, instinctive behavior; that you might no longer keep yourself oppressed. That you might begin to feel good in your skin, in the flow of your emotions. That you will integrate that which one calls the female element, so that you don't have to cling to "female" figures in your environment, or react against them because you feel threatened.

Possibly, you oppress yourself in situations where you have to CHOOSE when you don't see how to choose: will you choose in favor of what you *feel* and in favor of your well-being, or will you "give in" to your partner, to the wishes of your parents? Or do you have to choose between two kinds of relationships? Between two people? The lesson here is that you can't love your fellow man if you don't first take care of yourself, in Self-love. But you mistrust yourself, and you make yourself emotionally dependent on another or others, so that you can't choose in favor of YOURSELF. And that is what really matters for your liberation: now choose inner freedom and don't keep yourself "stuck" any longer. In this way, you

won't "enslave" yourself in oppressive ties any longer. Love has nothing to do with any of this — free yourself, and live like a human being who is inwardly Free.

The female aspect forces itself emphatically on you, inside you as well as outside: whether it is by compulsively being sexually attracted or by being flooded with emotions. Emotionally, you can then be tossed back and forth: "What do I do with my anxieties, with my feelings?" The symbol of "the woman" might be pursuing you. In an extreme situation, you can't control your emotions; you have no perspective on them and don't know how to direct them in an harmonious way. You then place yourself in a position of Powerlessness regarding these feelings — the female, the free life-powers in yourself.

It seems that under this authority you are sliding away, out of control. It seems to you then that you are no longer in charge of your own life: you'd prefer to hide in a mother's lap — you don't want to see anymore! But this is anything but a solution. You deny that deep source-power in yourself.

Trust those life-powers which flow through you and let yourself go: surrender to your great Self, to Life in yourself. Your emotions know themselves to be safely secure in that strong, carrying power of your Self. Externalize! Bring out those living powers and allow your feelings to flow freely! Don't grasp at another person, outside yourself, but come now fully into your own being. Now, cut off those dead branches! (the roads that don't lead anywhere but to death — read the book *New Days*) No longer hide your "I" behind someone else, behind a partner or behind a sexual relationship to which you've tied yourself down. Don't lose yourself in another or in anything else.

When you "let go," you are being confronted with yourself, with your feelings: you now need to avail yourself of these feelings in a constructive way. Now, don't SUPPRESS your forces, your feelings, so that they don't overpower you, so that you don't need to look for an outlet for what you hold on to (in sexuality, in a flood of tears, in incontinence, in ejaculation . . .). Your feelings, your life forces, ask to be permitted to EXPRESS themselves, to LIVE fully, to exist freely! No more "stifling," no more outlet valves: don't suck yourself onto things or people anymore, but bring yourself outward! Don't experience yourself as being small and weak compared to the great-femininity that is outside you — which possibly you have placed upon a Throne. Instead, integrate this femininity into yourself. EXTERIORIZE — with a centrifugal force, from out of your inner Power-source — all worthy energies and feelings. Become yourself in an active way, without hesitation. Speak, if you have something to say; express yourself! Don't allow those spontaneous forces to accumulate inside you! Go out into Nature: into your nature, and feel good in it. Trust in your Self, without having to ask questions in a worried way regarding your content, regarding life. You know that you, yourself, determine the path of your life according to your convictions. You are taking your life in hand, without anxieties.

You will find out that if you remove the "plug" that blocks your flow of feelings, your feelings will spontaneously resolve themselves and won't be as overwhelming as you feared. So, express yourself, don't hold back, no longer put the brakes on life; be spontaneous, sing and laugh, be yourself in your Feelings! If you want to weep, then look at your sadness and resolve it. Only you can make yourself happy: the circumstances in your life now are only the result of your attitude to life. If you don't like those circumstances, then bring about change inside yourself so that your surroundings will undergo changes as a result.

Sadness only indicates that you are not yet really HAPPY about yourself, that you don't yet LIVE in the feeling of Thankful-

ness about your "I," about your Being. You will be happy if you don't put Conditions on life: "I will only be happy if I have this or that. . ." On the path of "wanting to have" and desire, you will never find happiness. If, however, you come into your joyful Being, everything that is good for you will appear on your path. Therefore, TRUST, believe in your goodness and in your spontaneous energies, and let go: only THIS will definitively dry up tears, because you are content in yourself. Connected with your Inner Source, you will know how to trust your Intuition, how to trust what you *feel:* every Anxiety, every sorrow, has now disappeared. New, optimistic perspectives are opening up to you!

Your emotional forces are not being suppressed; you express yourself in a creative way, living life to the fullest. You now dare to fully swim in the waters of Life and enjoy its warmth, because you now feel safely sheltered — as an Autonomous human being — in the womb of your Self, which is full of love. A life in Joy!

(Regarding suppuration, read the category Suppuration.)

RIGHT EYE

Ailments, in general;
tearing, possibly discharging pus

An urgent call for a Solid Grounding of yourself. With the force of the "right side" you push yourself, as it were, very strongly into yourself. With assertiveness, energetic action. . . . Now you decide to plant yourself resolutely in the Earth!

If your right eye tears, then this means that the life energies in you want to strongly "pull you into yourself." Don't cling to Authority or Structures outside yourself, but establish this Pillar solidly in yourself: concentrate these life-powers in yourself, in your body. Take yourself in; don't grasp at other people, don't try to "pull in" other people.

Don't *allow* the life-powers (and the feelings) to "flood you," but integrate them solidly in yourself under the self-assured Authority of your Conscious "I." You need to designate a "place" in yourself for the water of life: you need to Steer this flow! So, deal resolutely with every feeling (with every conviction) of being Unable to Lead yourself, to put all life-powers in yourself under your Authority.

You want to purify your Eye in order to be able to see more clearly: "Which convictions are still living in me, because of which I again and again have the feeling that I can't really get a 'grip' on myself? Who am I? Where am I going? How can I direct my life?" This uncertainty now requires a breakthrough of self-awareness, a decisiveness: that self-doubt may now cease to exist!

No longer look in a weak or emotional way at yourself, at your life — you're not at all a sad, incapable child. SEE CLEARLY! THAT FORMIDABLE, DIVINE POWER in you calls for acknowledgment. Here, we're talking about the self-core, which knows that Life means JOY when you see clearly into yourself, into your ability to create your life yourself. If you become aware of this Content, then you won't weep one more moment.

You see as through a haze, unclearly — as long as you maintain in yourself the lie which says that happiness is not meant for you, and that joy doesn't really belong to this Earth. You need to destroy this Counterforce in yourself.

(Read the chapter regarding this subject in our book *New Days*.)

Originally, what was meant by the term "water" was primitive or animal energies, which now require that they be used in a human, correct way: it's up to the human being to rise above this "unconscious" state, to become, as a Self-aware "I," master over these magnetic powers. Certainly not to remain stuck in a feeling of "desires," longings. . . . If uncertainty about one's own Basis still exists, and there are anxieties regarding this — and also anxiety about loneliness — then one instinctively begins to desire, to grab

hold. The Self-aware Human Being lives with clear Insight and in Trust.

In uncertainty, one clings fast to a Basis outside oneself; one would leave, as it were, one's own base! This actually has to do with a "sadness" about not being able to come closer to one's own Core, one's own Basis, because one doesn't Believe enough in it; as a result, one anchors oneself in another; but in this case one also might feel sadness because one has the feeling of being unable to come close to another: then it has to do with a projection of one's own inability. Firmly make that unifying bond with yourself!

Enormous powers radiate from the lowest vertebrae, the lower abdomen, and the thighs; as long as they don't have a Self-assured "I" at their Basis, however, they can't exist sufficiently freely and creatively; but instead they are subjected to the influence of anxieties and the feeling of being without structure, not solidly in oneself as a human being. One has the feeling one is dangling somewhere in the empty, dark cosmos, and is about to fall into Nothingness. . . . Instead of being able to exist in a state of gladness, these enormous energies are being called into question: should they be allowed to be there? Is it possible that the person concerned is Angry with these powers in himself, or with the Body into which they have cast themselves?

Allow the bodily forms and the energies represented therein to exist Freely! Arrive at your own Power and be proud of yourself!

Allow these energies to blossom in the Light of Life! Let go of others and pick your own fruits! Look at that which is beautiful, the beautiful in yourself. Keep that radiating Joy in yourself going: for yourself! As an autonomous being, direct your emotions, your powers, in certainty and trust. Don't place yourself UNDER someone; don't hang on a partner; left and right in balance, the partnership in yourself! Put all power over your life in yourself. Don't let another lead you away from your Joy. . . . Don't be sad because This or That is not in your life the way you WANT IT TO BE, or because your partner or your parents or your children don't give you what you "EXPECT" from them. Now you know that if you trustingly decide TO BE — if you no longer "desire" something or expect something from others — then everything that is good for your evolution will appear automatically on your path. Such desiring and the related disappointments make your eyes tear. You can only make YOURSELF happy — let go of others. Now, come closer to your own joyful soul-core, after which you will automatically come "closer" to your fellow man. Now be convinced that no sadness need make your life miserable: CHOOSE Joy, so that ultimately you no longer attract sad circumstances.

Crawl DEEPLY INTO YOURSELF. Love the Flesh, which your body is! Great powers require a RADIATING activity: don't expect anything from others, or your eye will keep on weeping because of your feeling of having been treated badly or because of unfulfilled longings.

Burst open, in full life, and take up your powerful leadership role; take good care of yourself. Enjoy, eat well. . . . You enjoy your own being.

Look at death: what binds you there? Nothing! Now, you live from out of your Central pillar, from out of your Center, not dependent on others. Sadness and anxiety indicate that you aren't yet on the True Path to Life.

The impelling energies in your eye indicate the fire of the unborn child, who is ready to burst into flame, to be born! So, radiate these energies: Live! Enjoy! Action! Assertiveness! Manifestation of the "I"! Say "Stop!" to the old, compulsive energies and elevate them. Send back to the sender those problems which are being worked off on you by certain people.

The water in the eyes indicates that many energies now are waiting to be blared out. Vul-

canic powers are bubbling from out of your depths: forge in yourself that which is most beautiful! Throw away the cross-of-suffering! Firmly grasp that which is productive; strengthen the "masculine" aspect in yourself, so that your fruitful stream has secure embankments. Now, deal firmly with desires! Go and sit on the throne of worthiness. Become master of those lion-powers in yourself and submit them to your Authority.

Don't keep your eyes in mist, in the underworld spheres of death, where water can only mean sadness. Go one step HIGHER and come to Insight, into that which is *truly* beautiful. As long as you are caught in the mist, you can never gain Insight into the true beauty of Life. Arrive at the Level of Life, of BEING, not of WANTING TO POSSESS. LOOK AT EVERYTHING FROM ABOVE, from out of your Mastery: then you won't bear a cross; then you won't allow yourself to be dragged along or be overwhelmed by emotions.

In a large way, take up all your place on earth, in your body. Feel how those enormous, positive powers find their home in your body. You don't want to "possess" another: you ARE yourself.

Dig ever more deeply to your IMPENETRABLE, powerful CORE. There's a "nuclear power" in it which you must direct lovingly. You're not dead, not suffering — even if in your conviction world this sometimes seems to be so. You live! Be happy for the juicy, red, earthly Fruit which you are, and enjoy it: stop looking upon yourself as rigid, old or stiff!

In the case of the eyes discharging pus: feelings of powerlessness, sorrow and anger — because one doesn't immediately succeed in getting a real hold and a perspective on oneself — will be stronger than in the case of the eyes tearing. Anxieties, looking gloomily at oneself, at Life, indicate that the person urgently must deal with the Lie as mentioned above. (Read the subject Suppuration) The person needs to clearly gain insight into the fact that there is no reason for sadness, anxiety or anger: the discovery of the Gladness of Living, of Being who one is, wipes away all tears. If a human being ignores himself — his worth, his Fullness — then he weeps and tries to "fill" himself with things or people outside himself, in desire: if these longings are not being satisfied, however, then he feels wronged, undervalued or shortchanged, sad, misunderstood or lonely. In short, a dead-end street. If man acknowledges his Mastery and "fulfills" himself, giving himself in Love, then nothing or no one can destroy this Joy, and all tears will be gone forever. He no longer expects or desires anything from others, but takes good care of himself from out of his Autonomous power. As long as he, himself, constantly nourishes his Joy — and this doesn't depend upon how other people behave toward him — then he can no longer be sad or disappointed. He is now *very* close to himself and knows that everything that is good for him will appear on his path. Above all, he has banished death so that there is only the Gladness of Living.

LACRYMAL CANAL AND TEAR-SAC
(See also Childhood illnesses, Lacrymal canal)

Ailments, in general

Sadness, powerlessness, insufficient trust in yourself, not really aware of the power of earthly incarnation; you don't actually realize that your Consciousness can influence your body. Cut off from your own divine core, you feel lonely, sad, and without real perspective in your life. Anxiety, sometimes panic; nervousness, afraid of death, getting no grip on life. You are afraid of not being good enough, or of doing things wrong, be it to fail, to collapse, literally or figuratively. You'd run away, but you don't really know from what; anxiety and coldness are pursuing you.

Become aware of your worth. Feel your warm heart, and know that you are safe in your deepest soul-core, where death doesn't exist. Calmly dare to bloom in earthly life as a worthy human being. Don't run away. Know yourself to be welcome in your body. Sadness is a lie: become master of your existence and create your life in joy. Full of self-confidence, partake in incarnation: the growth of rich awareness in an earthly body. Feel good in your skin, and enjoy that which is beautiful, the sensory. Warm yourself with the fire of your heart.

Astigmatism

Sad, broken, lonely, anxious; clinging to the past, to others; self-doubt. You have no perspective, no grip on yourself: "Who am I?"

You are knotted up, estranged from yourself, probably brought up in an environment in which you could not at all be yourself. Inwardly split: you experience two parallel lines in yourself. One side calls for love, and the other rejects itself. Longing-pushing away: this is reflected in relationships with others.

Because you can't be nice to yourself, you'll attract a partner who will make you angry or will make you feel sad.

You seek too much outside yourself; you identify yourself with others so that you experience yourself as "empty." You are afraid of yourself; you're not really aware of your Worth!

Do you feel desperate because in a relationship you can't really come lovingly close to your partner, or because your relationships always go wrong or break up? Then the cause here lies in you: as long as you don't dare to completely be YOURSELF, don't dare to discover and appreciate yourself in love — as long as you don't experience yourself in oneness — it's impossible for you to live in harmony with a partner.

You turn away from yourself, possibly from your body; you consider yourself a silly goose; you nervously and confusedly look for a way out; you conceal yourself in others. You feel dulled, cut off from your deepest Self, from your heart, because you don't really believe in your autonomous worth, because you don't at all see who you *are*.

Unfold, discover, illuminate yourself — with regard to soul and body. Take another road: don't allow your being to merge into the being of someone else, but come to fullness in yourself.

Become aware of your specific worth and possibilities! Be good to yourself, look deeply into your rich emotional world, transform all your potential energies into creativity, live from out of your heart, feel your longings, enjoy earthly beauty, stop belittling yourself!

Be faithful to your nature so that those people who really fit with you are able to come to you.

Grow toward oneness in yourself, offer your heart that which it deserves, and in this way you will make warm contacts with others.

Honest openness toward yourself, and no longer "filling" yourself up with others, but with the richness of yourself.

Don't degrade yourself: be proud of yourself!

Bleeding in the eye

Wanting to keep your hard "I" firmly standing, suppressing your gentle feelings.

From fear of losing your freedom or fear of others "catching" or misusing you, from fear of being submerged by your feelings: you suppress the gentleness, the feminine, the yielding, the supple, in yourself.

A stubborn, hard, obstinate attitude — hardened muscles, petrified neck, tense sorrow — holding in feelings in an iron cell. "I close myself off; my inner feelings are no one's business." A refusal to allow feelings to flow flexibly; you hide your sadness and anxieties. You surely won't cry! Utter ten-

sion; water looks for a relief valve; the pressure becomes too great; suppression demands its toll.

Inner conflict: you want Freedom, separate from everyone, independence, pushing away leadership and others — on the other hand, you don't know what to do with your feelings. Unconscious anxieties lie at the base of this "rejection" of warm love, of others. Anxieties, because you don't truly love yourself: Why do you push yourself away? Why do you disdain your warm, gentle sensitivities? Do you have no right to them? Do you have to be tough and hard in order to be accepted by yourself? Perhaps this inner conviction also was confirmed in your upbringing.

In a relaxed way, be open to yourself, to your feelings, to warm communication with others. Acknowledge your worth and allow your feelings to come through like worthy content; don't hide behind a hard mask. If you do, you hurt yourself and your fellow man. Allow your heart to speak, express your feelings in words, in song, in art, in creativity. Don't be afraid to be yourself: the more strongly you come into harmony with yourself and allow the "feminine" aspect into your life, the more joyful your life will be. Dare to express your feelings spontaneously, to cry when necessary; no longer close yourself off from yourself, from others. Don't belittle yourself: become aware of your possibilities, of your talents, and stop pushing yourself to the side. If you don't love yourself, you will be sad and unhappy, and contact with others won't go the way you want it to. Open your gentle heart; no longer let it bleed; come to love and gentleness.

Blepharitis
inflammation of an eyelid

Aggression. Somewhere you'd like to get through, but you hold back. Inner conflict and doubt: yes or no? You feel stuck, but you are filled to the brim with energy; frustration. You are insufficiently present in yourself; you smother yourself in a space which is too small; you withdraw instead of allowing energies to blossom! Hesitating to go on; powers are being suppressed too long, you don't see clearly what road to take, what action you will take: pent-up, healthy aggressive powers can now attract to you situations from the outside world, which can make you very angry or which contribute to you "opening up" or going on.

You are too cold toward yourself; you run in place because you don't really build upon your deepest Self. Too afraid to go straight ahead. This can lead to powerless anger toward yourself, or to circumstances which you have attracted by your hesitating attitude.

Don't put the brake on your energies, allow yourself to spin like a top; a joyful radiation which comes from a self-assured, loving core. Express yourself, Live, create without hesitation. Don't tie yourself down any longer; relax, discover the warm comfort in life, make a feast of life, trust in your extremely solid basis, your inner Self and build up your life actively the way you want it. Don't frustrate yourself by bottling up powers and feelings: speak and act, go on !

Blindness — becoming blind

An unconscious refusal to be born in yourself. You can't, or dare not, shine light into yourself and your life; you have no clear view of yourself; possibly, you closed your eyes because of painful and sad remembrances from the past, but you don't wish to see how your inner convictions regarding yourself were the causes of these sad experiences. You run away from your deepest Self. Possibly, there's not at all an harmonious correspondence between the life you lead in society and how you inwardly feel: you are then blind to the true needs and longings of your Self; possibly, there is an inner conflict,

whereby you again and again choose in favor of the outer world instead of for your inner self. Do you prefer to close yourself off from the truth inside yourself? And do you live exclusively oriented to the outer world? You close yourself off to your true inner "I," to your true natural being. You flee from yourself, or you play ostrich. Dependence: you take the freedom from yourself.

Instead of building your life upon inner wisdom and autonomy, you run away from yourself, pull the wool over your own eyes. Are you afraid to walk independently through life? Don't you dare to accept confrontation with your true nature because you are afraid to discover something inferior, something that is not worth living for? You cling to something or someone, a partner or a situation, which you don't want to let go of, despite the fact that in this way you imprison yourself. But you don't want to "see" this. You don't live from out of your true Self; in this way, you stand still, you can't truly transform. You keep on living off the remnants of the past; you don't really dare to go on.

With regard to the genetic predisposition to develop blindness, genes follow the conscious and unconscious convictions and programming of ourselves.

If you are inwardly convinced that there's no other way out than becoming blind, then you *allow* yourself to "be lived," then genes will follow their negatively programmed path on a physical level, and you will become blind. We direct every element of our bodies, including the genes, with our Consciousness.

When you refuse to listen to that voice deep inside yourself, when you refuse to live an autonomous life or to listen to the wisdom in yourself, and prefer to listen to what others have to say — what the outer world tells you — when you live on the surface and refuse to look into your own psyche for every cause of every physical ailment, then you are closing your eyes to the truth, and your living Self calls up a blindness so that you might enter an honest confrontation with yourself. So that you not hide any emotions anymore; so that you can bring out all the potential that is in you; an inner liberation. So that you might see clearly into your deepest Self and put all Authority in yourself; so that you might no longer make your life dependent on others, on an Authority above your head. So that you might dare to enter an independent life in a way that is honest with your unique nature.

Becoming blind also means hindering yourself from looking at the outer world any longer; it also means not having to look at yourself in the mirror. It's precisely because you insufficiently believe in yourself, because you insufficiently love yourself — outwardly and inwardly — because you've made yourself too dependent on the eye of, the word of, the knowledge of, and the authority of the outer world. Becoming able to see means, therefore, freeing yourself from all this and, in love for yourself, being open and listening to the longings of your heart; autonomously, in complete self-trust, daring to express your true nature and not allowing yourself to be misled from your true path by anything or anyone. No "must" anymore, but daring to clearly look yourself in the eyes, because you are faithful to your true nature, independently of others. Allowing yourself to be born, standing on your own feet. As long as you stick to the conviction that you are a victim of a situation which simply came upon you, you are putting all responsibility outside yourself, denying power and mastery in yourself over your life and your health, and you won't recover. When you reverse this and become aware that life and health are waiting for your mastery, then you can heal your eyes: reality will follow your inner convictions without your having to practice positive thinking for entire days! Believing is enough; the body will follow. Seeing clearly into the reality of life will free you from anxieties and sadness because you will see how you are the creator of your world.

And. . . . you consider yourself good, beautiful, and full of love, living according to your highly unique nature. Yes, you like to see this!

Born blind
(See also Blindness)

Babies are born this way with the unconscious conviction that in this manner they will get a better and clearer perspective of themselves, so to be able to free themselves of their anxieties, their insecurities. With the sight turned inward, an inner voyage of discovery begins which can lead to true wisdom.

On the one hand, one is afraid to be confronted with reality, because one doesn't trust, because one is afraid of that which is bad or ugly in oneself, of sadness in the outer world; one feels like a prisoner of anxieties, of limitations one puts upon oneself (such as not daring to be oneself, because of dependence on others, not believing in one's own autonomy, one's own creative-power). On the other hand, one wishes to free oneself from this, to deliver oneself from one's anxieties, to confront oneself with the truth regarding oneself and life, making an end to sadness. These people wish to begin seeking their content, their inner senses, their true feeling, independent of the outer world. It is necessary that they don't, in sheer dependence upon others, flee any further from themselves — that they don't just cling to the outer world and, as a result, ignore their own deepest nature. Actual transformation is necessary, truly going on, daring to look deep inside oneself, freeing oneself from a dark, fatalistic outlook on life. Self-liberation; they can proclaim this message of inner freedom and true wisdom to those who seem able to see, but who also are blind to the richness in themselves. A voyage of discovery, to joy, light, power, and wisdom in oneself. Concentrating on the essence of life, a fascinating search for the core of oneself. And. . . . "seeing" in other ways than does the average human being. The richness of this!

Cataract

You don't dare manifest yourself outwardly; you withdraw into a hiding place; the world appears to you as threatening and hostile.

You withdraw, fearful: afraid of your father, of your mother, or of one or another abstract Authority.

You have such a dark outlook; you stick your head into a dark bag so you don't have to look anymore — like an ostrich.

You hide yourself from your own feelings — you are afraid of them — until they flood you.

You are afraid that an angry, threatening figure might suddenly pop up; you are afraid of the reactions of others, afraid that the wolf might gobble you up, just like Little Red Riding Hood.

You don't dare. You feel pain. You get angry because of your powerlessness. Being too much "spirit."

You "need" others, but you are afraid of others; so you crawl into a hole, lonely and deserted, because you created this situation yourself.

Incarnating, becoming truly human: landing with both feet on the ground, feeling in contact with your body.

No longer withdraw into an anxious, spiritual state of being, but dare to fully come into life; discover spontaneous joy: feel safe among others and throw those imaginary spheres overboard. Revelry, like in a Bruegel painting; freely dancing in the wind, sounding the trumpets.

Taking up all your space, freedom, and happiness! When you experience reality here-and-now, anxieties will disappear because sadness and powerlessness are the consequences of not truly being in yourself:

come into contact with your heart, with your deepest Self; wake up from dreaming sleep and live intensely and happily NOW. Sad memories from the past can be looked upon as a consequence of living too unconsciously, full of negative and anxious anticipations.

Change this, and be convinced that life offers you that which is most beautiful if at last you, yourself, begin to create your life in a self-aware way. Come out, descend from out of these dark clouds; be critical in a healthy, optimistic way, and develop yourself in joy.

Color-blindness; Daltonism

Strongly suppressed emotions, removed to unconscious regions, lead to you no longer seeing things as they "objectively" are, to you lifting yourself far above the earthly, and from this height you no longer wish to take advice from anyone. You might even coldly turn up your nose at them.

Possibly, you've been brutally treated by one or another authority (in this or another life). You've been forced to accept certain things; someone has approached you aggressively; your senses were forced to see, hear or taste certain things. Your anxious powerlessness was the cause of these experiences. As a reaction to this, you develop a strong Authority in yourself, possibly also toward others. Now, you don't want to see certain things anymore; you refuse to listen to others any longer; you look down and spit on the world below you. Duality inside you asks for a solution: on the one hand you are that dependent, wronged, mistreated, anxious little one — on the other hand you possibly put up a big front and are arrogant, cold, and distant. "I know it and no one has to tell me"; false pride, aggressive, nasty to others, clawing.

But you are so afraid of a claw crushing your head, afraid of something awful, of which you don't have a clear view; you escape into a false posture, more or less.

Descend from that high mountain and show yourself the way you are; you are good the way you are.

Arrive at higher awareness, at true wisdom, and look at everything from different sides, don't limit yourself to a narrow point of view. Realize how you react to experiences from the past; first of all, arrive at clear Insight in yourself and grow in trust toward your Self. Don't close yourself off; turn toward the many aspects of life; come out of your ivory tower and listen to your intuition, to your inner wisdom. True mastery over yourself, unalloyed pride about your Being, power over yourself and not over others. Replacing blinders and self-righteousness with a very broad perspective and loving openness toward yourself and others.

Conjunctivitis

A cold, reserved, aloof, distant attitude toward life, toward others. A coldness which keeps you imprisoned; you aren't really present in yourself, in your body; critical and remote, not warmly participating in life.

Outwardly you perhaps wear a crown of gold and sit on a high throne, but you push others away with sharp aggression: "Stay away from me!" A railing between you and earthly life; you think, dream, or float away as if you were lifeless.

You look down, disdainfully, critically, without love, upon life and what happens around you, and you take distance from it.

The deepest cause of this attitude is Anxiety. Your heart is cold because, first of all, you insufficiently trust your deepest Self; you keep to the surface. Cut off from your own soul-core, from your own warm heart, you don't truly feel part of earthly existence. You refuse to allow your Consciousness to exist intensely, like a warm motor in your body. Because of anxiety and unsureness, because you keep yourself cut off from your solid Basis, you don't take up your place. Your energies, your powers, your feelings,

are thus being contained, and so you burn yourself up.

With your feelings and thoughts, you remain stuck to your most sensitive or painful remembrances. You are so afraid that other, new experiences might crush you, that you again and again flee into higher spheres, withdrawing ever further into a nostalgic, romantic dream world, into a foretell palace. But to the same degree, anxiety increases, and your Conscious grip on your life, here-and-now, becomes less and less.

You might also project the dream into reality; you don't really live with your feet on the ground. Ultimately, you hang your head with despondency, for resistance to life isn't of any use anymore; you can't take it anymore; heart pains and sorrow, as well as heavy, morbid thoughts or anxieties about death, flood you now.

Make an end to your anxieties, your chilliness, by experiencing yourself intensely, here-and-now, in a Conscious way. Nice and warm with regard to yourself, forthcoming to others.

Close the book of the past; don't flee to imaginary spheres, but come with both feet solidly on the ground. Know that you are the cause of all circumstances in your life. Are you convinced that you don't deserve love, that others always will hurt you again, that everything in life and in relationships will go wrong again? Then, indeed, you will actually attract the confirmation of this. So look very closely to your inner expectations of your existence, of your future: see how you let yourself burn away. Change these negative convictions; seize life with both hands and create your existence yourself instead of being an observer. Self-aware, resolute participation in life, with love and respect for the sensorial, the physical, the heart of yourself and others. Descend onto the warm earth, become intensely present in yourself, make an end to your sadness, which was a consequence of a denial of your reality and your creative possibilities from the NOW.

Inflammation of the cornea
keratitis

Extreme anger, an urge to aggressive deeds, as a consequence of an enormous feeling of powerlessness, of sorrow and pain, of deep anxiety.

Deeply hidden sadness makes you sharp-edged and hard; you are so afraid. "What am I going to see now?" You don't trust your nature; you feel cut off from your deepest Self.

You feel imprisoned in an iron frame-work; others can X-ray you and hurt you as much as they want, and you are afraid of the pain that someone might want to inflict upon you. You feel like a powerless insect on its back; you'd like to grasp, with claws, and push through with all power, but you don't know very well where to direct your aggression. . . . You hold yourself back from actually achieving wholesome self-realization, from developing your creative energies, from allowing your feelings to exist freely, no longer suppressing them in a suffocating framework which will lead to volcanic out-bursts of powers that have been pent-up for too long. You push away an important, natural part of yourself!

Make yourself welcome, no longer push away, but allow your feelings and your ener-gies to flow freely; don't stop yourself with a hard barrier. Step through, and no longer block yourself. You shouldn't be afraid of your feelings, of your nature: you aren't bad; acknowledge your beauty! Now come to rest, feel peace in yourself, be good and gentle, allow yourself to grow, accept those enor-mous potential powers in you, and flexibly transform them into action! Place trust in your deepest Self, feel safe, take good care of yourself, allow peace, relaxation.

Allow it all to come in without resistance; open yourself in gentleness, discover humor and flexibility, GIVE your love instead of cherishing negative expectations so that in this way you will attract that which is beau-tiful.

Cross-eyed
weakened eye muscles; alternating strabismus

Anxiety, a feeling of insecurity, loose struc-ture, unstable ground under your feet. In anxiety and uncertainty, in sadness and igno-rance, you cling to your parents, a person, a group, a system or a religion; you don't ac-knowledge the Authority in yourself. By doing this you deviate from your own Direc-tion

You seek in various directions; you hesi-tate; you turn again toward another path, etc.: you don't see it all clearly because you again and again look for it outside yourself. You feel dependent on others, perhaps lonely; you observe everything in a confused way, in chaos — as a child, you possibly are thrown back and forth between your father and mother, especially if there's a matter of disa-greement or divorce. With *one* eye, you fix-ate yourself as you hold on to *one* safe point outside yourself (a person, etc.): from this point only do you dare to turn around and explore in the world. Because you are on guard, perhaps even suspicious, anxious that they might hurt you.

Nor do you emotionally see a way out; you are afraid of negative powers which might be inside you. You don't trust your own nature. You remain too absent: like a shade; a vessel full of emotions, where Lead-ership of your Aware "I" is lacking!

You "don't anchor yourself" in yourself; sometimes you don't care anymore; you bot-tle up sadness, and you peer at the hostile world — because you don't believe in your own Basis, because you consider yourself to be just an insignificant, inferior being.

With a feeling of powerlessness, you look for a way out: in reaction to your own impo-tence and your dependence on others, you'd aggressively revolt! This anger, all your emotions, seem threatening to you because after all you feel so unstable. Possibly, you reject yourself, or you find your body ugly: this is only a consequence, a reflection, of a general "self-denial."

Don't close yourself off from that which spontaneously comes up in you, from your aggression, your emotions: allow them to come through and don't experience them as threatening. Look at them and know that they are the consequence of your convictions regarding yourself: so, turn INWARDLY, not toward others.

As a child, you were strongly influenced by the contradictions in your environment; perhaps you identified with your father or mother, who thought they were not at all worthy and experienced themselves as "bad" and therefore poured out their gall at their partner. Look then in that mirror! Which conflict do you have to solve inside yourself?

Arrive with both feet on the ground, here-and-now: find stability in yourself. In friendship and trust, open yourself to your deepest "I" and let your ears hear only this; you are good. You are worthy: acknowledge your inner beauty, your talents — don't degrade yourself, don't elevate yourself: take a good look at yourself; don't pay attention to what others say about you, but get hold of yourself and look closely at your content. Don't run away from this treasure!

If you allow your feelings to flow freely, they won't start to dominate you; but also acknowledge rational thinking, the Self-aware mastery in yourself, and allow your emotions to exist in freedom under the guardian eye of your "I."

A balance is necessary in yourself between the unconscious-intuitive-emotional-aspect on the one hand and the rational-conscious-aspect on the other. The "male" way of manifesting and the "female" way of listening in harmony: right-eye and left-eye in balance.

With new eyes, from your personal point of view, observe yourself and also your body: that which you feel spontaneously is good; don't let yourself be misled by the opinions of others. Discover love and affection; live NOW, let go of the past. To achieve straight eyesight you will have to find the Unity in

*yourself! Your mastership; **one** straight Path!*

No kaleidoscopic totality of fragments picked up here and there, but a life based on rock-solid Belief in yourself, in your unshakable Basis. Relationships, friendships, are enriching, if you are firstly completely in your Self. Then don't lose yourself in your surroundings, in others, in far-away dreams. Live from out of the balanced, strong Center Point of your Living "I"!

Exotropia
divergent strabismus

Deep fundamental anxieties about unconscious powers in yourself. Threat. Needless, however.

Anxieties about that primal-power in your Self, about your deepest emotional content; you feel yourself to be on unsafe ground; you think there is, as it were, a sort of monster inside you, and that you can't at all trust that "devilishness" inside you. These are only "convictions."

Dark, threatening, aggressive powers are being reflected in the world around you. You don't get a perspective on reality, not on yourself, not on the world outside you. Fear of death, as long as you don't surrender to Life in yourself.

In fact, you still have to be born in Life: you keep on holding on to unconscious realms, to dreams, and to your sleep of death. With your Consciousness you can, here-and-now, become master over your unconscious emotional-world: imaginary anxiety visions are just a consequence of insufficient trust in your "I"-awareness.

Surrender to your deepest Self; allow lighter energies to come through; give space to life; don't remain stuck in the dream, in the sleep, in not daring to be "I" on earth.

Achieve clear Insight in Life, discover the joy! You don't have anything deep in you that is threatening. Allow your emotions to flow freely, observe them, and deal with them; don't be afraid of them. Only if you stop visualizing your dark "lies" will you discover the peaceful light of your deepest soul-core.

The most misleading lie you can maintain as a human being is the voice of doubt, the conviction of being a victim, or worthless.

Eyelashes, falling out

An anxious, expectant atmosphere. Fear of totally disappearing, of being swallowed up in your emotions, in intangible, unconscious streams. Horrified, you conclude that you can't go back anymore, that you can only count on yourself, and not on others. High in your tower, isolated, you experience the threat of humanity, of the group; it's as if your fate is sealed, as if others make decisions about you.

You are now driven into a corner, so that you will come to the realization that only you can live your life, that it is you who has to orient your existence and make decisions, that you no longer may let your life be led (misled) by others.

You don't trust others, but still you listen to everyone; you think you are locked out. A suffocating feeling; you don't see any way out anymore; you are now searching in panicked anxiety.

The masses don't compose a threat for you; it's your emotions that threaten you so.

Push things away from you; allow your own energies to blossom. Make yourself welcome in life, enter the group; you ARE accepted on the condition that you no longer reject yourself; you have to decide about yourself. Take your fate in your own hands: create your existence in a self-aware way. In that Basis of your deepest self, you are always safe; anxieties are needless. Anxieties indicate that you are choosing the path to death; turn now toward life by acknowledging all authority and worth in your Self. Your consciousness is able to guide, to change, to heal your body. No longer withdraw anxiously into yourself.

Allow that emotional stream in you to come through, and accompany it in a friendly way, just as eyelashes accompany moist eyes. Be proud of yourself!

Glaucoma

You can't comprehend it (any longer): a feeling of being overwhelmed; you can't bear it any more (can't look at it any more). You'd like to let go of the past, but you can't. You see everything with insufficient nuance, too much in black and white. You understand only your own point of view; stubborn sadness, anger. You stand there stiff-legged. You hold on too stubbornly, too forcedly, as if made of stone; you can't forget something and probably also feel hurt. You refuse to look at everything in a bigger picture; you refuse to accept.

With grasping claws, you stiffly retain certain happenings or sad remembrances, so that you become extremely tense — until at last you collapse.

Frustrated, you don't go on in life; you block yourself completely.

Liberate yourself: in the past you have attracted circumstances in accord with your convictions and your expectations from life. So, look inside yourself and let go of everything! Don't get stuck in the past. Discover now a new life on the basis of joy because of yourself. First experience your autonomy, your independence, your productive possibilities, and don't cling to things or people outside yourself. Only when you let go of this enormous burden can you begin to feel free and happy and experience your life intensely in the here-and-now with new, optimistic expectations.

Eye inflammation, in general

Anxiety and powerlessness: this leads to aggression, anger. You can't let go of a certain thing: you fixate, almost compulsively, on a certain object. Even if you destroy yourself because of it, even if it would mean the loss of life, you keep stubbornly holding on.

You are sad, you have heart pain; maybe you've been severely struck by a certain happening, by something that now appears to completely control you or take possession over you.

You only "see" *that;* it might become an obsession. You develop deep anxieties and dark thoughts, anger, and perhaps even vengeful or sadistic feelings — but in fact we're dealing here with an angry powerlessness about yourself. That thought or this happening — which appear to you to be threatening — harden you: fiery, cutting energies, deep emotions, radiate intense redness. But you don't see clearly, or you refuse to see the truth before your eyes, the truth which lies inside yourself.

Softening and suppleness: realize that the true problem is your own powerlessness. Achieve clear Insight as to why certain happenings now occur; you have, by your expectations from life, unconsciously called up every situation in your life. Now, acknowledge that self-aware sun-power deep within you; don't blame others, but turn inward, observe your emotions. Let go of that which hinders you from living happily; look beneath the surface and discover your deepest Self. See how you can renew everything in your life, how you can build in another direction. No longer ALLOW yourself to be led by obsolete values from the past: don't fixate on anything, let go, so that the path lies open for that which is truly good for you. No longer shoot arrows; no longer sorrow yourself; become master over the situation. Inner peace, Love for yourself.

Iris inflammation
iritis

Aggressive revolt, radical resistance, a cry for more freedom, for more space.

You feel deeply hurt; you have to allow something to pass through or you have to accept something in your life that you don't like. Someone hurts you; you want to get away. Possibly, this is an enormous reaction to incomprehension and pain with which you are confronted in the parental home; you feel misunderstood. You want to break out, or you'll explode. The deepest reason for aggressively contrary behavior — "Me first!" — is a profound anxiety, powerlessness, being stuck in your own unsureness; you don't really love yourself. You ignore the power of your deepest Self; you don't offer yourself warmth or love. You flee from your anxieties and from your pain, and you oppose others. You, yourself, stay rather immobile, passively stuck, frustrated and furious because of your own powerlessness. Dark, accumulated feelings, until you burst apart.

You don't really SEE clearly into yourself; you search through the depths, but then again you become afraid of your emotions and flee to the surface again — a flight away from yourself, gasping for breath. You are cut off from your deepest Self; you get lost.

The path toward your liberation lies in your deepest, divine Self; turn toward this inner core, feel your solid basis, and don't look for a handhold outside yourself; don't expect anything from others, and don't blame others because you ignore all love and wisdom that are in yourself. Discover that which is beautiful in yourself, the richness of color, and that in your existence which pleases the senses: feel connected with the pure, radiating, gentle forms and lines in your soul, in your environment. Certainly and purely determine your direction; a clear balance in your life, a purification of negative thoughts, of destructive feelings. Discover your noble talents, your sensory power, your body, the sensual nuances in your existence. Don't use only the black paint of your palette, but paint your life in all colors of the rainbow, in joy and optimism. (Iris is Greek for rainbow.)

No longer bottle up your possibilities, your powerful energies; be faithful to your own nature and don't expect others to understand you. Dare to be yourself, fight your way to inner freedom, achieve active devel-opment of your total personality, let go of the past and go on resolutely. Experience your-self as a Unity: an earthly existence based on the fundamentally strong foundations of your eternal Self.

Long-sightedness, hyperopia

A flight, *away* from yourself; fear of con-frontation.

You have no clear perspective on yourself or on your situation. Cut off from your deepest, intuitive emotional ground. Anxiety; you jump ahead, fleeing, away from the "I." "Over there, in the distance," nothing can happen to you.

You don't dare look very well into the here-and-now; you think something threat-ening is hanging above your head, from which you'd like to flee into the distance.

You feel unable to manage here; you'd rather jump over your emotions than confront yourself with them. You flee from your emotions, you feel constrained and Now shut off from true joy. You can't get a true grip on your life; you'd rather let yourself float on the stream of life without really steering yourself in the direction you wish to go. You hang your head with despondency; you are insufficiently aware of your worth. Don't you dare to have a good look at your situa-tion, at your feelings? Do you flee from yourself? From others? You feel chained; perhaps you are afraid of death. You don't really trust the roof above your head because you don't really have a true view of your deepest Self. Because you look for a hand-hold far outside yourself, instead of in your deepest Self. You try to "anticipate" every-thing far in advance, because you insuffi-ciently trust yourself, your intuition, here and now.

Now, turn inward and no longer run away from your deepest "I," from your uncon-

scious emotional world, and from the situa-tion in which you find yourself. Feel safe and sheltered in the here-and-now, and don't project your life too far into the future, but observe all that is beautiful in your life NOW. Confront yourself with anxieties and problems; don't flee from them, but work them out. Take these hands away from your eyes and look around you! Don't be blind to yourself in the present. In the power of the Now-moment you are able to create life in the direction you want. Self-awareness, joy, and trust in your spontaneous nature. That which hangs above your head is not sinister, but is a projection of your anxieties. Solve that darkness in your heart by listening to the inner wisdom, which no one can teach you; follow your inner eye, your intuition, and know yourself to be safe inside yourself. Al-low transformation!

Myopia, near-sightedness

You already feel uncertain and unsafe here and now, and therefore you don't dare to really go forward and are afraid of the future and of that which is far away.

You anxiously protect yourself; some-times you'd prefer to go back to the past. You are rather closed up, turned inward, and would rather attract things to you than have to come out of your shell and go toward things yourself. Sometimes you stick your head in the sand, refusing to look further; you concentrate on the present problems in such a way that you withhold every optimis-tic perspective from yourself.

You feel weak; your self-awareness is in-sufficiently developed; you feel hurt by oth-ers; you have pain and sadness; you feel de-pendent on others; you insufficiently believe in your inner, divine Self, which is able to build up a safe and happy existence; you un-dervalue your power, your wisdom, your possibilities. If you don't want to see the power in your SELF, if you don't trust your inner Self, then you'll have no confidence in the world around you; then you'll look at the world, the future, with suspicion and from behind the shield of your glasses.

You don't really go forward; you are stuck; sometimes, this anxious powerlessness really makes you angry. Also, your dependence on people and things outside yourself sometimes leads to aggression against others.

You are on guard; you are peering through a loophole; you mostly choose to take byways instead of that main road which lies in the extension of your true nature. You doubt your worth; you limit your room to move, although you ache for freedom.

Feel warm, safe, and protected in yourself; honestly look at your inner depths, at your feelings, and express them. No longer hold yourself back; give yourself all freedom in wide spaces. Don't be afraid; come solidly with your feet on the ground, and straighten up proudly: become aware of your worth, achieve peace in yourself, and experience this joy of life from out of your deepest Self. No longer doubt the possibility of every man to create his life himself; nothing threatening "just" happens. Every occurrence is being created by the expectations that are present in a human being.

Build up a strong structure, let go of the past; observe everything from your higher awareness; don't get stuck at the problems of today, but in optimism create a positive future: put things in perspective and go on without hesitation! Look beyond; resolve duality in yourself; put things in order. Don't get stuck in a problem, but look for a solution and let go.

Night-blindness

A powerful urge for self-manifestation is being suppressed. You don't give in to aggressive powers in yourself; enormous energy asks for a breakthrough; you suppress it. You *let* yourself "be lived"; you don't really dare to live from out of your spontaneous feelings, from out of your intuition; you block the passageway of the inspirational fire

that seeks its way up from out of your inner core and asks for your creativity — your acknowledgment of your valuable possibilities; but you limit yourself, perhaps to sheer material or earthly occupations without stopping to think about your greater possibilities, about your intense emotional world, which asks for acknowledgment, about your true worth. You deny a great part of yourself; you are blind to that which lies below the light of the surface; you prefer to keep all this dark and untouched.

You keep covered the pot of your unconscious powers and talents. You are like a king who doesn't acknowledge his kingship; perhaps you keep your outer Face proud and stiff while behind it natural powers are being held back. You have insufficient trust in your deepest Self; to you it seems dark and unknown, perhaps threatening, and it makes you anxious. Therefore, you don't allow yourself to live from out of the most beautiful depths of your inner Self; therefore, you close yourself off from your inner senses, from the intuitive channels, and you direct yourself too much toward the outer ego. From fear of being yourself, do you imprison yourself in the clutches of another?

Acknowledge the leadership of your deepest Self, and unblock yourself: allow feelings, powers, and talents to go free. Cut yourself off no longer from that which is deepest in yourself.

Don't be afraid of your inner sunlight. Were you taught not to trust your nature, to keep your emotions covered? Are you afraid of truly being yourself? Acknowledge this worthiness in yourself and trust in your intuitive powers; dare to go on; acknowledge the leadership of your inner Self, allow your spontaneity to freely exist as your personal identity. No longer keep yourself imprisoned; don't allow yourself to be strangled in the grip of another: be yourself!

Deep anxieties and mistrust of your own nature have perhaps been the reason why you hide behind another, behind a part-

ner: come out and feel safe in the darkest night, in the darkest depths of your being, where the Light never, in fact, goes out, where death doesn't exist.

Optic nerve, inflamed

You feel powerless to get a grip on something; you want to force something, something impossible. You want to get a grip on a situation, but you don't have a clear perspective on it; perhaps you want to rescue something, but you don't see how.

You want to comprehend something, understand something, but you feel powerless.

You fixate with glowing attention on a certain thing, but "it doesn't want to work." You don't get any further; perhaps you get angry; the aggression pushes inside your eye. Because of insufficient trust in your own Power, you don't believe in your ability to achieve something, so you either start to force things — things it would be better to let go of — or you fixate on something which you think you will mess up again anyway. That which you can't "grasp" constantly occupies you. Other energies are being blocked, so that you block yourself.

If you spontaneously followed your nature, you would think you are not good enough; so therefore you'd force yourself by choosing a path that is not good for you at all. Frustration; insufficient self-confidence.

Come to clear insight in yourself: be happy to be who you are. Show your true being in all openness; you are good the way you are. Allow all your energies to break through with volcanic power; dare to go on, to develop yourself in all possible directions, while listening to your nature, your intuition. Observe the situation in which you find yourself; believe in yourself, have contact with your inner self. Now follow that path which you intuitively sense to be the right one; let go of that which "has to be". Give yourself all opportunity to be flexible in life, to slowly but surely build up a solid structure in which you easily will be able to comprehend and

assimilate everything. In self-confidence, seeing more clearly, and transforming energies into action. Peace, harmony, certainty in yourself.

Photophobia, shunning light

Ignoring one's own Light causes one to shun the other light.

You live according to norms, laws, because that is how it's supposed to be, because it fits within this or that structure — not because you feel it all from within.

Interruption of the contact with your deepest "I," cut off from your own white source, your deepest Self, your consciousness-core, which lies at the base of your earthly existence. You feel too little connected with it; you are looking for a hold outside yourself.

You don't see your own sun-core!

You ignore an important part of yourself; perhaps you think there's something dark and bad living in your nature. You don't dare trust your spontaneous nature because you don't really believe in your nature and your feelings. You consider yourself too inadequate, too awkward, too clumsy in your feelings — you push them away.

Are you afraid that if you allowed your natural feelings to flow then everything would go wrong? Do you therefore stick yourself in a "structure" which doesn't offer you a chance to experience your total self, to express yourself the way you feel? You hide your warm sun-center; you underestimate your worth, your spontaneous possibilities. You don't truly live from out of yourself. . . .

Go and search for that inner light, for that intense, happy joy in yourself.

No longer keep standing still, allow your energies to flow freely, acknowledge these powers in yourself, discover your real nature, and follow your path spontaneously and intuitively.

Radiate your power, your worth, your love, to others and make them happy, too; no longer lock yourself up inside yourself, in armor; don't live according to the rules of others. Feel your heart and the light of the warmth in your heart. You are the center of your life; don't let yourself "be lived." . . .

Red eyes

You vigorously defend yourself against the grip of emotions in which you feel imprisoned.

You keep at a distance from your feelings; you push away certain anxieties and sadness or pain; you don't allow certain feelings to get the upper hand on your "I." You fight against your feelings because you're not really strongly rooted, and these emotions could be a threat. You put up a bold front, presenting yourself as sharp-edged, while your heart is so soft and fragile. You'd even conceal that you have a good and big heart; you don't dare show your "female" aspects. On the contrary, you resist, in a Mars-like way — in a rather aggressive way — your own feelings. You fight to remain standing above sorrow or emotions; inner tears or tensions are being repressed, controlled.

Allow your bold, "male" aspects to integrate with the rest of your being; dare to experience yourself, spontaneously, don't be ashamed about your feelings, don't be angry because of your pain, experience the Power of your inner self, develop your life in a Self-aware way, allow your heart to radiate outwardly, be yourself without doubts.

Know yourself to be secure in your own Basis. Don't live like a wooden plank; allow your feelings to express themselves via your body. Don't brace yourself, don't force yourself, become master over your existence and give yourself the freedom to also be flexible on the emotional level. Don't suppress your gentleness!

Retinal degeneration

You flee into the Neptunian spiritual realms; worries have been a heavy load on you, and you now feel old and unable to really keep a grip on your life any more, on the problems. Now, you let it all slide through your fingers because you don't feel able to comprehend and deal with experiences, emotional impressions, sadness, or worries. A longing to be delivered, freed, from experiences you can't handle very well, from earthly burdens: you lift yourself above the world; you feel you are in a vacuum — you have withdrawn. You want be absorbed into the ALL. You come out of a dark tunnel, with heavy thoughts and feelings; now you look for liberation in a de-materialization of yourself. In the "spirit" you no longer have to see what lay so heavily upon you. You take everything too sternly, without putting things in perspective, without acknowledging the cheerful things of earthly life. You are not really present with your consciousness in your body.

Individualization; allow your consciousness to become master over your body and your life.

Don't let yourself be overcome by things, but self-awarely create your existence. Here-and-now, being present on earth and enjoying; allow your spirit to act on matter, allow your body to grow beautifully, create the circumstances around you. Take that lemon out of your mouth, feel that iron solidity of your deepest Self; with joyful expectations about life, you will attract beautiful situations. Become aware of the spirit's power on matter, and form that matter with the power of your longings, your feelings, your thoughts: materialize, regenerate!

Retinal detachment

On the basis of negative experiences from the past (at whose foundation, however, were your negative expectations), you don't at all trust life anymore.

Even behind that which is the most beautiful, you suspect there lies the strongest poison. That which now serves as your life-preserver or handhold can later on cause you to drown because it proves not to be *authentic;* the human being you now love can later on hurt you and reject you. What is underneath that cover? An explosive? Or just a plain ball?

On the one hand, you bubble with enthusiastic longings for life; on the other hand you are afraid of falling.

You see the world "dualistically"; you experience yourself as being dubious. "Am I good or bad? Is there something devilish in me?" Feelings of guilt regarding experiences from the past can play a role here.

You are angry with the past, aggressive and hurt in your worthiness; dark remembrances eat at you; you hinder yourself from enjoying that which is beautiful because you immediately pull it down. You no longer dare to truly, spontaneously, experience joy, because you automatically begin to rationalize with your mind in a pessimistic, reserved, proud way. Someone has hurt you, and now you no longer trust anything or anyone. Outwardly, you may even appear proud and cold, your feelings deeply hidden. Nevertheless, you long so much for that which is beautiful, idyllic; you dream and long — until you again see the negative and again "detach" yourself from that which is beautiful — and in this way you don't find a hold anywhere in life.

Don't reject any part of yourself; come to full integration: consciousness, body, feelings. Make an end to the duality of black-white, and know how you, yourself, have attracted life situations. Now create the life you wish; negative expectations bring sad happenings into being: destroy the pessimistic philosophy with which you've been dealing so self-destructively. Now let go of the past and go on. Don't be afraid to fall in life: stand sol-

idly and count on the creative powers of your deepest Self. Trust the flow of your spontaneous nature, of life and love-energy, and open yourself to this.

Don't let go of life, of joyful dreams, of those happy expectations, because of negative experiences from the past. Believe in yourself, put your trust in others, don't disparage everything, give yourself every chance for another new, happy existence.

Stinging eyes

Here, it's not about a sudden emotional turmoil, but about a constant, irritated feeling. Your head is filled to bursting with emotional impressions; you feel pain and sorrow; you recall painful experiences; you are stuck with an overwhelming amount of energies; your heart is hurt; your aggression is being softened by your sensitivity. You insufficiently experience your solid basis; you don't really trust in your deepest Self; you don't feel as if you have the power to really do what you want, and you long, or desire, very much — emotionally, materialistically or sexually. You can't put the person or the object of your longing out of your mind, until it becomes too much for you. You'd like to force certain things because you experience yourself as powerless. You try to keep your feelings and your longings under control; you think you have complete command over yourself, but you are afraid that this bridge might suddenly collapse.

Anxiety and pain, a feeling of being pinched together, not being able to fully live the way you'd like to, a self-suppression. You try to stand above your emotions! But your feelings call for acknowledgment, for an actual breakthrough in your life.

You are too much in your mind with your feelings and actions instead of truly bringing them to realization and actually experiencing them.

Calmly, gradually, unfolding your feelings and longings. Don't force yourself; don't overburden your head any longer, but DO, experience, create; don't bottle things up; allow a free flowing of your inner powers. Allow consciousness and body to merge; don't take distance from a part of yourself. Let go of the past and develop your creative energies in a steady way; express your longings and don't remain stuck in yourself. Feel solid in yourself, with both feet on the ground, and don't direct yourself toward unimportant details. Live from out of your sun-center and don't hold back energies — but don't outrun yourself; live here and now, step-by-step, steadily. Control your accelerator without being over-hasty — in trust. Be thankful for today and don't cry about yesterday or tomorrow. You are the creator of your situation.

Sty, hordeolum

Unsureness, insufficient self-confidence, fear of falling, insufficient feeling of security in your deepest Self. You don't really feel master over your body: you can't yet stand on your own feet. You are too much stuck in yourself; you withdraw; you close your eyes, as it were, to fully living; you'd rather hide behind others or in unearthly dimensions; you don't completely come through. You don't yet dare to. You quietly stay where you are; you allow yourself to "be lived," unaware rather than aware: you don't take responsibility for yourself — you'd rather leave that to others. Fear of pain; you feel safer when you can put yourself to rest in the radiating sun-warmth of another, because you feel too small, too anxious, and too cold.

Development of self-confidence, feeling the safe basis in yourself, making yourself master over your life and your body; allowing powerful energies from your deepest Self to freely blossom — a gradual growth toward Self-awareness and acknowledging your own worth, your personal creative powers. Feeling the warm heart-center in yourself.

Eyes, tearing, watering, sticky, possibly discharging pus

Thoughtful, slow, careful, RE-STRAINED.... Not truly coming outward with energies with which you are full. You (unconsciously) hold back from shooting forward. You don't really get a grip on reality; you still live too much in the unconscious or vague spheres of yourself. The feeling of living in a dream-realm and not being able to transform this into reality. As if in a slow-motion movie, as if in a dream: you can't really "reach" it. You keep on going in circles, in thoughts, in longings, in desires, in energies — "Let's wait a moment." You hesitate going onward from out of your "I." This gives you a feeling of frustration, of being locked up. "I want to get out of here!" Yet you remain where you are, you don't do anything, you don't really come through with your "I" in the here-and-now of reality. Nevertheless, the water of life calls out, asking to stream freely in a beneficial, creative way.

Allow energies to flow! Start! Do! Action! Letting off steam, like a Bull that snorts through its nose. Deal firmly with your feeling of Powerlessness — "I can't" — with your convictions that you will become older and degenerate in the sense of being less active or agile, of being less able to do what you want to/have to do for your own well being. Confront yourself with those negative convictions regarding so-called "weakness" in you, to which convictions the body definitely reacts with braking signals, with physical symptoms. Energies stagnate. So take up the gauntlet of Life! Don't procrastinate! The watchword is: take things in hand! Feel solid in your body, very close to yourself, with a strong Backbone. Be involved in things and feel good, strong in the flesh, and mobile. Don't flee from your body: the spirit-power in your body; you are a unified being. Make short work of listlessness and self-doubt, and arrive at the physical work that is good for you: whether it has to do with cleaning, writing, stonemasonry or dancing — allow these energies to circulate in yourself and don't stop them any longer! Don't keep living in "thoughts." Live, speak, be creative, do! Active involvement in life, in your body, in yourself. Don't dream yourself, but come with both feet on the ground, in the reality of the here-and-now. (Read further: Left Eye, Right Eye)

BLACK EYE

Inwardly, you are angry, aggressive, and you close yourself off! You refuse to SEE that you, yourself, are at the basis of a situation that has gotten out of hand. Your aggressive emotions are bubbling up and attracting similar vibrations: an angry fist or an aggressive beam.

Look clearly into yourself: you are angry because of your own powerlessness, and you project this to the outside. (See Bruises)

Hatred, aggression, dislike, wanting to push away — having these feelings calls up the same in others!

Direct your feelings, in self-awareness, in powerful, creative channels. Cordiality, warmth, community spirit, acknowledging yourself and bidding yourself welcome, openness toward yourself and your relations. Don't shut your eyes to the true cause of your aggression: suppression of your own powers and possibilities. They are your aggressions and frustrations, which send electromagnetic impulses and call up unpleasant situations.

F

FACE

Psychological correspondence

Your face can be an open book, but it also can camouflage a certain content. Your countenance symbolizes a reaction-screen, where outer and inner worlds meet each other; your emotion-and-thought world are mirrored here. Your surroundings are there as a mirror of your convictions. Your countenance also. Your inner sensorial abilities to observe are channeled via the outer senses: you can radiate warmth that comes from the depths of your heart. You can also hide, hold fast, put on a mask. Do you achieve open communication with others?

Ailments, in general

Do you close yourself off via a defense mechanism? Why hide yourself? Do you feel threatened or "taken," hurt by others in your pride, in your outer ego? Do you feel your innermost being exposed, powerless, and therefore do you crawl away into a hidden tunnel? Does it have to do with an inner struggle, doubt? . . . Do you not want to get to the essence of the matter? Do you stay on the surface? Do you live too much in "appearances"? Why act so tough? Do you just live for the eyes of others? Do you feel so ashamed or unsure? Do you not live from out of your deepest Self? Have you not been faithful to your true nature in order to satisfy the eyes of others? Is your countenance

"contorted" in a grimace of powerless anger because you don't succeed in developing your true Self?

Don't bind yourself so! You perhaps have let others take too strong a hold on you and on your weakest points. Now, be reborn within yourself and mark off your terrain safely. From here, you can radiate outward: self-expression, self-manifestation! Love yourself first of all, then you acknowledge your fundamentally strong foundation, and you won't experience others as a threat, nor judge them superficially. Of first importance is not the outer form, but how people really feel. True worth lies deep inside every man. Be faithful to your inner nature. Don't live for the eyes of the outer world, nor for outer appearances or achievements.

Facial pain — neuralgia
(See also Neuralgia)

Anxiety, feeling threatened and unsafe. You will protect yourself against this feeling — tense alertness, drawn in too tightly, stern structure, girdled closed. At last, you lose real contact with your Self and your nature. So, then, you also consider the Earth and people to be strange, unknown, encapsulated in a metallic robotic structure, with whom you can't have any real human contact, just as you can't with your deepest I. You suppress your spontaneous, natural feelings. Then the unavoidable reaction: "I'm breaking out of this!" with fist held high. Sometimes, exaggerated self-manifestation after a long self-suppression. Often, you have the feeling that others hinder you, condemn or punish you; and you wonder, "Maybe I deserve it?"

An inner urge, wanting to climb higher and farther on high mountains, despite heavy burdens on your back. Or, because you fear you'll fall by the wayside, you want to be the first to get somewhere! Sometimes, this can get to the point that you go beyond your own limits, neglect to respect others and every structure — a reaction to the repeated suppression of your own life-Fire.

Anxieties, dream-castles, and unrealistic ambitions can then go hand-in-hand.

Do you clamp yourself closed? For fear of the reactions of the outer world, do you not show your inner feelings? Do you try in a tense and cramped way to satisfy the Eyes of others? Resistance!

Ease off the gas pedal, and first of all peacefully come to yourself. Be aware of your true, safe center and your worth. Let the bubbles pop; your anxieties, too, are in such bubbles. Trust: nothing "just" happens in your life, in world events.

Steadily erect your structure in space and time, step by step; don't allow yourself to be suppressed by the fear of totally being yourself.

Break through the harness and enter the warmth of your safe Self; so that you will also meet the heart of others and come to real contact.

The structures in which you feel imprisoned, you have built them up yourself, though it be unconsciously. Now follow your true nature. Let the dynamic powers push steadily through, without self-blockage.

Facial palsy

Paralyzing anxiousness to "see" your own feelings. Afraid that if you would open the floodgates a deluge of emotions would crush you. You don't trust your feelings. Thus, you also hide from others, often in order to maintain your "dignity" or "worth" in front of them. You condemn your feelings or you

are ashamed to express them, and you believe you have to conceal everything under the authority of rationality; this sometimes finds its reflection in fear of paternal authority and of severe authority in school, at home, at work. . . . But, in fact, it has to do with constantly calling yourself into line, so that your natural feelings stay blocked up.

Don't hide yourself; sooner or later, your feelings will break through. Let everything grow, don't cause your own nature to stagnate. By themselves, emotions never form a threat for you, but if you keep suppressing them, they will. Accept your feelings: when you let them flow through, one emotion will flow into the other — only then it will be clear where the deepest anxiety or problem lies. Observe it, don't run away from it — and solve it. Your nature and your feelings are not your enemy, but are the strong motor for a life in progress. Allow a natural flow of your life-energies — a flow that emanates from your Being, not from Desires. Don't keep on placing yourself "above" your Nature, in a tense way. Surrender to your heart, to your deep life-core.

FAINTING

You withdraw; you can't handle it anymore. You are afraid; something is beyond you, a shock. You are burning away, right there, where you are standing — because you are not taking the path you should be taking. Your life is directed toward others, onto side-tracks: so, first choose in favor of yourself, the main track! The side-tracks then will be met in good time.

You were too much a shadow, too absent in your life; you've compelled or forced yourself too much to go in this certain direction, although it was not at all good for you. You struggle against having to truly evolve

— because you feel too small, too powerless. Your deepest Self might call up a certain happening in your life that makes you stop and contemplate your being, and it shakes you awake: this can be the beginning of a more-aware, new track. Were you on the wrong track? Then back up a little, review your life course, and go on with new energy. So get in very close contact with your deepest "I," with your true nature, and find there the solidity, the certainty, the safety: this drives away all anxieties. Be strongly present, here-and-now, and listen to the signals that you unconsciously have called up. First consciously choose your own life and resolutely push away that which — in an exaggerated way — blocks your path. First of all, a loving presence in yourself is necessary; only then can you live in love with others. First and foremost, take care that you find yourself free space to breathe in.

FALLING BACKWARDS

Fear of evolving, or of letting go of obsolete insights. You don't dare fully reveal the way you feel inwardly to the outer world; perhaps you attach too much importance to what others think or say instead of staying faithful to your own personal feelings. True kingship is not worthiness in the eyes of others, but the worthiness you attribute to yourself.

Do you build your life on uncertain values? Perhaps the scepter you bear doesn't represent inner sureness? Are you stuck in limited religious or philosophical concepts? Do you forcefully cling to old habits or structures instead of honestly confronting yourself with renewals that are necessary? Do you feel "touched" or hurt in your essence? Do you feel threatened, pushed off your throne? Then your life is built on uncertainties.

Time for transformation! Don't resist. Let go. No longer offer resistance to real evolution, so that you don't unconsciously instigate a revolt by the renewing energies! Don't cling to out-of-date values; follow your deepest intuition; even if you are confused, your deepest inner Self knows what's best for you; so don't resist new ways that you've already unconsciously called up. Solid grounding: here-and-now, in your body, not always distant with your thoughts. Don't live for the eyes of others, but from out of your own basis. Listen to the Uranus powers inside you.

FALLING, ON ONE'S BOTTOM, CAUSING PAIN

You wriggle, getting angry, like a cat caught in a bag, instead of jumping out and going on. You've run in place for too long, without making any progress; you go around in a vicious circle. You place power over yourself in the outer world, in others, in authority outside yourself. You don't dare to really spontaneously live from within. You question too much how you appear or what you "have to do" to be accepted or acknowledged by the outer world. You insufficiently allow your inner powers to come through, because you don't truly feel safe in your deepest Self, because you doubt your worth, because you aren't nice enough to yourself, because you are insufficiently rooted in yourself. Moreover, you smother yourself with a head that overflows with "thinking." Pure Mars-powers are turning inward, are being suppressed by the rational. You don't really dare to surrender to your feelings, to your impulses. Because you don't really believe in yourself, you present to others, to the outer world, a bearing that is proud, stiff, and tense while you are suppressing primitive powers and emotions. In order to cast off every armor in honest confrontation with yourself, you first have to be lifted off your platform or whipped out of your saddle.

Only you must have power over yourself; it makes no sense to live for the eyes of others. Don't betray yourself; allow those pure powers and emotions to come through. Spontaneously dare to be yourself, without forcing anything. You are good the way you *are,* without having to assume a certain posture. Pride, self-respect, self-realization: spontaneous realization in accord with your heart, with your true nature.

No false or outer pride to please anyone; but an honest and open "I"-experience, in friendship with, and appreciation for, yourself. Stand solidly with both feet on the ground and know yourself to be safe in your deepest immortal Self. Trust; flexibly being yourself, without minding what others think of you. Stopping the turning windmill in your head, and calmly arriving at your feeling and intuition.

Enjoy life; don't hold back impelling forces anymore; be faithful to your nature. It is not the external that is important — neither what you achieve, nor what people say about you or expect from you — but what you feel and what you *are!* Put Authority in yourself; don't allow anyone or anything to get a grip on you. Determine your direction yourself, and go onward without delay.

FAT

Fat, by itself, is Good and Healthy, Soft and Beautiful. Western society, however, is oriented toward the notion that fat is ugly and unhealthy.

Many people — and especially women — are slaves of this destructive conviction, and they violate themselves just to make "fat" melt away. This is unnatural and unhealthy.

Feelings and potential possibilities for Creativity — which are extensive but don't have to be transformed right away into action and realization — are Energies. These energies seek to be solidified into Fat. Fat cannot disappear so long as it is necessary for the human being that these energies remain solidified.

Fat symbolizes Energy, Power, Potentiality, Self-cherishing, and Gentleness. Without a physical reception-base for the enormous energies that are present in the nature of certain people, these people would become ill or insane. (It's completely normal that most people who begin following a "diet" will begin to suffer from one or another ailment.)

The balance between Energy (feelings, potential creativity, etc.) and Body, between spirit and matter, constantly needs to be maintained in a natural way.

Therefore, you are fine the way you are at any moment in your existence, so long as you don't mold yourself into an artificial corset!

Follow only your inner Authority, which gives you the body that is ideal for you at this moment. Fat is not ugly or bad. As long as it is needed, as long as it is good, fat will stay. Don't fight against it, but be in solidarity with your beautiful, soft, warm, powerful, downy body, which retains its muscles and layers of fat where they are needed for your health. No longer doubt this perfection of your nature: no longer look at fat through the eyes of a society which only lives superficially and doesn't know true love. A society in which the woman is being proclaimed as a skinny, drawing suction-power instead of as a representation of full love that *gives.*

Listen to your heart, to your body: don't listen to superficial counselors who can't get to the bottom of things because they, themselves, are swallowed up by these destructive convictions.

A body shape reflects the individual nature of a human being. No one's too fat or too skinny. The ideal weight doesn't exist. Certain "fat places" make it clear to you why it just has to be *there:* and it is good. It doesn't have to disappear. Fat is not "ugly" or "bad" or "unhealthy": this is only being proclaimed by people who mistrust their own Nature, their Body, because they are taught that way. . . .

Break with this lie; express who you really are, and don't hide behind the false "suction-mask" of a "diet, massage," etc. And *if* the fat at some point should disappear spontaneously, just like that, then your deepest Self will know that this is also good. And should it spontaneously come back at a certain moment, then that is also good, just as healthy, and just as beautiful.

Don't live for the outer world, but from out of your deepest Nature, from your true Being: then you will see where it is good to have fat on your body.

If you don't "lie" to yourself by, for instance, "losing weight" — whereas actually it's your nature to be round — only then will you meet a boyfriend or girlfriend, a partner, who loves YOU and not a FALSE IMAGE.

If a boyfriend or girlfriend "takes" you because (and as long as) you meet the requirements of that skinny-form-without-fat, then there's no question of genuine love for your Genuine Being. Let go; no longer throw pearls before swine; open yourself in love to those friends who wish to truthfully share that golden treasure in you (the heart, the fat, the love, the gentleness. . . .).

And discover round beauty.

CHRONIC FATIGUE SYNDROME
M.E., myalgic encephalomyelitis

Your destructive outlook on life kills you.

You too much consider life as being a coincidental, superficial happening. Possibly, you do experience the psychological problems, but you cut yourself off from *this*

source in you which can show you a way out of this close-to-the-ground life.

Emotional death. You feel squeezed like a sour lemon.

With nervous thoughts you plan this and that; you don't trust your intuition. You build your life with rational thinking and planning, but your deepest Self, your heart, your feelings, aren't being integrated into your existence. You do Want to, and you do make Decisions, but you sometimes fight a desperate battle because you don't listen enough to your intuition, to that inside yourself which tells you: "Stop! You're busy with the wrong thing here; you put your energies into needless things, in a direction that is wrong for you."

That which you absolutely Want is not always the best for you: listen to your feelings, to your deepest Self. You can't handle it all anymore! But in this way you don't *need* to handle it anymore: your Living Self shows you that you're on the wrong track! Do you too much live directed toward the outer world? You have to step out of your old situation. Live on the basis of what you feel deep inside, honest with yourself. First task: stop considering yourself to be a negative, unloved, tiresome, failed being. Second task: put yourself in contact with your heart, with your deepest Self, and no longer fight against the path that you, yourself, unconsciously call up as being the best one for you. Now, don't cling to material things; trustfully surrender to your Self. Stop degrading yourself and mankind to a powerless insignificant being, and place the Crown on your head.

Finally, acknowledge your autonomous Worth and the ability of a human being to create a new life *himself;* no longer doubt those inner powers. Stop wasting energies on useless details, on a future which you rationally can't "pin down." Don't expect the solution of your problem to come from others! Not from diets, not from therapies — although profound communication with others can be beneficial for you, and this is okay of course. But you have to do it yourself!

Create your life in thoughts; long for that which is beautiful, but let go trustfully and don't tire yourself with positive or negative "thoughts": if you believe in this life-process, then that which is best for you, you'll attract. Even a cactus finds nourishment in the dry desert: thus, only in the inexhaustible Source of your deepest Self will you find all the energies you need to be healthy and fit. Self-aware, wise guidance and intuitive trust will go hand-in-hand; building upon that inner Power source deep inside yourself — a give-and-take between Intuition and Self-resolve. Build upon that eternal energy in yourself! Don't cling to a limited Self-image, to one-sided rationalization, to "this *has* to be so," but be open to that which offers itself to you on your path. Be flexibly open to innovations! Also, don't let yourself be sucked empty by others; don't let yourself be squeezed out. Don't fix yourself into others.

Protect yourself; become aware of your worth and border off your terrain. Feel safe in your deepest self, and don't live for the outer world. Don't be creative just in order to gain respect and appreciation from others. . . . Don't build up your life for the sake of outer appearances, as an image, or in order to please the outer world; but only live on the basis of what you Feel, of your inner Source, of your Core.

Don't deny your feelings: go through them, fully experience them, express them; don't live for the eye of others — by doing so you cut yourself off from that deep energy source inside you!

Live in harmony with yourself: be faithful to yourself so that you no longer needlessly tire yourself in order to satisfy the expectations of others. Live in Unity with yourself: don't divide yourself in an exhausting rift by which you execute a task, take on an attitude, or perform a function which goes against your inner nature but fits into the outer framework.

Don't play a role, but play *yourself*. Are you so afraid to be yourself? Do you experience life as being senseless? Do you try to fill your life with loveless sex and purely material things? This isn't life; this attitude results in death.

Now open yourself up to that fundamental power, those atomic energies from out of your deepest Self: in the electrical socket with yourself, you'll receive energy. If you refuse that communication with your Living Self, then you won't be provided with energy.

THE FEET
(Also read the categories Ankle and Toes)

Psychological correspondence

The symbol of knowing one is being carried joyfully by harmony and love. The symbol of being open, in Trust, to yourself, to others.

Thankful acceptance of Life, of everything we encounter on our path.

A flexible exchange between the intuitive, emotional aspect and the more mind-oriented, active part of yourself. The reconciliation in yourself between the receptive "female" and the assertive "male" aspect.

Being solidly anchored in yourself; being master over your emotions in a self-aware way, and full of self-confidence, allowing these feelings, not blocking them. A light-footed, joyful, warm existence, if we build on our deepest, divine Self: standing on your own feet, in balance.

The symbol of naked honesty toward ourselves. Honest confrontation with others, without going beyond your own limits: respect.

Ailments, in general

You carry loads that are too heavy: unburden yourself.

You try to force something, you trust natural evolution too little, you'd "twist" certain things, violate them: let go, let everything and everyone go its course; direct yourself toward yourself!

Because you are too little grounded in yourself, you strongly direct yourself toward others; perhaps you become meddlesome. You feel stuck: solve this problem in yourself!

Don't work out your problems on others! Do emotions weigh too heavily?

Don't look for the cause in others.

Foot problems often ask for a radical break with habits from the past. Have anxieties hindered you from going onward on your life-path? The cause of problems, sadness, and misery is mostly looked for in others; begin now, however, by observing yourself, in all honesty, in the mirror, as it were. Confront yourself with your deepest Self: beneath your problems lies a blissful core; discover it. Let go of others and turn inward. Now, give in to your beautiful feelings, to your longings, independent of others. Bring yourself to realization and dare enjoy every moment: life for life itself, thankfulness! Go onward on this path of joy; when you find happiness inside yourself, then your surroundings will change also. Don't try to change others: evolve yourself, transform. Only in this way, by standing on your own feet, by letting the prime feeling of happiness come inside you and by resolutely going your path, and by allowing others to go their way — then you'll experience being relaxed and joyful.

Don't let yourself be misled or towed along by others: go *yourself* and choose the path that best suits your true nature.

Don't do anything that goes against your nature: be faithful to yourself; don't allow yourself to "be lived"! Don't let yourself be demolished by foolish, so-called, obligations: be good to yourself and make yourself happy. Comfortable, warm, blood-circulation in your feet: magnetic contact with the earth. Don't fly away from yourself; experience your fullness in your earthly body.

Blisters on the feet
(See also Blisters, in general)

Perhaps you walk a lot, but actually you don't really go forward in life! You hide your feelings behind a proud mask; you want to keep your outer ego in high profile. You trust neither yourself nor others; you live a little in fear, on guard. You restrain too much: emotions, spontaneous aggressive powers, healthy impulses — you aren't completely yourself! With your rational thinking, with your critical mind, you block the healthy flow of spontaneous energies. You aren't good to yourself; you are too hard, too inflexible with yourself and your feelings.

Possibly you look for affirmation in the outer world, in deeds, in achievements, because you don't really value yourself enough. In this way, you might make yourself suffer needlessly, because you think that is how it's supposed to be, that you have to play the victim. You'd even cry about another's sadness; no one's helped by this. You know yourself to be protected in the armor you put on; you live too much on edge, standing on tip-toe, ready to shoot, because you don't really believe in immunity, in the security of your deepest Self. You make your skin too hard, but inner feelings get the upper hand. Outwardly, you present yourself as being tough and strong, but the self-aware authority which you are lies hidden — your sensitivity dwells hidden away. Troubled thoughts hinder you from being receptive to the honest language of your body, of your Self.

*Be gentler to yourself. Let intuition and rationality go hand-in-hand. Trust those spontaneous impulses that come from your innermost being; listen to what you **feel**. Needless suffering from being hard to yourself; dominating your life with your mind, without listening to your body, to the longings of your nature — stop it: respect yourself. No one benefits from your appearing to be stronger than you really are, from your hurting yourself. You have a built-in security* system on which you can blindly trust. Descend with your "spirit" into your body and no longer be critical and demanding toward yourself. Allow spontaneous energies and feelings to come through freely; no longer resist the language of your body, of your feelings. You don't have to be on guard at all. Trust in yourself! Let go of worries; surrender to yourself!

Chilblains, and feet that are always cold

The cause of chilblains lies in hesitation, even in the refusal to stand completely, as "I," with your feet on the ground. One hides somewhere. . . . There's a sort of "indecisiveness": one doesn't really manifest one's "I." One still lives partly hidden in the anonymity of the mother's womb, of the serpent-energy. It seems a bit like cowardliness, like betrayal: one doesn't really present oneself as an Individual; it's as though one is afraid of being reprimanded if, in an honest way, one began to manifest oneself — completely and extremely personally — as an "I," with all one's opinions, one's feelings, one's thoughts, one's character. One stays meekly behind the screens of the ALL. . . . One DENIES one's true "I," or better yet, doesn't manifest oneself in a straightforward and honest way.

One is a little afraid. . . . One would prefer to stay "unknown" and thus not be punished, not be seized, not be judged, not be rejected by others. . . . Perhaps one nods "yes" when one inwardly feels "no," even if it's only in order not to reveal oneself. The human being is afraid, anxious, and sometimes somewhat "cowardly" because he refuses to take full responsibility for himself, for his true "I"!

When someone has cold feet, he already pulls in his toes, as it were, before having put down his foot; he pulls in his feet before anyone has a chance to see his toes, let alone have a chance to step on them or give an opinion about them. This person doesn't choose a direction, from out of inner Authority, with the full warmth of his heart. He waits — for what the other is going to say. He holds back. . . . He doesn't really go straight ahead. He assumes an attitude of dependence, waiting to see what the surroundings will do, what the outer world will say, or what the Authority which he puts above his head wants from him. . . . He doesn't want to let it be known who he is. He doesn't truly believe in his inner Power, and he carefully conceals himself.

The person with chilblains on his feet sometimes totally withdraws, as it were, out of his feet: he does NOT take up his space. Actually, he unconsciously expects that someone else or something else will Guide his life for him so that he might observe things from "behind the scenes" of himself.

Cold feet indicate the inability to warmly welcome oneself into one's body.

This person will work at becoming *one* with himself, with his body. Taking up total responsibility for HIS "I." He may not scramble back, doesn't have to hide himself nor be ashamed nor reveal only a "certain form," a certain view, of himself. He will come STRAIGHTFORWARDLY, in an honest way, into his body: he will no longer try to escape from himself. He will STEP INTO LIFE, into his body, without the slightest hesitation. He will push himself into life and exhort himself to honestly manifest his Content, without camouflage, without holding back truth-energies.

If he holds back, if he doesn't dare bring himself into Life as a unified being, straightforward, then he hides behind a death-mask. He shows but an unreal, lifeless image of himself. He doesn't really bring himself into life: he stares at life without really participating in it. His feelings stare woodenly; his longing for Life remains dangling — but it seems he can't really reach it — possibly, he fills himself up with pseudo-things, which have to replace "life": possibly, he warms himself on all kinds of things/people outside himself, which is supposed to compensate for him not totally engaging himself in life, in his body, from within. He has to come to an absolute SURRENDER to himself! He will have to stop holding himself back at the border of life. From grateful awareness of being able to Live as "I," he will allow himself TO BE COMPLETELY in his BODY with all his delightful FEELINGS. He needs to open his HEART to himself, to his "I" as it is, without compromise. He has to dare be himself, taking up HIS place without asking himself whether this is allowed, whether he is good as he is? ... If he takes himself in with warmth, he won't have to look for compensation in pseudo life-sources anymore.

It is important that this person doesn't hide behind anything or anyone: behind no mentors, no parents, no partner, no system, no doctrine, no conventional structures, no schools.... He now has to take RESPONSIBILITY for his "I" and dare to express — in a very honest way — his true nature. He stands with both feet warmly on the earth because he allows himself to Be in LOVE the way HE is in heart and soul. In this warm Self-love, he is no longer afraid of anyone.... Love chases away every anxiety in the heart: now, he dares be himself — honestly, openly and freely. Everything which thus far has existed to compensate for that inner coldness can now disappear. He doesn't expect ANYTHING from others anymore, but knows how to give himself the warmth he needs. He no longer FLEES away from himself, no longer fears to fully take up that highly personal place that is his own! He pushes himself down onto the earth; he takes up the space of his Body right to the tips of his toes: his body becomes an inseparable unity with his content. In Gratitude, he now takes possession of his body. A total integration.

His BODY is no longer purely functional, A HIDING PLACE, a storage space, a place in which he could hide himself and where no one could really find him — but, his body is

a POSSIBILITY to ALLOW his "I"-being to be BORN on earth in a very pleasant way, a possibility to let his Love Exist! And he now manifests himself in a warm, heartfelt way. He pushes himself down onto the ground with both feet: he LIVES! He feels connected with himself in a warm, heartfelt way: he radiates this oneness (soul-body) in a happy, expressive way. He no longer refuses to go in his own DIRECTION: he chooses the direction of the honest life in himself. He feels it; he knows it now, deep down in himself. He now is RESOLUTELY present in life. He no longer feels shortchanged, hurt, hit, pushed aside, unacknowledged by anything or anyone — because he now Robustly takes up his wide PLACE. He no longer can be pushed from his place by anyone: I AM! He now also enjoys more the full-blooded sensuality that flows through his earthly body; he enjoys BEING in his body. He LOVES himself, his living body. He no longer looks down in a chilly way at his body: he is GRATEFUL for his earthly Self and no longer desires anything. ... This Gratitude for his physical existence brings about a warm healing flow. ... He no longer stands with his head at a distance from his body: from out of his warm feeling, he becomes *one* with his body.

Heel pain

You hold on to certain things, habits, and structures from the past. You carry loads that are too heavy. You are too severe with yourself or you allow someone else to be too strongly authoritarian with you. You don't go along with your feelings; you don't listen to your nature; you dutifully fulfill your tasks; you bind up your emotional world in a structure that is too tense.

You try to sustain it; possibly, you act as if it's all easy for you to do, but by doing this you are no longer able to carry on. You feel as if you are but an inferior, forgotten, worthless human being. It's as if your neck were being squeezed, because you deny your own fruitful qualities, your true nature.

You cut yourself off from your Living Self: you live superficially; you can't throw yourself, heart-and-soul, into something because you don't very well know "who you really *are*." Where's your content? Where's the person behind the clown mask?

Therefore, there's no question of advancement or real evolution; you don't truly live from out of yourself; you *let* yourself "be lived"; in this way, you might feel yourself to be the victim "of" — but it is you who doesn't stand with both feet solidly on the ground, it is you who are not fully in solidarity with your feelings, with your heart.

You restrict your life; you don't allow yourself any joy; your burdens weigh too heavily, because you don't listen to that voice in yourself. Are you dancing on hot coals? Do you possibly flee from yourself or hide behind an "inferior" role?

You don't only have duties, don't only carry burdens, but first and foremost, you have rights: you may take up your space on earth, anchor your heels very solidly in the ground. Feel that secure Basis of your inner Self: you are master over your existence. Place yourself in the center and listen lovingly to your heart, to that which your nature, your body, spontaneously ask, because it's good for you. Go on, let go of the past. Take your life in hand and don't be too hard on yourself. Now, look inside yourself and discover your worthy content.

Put the authority in yourself; don't degrade yourself; carry your life in joy and allow yourself to flow with the stream of your nature. No longer restrict yourself emotionally!

Are the stones burning under your feet? Take your life in your own hands; don't let anyone else put pressure on you; bring about changes in your life; don't pay attention to the expectations of others; first of all you owe love to yourself. Come forward honestly with your true feelings so there's no conflict

between what you feel and what you bring out: this, after all, hinders an open, joyful exchange with your surroundings, and as a result you become estranged from yourself. Don't turn away from yourself: "rehabilitation!" of yourself.

Heel spur

Anxieties, a feeling of insecurity. On the one hand you allow others to treat you as they like; you listen to an authority outside you because you are afraid, insufficiently present in yourself. You only follow the footsteps of your father or your strict teacher; you don't really live on your own solid foundation. You don't honor yourself; without daring to push your unique personality through, you remain rooted in regulations, habits, or systems that have been taught to you.

You allow yourself to be crushed, suppressed; you do what someone "tells" you to; you allow yourself to "be lived," allow yourself to be wedged, without resisting. On the other hand, you are stuck with a lot of sadness; also, you cling to others because you don't dare to build upon yourself.

You experience yourself as a prisoner with a ball and chain on his leg; you make yourself stuck. You feel weak and vulnerable; as a defense you lock yourself up inside yourself.

Introverted sadness; sometimes you don't see the sense of it anymore. Inwardly, you sometimes become angry, but it is you who throws out the anchor into someone else's basis; it is you who refuses to lead a fruitful and highly personal life in a self-reliant, independent way. You don't listen to yourself, to your heart; you ignore your possibilities of self-realization.

Strong resistance to self-affirmation, to fully experiencing your feelings and sharing them with your fellow man — simply because you feel so vulnerable. You "hook" yourself onto someone else instead of sending out your own roots into the ground. You stay in a situation that doesn't offer you free breathing space. Your consciousness-energy, your "spirit," has no full "impact" upon your body because you are partly *absent* from yourself. Desperate, sometimes fatalistic.

Concentrate your powers in your body and stay close to yourself. Listen only to the authority in yourself. Break with old laws and habits. Know yourself to be secure and solid in your deepest Self. Build a solid structure for yourself; count on yourself and be faithful only to your heart, to your true nature. Break loose from ties that are suffocating you; free yourself, and don't be afraid to take a totally new turn in your life. A path to independence, to self-appreciation and love for yourself.

Only if you are in harmony with yourself will you be able to share feelings with others, in trust, freedom, and openness. No longer hide yourself in the shadow of someone else: live from out of yourself!

Sweaty feet

You come out of an abyss, and you are afraid of sliding back into it. Anxieties. Inwardly, you feel unsure; you don't really know where you are going. You don't have true Authority over yourself; you give others, the outer world, too much power over you. Possibly, you achieve a great deal in order to prove yourself — to them. You are dependent on others because you feel uncertain and unsafe by yourself. You are afraid that something sharp, something hard, might hit you; mortal fears. You go through life in a mistrusting, anxious way. You do *not* really believe in the inner Powers of self-realization of your "I." You exert yourself emotionally in order to be accepted by others. It's as if you are afraid of yourself, of phantoms, and of your deep feelings. You ignore your possibilities; you experience yourself as only a weak being. Emotions direct your life, but you anxiously run away from them. You just think and fret tensely.

Don't grab anxiously onto anything, let go of everything and surrender to your Nature, to your feelings. Every human being has an inner indestructible core which, when you give it your trust, will take care that nothing negative can happen to you.

Turn away from death and submerge yourself in life; don't be afraid of your emotions. Full of self-confidence, experience your feelings; you are strong and immortal. Anxieties only indicate that you've not yet found the path to life, the path to self-aware creation of your life. Cheerfully build upon your Nature! Self-confidence.

FEVER

There's a tense, sickly thought-kernel present in you; anxious brooding, anger, nervousness — and as a reaction to this your healing energies are now being called up.

Chaff and wheat have been ground together in your head, in your confused feelings; it is time now for sifting and purifying. Your blood becomes too heavy, as it were, because of the burden of oppressive energies, which are the result of too-intense seeking thoughts.

With your consciousness, you are *there* where your thoughts are, with a person or at work etc.; you are feverishly busy with everything but the peaceful here-and-now.

Your core is, as it were, outside your body: the fever calls you back here. Now, you are too little aware of your basis, of your connection to the earth, of the joy about your total Self.

Grounding! From the here-and-now, set to work on your problems and your evolution. Don't drift out of yourself with your thoughts. Don't lose contact with your deepest Self, where you can sense intuitively every solution. First, root your own "I", your sun-

center, solidly into the Earth; you can gradually build up on the basis of this sureness. In self-assuredness you don't allow yourself to be rushed by anything or anyone, because it was actually you who rattled yourself. Look at your unrest, at the busyness in your thoughts, at the needless nervousness: come back into yourself; the cause lies in you. So don't be angry. Old, soiled energies will be led away to make room for new life-power. Trust, rest, letting go — instead of feverish "thinking."

ties are unnecessary in the light of your creative possibilities. You really can count on yourself one hundred per cent; just share with others in love, don't grasp because of a feeling of "need." No longer carry needless burdens, undo the chains, and live on lightheartedly; then, altered vibrations with magnetic power, propelled by the trust and belief in yourself, make the growths gradually disappear. No longer hold on! Free yourself from every burden!

FIBROMAS
benign tumors of fibrous tissue

You experience yourself as being too weak, too powerless, and as a result you try to get a "grip," or power, over certain situations or persons. You cling to persons or things outside yourself; furthermore, with your thoughts you constantly stir up the negativity of life, of your past; your feelings weigh heavily — you carry enormous burdens; your thoughts circle around — you don't let loose! You allow yourself to be blown over by happenings; you determine your own life much too little; you allow yourself to be influenced; you doubt. You don't resolutely choose *one* certain direction.

Powerlessness, anxieties, and unsureness lead to somberness, power, and aggression.

Now let your Conscious "I" self-determine a path, in wisdom and insight; the rest will then follow. Be faithful to yourself and don't cling to things or people outside yourself; do only that which lies in the projection of your nature. Be creative and fruitful; produce! Allow all your energies to come through freely, and resolutely aim them in one direction. Let go of the old. You are stronger than you think: become aware of your power and possibilities. Black thoughts and anxie-

FIBROMYALGIA

Standing still, refusal, "No," not wanting to go on nor grow, nor live. It's now been enough; you don't want anything to do with it anymore. You overflow with accumulated emotions, sadness, sorrow, wistfulness, painful remembrances from the past. You brace yourself, "angular" resistance; the child in you suffers and longs for sweetness, warmth, the earthly, love. But you've already gone through too much pain; you now become like stone, as it were; you cut yourself off from your gentle feelings; you don't give sweetness to yourself because you expect too much from others. Powerful streams of inner energy wish to flow through in creativity and productivity, but you resist this natural flow. You are hard to the child in yourself!

You are sheltered securely in yourself; make yourself warmly welcome; don't expect from others that which you deny yourself. Shower yourself with flowers and enjoy juicy earthly fruits. Experience yourself as a fruit ripened in the sun; enjoy that warm sun-center in yourself. Enjoy the sensually beautiful, tastes and fragrances, your body, the colors and sounds that are pleasurable to the senses. Allow yourself to grow up, and adore the child in yourself with a clearly awake consciousness. Allow sweetness in your ex-

istence. *Produce and harvest, go on and create your existence. No longer hinder that warm emotional flow in yourself: warm those places in yourself that feel cold and hurt. Relax, and enjoy the light of the sun; no longer cringe; open yourself in love toward yourself. Discover joy!*

FINGERS

THE THUMB

Psychological correspondence

The thumb, as a radiating energetic source, externalizes to what measure we become Aware of our Worth without sinking into anxiety, sadness or nervousness.

The thumb indicates the powerful presence of primal powers, of sensual longings, of primitive emotions, of needs; it indicates attachment and the secure womb, self-gratification, instincts, and sexuality. Even more strongly, however, it indicates transformation: the conversion of these primal-elements into Consciousness-raising! The extremely strong fundamentals of your Self. You know yourself to be safe and protected in your nature.

Shelteredness: the child in you knows itself to be safe under the Authority and power of your "I"-consciousness. You reach only for a hold IN yourself.

You handle your primitive powers and feelings; you satisfy your sensory and material bodily needs. You take care that you lack nothing. Primitive instincts are being transformed into conscious experiencing of reality: you provide yourself with joy and happiness. You take up your central place. You acknowledge the Worth of yourself; you do that for which you have talents or have a calling.

You allow yourself the pleasure of earthly enjoyments; you don't punish yourself by following severe diets. You don't sacrifice yourself for an ideal, for a person: you listen first of all to your own longings.

You occupy the total Space you need to occupy! You don't smother yourself by exerting yourself for someone else — neglecting yourself — or by aggressive, possessive behavior to guard your "possession" or your partner; doing this, you would get yourself stuck.

As long as you look for a hold outside yourself — as long as you experience a "need" for "receiving" from others — instead of providing for yourself, you limit your space, you aren't free.

Do you demolish yourself with Negativity? Or, do you completely seize power over yourself and gallop along strongly on your own Basis?

Do you dare to enjoy? Do you build upon your fundamentally strong powers? Do you feel warm and secure in yourself? You radiate like a Sun; you move Freely, the way you *are,* you dare to voice your opinion. You radiate and *give* instead of absorbing, seizing; you warm yourself; you let go of those emotions that are too much for you.

You are born out of yourself; now you provide for yourself, the umbilical cord is broken. Also, in the area of life-philosophy and thinking programs, you are not a follower; you think for yourself, not according to your parents, your mentors or your teachers.

A healthy thumb also indicates quiet brain activity, by which a balance is maintained between sober, logical thinking and the feelings, the intuition.

In the sureness of the safe Basis, your deepest Self, there's no question of anxiety and sorrow, of worried thoughts, of nervousness: your Head is not overloaded if you are not pursued by anxious, nervous thoughts.

From pure, self-assured Awareness, you can push away things you don't want, which only burden you. You are master of your existence: you determine who you allow to come in. You don't allow yourself to be threatened, nor to be suffocated by others. You don't allow yourself to be "seized" by a teaching or a person.

You are good and gentle to yourself. From out of the pure joy-center in your heart, you radiate loving energies in all possible directions.

You take care that the Rest in yourself is maintained, that your thoughts, as pure yellow powers, are not burdened with sadness and anxieties. You experience a unity in yourself between thinking and feeling, because ultimately your all-embracing, Conscious "I" is master. The thumb can indicate just how much you remain stuck to sorrows from the past, and it asks that a break be made with certain things, that heavy emotional burdens be let go of in order to keep your head cool — that you don't go on in "thoughts" but truly go on in action with your total being.

Ailments, in general; causes

Anxieties, nervous thoughts, insecure dark feelings. Sadness. Unsteadiness, instability, imbalance: emotions are suffocating you; they don't allow you to think in a healthy and sober way. Heated brains; you plan a lot in your head rather than actually carrying things out. You carry heavy loads; you can't let go of the useless things from the past.

Aggression; angry, frustrated emotions and thoughts fill your lungs so that you hardly have any free breathing space for yourself. Instead of taking care of yourself, you live for others; you seize them or you feel they should fulfill your expectations. Because you don't believe in your own powers — don't believe in your worth — you are sometimes like a grownup who still lives in his mother's womb or has to hold on to his mother's hand.

Or do you try again and again to satisfy the needs of others? Don't you completely live the life you'd like to lead? Do you let yourself be scorched by the sun, by the authority outside yourself, and do you see life "double"? Don't you act out of unity in yourself? Instead of honestly enjoying the earthly, your feelings, do you perhaps refuse to truly live from out of yourself? Do you almost throw up because you hold on to so much, emotionally and in thought? Are you nauseated because of yourself, because you refuse to evolve onward, because you again and again are stuck at the same braking ideas, because you refuse to transform your primitive powers into consciousness, because you limit your life to brooding, to sexual or aggressive thoughts?

Possibly, you stand still; you rear up; you feel seized by anxiety, possibly by panicky fear. You feel cold and naked, unsafe in yourself; you are afraid of those primitive, unconscious powers in yourself. You run away from your own emotional content because you don't assume mastery over yourself. Possibly, you feel helpless, without oxygen; you are so afraid of dying, of not being able to keep yourself under control, afraid of yourself.

You overload your nervous system with sad, nervous thoughts; you insufficiently trust that deep emotional ground in you, your intuition. You absorb too much; you don't protect yourself. You exaggeratedly take in everything and everyone, information and experiences, because you don't really respect yourself, because you aren't Aware of your sun-power!

A feeling of suffocation: you stuff yourself with the ideas of those who bring you up, of your friends, because you feel so small, powerless, unsafe in yourself.

Open up your lungs! Let your head become lighter; free yourself of needless burdens.

Move Freely, direct your inner powers outwardly; warm yourself in love and acknowledge, in trust, that worthy, masterful Consciousness-source which you are. Build on these fundamental powers in yourself and allow transformation, evolution. In a self-aware way, become master over yourself, your deeds, your thoughts, your emotions.

Fracture of the thumb

You feel your back's against the wall; anxieties and psychological suffocation.

Aggressive confrontation with someone (or with a situation). For far too long you've bottled up your powers; until now, you haven't truly built your life on yourself, on your true, real core. You can't really go on the way you've organized your life until now.

You will begin finding your security only in yourself; you will free yourself and transform your anger into self-realization. You break out of your oppressive situation; nervous anger, anxious, dark thoughts.

Let this be a signal that you may "break" with habits that have a suffocating influence on you. (See Ailments, above)

THE FOREFINGER
index finger

Psychological correspondence

Me first.
Acknowledging the wisdom in your divine Self; knowing the worth of your "I."

The "I" stands up for itself. Body and spirit, emotions and "head": in unity together.

In Your life, you are in first place. You feel strong and secure in your Self.

You flexibly surrender to your nature. The freedom to be yourself, without anxiety, trusting your own Authority. You are proud of yourself; you demonstrate this pride outwardly, in calmness and dignity. In wisdom, you point things out to yourself and to others. You don't let yourself be pushed aside; you don't feel undervalued or pushed into a corner by others — because you, yourself, create your large space; because you, independently, without the help of others, in an autonomous and self-assured way, indicate your path and place all Power over your life in your Self.

You don't tolerate someone else stealing the food from your plate or someone hindering you on your path toward a certain goal or ideal: "Leave me alone!" You don't lock yourself up inside yourself; you come forth, in a relaxed way, proud and self-assured, building on that inner Authority; you dare express your opinion in words, dare to show your true nature; you feel free to show your emotions without fear, to proclaim knowledge based on inner wisdom, without becoming pedantic or minding other people's business thereby. Here, one chooses either wisdom and inner power or (because you feel inwardly anxious and unsure) priggishness and the desire to seize power over others.

You can see things in a very broad view; you are able to put things in perspective, to be tolerant, to leave free or to show understanding of others, because you are so *Sure* of your "I."

It doesn't bother you what others think of you, because you are sure of yourself.

You allow yourself to blossom in all possible directions; you constantly enlarge your life's space. You don't tie yourself down by wanting to "grasp" everything with your rational thinking: you trust your intuition, your feelings.

You don't carp about things, you don't criticize, but you strive for beautiful ideals and goals. You don't constantly blame or reproach others, but you go on yourself; you push back your limits again and again. The path to self-realization and wisdom is without end. You allow yourself to be reborn constantly; you take care of your inner and outer aspects. You stand up for your joy; on your path, the spectrum of colors and odors expands. You choose to experience life like a feast.

Now, first of all, point your finger inward, at yourself, at your heart, at the light of life which burns inside you. You are silent when you feel you should be silent. You are silent in wisdom; you speak in wisdom. Ever and again you look for the cause of "what happens to you" . . . in yourself.

Ailments, in general

Do you tensely want to outwardly keep up your Authority because inwardly you experience yourself as powerless and unsure — because you are cut off from your own feelings, because you don't really get a grip on yourself, because you don't really believe in your own worth? Do you perhaps feel passed over by others, or undervalued, or perhaps even dominated? These are only the consequences of self-undervaluation. Or are you a "know-it-all"?

Do you want people to listen to you? Then first listen to yourself. If you remain stuck at the surface of your existence, if you don't listen first of all to your own deep, inner Authority, then don't blame others, don't expect anything.

Are you sad? Do you want to be in *first* place in someone else's world or in the outer world? And don't you manage to do it? Do you stubbornly fixate your thoughts on certain things outside you, while you are feeling so powerless? Let go, and turn inward!

Or do you expect someone else to tell you what to do, or where your path lies? Do you get inwardly angry because someone doesn't do what you say? Do you emotionally isolate yourself from others? Do you create a barrier? Then this is a consequence of the fact that you really don't accept yourself, that you really don't put yourself in the first place; that you still always look to the outer world for an affirmation of your existence. And this, of course, you can't do. Make yourself welcome, and listen to your longings.

Do you feel like Don Quixote? Do you feel so powerless, so cut off from your divine Self, that you are afraid of something threatening, of something very evil deep inside yourself? Do you fear being "seized" by something or someone? Something that would invade you and threaten you? Does anxiety choke you? Do you trust so little in your deepest Self? Do you have a dominating, critical, judgmental, bossy attitude regarding yourself, regarding others?

Do you run in place without making any progress? Are you furious, frustrated, because you don't realize yourself the way you would like to, because you've placed all power outside yourself? Do you place thinking, your head, so centrally in your life that there's too little place for earthly enjoyment, for feeling and intuition? Your head can become a nervous, insane grinder. Possibly, you hinder yourself from transforming powerful energies and aggression into action and hinder yourself from going on in a self-aware way. With thoughts, you block yourself. You are stuck. You put up blinders. Possibly, you fixate your attention on Image, on Outer appearance or on the negativity of others. In these circumstances you overlook the worth and power of the "I." Or, do you lock yourself up in yourself in a claustrophobic way? Do you only listen to that which others expect from you? Until it all becomes too much and you don't accept or tolerate anything anymore. Possibly, you then stand up for yourself in an enormous, abrupt manner, after a long time of sustained frustration: you want to free yourself! But for you true liberation lies in solving anxieties, in taking away this feeling of powerlessness by working out the doubt regarding yourself, by acknowledging the Power in yourself, by building up your life in a self-aware way and acknowledging fully your "I"! By taking good care of yourself and not longing for the acknowledgment of others.

Make it possible for you to be freely and flexibly yourself, so that you, yourself, choose your direction, so that you stand in the center of your existence, so that you put true Authority in yourself.

Enlarge your life space; open your lungs wide; move your limits; be born in yourself.

In pride, acknowledging your Self, outwardly manifesting your true Nature. Don't point at others; look inside yourself. No power-game; acknowledge the power in yourself.

Fracture of the forefinger

Anxiety about losing power over yourself and your emotions. You hold on to certain situations in a, sometimes, child-like way; fear hinders you from letting go. You are afraid of drowning in your emotions; you row and row, but the boat sinks. You should let go instead of frantically rowing on in a waterlogged boat, in a situation.

Because you want to seize and hold on to too much: just as well outside yourself (people, situations) as inside yourself (you want to place your nature under control, pushing your feelings in a certain direction), because you want to seize power over something or someone, because you feel so powerless and stuck in yourself, seized, in the power of others or of circumstances. You might revolt, might want to anxiously run away, but you aren't really able to build your life in a self-aware way because you don't listen to the wisdom IN yourself. You run away from that which is most beautiful in yourself. You fight *against* others, *against* situations, instead of letting go and resolutely building your own life. Emotions are piling up in such a way that you can't keep suppressing them. Nervousness, anxiety and panic. You don't believe in that divine wisdom in yourself; possibly, you get mixed up in power-games, or you get involved in a game of sexual-seduction and power. This is because you refuse to acknowledge the power and mastery over yourself that is in your Self. As long as you ignore this, you will anxiously run away from everything that has you in its power, but in fact you run away from your most beautiful Core. You feel bound hand-and-foot. Conflicting feelings ravage you: attracting-rejecting, because it's this very game that you play with yourself. A question

of power - powerlessness, of wisdom - denial of your wisdom; eye-blinders. You'd like to break out in aggressive fury! An honest confrontation with yourself, an acknowledgment of your inner Wisdom, self-contemplation: here, the solution begins, not in rebellion against others, against circumstances. Peace lies in you.

THE MIDDLE FINGER

Psychological correspondence

You plant yourself solidly with your feet on the Earth. You know yourself to be protected within a safe Basic Structure. The middle finger indicates the long path you have to go in your life. The middle finger is like the guard at the threshold inside you, the guard who sees to it that you don't run away from your task and your responsibilities, that you don't get "derailed," that you stay within *these* lines — the lines which are necessary for the realization of your task, your goals. The middle finger represents the possibilities you plan — the work, the productivity — so that you can reap the harvest later on.

You do what you have to do; you organize and make plans with your common sense.

You trust that patron saint in yourself; you operate and function smoothly; you seek, and always find, your way; conscious of your goal, you walk in a certain direction.

You look out; you are sure of your ground; you feel safe and sheltered in your Basis, in your deepest Self. You are building a solid house, a solid structure, with thick walls; you feel safe in your deep hole.

You always look forward; you don't remain stuck in the past; you don't stand still, twiddling your thumbs. You allow creative energies, healthy aggressive powers, to blossom freely; you produce; you are fruitful on many earthly levels, including in artistic matters. You direct the childlike energies and the active powers in yourself in a self-aware way, but with care, within structural order. With respect, you take care of yourself, and of your body.

You don't linger over trivial details, nor over outer appearance. You resolutely go on; the leadership of your life rests with you. With a wise, calm, clear eye, you are faithful to the higher rules of morality — to rules which contribute to respect for yourself, for people in general.

You scatter your seed over the earth; you feel responsible, including responsibility for others.

You are willing to "learn" and to grow and to give the necessary effort needed to conquer the required obstacles. You don't believe in Fate or coincidence, but you work, you create your life path, in a self-aware way. You conquer the negative, the devilish; you don't offer resistance to your evolution. You stand solidly, you let go of that which is superfluous.

Ambition here means self-realization, not the urge for power, not the pursuit of careers or the pursuit of stars. You are ambitious to make, ever more strongly, your life fulfill its Worth, more and more to enrich your Self, to produce in fruitfulness.

The middle finger indicates how you find your way in earthly life; how you deal with emotions, sexuality, earthly things and techniques in general. How you find your way to other people. How you resolutely make yourself a path through the emotional world. You are multi-functional. Active and full of courage in fulfilling your task, your ambition, your plans. The Bull that plows furrows in the earth. The Capricorn that climbs the mountaintop in a well-planned way.

The "practical" cares of a mother for her child. The farmer who sows his field.

Ailments, in general

Anxieties, emotions, can flood the secure basic structure if you're not really present here-and-now in your earthly being. You think, you float, you fret and brood, you exist in your "head" too much: your conscious "I"

has too little grip on your body, on your life, because you are too much "gone" — in thoughts, in dreams — instead of actually building up your life in an active and concrete way, transforming your creativity into productivity. Frustration, anxious aggression, block your passage.

Self-degradation. "But who am I?" You withdraw into yourself, passively, because you don't really believe in your consciousness-powers. Thus, as a consequence of your feeling of inferiority, the large array of talents and creativity in you can be limited to sexuality or to sexual thoughts; or you limit yourself to a modest role; possibly, you mock yourself while looking down on yourself. You ignore your worth; you avoid the responsibility of building yourself a fruitful life. The angels or the gnomes will do it. . . .

Two possibilities: either you withdraw, you hesitate, standing still on your path, not taking your life into your own hands. Or, inversely, you try to — and absolutely want to — push ahead upon this path or for that goal. You don't give up, you force things, you don't slack off, even if outer circumstances indicate to you that it would be better to let go. Neither extreme is good: not effacing yourself in a forgotten background, nor the exaggerated "wanting" too much — nor an exaggerated accentuation of structural laws and requirements, of career, of an aggressive urge for power. Being hard on yourself.

Respect for worthy morality — not according to the letter of the law — a morality that has grown from inside and is not put upon you from the outside.

Respect for that which is beautiful, for that which is valuable, with style, but without getting stuck on an exaggerated sense of protocol and solemnity; a Structure which naturally suits the Content. Healthy pride, wholesome labor, and creativity.

You don't stick your powers and talents in the ground. You spread the seed over the field. You don't frustrate yourself by keeping these powerful energies in, whereby an outlet will be sought in sexual experience — not as an expression of love, but as compensation for the "emptiness" in yourself, because you refuse to make use of all your possibilities in a broad field. Acknowledge yourself, discover your worth, and go on without hesitation. Get a hold of your life, try to see clearly into yourself, and don't place the Ideal outside yourself.

Be fruitful, self-aware, active, proud, resolute, sure of yourself. Don't lose yourself in details.

Don't wait until pent-up energies explode in an aggressive or sexual bomb, but allow your powerful energies to unfold themselves gradually, within a specific terrain, a structure, or the lines you, yourself, place. In this way, you keep everything going beautifully, without emotions getting the upper hand.

Calm, balanced labor, without stress, without being too harsh with yourself.

Fracture of the middle finger

You feel *too* stuck; you want more and further. Repressed aggressive powers break through. Revolt. Possibly you want too much in matters of career or ambition. Or are you too severe with regard to structural limitations, to the exercising of power, to laws and duties? Perhaps you declare war; with giant cannonballs you'd like to gain ground or take a position. Aggression can come out in several ways, in word and deed.

For too long you've limited yourself, because you've paid too little attention to your deeper worth. Have you been concentrating your thoughts for too long a time on Image, matter, sexuality, superficial Rules — instead of giving room to content, feeling, and creativity in many areas? You live too much stuck fast, too hard: shake yourself looser, and build Calmly and steadily toward a beautiful future, without forcing. Don't push yourself into a corner, don't let yourself be pushed backward until a backlash follows. Don't reach further than the next step; don't

"want" more than that which is good for you NOW. Don't be anxious; build on the solid Basis in yourself.

THE RING FINGER

Psychological correspondence

How do you relate to yourself: are you good and loving to yourself? If you don't "retain" or "hold on to" something or someone or seize "power" over them; if you place the golden nimbus like a solar crown on your head; if you are Conscious of the worth and beauty of yourself and Life — then you experience the power, the fullness of your Self, then you are open to higher Consciousness-energies.

Death is being led away: here, there's room only for Joyful Life! Your head and your body are sensitive, receptive channels for your Spiritual Awareness.

The "sacred covenant" with yourself: in self-trust, in Love, you acknowledge the warm Sun-center in yourself.

You feel Free: you can count on your deepest core; you don't have to worry about anything. Optimal communication between body and "soul-awareness."

The relationship between the moon-aspect and the sun-aspect is harmonious: the warm, comfortable, secure arms of the Father in you comfort the child in you when it feels sad or lonely. In this unity of yourself, you *can* never be left out in the cold, you can never feel lonely. You can share this love with a partner, but the Ring indicates, first of all, the most beautiful seclusion, the fullness of yourself. You cherish yourself with reverence and respect.

You are well aware of the sanctity that every human being carries inside: Life itself.

You are aware of your worth; you are good and gentle to yourself. You love yourself. The ring finger indicates, therefore, to what degree you approach the Core of life, to what degree you live in harmony with the deep wishes of your Heart; you don't live at the surface, nor like a wooden doll. Your feelings are allowed to exist freely: you don't bind yourself down; you don't pose obstacles to life. Peace and reconciliation, harmony and safety, deep in yourself: you solidly stand on your own feet. You don't say No to the power of your Sun; you don't cling to a partner.

The Ring Finger indicates to what degree you put yourself in the shadow of someone's else's sun, to what degree you *need* others in order to compensate for the denial of the Sun in yourself! A relationship with someone else will give joy if you both, in reciprocal respect, ally yourselves to each other as equal partners — not when one's own Identity is being destroyed in the relationship.

In this sense, the Ring Finger is a paradoxical symbol of both Freedom and Union. A fundamentally strong Trust in yourself. A feeling of ultra-security. Nothing can go wrong. You don't lose your life in details, in outer futilities. You know yourself to be protected in yourself; you completely take up your space. Proud as a lion, free as a bird. Living fully, experiencing your nature and your feelings. Suppleness in emotion; solid on your Basic Structure.

The gentle, the "female," is led by the "male," the self-assured aspect in you. You don't flee from sadness, from emotions: you work them out; you solve emotional problems in the light of love for yourself, in the light of a pure Self-awareness. You hold on only to your Self: you put in yourself all power over yourself. You warn others when they hinder you in your own free being, when someone wants to threaten you, wants to restrict your space. You are the guardian of the golden treasure chest in yourself.

You don't "tie yourself down." Via fine "antennae," the electrical network in you — the nervous system — is tuned to messages from your deepest Self, to awareness-signals; you constantly translate impulses from your inner Self into your earthly being. Freedom exists in not trying to "comprehend," to "grasp," with your rational mind, with your hands, but in being open ever again to new experiences, new impulses, new information. A future-directed trust in the Now, in your Self. The sacred alliance, the unity with your Self leads to Freedom, openness.

Ailments, in general; causes

You feel pain; you don't offer yourself trust, love and freedom; this can then lead again to relationship problems. You don't get a true grip on yourself, and therefore you try to hold on to people and things outside yourself. Anxiously, you try to hold on to power or to grasp it, but sooner or later you have to "let go."

Possibly, you feel painfully hurt; others can still hurt you, because your feelings are insufficiently cherished by your warm heart, by your self-aware "I." Your joy is still dependent on the reaction, the attitude of others! The cause of your sadness, your pain, doesn't lie in others, but in yourself: You attune your life insufficiently to yourself; You are too pliable, perhaps too docile, or too dependent on someone other than yourself; but you are too cruel, too hard on yourself. Don't you love yourself? Are you sick of yourself: don't you think yourself to be good at all, and are you destroying yourself, are you killing yourself?

You think danger is hanging above your head; you feel anxieties and threats: here, we're only dealing with the suppression of your own powers! The danger doesn't lie outside you.

Do you ignore your talents? Do you restrain beautiful energies? Then, you live angry and frustrated. Do you spit out your gall instead of acknowledging yourself?

Don't you give yourself room to exist; do you suffocate yourself? Do you cling to a partner instead of giving freedom to yourself and to your partner? Are you hard, angry, sarcastic, merciless, desperate? Are you sick of everything? Would you like to spit it out?

Do you say "no " to that Sun-power in yourself? Do you allow yourself to drift along on a sea of emotions, while you aren't directing your life in an Independent way? Do you revolt against a situation, against a relationship in which you've positioned yourself like a wooden doll, like a mannequin, without depth? Are your heart and deeper feelings, your natural powers, calling for acknowledgment? Aggression, nervousness: Do you want to free *yourself?*

Do you feel old, sick, looking for "support" instead of counting on your deepest Self?

Do you trample on your own heart, or allow yourself to be hurt by others? Do you live in a way that is too unearthly, too floating, too "spiritual," without taking into account your body, sensory enjoyments, earthly joy? Would you sooner live toward death than life? Do you leave yourself in the cold and then expect others to warm you? Do you refuse to stand on your own feet? Do you live too much on the surface of existence? Do you attach more importance to outer worth and Image than to your feelings and deeper values?

Are mortal fears throttling you? Do you not dare to be nice, to express your warmth? Do you not dare to outwardly manifest your energies, your Individual qualities? Do you not really look at the core, at the essentials of life?

Fracture of the ring finger

You are revolting against a situation that doesn't please you: sadness and aggression have piled up. But even if you now say "Stop! No!" to a partner, to a certain situation that has been going on for too long, you should know that the deeper cause lies in the fact that, in the past, you really were fighting against your own Sun-center, that you denied your Self-aware "I," your worth, that you lived too much for someone else, that your deepest feelings were actually never given the room that is so necessary to live freely

and joyfully. You were busy suffocating yourself or allowing yourself to be suffocated; now, you revolt, also against authority — the sun outside yourself. You are tired of not truly being able to Live! Only if you are directed toward yourself, in respect and love, will you no longer attract painful experiences. Someone else can't hurt you, can't shortchange you: you can shortchange yourself by not being faithful to your heart, by not listening to the voice of your heart, which asks for freedom and joy, independent of others. Wholesome energies have been blocked for too long, and they ask for a breakthrough, outward, into action, creativity, and self-realization.

THE LITTLE FINGER

Psychological correspondence

Represents correctness, integrity, purity, clear openness to the inside, toward others. Inner knowing, divine wisdom, the Ability to assimilate everything, to gain knowledge, to calmly open yourself in flexibility. Wisely knowing, calm trust, being aware of your divine worth as a human being.

There, where heaven and earth touch each other: the manifestation, in a clear earthly structure, of divine Awareness-energies, of wisdom. A balance between intuition — inner knowing — and the rational, healthy mind. Being honest with yourself; an honest megaphone from your personal content to others.

You work out new experiences and information, you put things in perspective; you easily assimilate, without fear, because you feel Peaceful in the divine Knowledge.

Bringing out your Content, your message. Taking care of this content: you know yourself to be protected in the wisdom, in the knowing, in your Awareness.

Also the symbol of flexibility, suppleness, by which you adjust to new circumstances, to other people, without having to behave differently from how you feel inwardly. You are a human being, unified and straightforward: open and clear as pure water, you are aware of the worth of honest gold in yourself. You don't doubt your wisdom, your ability to reach sensible decisions, to go on in a self-aware way in *that* direction which you, yourself, point out. You live in balance, in self-assuredness, without the fear of failure. You feel calm on that large Basis of your Individual Being; you feel peaceful under the roof of pure and beautiful Awareness.

Your life is not built on that which your parents taught you, but on wisdom and knowledge that you acquired yourself. You don't let yourself be pushed around. You don't want to go, confused and nervous, in a hundred directions at the same time. This is because you, yourself, determine your life, undisturbed — because you don't build your life on superficialities, in self-doubt, but on the certainty of your personal Insight. You don't allow yourself to be indoctrinated or intimidated; you feel yourself to be free — open, honest, spontaneous, natural, unconstrained, curious, hungry to learn, as original as a "fool." You adventure through life; you flexibly look in many directions without blinders on your eyes! Thoughtfully observing, gathering your energies in order to then go on in full force.

Ailments, in general; causes

You ignore your wisdom; you don't use your brains; you don't really build up your life yourself. You let your parents, your friends, do what they want with you. You don't really dare stand up for yourself; you don't really know how or where to go, because you are afraid or cowardly. Possibly, you blow with the wind, or you don't build your own path, and therefore you drift and you talk this way one time, that way another time. Sometimes this appears to be dishonest or hypocritical, but in fact it's your indecisiveness, your nervous unsureness: you don't very well know what you want; you look for a grip outside yourself; you withdraw anxiously

into a hole; you don't dare manifest yourself the way you really are because you don't believe in that divine beauty and wisdom in yourself. You degrade yourself and humanity in general. You don't honor the divine in the human being; you feel, therefore, anything but peaceful and full of trust. Nervous, agitated, seeking, fretting. ... Ultimately, you remain standing still; you let others "beat" you because you don't really see where to go; you bend in exaggerated pliability. Possibly, you want to be on good terms with everyone, and so you use flattery. Do you withdraw? Are you silent instead of speaking? Do you refuse to give voice to that which is most beautiful in you?

You burn away on the spot. Do you refuse to take the reins in hand? Don't you care about anything anymore? Does anxiety paralyze you because you cut yourself off from that which is profound, intuitive, and from your deepest Self? Do you restrict your brain activity to fretting, to thinking, to rational or intellectual worries, instead of trusting inner knowledge, intuition — trusting that which rises above rationality? Your path doesn't run straight; you walk bow-leggedly, as it were, because you hold yourself back, because you don't believe in those beautiful powers deep in yourself. Possibly, you get involved in a "marriage of convenience," in whatsoever area, in order to keep the peace, because you refuse to find that Peace inside yourself; you close yourself off from that pure, divine source in you. You don't take up psychological space; you have, as it were, a shortage of oxygen. You make your life oppressive. Self-liberation, openness, and wise insight are necessary for you to experience joy.

Fracture of the little finger

You want to free yourself. You no longer participate! You throw off the pressure on your head, the burdens from your shoulders. You revolt against those who, until now, have determined or directed your life, against those who exercised Authority over you. Nervous, aggressive powers break through; no more question of flexibility. An urge toward inner liberation, to becoming completely faithful to your original nature, without compromise, without suppression.

Arthritic fingers

No matter what the cost, you want to push the flow into a certain direction. In vain! You try to get power over a certain situation or person, and you want it absolutely so, and there is no other way. Holding on. "We will see who is the strongest!" In this way, you totally cut yourself off from all light and freedom! Also, proud resistance, sometimes against others who want to help you. You constantly clash: reproach, criticism. You keep yourself within an iron structure; hard and ruthless. The true deepest cause: feeling yourself to be painfully tied down, seized and held by your nose in extreme . . . powerlessness. In fact, you are not able to depend on your own authority; you don't acknowledge your personal authority and long for others to acknowledge you.

Of course, your relations and life circumstances confirm your personal conviction about yourself. Do you experience yourself as being powerless? Then you will end up in a relationship, in circumstances upon which you seem unable to get any hold. Change your opinion about yourself. Realize your worth and then there will be changes in your surroundings! Let everything and everybody go free: one does not force love or change! Transform yourself, come close to your essence and gain power over yourself. In this way, you will no longer feel powerless. Be gentle toward yourself and resolutely direct your life — not that of others. Digest, produce, and let everything go. Trust the life process.

As soon as you let go of, and give freedom to, everything and everyone, then and only then will things and people automatically come to you in a way which will make you much happier.

Crushed finger
(See also the finger concerned)

In what situation — by whom or by what — do you feel "crushed"? Between your work and your private life, for instance? Between this or that person? "Who, or what, will I choose?"

You don't feel safe and protected in yourself; you place Authority, the Sun, outside yourself, because you feel anxious, small, and powerless. This impels you to tensely hold on to everything you possibly can, to stand up for yourself in a forced, sometimes dominant, way; you are afraid of losing what you have, including the outer ego, Possessions, authority over others. . . . You exaggerate in order to keep yourself on your feet. Possibly, you fanatically throw yourself into a job, a system, a religion, an achievement — but you burden yourself much too much! You try to embrace everything, to stay in charge; structurally, you are too hard or too severe on yourself. Are you afraid that someone will take something away from you? Do you feel so threatened? Because of this, spontaneous natural and aggressive powers are being suppressed! You restrain your nature; you can't really live your life to the fullest, the way you *are*. You crush yourself, although you *feel* crushed under a structure — the Authority of someone else. Do you let yourself be wrung out like a rag by someone else? And are you now inwardly smoldering with anger and accusation? The cause lies in you.

No longer tie down your nature, your feelings. Feel secure and protected in yourself. No longer force yourself; say what you have to say; don't bottle up aggression; show your teeth, if necessary. Count on those funda-mental powers in yourself; feel that strong central pillar, the authority, the self-aware Sun-power in yourself!

Don't let yourself be pushed down or in-fluenced by the outer world, but determine your life *yourself*. Don't hold back for any-one: always honestly be yourself! Express your anger and see then how you've bottled it up for too long because you don't dare be yourself! Make an end to anxieties and frus-trations: break through. Handle those inner energies with mastery; don't wait for the fiery flames to forcefully shoot out. Let go. . . .

Don't exaggerate in physical activity in order to satisfy; don't pin yourself down to a nervous schedule. Take the time to live, to enjoy; relax, feel strong in yourself. Don't put the power over your life in the outer world, nor in another, in a job, in a function or in a social system — "This is how it has to be" — free yourself from this and be faithful to your Nature! Fulfill your tasks with love, in respect for yourself and for others.

FISTULA
(See also Anal fistula)

Anxiously pinched, closed up. Inwardly afraid, holding feelings in.

You don't radiate outwardly, but you draw in, you pull everything into you; your emotional world slumps deeply away, timid and hidden. Nevertheless, the longing exists in you to go outward and fly open! But you fold yourself up, as it were, afraid of pain, because of self-protection. You don't let anything escape, you don't allow yourself to evolve.

Get a solid grip on yourself from out of your self-aware mind and stand firmly with your feet on the ground. Awareness of the power

of your conscious mastery over yourself will allow you to live freely and openly, to let go of everything. Feelings are then experienced and guided under the higher Authority of yourself. This power in yourself undoes fear and deep sunkenness: self-aware, grasp the reins! Head and heart are the physical con-ductors; your anxious feelings are but dust that can be swept away; don't allow your life to be dominated by feelings, but thankfully make use of them, and transform negativity into productivity, action!

FLU
(See also Infections)

Do you still believe in the system of "accidental contagion" by someone else? Know, then, that when you are not attuned to the vibration of the flu virus (see continua-tion of this text), you cannot be "infected" by it.

Unconsciously, you call up a time of rest for yourself, because hectic, stressful life is so demanding on you. It becomes too much for you, as does the busyness around you; you'd like to be peacefully alone for a little while — a flu will permit this. You throw out the anchor.

The outer world seems threatening to you; you wish to withdraw into a safe shell. You feel like a slave in a social, or other, system; your personal feelings are not allowed to count — tension, frustrations, sadness. The outbreak of flu hinders more serious illnesses from developing themselves. (Just allow a cold, fever, or flu to come through, and don't suppress it.)

Flu, therefore, is like a pair of tongs which seize you and simultaneously offer protection. That is what you prefer to look for: a safe shelter, rest.

Accumulated energies (emotions, thoughts, creativity) seek a way out.

Flu is often an indication that you are unsure and afraid; "Am I doing it right?" You're perhaps afraid to take total responsibility regarding a certain task; you're afraid of reprimand. Fear of failure; possibly, we're dealing here with an overload. You fiercely use your elbows, but you fear that it's not all going to work out — you feel like a SLAVE.

Feelings of oppression, insecurity, and anxiety, not trusting in your own Basis: this all breaks down your immunity.

Are you allowing yourself to be influenced too much by your surroundings? Do you refuse to live autonomously, "from out of yourself"?

Live YOURSELF, not trained like a circus animal. Clearly determine your limits, full of self-confidence!

Experience your inner powers, your immune system, the cheerfulness and warmth in your original nature. Feel welcome among people, dare to enjoy; know yourself to be safe in your Living self, and don't let yourself be rushed by anything or anyone! Becoming infected only happens if you unconsciously ask for it (to bring about changes in yourself); you are naturally immune.

Don't allow yourself to be influenced by negativity in your surroundings: be faithful to yourself.

FLUORIDE
Deficiency, insufficient assimilation of

You feel insufficiently supported by yourself. Powerlessness, which can lead to fury, grinding of the teeth, nervousness. You worship certain things outside yourself, but you ignore your own strong basis. You are loaded up with feelings; you hold on to material values, or to spiritual goals outside yourself.

In this way, your personal powers are being blocked: you don't truly live from out of your center; you are not aware of the divine power in yourself. Frustration and accumulated aggression can be the consequence. Are you "bad," and do you think you have to do penance?

Free yourself now from all useless burdens: throw them from your shoulders; let go, and be proud of your unique being. Allow new impulses and energies to come through freely; don't hold on to old things, or to a god outside yourself; place joy, optimism, in your deepest Self and feel gratitude for life, so that you feel lighter, unburdened by guilt and penance, and open yourself up to higher consciousness energies; don't cling to material things, nor to one doctrine or another. Live from out of your heart and your longings: inner peace. Don't doubt yourself, your content, your possibilities, and come now to powerful self-manifestation!

FOOD POISONING

Where are "you"? You habitually do what you have to do; you play your role in the community; possibly you attach much importance to outer appearance — "Am I stalwart enough or beautiful enough?" You pay too much attention to outer, or prestige-directed, values. You live like a perfectly oiled machine, but where is the Human Being? You are insufficiently in contact with your deepest, divine Self. Your true "I"-power, your spontaneous, active Mars-energies, remain suppressed. You are too little aware of your own worth and of your inner Power as a human being. Your total personality can't come through; wholesome energies, consciousness-powers, have been suppressed for too long beneath the surface. You feel imprisoned in a system, but you don't do anything about it. Instead of ac-knowledging the Power of your inner Self, you feel "in the grip of" others, of an Authority outside yourself.

Step out of the slave-like herd-pattern and place the mastery in yourself. Only you are able to direct your body, your life, to guide it toward health. Heal yourself; drive away strange intruders, chase away the authority above your head, and resolutely take your life in hand.

Step outside, starting from your true Self:

a rebirth, transformation. The way a snake throws off its old skin is how you now say goodbye to your old, artificial existence. Allow those consciousness-powers to come free; deliver yourself from those oppressive ties. Unroll those energies, those feelings that are very deep in you, and create an original existence, not for the eyes of others, not to satisfy the expectations of society, but in Love for yourself. Throw the burdens from your back: free yourself from unau-thentic existence. Discover your beautiful, pure "I" deep under the surface.

G

GALL BLADDER

Psychological correspondence

The liver and the gall play a role in the metabolism process; the gall drains substances to the intestinal tract after decomposition in the liver. While the gall does its task in the excretion of poisonous matter, the psychological mirror of this process is a "purification — the draining of poisonous experiences and emotions, the excretion of negativity; free digestion and flow of energies and emotions."

Bitter pain and sadness are being worked out and propelled onward, let go of, and buried in the earth. In a positive sense the Gall symbolizes the ability to actively work out experiences, emotions, and longings in a powerful, energetic way. Daring to openly stand up for yourself, without self-limitations, and bringing your talents to realization after eliminating hindrances or emotional-blocks such as: unsureness, "I don't dare to. . ."; anxiety; not daring to exchange your feelings with others; passiveness, self-isolation. . .

Action — being earthbound — emotional dynamism — spontaneous, healthy aggression, "doing" — exuberantly experiencing feelings — in love, communicating with others — manifesting your talents in awareness of self-worth — letting go of self-destructive feelings and self-poisoning memories.

Ailments, in general

Powerless anger, mostly not expressed.

Do you feel so burdened with a mountain of sorrow that you just want to hide in a deserted place? Hurt, powerless, and melancholic: something's brewing in your inner being. Sorrow and anger make you hard.

Do you live in frustration? Don't you dare to show yourself as you are, with feelings of inferiority, afraid of being mocked by others? You would like to experience your feelings to the utmost, casting your powers abroad, with lots of pent up energies. You would like "to do," but you remain stuck in your shell or in your passive situation. You don't move. . . . You experience yourself as being completely unable to realize yourself and rise above all negative emotions; you become ever more frustrated. It makes you furiously aggressive, but you don't express this powerless anger. Perhaps others are constantly hurting you, but you remain silent. Inability to communicate; you possibly experience little love and understanding from your environment; this makes you aggressive and desperate. You feel "seized" in the claws of others, and you aren't able to consciously become master over your vat full of feelings. Inner energies pile up in a threatening way: black clouds hinder a breakthrough of your sun-center, your self-esteem. Self-underestimation.

Your outer ego-manifestation and your relationship with others only exist in a fog, because you keep yourself hidden. You don't have contact with your deepest Self, don't stand with both feet on the earth; feeling of insecurity.

Take up your scepter in a self-aware way and lead your life yourself; produce, and be creative; bring your talents into realization, say what you have to say, don't bottle things up; don't allow yourself to get hurt; free yourself from authoritative or oppressive ties and become yourself. Dare to be yourself, the way you truly feel, and don't create a barrier between yourself and others. First of all, come closer to yourself by being faithful to your own nature; only then will you also feel satisfaction in other relationships. No one can tell you what's good for you: so, stand up for yourself with self-confidence, steadily, with both feet on the ground! Say it, express it, don't be afraid to fully experience your emotions; don't be ashamed to show your true feelings. Dare to accept your gentle, sensitive side — dare to experience it, to share it with others. Your sadness and aggression are only the consequences of self-underestimation and powerlessness. Manifest yourself, express yourself, work out your emotions — so that the bile drains away the poison, and sadness moves aside for light, joy, and gentleness.

Biliary colic

Being totally stuck; you can't get out of it; anger, panic, fear! With great endurance you've been keeping it up for a long time, but now a repressed energy rises up with bitterness because of all the suffered pain! Nevertheless, you are so anxious about making changes in your life. You feel weaker than you are; you deny your powers and possibilities, clinging too much to a person or a situation from your environment — you are bound to it, and stuck! Powerless fury. A heavy burden rests on your shoulders; pain and sadness "caused by others" is hard for you to digest: you don't realize that first of all you have to communicate with yourself! Don't cling to those who deny or belittle your worth; finally acknowledge yourself. Let go, and enter a new life. You see everything as being black because you

build your life on everything but your basis and your talents! Are you angry with someone of whom you expected love and didn't receive it?

No longer be aggressive toward others, but turn now in gentleness toward yourself: offer yourself the appreciation and love you deserve; neither expect nor reproach. Transform your pain and sadness into action! Live from out of your deepest inner being and feel that joy in yourself; let go of your relationships and know that on your path will then come the person who is ideal for you as a friend, partner or. . . .

Self-confidence, letting go, freeing yourself from your imprisonment. No longer cling to anything or anyone, using them as a stepping-stone or a "clothes-hanger"; cut those parts that don't belong to you out of your life, no longer make yourself angry. Live, one hundred percent, without holding back! Dare to build on your own foundation; let go of the past. In this way, new things and people can enter your life on the path to peace and happiness. Stop vomiting anger, and "do"!

Gallstones

In a surrounding in which you don't feel secure — in which you don't feel accepted lovingly and with understanding — you will not show your true feelings, will not be aware of your talents, and will withdraw into yourself with a feeling of inferiority. Especially with women, the active form of self-manifestation has often not been encouraged; it wasn't permitted for them to outwardly show natural aggression or anger, and no confidence was placed in their talents or ambitions: mothers showed this example of suppression and complexes to their daughters. As the female and male aspects in men as well as women are becoming equalized, the woman will be able to manifest herself with all her possibilities on the societal level. The basic cause of why someone attracts a certain situation wherein anger, powerlessness, and suppression play a role, lies of course in the personal nature and conviction-sphere of the woman herself.

You would like to tell and "do," but because of feelings like "I am just a nothing," you can't express yourself in energetic action. The gall takes care of tension that is too great; gallstones are crystallized talents, which were not used. An enormous power piles up inwardly. You don't realize what possibilities you carry inside you, nor do your surroundings encourage you: the gall bladder becomes a piggy-bank. Unused possibilities transform into anger, pent-up aggression, fury.... Your true nature doesn't dare to show itself, you stay deeply hidden, because someone might even hurt you more; you are afraid of condemnation, because you give too much importance to the judgment of others.

Your nervous system is under great pressure — you don't dare to be yourself because you feel so threatened by your surroundings; you are silent, you bottle things up, and once in a while you may release uncontrollable outbursts because of not-doing, not-being, for too long.

Not being able to be yourself the way you feel inwardly leads to anger, even to hatred and to harsh reproach of those who hurt you or who allegedly hinder you from being yourself.

In fact, the cause lies in you: no longer be afraid of others; become aware of your talents and dare to show yourself, to express yourself as you are. Allow yourself to go along with the natural flow of your feelings and don't block them because of fear; don't hinder your own growth and don't poison yourself with sharp feelings. Build your life the way you wish; don't let yourself be hindered by others; dare to stand up for yourself. First of all, come to peace and gentleness in yourself and, in an active energetic way, realize yourself, no longer staying stuck to emotional situations from the past.

Work out your emotions, transform aggression into action, transform talents into creativity, transform hatred into love toward yourself. Flexibility in dealing with experiences; appreciation of yourself. No longer clash and fight. Dare to go on and truly live from out of your deepest longings, from out of your true nature!

Softening!

Vomiting bile

You are tense, you offer resistance, you revolt, you vomit: because you bend too much toward something that doesn't totally suit you — you go along in a situation where you can't truly be yourself. You give in too much, while you don't really want to. Ultimately, you can't keep this up. You even flee from yourself; you don't really live with your feet on the ground any more. You are absent; it makes you vomit. Your breath is being cut off in some life situation in which you feel bound hand-and-foot; you hurt yourself, or allow yourself to be hurt because you can't rise above the situation. Powerlessness makes you aggressive: in this way, you hurt only yourself.

Thus, acknowledge your own nature, your worth, and protect yourself: clearly mark off your terrain and don't allow anyone to pin you down or hurt you. Also, in accordance with this, be honest with yourself! For instance, don't hold on to certain situations or persons that do you more bad than good, but to whom you hold on because of unsureness. Now, calmly withdraw within yourself and look at the situation from above: bring into realization your leadership over your life and determine your limits; follow these signals from your body. Be more gentle to yourself and change directions if you have to force yourself in the present situation. If you carry out your tasks according to your own responsibility, if you live in love and thankfulness, then you don't have to revolt against others.

GANGRENE

Bitter, sarcastic thoughts of death; crushing aggressiveness — self-destruction.

You let yourself droop, becoming totally passive. You've lost mastery over yourself, can't at all get a grip on yourself, on your life. Your life energies flow away, decomposing as it were; life is ebbing away. There's no longer a concentrated presence of your conscious "I" in your body: your "I" is no longer leading your body. Like a victim, you allow yourself to be tortured. In this way, you can at least still *feel* yourself! This way, you still have the attention of others, for you would in fact like to feel others in your grip because you experience yourself as being so powerless and fragmented.

In your martyrdom, you are full of destructive feelings; you would cling, reach out your power-claw, to others, in aggressive powerlessness. Embittered with life itself, a biting self-mockery; insane, deadly self-poisoning.

Become master over yourself and make contact with your deepest divine Self: let joy and powers flow through your body, ban death from your life. Put all power in yourself, and appreciate, in love, your Humanity. Build up instead of breaking down.

Ignoring your deeper divine core leads to insane thoughts; concentration and trust in this center lead you to rest and joy.

GASTRO-ENTERITIS
inflammation of the stomach and intestines, causing vomiting and/or diarrhea

In anxiety and unsureness you flee from yourself. You don't follow the spontaneous guidance from your inner Self. You'd sooner live according to laws and norms placed upon you by an Authority or a social structure. Because of your inner unsureness you might too much want to hold aloft your outer ego, might even force yourself in order to find affirmation or appreciation outside yourself.

You live too much according to structures, according to a mold; your emotional world isn't allowed to flow freely. "That has to be so; that is supposed to be so. . . ." Also, tension governs your thought-life. Your own deeper nature can't express itself; for that reason, restrained energies strike inward in a destructive way. You cannot and may not truly live.

You feel sorrow and pain; you are hurt, and you don't dare to fully acknowledge or experience your own power and autonomy; you possibly allow yourself to be hurt by an authority that supposedly stands above you. Because of the fear of not being loved or acknowledged by others, you might go too far this way, might give in too much. You are not faithful to your own nature. You follow the laws of the outer world.

It all becomes too much for you; you no longer can handle it — your deepest Self now asks for acknowledgment!

Don't flee from your "I": dare to open up in a more relaxed way, and dare to truly Live! Don't be afraid: you are good the way you are. Accept yourself, honestly manifest your true nature. Don't expect to be accepted by the outer world; don't exhibit a "false self." The external structure should not be a camouflage laid over you: your structure will automatically build itself up in accord with the energetic blossoming of your natural disposition, your content. Trust these deep powers in yourself and allow them to come through freely.

It's only your false "I" that nauseates you: now, come close to yourself and dare to free yourself, dare to live in full openness; no longer be hard on yourself. If you love yourself in this way, you will automatically at-

tract those people who will offer you just as much rich content. This honest contact with your Self drives away anxieties and unsureness: allow your personal breakthrough to occur.

GLANDS
(See, separately, Lymph glands)

Psychological correspondence

The endocrine glands as well as the exocrine glands secrete substances as a consequence of inner messages. When there's a question of psychological unbalance, then it lies in the nature of the Life of a human-being to recover the balance as quickly as possible. Thus, with regard to feelings of anxiety and powerlessness, for instance, the glands will react with the secretion of certain substances (mostly hormones). These will cause certain physical sensations, offering the possibility of conscious contemplation, in order to be able to bring about changes in the psyche, thus restoring harmony and relaxation. (See further in the categories endocrine glands and their hormonal secretions: genital glands, adrenal glands, thymus, hypophysis, epiphysis, thyroid, parathyroid glands, pancreas; the exocrine glands such as tear-glands, salivary glands. . . .)

Glands represent the person "being governed" by his Living Self-Core.

Glands are energy centers that immediately react to every change in our psyche.

On the basis of our deepest convictions, on the basis of deeply embedded memory and emotions, we will attract certain situations in life.

Nothing just happens. Nothing is predestined. Also, in accordance with our convictions regarding the world and ourselves, we will experience these situations again in a very specific way.

The glands also listen to that which is "printed" by the brain, received from our Consciousness, from the Living Self.

Every gland has a specific function, but they all work in accord with one another. Depending on the message that the Consciousness sends out, this or that gland will function more weakly or more strongly.

It is good that, here and now, we very Consciously create our reality, so that the glands will react not only to unconscious impulses, to unconscious convictions: as we live more Consciously, we will get more of a grip on ourselves and on the functioning of the glands.

After all, the glands constantly react to conscious or unconscious commands from our Self.

You create your own reality!

When, in Self-awareness, we create our own lives, then future desired realizations or materializations will occur more quickly. (Not to be confused with so-called positive thinking: see Part I; Positive thinking?) We then consciously create our reality: brain, nervous system, and glandular system send out electromagnetic waves as a reaction to our conscious or unconscious longings. The more intensely we long for (and are convinced that we deserve) a positive future, the stronger the glands will react as true atomic-power centers; they produce energies which, together, are at the origin of "manifestation in matter" of our expectations. That which we believe deep in our heart — of which we are most deeply convinced — that will be the touchstone, the sieve, by which we will or won't attract certain situations and happenings. The better we get to know our silent wishes and convictions regarding ourselves, the stronger will we realize why we have attracted this or that situation or happening into our lives.

Unlimited Consciousness

By building up a very conscious, creative life, we get a grip on our existence; we are not victims who are subject to Destiny or to predetermination. The more strongly we become conscious of this, the more strongly the glands will produce — in accordance with what's needed for the desired reality.

Glands receive and translate inner messages. From out of this earthly existence, we are able — especially via the glands in our head — to experience reality beyond the borders of space and time. A powerful ability to see things very broadly, unlimitedly. In openness, our Awareness can go in all directions.

It's thanks especially to our glands, brain, and nervous system that we are able to experience, as a unity, our material three-dimensional world *and* the world of consciousness which lies at the foundation of it — hooked together, as it were. Thus, glands tell us about the unlimited possibilities a human being possesses. The divine wealth in ourselves, which will blossom. Glands symbolize the resilient, psychological leap of the human being out of his non-material world into earthly existence.

Ailments of the glands, in general

One's own Authority is being ignored and put outside of oneself.

The eagle who considers himself a sparrow.

A human-being who ignores his wealth and encapsulates himself in a shield.

When he denies his humanity and, without questioning, surrenders to unconscious impulses; when he refuses to live his life creatively in a Self-aware way.

A passiveness, not doing anything, feeling oneself to be a stupid and helpless victim.

Not using one's own powers. Refusing to surrender to oneself. Being convinced that the human being is born as a powerless being that has no say about its life, that is here to suffer and die; a being that is cut off from its deep inner Source, its divine Self. He lives superficially, fatalistically, or is directed toward the sheerly rational or material. Blindly being stuck.

Giving up; constantly being on guard against others, against a supposed evil. A feeling of insecurity and, as a result, nervous anxieties.

Daring to penetrate into your Core, and opening yourself up to all feelings and energies that wish to come through. Creativity, development in all possible directions, concentration in yourself, and gradual enlargement of your being. Productivity! Allowing an active Mars-energy to flow through, without fear or self-degradation. High-spiritedness about yourself, pride in the ability inside you, in being able to create your reality in a self-aware way. The joy for Life itself!

Not allowing your life to be dependent on others, on an authority outside yourself. Trustfully daring to take up your large space: daring to inhale life with all your senses in a very earthly way, with your feet on the ground. Strive after optimal unity between spirit and matter, between awareness and body; no one-sided development, not of the spiritual nor of the physical aspect; a loving marriage between soul and heart. A warm, earthly experience, directed by your Conscious "I." Calmly, securely, relax in yourself.

Gland inflammation
adenitis

You thrash about like a devil in a font of holy-water.

Aggressively, you show your teeth, but it is only for self-defense. In fact, you are very self-destructive: perhaps someone has hurt you; you feel powerless because you feel cut off from that powerful Core in yourself; you defend yourself furiously, but you don't get one step further with it.

Frenetically, you seek. You fight, you go around in circles, with your thoughts sharply tuned — aggression toward yourself because you don't really know who you are?

You are hard on yourself, reproachful toward others. Your pride is gone. Perhaps you've even suffered painful humiliations because you deny yourself so or because you cling to outer achievements and you have failed in this regard.

Achieve creative self-development from within your deepest Self! Transform aggression into real action; indulge in those things that are in the line with your true longings, with your specific nature, and don't put your life in the hands of false pride, image, outer display. Make contact with yourself in an affectionate, heartfelt way. Be gentle with yourself and others; open your heart in tenderness. You don't have to defend yourself: turn inward and bid yourself welcome; produce fruits from these powerful energies, which ask for a resolute breakthrough; stand still no longer! Opening up to your deepest Self will lead to a true presence in life, NOW: concentrated, motivated, and joyful. This will not work using only your rational thinking: listen to your feelings, to your intuition, and to those happy messages in your environment, which after all you have unconsciously called up; no longer direct yourself in a self-destructive way toward yourself or others.

Glandular tumor
adenoma

Your inner self wants to push through with a creative fire-power! But you are not open to these impelling energies; you hold back these powers by simply not believing in them, by underestimating yourself and limiting yourself to the physically superficial or the "thinking."

Your earthly "funnel" is too small to allow your awareness-powers to be born in your physical-being: you limit yourself, imprison yourself in a living-space that is too confined; you are cut off from your deeper, divine creative powers. Therefore, energies that glow like fire impel your earthly-being in order to weld it, here-and-now, onto a deeper reason for existence: these energies puff up, irritate you, wake you up from your superficial sleep.

Perhaps you feel inhibited in your "active" life-course by an anxiety, a sadness, inflicted upon you by others. . . . This is only a consequence of not placing the Authority in yourself; you allow your life to be too much dependent on the behavior of your fellow man, without really making choices *yourself.* You refuse to see clearly; you base yourself upon book-knowledge or the words of others, not on the strength of your inner Wisdom. As a result, you don't have things in perspective: you can't distinguish important things from minor things, and you cling to details. "Which path shall I follow? I don't know." You don't open yourself up to your inner knowing, your intuition. Possibly, you block yourself completely by fretting and thinking in a worrisome way, by accumulating emotions. You keep on running in place; resistance to truly growing into adulthood.

Be sensitive to the powers of your deepest Being in your body, in your palms. . . . Now allow your creative energies and accumulated emotions to flow freely! Offer a flexible passage to natural impulses: give in to your spontaneous feelings; no longer tie yourself down. Become aware, proudly, of your unique powers, and feel that solid, secure Basis in you. Don't listen firstly to others. In trust, allow the child in you to grow up toward Self-aware authority.

GLANDULAR FEVER
infectious mononucleosis,
caused by Epstein-Barr virus

"So if I am not good enough, then I have nothing to lose; you mistreated me! Pay attention or I'll shoot!" Extreme nervousness, active energy that has been held in too long, will ultimately lead to rage and exaggerated, uncontrollable aggression; you no longer know when to stop. Sparing nothing or no one. . . .

The real cause of this: you can't reach your self; you think you are "bad" or you feel anxiety about your deep "I," about a series of deep emotions and powers in yourself which wish to come through. You suppress them, and you look at them suspiciously; also, you don't trust the people around you. You are constantly ready to defend yourself! You suspect others of condemning you or mistreating you, but in fact you are constantly on guard against your Self. There's a duality in yourself because you especially long for acknowledgment and love. But you think you are "not worthy of it." Because of this nervous state of anxiety you'd like to tear yourself free from all ties and relations; you are angry because of your condition of being tied down: but in fact it has to do with anger at a part of yourself which you don't at all like, and which you'd prefer to crush. Possibly, you vent this at your relations, your colleagues, etc.

You end up in a nervous breakdown because you don't trust, and you can't let go of anything or anyone; you claw things and persons into your grasp; you magnetically draw toward you; you are sharp, hard, aggressive, and full of suspicion.

With enormous power you ultimately drive everything into the ground — yourself and everything around you: (self-)destruction because of powerlessness.

Become Conscious: you are good. Allow your emotions, your unconscious feelings, to come up calmly, and look at them. No longer keep yourself imprisoned: via dealing with anxiety, sadness, and hatred, you can achieve joy. Come to the surface, break through with your powers in positive action and creativity; now take up ALL your space. No longer seize — let go of everything, but be Master over your life and direct your feelings into the right channels. Solve the duality in yourself by wholly accepting your-self in every way! The unity in yourself; nothing is wrong or bad in you; know yourself to be safe. Your powers, emotions, energies, require leadership from your Self-awareness: your possibilities of creation are boundless. Nothing has to be defended, not regarding yourself nor regarding others. Now come to full, active self-realization, whereby your "I" chooses certain directions very consciously. Put all power over your life in yourself, build calmly — no one's rushing you — don't get excited; come to peace in yourself. Trust, let go!

GOLD
Deficiency, insufficient assimilation of

Self-negation, absence, under-appreciation of yourself, self-suffocation, self-limitation. You no longer can handle it all; you let yourself droop; you are at the bottom with your feelings. You have no confidence in your "I." You have no hope, no expectations. Energies are being suppressed, until you are completely paralyzed. Many emotions have been bottled up; you see your future as being black and morbid.

A pure, strong genesis of your "I": self-confidence!

The triumphal bells of life are ringing; joy! "I AM, I can, I know myself to be secure and protected in my sun-center." Just let the wheel of life keep turning: a stream of powerful energy-development. You create your life in a self-aware way. Self-affirmation in harmony with your inner feelings.

GOUT

Wishing to build up a position of Power in order to be able to conceal your sensitivity.

You hide your powerlessness, your feelings of inferiority, behind a shield of toughness. You anxiously guard your private psychological domain: "That belongs to me! No one's allowed to touch it." Possessive, showing off your power; judgmental of others — because you experience people to be threatening and unauthentic; because you don't really show yourself the way you are (sensitive, fragile), and also because you consider yourself partly "bad"! You condemn yourself: "I am just —" And you still try to prove yourself with your outer appearance: you will "measure" yourself, perhaps will submit yourself to severe rules, because your badness has to be brought under control!

And, in the meantime, you will criticize others about those things which you suppress in yourself: physical enjoyment, play, spontaneous joy. . . . The more powerless you feel and the less a grip you have on your own emotional life, the more intensely you will try to maintain this power-grip. This is not "bad," but it's a sad reaction to your own powerlessness. Becoming aware of this can set the healing process in motion. Doubt regarding yourself: all feelings tied up, a militaristic attitude toward yourself. Seeing life in black-and-white; anxiously trying to destroy everything you see as black or bad, whether in yourself or in others. You believe insufficiently in that which is beautiful and divine in yourself; you'd rather be on guard against that which is "bad." You would strive for an ideal, but you don't see that the bad is only a lack of Insight, and that human nature and its feelings are completely trustworthy so long as one does not suppress them the way you do. You think you have to constantly "stand guard" over yourself. You don't put the Power in your divine core; therefore, you "fight" — against windmills. These complexes ("I have to be wary of my own badness.") lead to communication problems: you can't openly manifest yourself to others because you've already closed yourself off from part of yourself. You don't know joy anymore. You don't show your true colors. You retain and hold on to eve-

rything until you can't grasp anything anymore. Your reaction to all this can be blazing fury! Out of powerlessness, you would "swell up" . . . .

Enjoy your body, your total being, your sensuality. . . . Nothing about you is bad. Don't block the flow of your feelings: live life to the fullest, spontaneously and naturally, without fear. Let go of others and realize yourself: don't be hindered by destructive, severe programming from your youth, which still prevents you from daring to truly accept and experience yourself the way you are. Feel welcome in yourself, amongst people — no longer withdraw behind a shield. Give yourself the warmth and the love you so need. Don't cling so much to your partner. Give her/him room, and have faith; free yourself from this prison cell and develop your talents; dare to enjoy sensitive, beautiful things. Instead of wanting to seize power, feel the power-source in yourself; let go. . . You are not a powerless "victim!"

GROIN

Lymph gland swelling and pain in the groin area

You imprison your nature; not others, but you yourself take away your Freedom.

You feel imprisoned in a certain structure, which generally is self-created, be it an unconscious thought-structure. In a tense state of being, you rush yourself — to go, to run, to live, to jump further and further, broader and wider; you scheme and anticipate, but in the meantime you go right past the requirements of your body, of your nature. You don't at all follow the demands of your nature. On the contrary, you offer resistance to your nature, to your feelings, to the need for relaxation.

You dynamite your moon, your emotional world; you spit fire to keep others at a distance, but it is you who imprisons yourself. Sharp, aggressive, and natural creative powers — emotional currents — are looking for a way through, but you resist it because you only feel at ease in your head, in your thought-world.

You insufficiently listen to the longings of your nature. You want to break out, to go toward freedom — at least, that's what you think, but you won't find this freedom by running away from part of yourself, by resisting your earthly nature

Integrate the gentle Venus powers in yourself and allow your feelings to flow freely. Listen to your nature and no longer close yourself up in a tense way.

Liberate yourself from this cell; allow your nature to relax; don't force things with your thoughts; feel good in your body. Enjoy that which is earthly; descend into your body and give in to your feelings. Suppleness and flexibility with yourself and others.

Achieve peace in yourself, and now let the poison, those boiling energies in your head, escape. Don't push outward; come inside yourself and integrate those gentler feelings in your being. Raise that sluice gate and allow the water, your emotional powers, to pass through freely. Total surrender to your feelings: don't curtail yourself so! Action, decisiveness, but not separate from your total self; your head not separate from your body! Experience in yourself that unity of awareness / thoughts and body / earth; take up your total Space; shoot the arrow from your bow, free yourself. In this way you no longer will feel "imprisoned" in situations, in relationships. The prison guard imprisons himself. Open those windows to all regions of yourself: self-liberation.

Groin rupture

You've carried a burden for too long: stop! Unconscious resistance to the way you have lived thus far. Feeling of imprisonment, a call for liberation.

You've lived constrictedly, tensely, because you couldn't really be yourself: did you have a task, a job, a function which didn't really suit you? Did you hold out too long in a relationship, which completely oppressed you? If so, all this was but a consequence of the fact that you don't liberate yourself INWARDLY.

All possible energies — your creative talents, your larger and natural possibilities, your natural flow of feelings — have been pent up for so long, until this gas bubble will explode in a volcanic way! You no longer go along with it!

Outwardly, you perhaps have established yourself in a job or in a controlled attitude to life; maybe to the outer world you came across as being calm, but inwardly you started to revolt (like a horse that rears up), perhaps unconsciously.

Your deepest Self calls up this rupture in order to reach thorough transformation: so that you might throw off your burdens, so that you might start living from out of your deepest Self, so that original energies might no longer be suppressed. Perhaps you have positioned yourself as small and subordinate to a partner, to an employer. Have you behaved for too long as a nice, obedient child who did everything for someone else, but never lived or worked for itself? Sooner or later you experienced yourself to be crushed, as it were, under this authority. But it's you who imprisoned yourself!

An aggressive breakthrough, an unconscious urge for self-liberation is the consequence of this. The deepest cause lies in the fact that you remain "hidden" from yourself. Because you don't yet have a good perspective of yourself or you don't yet dare to become who you are, you hold on too long to structures — or to a situation — which are not good for you. Anxiously, you hold in your feelings, which are not allowed to flow freely because you want to keep yourself too much under control: this leads to pent-up emotional tensions. You don't give in to longings.

When you refuse to let go (for instance of a partner after a divorce or a death) then the groin forces you to do so.

You would fight to be free!

The others, however, are not depriving you of your freedom: you, yourself, are your own prison guard. Often, you are not aware of this inner problem.

Break with old, detrimental habits.

Eliminate this self-blockage and achieve surrender to yourself, to your deepest feelings.

Love for yourself and awareness of your worth and possibilities are necessary in order to discover a job, a partner, a lifestyle which really fit your true nature. Achieve this self-appreciation and let go of too much pressure and tensions; let go of relationships and tasks that burden you too much or don't at all belong in your life.

Surrender to spontaneous, natural impulses; dare to free yourself of needless burdens and of limiting, suffocating structures and traditions. Find rest and relaxation in yourself.

If you feel imprisoned, it is because of yourself: you are taken hostage by yourself; you put yourself into armor; your nature suffocates. Of course, you then attract outer circumstances that cause you to feel oppressed. First of all, free yourself from your cramped emotional life; dare to "let out" of your feelings instead of piling them up. Don't deny your emotional world and your longings: live your life to the fullest, allow energies and creativity to flow freely, and

don't put up any barriers. First, intuitively feel where your path lies, and then resolutely come to manifestation, to active development of yourself: a powerful revolving of the Wheel of Life, from inside to outside; inwardly and outwardly in harmony, without any reserve.

GROWTH HORMONE
(See also Acromegaly; Dwarfism)

Growth hormone:
insufficient production in puberty
or in a child; growth that is too slow

On guard, very carefully, you dare to walk into life. You are afraid: "What will happen now?"

You'd prefer to stay a child for a long time: then, after all, you are more "protected." Too afraid to grow, you hide behind someone, or behind your own mask.

For instance, you'll start to live according to the standards of someone else; you possibly situate yourself very much at the service of a certain person, as long as you don't really have to BE or to grow.

You feel threatened by your own emotions, by anxieties; you don't know how to deal with them, because you don't really feel your inner essence. Possibly, you might want to hide behind your body, your exterior, and then crawl completely into a hole.

Take up your space and stand up! Explore your life, don't be afraid. Allow your energies to blossom in all freedom, and acknowledge your worth. Enjoy all the sensory pleasures; don't close yourself off to all the earthly beauty. Acknowledge your possibilities, and develop them! Allow yourself to grow up in love — give trust to your Living Self!

Growth Hormone:
overproduction in puberty or in a child; growth that is too fast

An inner feeling of imprisonment: in a structure, under an authority, in emotions. The child has an unconscious urge to break out! It feels confined and struggles to break loose. Actually, it tries to escape from its feelings, its anxieties; it already feels that it's stuck in itself: every authority that is being placed on it in addition to this, is too much for it — even well-meant, motherly, oppressive ties are too much for it. Mistrust regarding its inner world; it doesn't assume leadership over itself; it doesn't give itself the opportunity for inner growth. It starts to run — away from its anxieties. Outer growth as a compensation for inner blockages.

"No, that can't go on this way any longer; I have to find a solution to this, I have to get out of this!" You push the cover on your head further and further away, you fight for liberation.

Take the strings in your hands and allow your wisdom to awaken: conditions here are daring to contemplate yourself, acknowledging your feelings, and daring to show them. No longer flee in such a rushed way; anxieties are unnecessary; take the time to discover yourself; observe your values with all respect, and cherish your content carefully and considerately. Don't be afraid.

Cut through oppressive ties; turn deeply inward; push away from yourself that which has to be pushed away, but no longer push yourself away! Live more calmly; trust in your personal Basis; arrive at self-assuredness: nothing or no one can threaten you if you don't consider yourself threatened. Freedom lies in the liberation from your anxieties, from the negative thoughts regarding yourself and your situation: bring about change in those convictions: your life will change.

GUMS

Psychological correspondence and Ailments, in general

In love and respect, holding your SELF; giving yourself the chance to grow.

Once you've "broken through" and — on the basis of inner will, wisdom and longings — have made the choice of a stable, straight course, then the tooth will rise solidly and proudly above the gum. If, however, you remain emotionally stuck in the past, in a previous stage of your life — don't really dare to go on, would prefer to crawl back to where you came from, are ashamed or feel guilty, are angry with yourself because you've been too flexible — then your gums won't solidly attach themselves around your teeth.

Yes/no — doubting. The insight is there already, but your feelings hinder you from going on, from breaking with something or someone of the past, from resolutely making a decision.

Are you afraid to stand up for yourself in a direct way? Do you hide yourself, camouflaging your true nature?

Contradictory feelings block evolution: Are you not basing your life on your own roots? The conflict which comes out of this is frustrating: Do I listen to others? Do I keep myself underwater? Repressed energies and repressed creative impulses as a consequence of doubting yourself, your Power, your worth! Or shall I, after all, stand up for myself?

Aggression, powerlessness, fury, despair, can be the consequence of the fact that you can't get a "hold" of yourself, can't live in Love for yourself, don't dare stand up for your qualities, your powers, and your possibilities! You "let go" of yourself, blow with the wind, aren't consistent with yourself, with your inner point of view, with the plans, the ideas and the decisions, which you yourself have formed. Do you flee from yourself because of fear, because you don't believe in the power of your deepest Self? Do you, again and again, keep bringing yourself into question? Do you not dare to cut the Gordian knot? Then this is because you don't really build on your inner wisdom, because you look too much at what others say or at "outer" factors, etc. Press your nose against the facts; listen to your inner wisdom and resolutely go on. Get a hold of yourself and build only on the power which is inside you. Act in love for yourself; don't force with your "mind" anything you can't handle emotionally; but no longer remain stuck to the past with your emotions.

Hold yourself in love, go onward without looking back: to the degree you surround yourself with loving care, to the degree you don't allow destroying doubts to gnaw at your Self, so will your gums solidly and securely protect your Teeth. A constant flow of powerful energies, of self-realization, is allowed to pass through freely: a direct and resolute allowing of your "I" to come through.

Bleeding gums

Frustration. Powerlessness to be yourself. You get angry because you don't really do what you would like to do; you feel limited, sometimes as if strangled; you have to walk in line too obediently, and you blame others for your feeling of limitation. You do what others do; you can't bring your Individuality, your specific uniqueness, to realization. You revolt against it! Suppressed aggression: you remain stuck; you don't succeed in truly bringing yourself to realization. Sometimes you direct your powerless fury at others as if they were the cause of your feeling of frustration.

Calmly look inside yourself and see the true cause here. You don't really believe in your worth, in your possibilities. You allow your

life to be too dependent on others, on the outer world. Seize power over yourself and feel those inner Forces.

Calmly surrender to your deepest Self; build your life in joy, without self-limitations. Realize yourself in self-confidence. Now, in love, bid yourself welcome; don't shut yourself out, but allow your unique "I" to blossom to its full expanse. Transform powerless aggression into action and creativity!

Inflammation of the gums
gingivitis

Inner aggression, powerless anger, standing still, being stuck.

Because you are actually riding in the back instead of steering yourself; because you don't succeed in being YOURSELF, in manifesting YOURSELF; because you doubt and are unsure; because you obstruct your own development — because of all this, powerless anger, frustration, and inner revolt are growing!

You'd like to go onward, but powers are wrongly directed; outwardly you appear tough, hard, distant, aggressive, or sometimes indignant, but inwardly you just feel small and unsure, dependent on others. Because you don't really believe in your content, in your worth, you don't dare to completely manifest how you really feel; in this way, you create distance with others and become estranged from yourself. You don't at all trust your spontaneous nature, although others can inspire awe in you. In short, you degrade yourself to remaining the lesser one. You might be angry with the Authority that supposedly hinders you from being yourself: the church, a religion, a partner, etc. — you might be angry with the hand that grasps you — but you are too fearful to stand on your own feet. Possibly, you criticize, condemn others, with your apparent self-assuredness, but actually you put yourself in the cold, without belief or love.

You suppress yourself! Pent-up energies are seeking their way, but you put a brake on yourself.

You are afraid to experience, to show, your feelings; you conceal your sensitive heart; you don't trust your intuition. You look too much behind you, at a useless burden of remembrances and facts that you cannot forget. You remain standing where you are.

Go on in flexibility and let go of the past. Trust your intuition, no longer hesitate, and come to self-realization; cut the Gordian knot where necessary; take the needed steps. Free yourself! Take hold of yourself and decide in what direction you will go; don't let yourself "be lived" by the expectations of others.

Feel that deep power and Love in yourself. Allow feelings and creative energies to flow freely now; no longer block yourself. Resolutely take the rudder in hand. Freedom and inner peace!

Receding gums

Your teeth contain many tears of powerlessness, which cause the gums to ebb away.

Powerless, feeble, unsure, inwardly aggressive, sometimes desperately weeping. You CAN'T bring yourself to forcefully live from out of yourself, to resolutely go in *one* direction; you drink from many waters, going one time to the left, then again to the right; you don't really get any further; you hesitate and keep lingering over the past; you constantly question whether you have done the right thing. . . . Your heart is being seized by a hard fist: Why do you doubt your worth, the Power of your inner Self? The duality in you, yes/no, is a reflection of the doubt about yourself; you don't unconditionally love yourself. You think you can't depend on yourself; sometimes you seem to be a chameleon, because you really don't openly dare to manifest your true nature. You hide your "I"; you live too pliantly, too flexibly, possi-

bly in order to be accepted by others. Do you weep about the past? But in spite of your sorrow, you don't give up: you go on!

Know that as long as you don't acknowledge yourself in love and trust, you will keep moaning, weeping or doubting about happenings from the past, or about your feeling feeble and powerless now. Let go of the past and now live on a self-assured basis: take your life in your own hands and create it in full, dynamic development! Go on and make an end to this self-underestimation. Be faithful to your true nature; LIVE according to your nature, without compromise, without wishing for affirmation from others. Manifest yourself the way you are; become aware of your worth and make an end to this "denial" of your inner power-center. In naked truth, unfolding your SELF toward the outside: daring to manifest yourself in expression, in emotional manifestations, which come directly from your heart

Suppuration of the dental tissue

You've imprisoned yourself; in powerless sadness, you've withdrawn into yourself; instead of really getting your teeth into it and going onward with all your "I"-power, you've looked for a hold outside yourself: in a person, an authority, a job, an outer world which is based on Image and achievement, etc.: your life isn't built on your Self, on your true nature. It's becoming too much for you; you are angry about it! Spontaneous, natural energies are being kept in; gentle feelings are being denied by you; you place yourself on an unstable platform because you don't base your life on your deepest, imperishable Self. You possibly exert yourself to please others, to outwardly play your "role" very well. You "reach" outside yourself because you don't believe in yourself, because you don't get a grip on your existence. You will accommodate your partner; you will keep your Image up high; you stay high and strong, seemingly in harmony with yourself, but in the meantime the powers which want to manifest themselves from your deepest Self are burning away. Your security is shaky and unreal; you are anxious; you don't trust yourself; you clamp on to something or someone in order to feel more secure; you hold on to people and things that you should have let go of a long time ago. Now, you feel bound to that, to this authority which you've seized, and you want to get out from under it! When you don't offer yourself love, then you make yourself dependent on the warmth others give you, but in this way you get totally stuck.

Your productivity, your emotional powers, pile up, but you remain stuck, frustrated, not really daring to go on.

Feel your warmth and your love being released from within and propel them outward like powerful, volcanic-streams from the heart: show your deep energies; express yourself the way you feel. Don't pull at others, don't draw them by some sort of suction force; don't pile up things from the past, but go on in a self-aware way; allow generous energies to radiate from your heart, for yourself and others. Become aware of that positive power in your Living Self and ACT in the name of love and trust. Break through, choose a well-determined direction, and don't hesitate! Being aware of the fullness, the worth, of yourself; it is not the outer world, but the way you feel that is of importance. Build a solid life on that fundamentally-reliable Basis of your deepest Self, autonomously, independent of others. Trust in common sense, in intuition; now allow all powers to flow outward; discharge your energies, go onward! Acknowledge in gentleness your unique person; bend in suppleness to your inner voice, and listen only to it. . . .

H

HAIR, HAIR GROWTH

Psychological correspondence

A strong, powerful concentration of "spirit energies" in the body; the pleasant, scintillating feeling that you experience in every fiber of your body. All powers united in your Center. Under the watchful eye of your Conscious "I," deep powers from your Self penetrate every cell. Powerfully governing yourself. Striving after a balance between the conscious and the unconscious and allowing a constant transformation: a conversion of instincts and primitive emotions into awareness and creativity. The growth of a human being: a supple growth of the hair, without exaggeration. The unity of man-woman in every individual.

Our conscious "I," here-and-now present on earth, has its roots in another dimension. The growth of hair on the body represents precisely the interlocking of these two worlds: of spiritual awareness in matter. The envelope that seeks its content and at the same time has developed out of it: a deeper dimension which lies behind the earthly. (This doesn't at all mean that someone who has no hair growth has a "shortage" of incarnation power. Here, it means only one of the so many symbols for it.)

The hair being rooted in the skin reflects the anchoring of Awareness in matter. The incarnation: an important path toward the manifestation of Love, symbolized by the Heart. A structure is being traced out in physical existence. The reconciliation of the "material" and the "spiritual" in a human being.

One feeds the other; awareness feeds the body. Hair growth comes to be as a result of life-giving powers, which rise up from another dimension, out of your deepest underlying consciousness, which again and again propels and gives form to your body. Hairs are fine antennae; they react very sensitively to impulses which you energetically receive or send out. Magnetic discharge, electromagnetic tensions, heavy-laden energy fields — thoughts, emotions, etc. — accumulate rather quickly in the hair. Hair, therefore, gives you a picture of how you handle the exchange between your "unconscious" and your "conscious" worlds: Do you allow a supple flow, in trust, or do you block this energetic flow by tension, by structures that are too tight, by stress, by limiting yourself to the "rational," the masculine? Do you feel the solid Basis deep within yourself? Do you dare build upon your roots? Is there a beautiful exchange between the intuitively emotional — as the translator of the "Unconscious" —and the rational thinking of your Conscious "I"? Peaceful harmony in this respect leads to healthy hair growth.

In a male, that which most of the time is led away to hidden terrain — to the "unconscious " — is mainly the intuition, the gentle sensitivity, the impulsive artistic creativity, the flexibility, the listening; in other words, that which has been labeled as "female." The unconscious, therefore, often is being looked upon as female; this is only partly true. By suppressing this intuitive side, by concentrating on the one-sided rational, by not trusting in the deepest Self, hair-loss or baldness can be the ultimate consequence. The balance between the so-called "male and female" hormones will also be disturbed.

Artists, women, hippies, certain philosophers all wear their hair long — for the most part unconsciously — as a symbol of the rich flow of unconscious, intuitive, spontaneous energies welling up from the inner Self. "Punks" refuse to listen to any authority — their inner urge for self-authority is shriekingly protested in all colors.

Samson did not place Authority in himself, but in his hair, in a God outside himself. Hair symbolizes unconscious powers, but someone with a bald head has just as much inner Authority as someone with a mop of hair. At all times, every person can become aware of his inner worth, his source, and can give himself to it in trust. As long as a Samson holds on only to the "outer Self," to an Authority outside himself, then he doesn't realize that the hair "symbolizes" precisely this Power of the human being: the ability of the Human Being to draw energy endlessly out of this inner divine source, which has its roots in another dimension and which he can completely trust — but which at the same time requires the responsibility to create his life with his Conscious "I," taking his life firmly in his own hands and having faith for the rest! The supple, gentle hair: the waves of constant materialization via the Power of our Core, which brings it about!

And . . . if the moment has come for the human being to be "bald," then this doesn't have any negative meaning. The "wise" person knows this for himself.

Baldness

Baldness doesn't have to be considered negative, neither with "men" nor with "women."

Growing bald indicates that the accelerator is being floored (with the right foot), *in order now to push through one's own "I" without frills. One longs (unconsciously) to experience the Essence of one's own being, and chooses this in an assertive way.* A revolt. Actually, one wants to leave behind the all-too-busy mind, the thinking and working, the having to walk and work under these or those terms. One throws off this pressure, as it were, and because of that the hair flies in all directions. One wishes to free oneself: one gets rid of that which is superfluous, of that which puts pressure on the head; symbolically, the Self manifests this as Baldness.

One longs to experience one's nature in an honest, free way, separate from obligations and laws, structures and work.

Most people don't listen to this language, and they further bind themselves to "having to" and to "systems," to habit-patterns with which they don't want to break: one of the reasons is that most people are still slaves of their desires, because of which they don't have faith in completely Being Themselves in a free way. With their rational thoughts, they try to keep everything under control, because they don't trust their intuition, their feelings. Tensions and emotions are being suppressed; one tries to keep a hold on the inner world. Growing bald indicates that this human being now is allowed to listen to himself in a flexible way, that the time has come to go through life in a relaxed way and to listen to the deeper feelings, without anxiety, to the creative and childlike energies in the Self, which possibly used to be suppressed by an (inner) dictator. A signal that now the spontaneous may break through the restrictive armor. . . .

Whether one has a lot of hair or is totally bald, this in fact has nothing to do with old age or degeneration, but it does have to do with the Language of the living Self (Read the category Gray, white hair).

It goes without saying that the inner Self-core of that person who has for years been putting himself under high pressure — for instance in a stressful job within a limited framework — will now urge him more and more to begin living his life in a different, more relaxed way! He unconsciously frees himself of the pressure on his head by throwing off his hair; it's a sign of the manifestation of the "I." If a person is annoyed by becoming bald, then this only means that he wrongly connects the balding with "ugliness" — in which case this person urgently needs to free himself of the naive, limiting norm-system within the Cult of the External Appearance. Or perhaps baldness is connected with degeneration or dying — which represents a complete Lie. (Read about this in *New Days*.)

Gray, white hair

Graying is a call of the Living Self to lead the "I" to total Liberation. The "I" lets itself be heard and now asks for complete attention. Often, this call for attention for the SELF is being resolved in the wrong way: one now begins to pay more attention to oneself by looking in the mirror at those gray hairs, or else one spends much time in "washing" one's hair with a coloring shampoo or at the hair dresser's — this, of course is not the objective of the Living Self! *True* liberation involves one really beginning to live from out of oneself, not always directed toward caring for others or living again and again for the sake of the eye of the outer world.... The human being is now stimulated to live in a relaxed way, from out of himself, without letting himself be prodded by others, without pushing himself in a stressful situation. Gray hair is not an illness: it is a signal that urges the human being to listen to his own Feeling. The rational mind seeks its path to Wisdom by joining in a marriage with the intuitive, with the deeper emotional world. The Time is now ripe for this. Have you lived on the outside so far? Then, the underground excavation now begins: don't worry about the outside, but begin now the transformation from within. The

mole now digs its tunnels underground and arranges its life there in a comfortable way. Has the limited Ego been in charge so far? If so, then the direction is now handed over to the great Master in the human being. It really makes no difference whether a human being has dark or gray hair, a shining mop, or is bald: that which goes on inside the head is what is important.

Gray, white hair is not a negative signal; graying only indicates that the time has come to dig INTO one's Self, to look inward, to transform oneself. Other powers now call; new powers ask to be heard.

Let go, and enter into your Greater Self, here on Earth; it seems that gray hair invites you: too bad that so many people feel this as a letting go of life itself, as the entering into the womb of a God, of a heaven or of a nirvana.

This is definitely not the idea!

Don't fixate on the external, but now direct yourself deeply inward, so that great changes can come about. All energies in your body will now put themselves in service of that which is new; it goes without saying that certain old elements will fall away, that for instance hormones will start working in function of the renewal of the body.

Gray hair tells you: it is Time now to direct yourself differently, to ready yourself for a fundamental transformation, where there will be no more suffering and death (Read the book *New Days*). Now allow the burdens from previously to slide off your shoulders, and direct yourself firmly inwardly; open yourself to the paradise inside you. The rest will then take place by itself.

Silver-white hair is the manifestation of the inner wish to bring upward, out of your deepest Self, in a joyful, exhilarating way, the inexhaustible stream of Intuition and Emotional-sounds (music, the feminine, water....). Here we are dealing with the silver-white, propelling forces in your Self: they are the threads of "the Original Child" inside you. These forces announce a change, a transformation: we are dealing here with a change of color; you "show your colors" to your feelings.

Out of this we hear the longing to lift yourself up to a deeper, richer, more spontaneous, happier emotional life. The inner wish to come to full Surrender to the Paradisal Source in yourself; a wish for truly being born in yourself. Super-sensitive, silver strings of the Instrument of Life, in no way connected with death. Now, acknowledge that inner Happiness. Time to step out of that limited Framework and to free yourself in such a way that life on Earth becomes total Joy.

A young human being grows up with blond or dark hair: his task is to discover the world, to explore himself, to open his eyes wide and, with all his senses, go and explore, in the world of promises; he needs to incarnate very strongly into Matter, on Earth, and to live on the gulf stream of his (mostly) unconscious Self. All of a sudden, a signal is given: the first gray-white hair is there. The human being is taken by the hand by his *inner Angel,* while the angel says: "You now have to take another direction; you now have lived enough in this direction. Now, for once, stand still — and then enter your next Life-phase." This silver-white angel will continue to accompany the human being until he is where he is supposed to be — in a transformed form in his new Life — and possibly his head of hair is then completely white, or possibly he is completely bald. This plays no role at all. If a human being listens to this voice of the living Self, then all suffering and death will disappear from his life. This inner voice says: *"Now be gentle to yourself, now be good to yourself. Now, come to inner peace. No longer work yourself to death. Enjoy life, and now, at last, start taking good care of yourself. Live the way you feel you should live, without constraint, without Time pressure, without allowing yourself to be rushed by others, by society. Listen to your deepest Feelings."*

Gray-white hair indicates that the human being is on the way to the deeper, underlying layers of life. It is symbolic for the Past, which constantly pushes itself away in order to come to new color in the NOW, directed toward the future. Acute shock waves from experiences or from problems, from sadness, can go together with suddenly turning gray: this indicates that the experiences a human being undergoes at that moment mark a Change. This human being will become aware of a call for transformation inside himself and will have to listen to this. If he submerges himself inwardly he will undergo spiritual growth. He will build up wisdom if he is now open to gain insight into the deepest regions of his Self: so that the human being can bring Light into the darkness of the being he used to be. *The journey* to the land of the masterful powers has now begun. Now, the brain is only working in service of that which is Good. The human being no longer imprisons himself in the straitjacket of Time, of that which Must be done. In thankful contentment he now cleans up all sadness: he chooses in favor of life, and knows that gray-white hair has nothing to do with life or death, but that it is *a Call* from the living Self-core in the human being, to enter a new life-phase, whereby first and foremost every tension and every sadness has to be definitively cleaned up, and whereby free passage is given to the intuitive, emotional flow which comes out of the deepest Self-core. *The next steps* which need to be taken on this joyful Path toward immortality will gradually manifest themselves.

If a human being is annoyed by having gray hair, then this indicates that he has an inner annoyance regarding the natural growth of his body; possibly he is stuck in the norms of the cult of external appearances; possibly, the fear of degeneration and death is behind it: this just indicates that this human being has not yet chosen eternal life; if he doubts this, then of course he has a basic fear which again and again pops up. He needs to free himself from this self-limitation! Also, gray-white hair is in harmony with life; you simply have to understand it in the right way. And it can be that the human being who, for a long period of time, has kept himself in a hard-working, stressful situation, turns gray within a short period of time. Then this is the language of the living Self, which now tells him it is time to turn "inward," to "give" to himself, to pay attention to the child within, to discover deeper regions in himself. He then doesn't have to "drop" that which is old just like that, but he will have to direct himself inwardly toward a new phase, in transformation, whereby — as a consequence of inner enrichment — the outer circumstances will evolve also toward renewal, in a constant movement.

Timeless powers of joy now propel themselves into the Angel-hair: the angel-man now surrenders to this and doesn't want to lower himself again to the world of desire and sadness. He now directs himself Higher and Deeper into himself and allows new powers — as beneficial streams — to do their work; he listens again and again to the silence in himself and no longer worries about the busyness of the world. He is wise and is silent now when he has to be. He enjoys his wisdom and chooses to place it at the disposal of an eternal Life on Earth.

Gray-white hair is a translation of a message from the deepest Self, which rings out: "Now enter into your Self, be welcome here, and feel that joy, that great happiness at being able to experience yourself, at being able to exist as an 'I.'" *Here, it's about these powers in the Self which draw you inside in order to turn you away from every stress, from every sadness — from every "lie" in this respect — and to begin searching for the Happy Child deep inside yourself.*

The result is inexpressible happiness: when you find yourself in this inner shelter of the silver mother. The vibration of gray-white hair is radiatingly powerful and joyful.

It says to you: *"Now, find happiness IN yourself!" And now allow the life powers*

to flow freely through yourself, without having to tensely restrain your nature any longer. Surrender to this spontaneous joy of being able to be yourself. Surrender, now, to that which is radiatingly angelic in yourself, and enjoy it. Don't turn your mind to the negative, to the problems, but to that which is beautiful. In your wisdom, you know then that everything will become only more beautiful and lighter. Listen to that invitation to Enter into your Great Self and don't offer any resistance by clinging to false, superficial, or outer values."

A flood of Silver Energies, which your deepest Self sends you: look at these loving rays inside your and respond to them so that the Child in you has the feeling of being loved and feels happy!

Hirsutism
that which one calls "masculine" hair-growth patterns in the "woman"

What is "masculine," what is "feminine"?

The black and white division into "men" and "women" and the (exterior) characteristics belonging to them is really not correct.

Many "women" would benefit in their well-being/health if they allowed the "male" element in themselves to unfold, and many men would benefit by developing the "female aspect" in themselves.

Unconsciously, humanity knows about this.

Why should a woman not be allowed to have facial hair?

Why should a man have hair growth on his chest? Etc.

The cult of the exterior makes no sense.

Every man-woman, i.e. every human being, does well when he/she allows him/herself to be whoever he/she is, according to content and shape, in a balanced way. When, suddenly, in a very short period of time, Hirsutism manifests itself in an acute, intense way, the woman can consider the following:

You stop yourself; you don't go on in a steady way — your life-course runs along in jerks and jolts, because you feel too insecure. Suppressed aggressive powers. Emotions oppress you; you can't work out certain feelings; you hold on to them — you feel blocked; you can't experience your feelings freely. . . .

Suppressed anger — toward others — but, in fact, it is you who doesn't dare go on independently! With your mind, you try to comprehend, to control everything; your female, emotional side is being suppressed; you underestimate yourself, insufficiently trust in your spontaneous impulses, in your deepest Self.

*Acknowledge the gold in yourself! Stand in the center of your life and make yourself a path through it in a certain and active way, without fear, without complexes, without reserve. Come into contact with your higher, beautiful energies and dare to trust in your intuition. Stop putting yourself under a glass bowl, and express your feelings completely. Go on, without hesitation, and spoil yourself in gentleness. Acknowledge fully this female side in you. Your anger is actually directed toward your "refusal to fully Live"; don't send out your frustrations toward others. Lead your energies in a self-aware way! Discover the balance, male **and** female, in yourself. Allow "hair growth" to be where your nature wants it to be. Don't divide humanity into "men" and "women" in a black and white way. Acknowledge the "god-man" in every human being. . . . Every human being on Earth is unique and original.*

Loss of hair

You too much limit your life within certain structures: everything in your life is being placed within a well-determined framework; you want too much to put everything into a box; it has to be "so." You lay obligations and strict rules upon yourself; you give yourself insufficient breathing space to let natural, spontaneous impulses flow freely — you

place everything under control; you take hold of your life in a way that is too oppressive.

You direct your life in *one* particular direction; you fixate too much; you hold on to things. You unconsciously refuse to look flexibly in all possible directions. Many hair roots wriggle to come through: many talents — free creative potential, higher energies, intuitive possibilities — ask for an outlet to come through, but you suppress or ignore all this. A transformation is required!

Achievements, ambition — these are good, as long as they go hand-in-hand with the joy of the development of your creative possibilities, but not when they bring on stress.

Stop carrying needless burdens, let go of everything, and trust. Open yourself up to broad experiences; be faithful to your true nature and don't force yourself at any level. Live in a relaxed way; don't put a damper on your head; allow your energies to come through flexibly.
Finally: little or no hair — that is of no importance. Now, come to wisdom; don't care about the "exterior." Hair does not at all have to grow "back"!

Profuse hair growth on the body

Rich hair growth on the body is *not* an "unhealthy" symbolism: it indicates enthusiastic life motives, outward-turning energies, produced by the Core, which is as strong as a Lion, as playful as a child, as original as an animal. These unconscious, fundamental powers can manifest themselves in a tough, strong, aggressive way if they aren't guided in a truly Conscious way.

If a human being *allows* himself to be led by his unconscious, instinctive powers — if for the most part he *allows* himself to "be lived" by primitive energies (which can translate into aggression, urges, emotions) instead of standing at the rudder in *self*-Awareness — then "abnormally" strong hair growth is possible.

Through awareness, all the bubbling-up powers will come through freely without being suppressed, and under the guidance of the Conscious "I" they will — in a healthy, transformed way — express themselves in creative, joyful energies.

Creative impulses in the fundamental uniqueness of every human being are represented by the sexual glands and organs: in these places we find the symbol of this primitive creative urge, which comes forth out of the unconscious: the hair; the transformation of potential into realization in matter.

It is of great importance not to reduce your existence, but to enjoy all your powers, in active, creative, emotional experiences, under the supervision of the conscious "I."

Don't let your life be directed by uncontrolled aggressive powers, nor suppress the spontaneous energies which come to the fore: let things flow, digest, create, transform.

Strive for a balance between the "mental and the emotional" in the awareness-experience where there is room for relaxation, enjoyment, work, and creativity. Also, a balance between the gentle, sweet, childlike and the Active, powerful.

The consequence of this will be a healthy hair growth.

Hair ends, split

You live too tensely; you close yourself up too much; you are too hard, too demanding, with yourself. As a reaction to this, you are angry: pent-up aggression because of powerlessness. Revolt against being tied down.

You feel in the grip of — in the power of — but in fact it is you who kills the child inside you; you refuse completely to choose in favor of yourself, to choose playful joy, true Life! You have Power over yourself, but you use it in a destructive way. Don't you love yourself?

You don't take the rudder in hand in a self-aware way: your emotions, anxieties, anger, disappointment, sadness, etc., all get the upper hand.

You flee from that which is earthly, from your body: you become more spirit, more thinking than truly daring to fully enjoy yourself, the sensorial, in the here-and-now.

You are a dictator toward yourself!

A split. A division into two paths: life or death?

Don't let yourself burn away! Come again into yourself and glorify all the beautiful things in your nature, in life! Open your total being toward beautiful energies: experience the sensorial, the physical, the earthly. Joy for existence itself! Dare to truly enjoy(!) your body, flowers, that which is delicious, all that is beautiful.

Humor!

Experience the concentration of awareness in your body; don't numb yourself, but learn to FEEL again; be content and happy, just because of being yourself! Allow powerful energies to blossom, without severity. First and foremost direct your love in gentleness toward yourself: don't condemn and punish yourself like an executioner. Make your Self, your body, fully welcome. Opt for YOU; no longer flee onto a second path, where, perhaps in fanatic idealism, you waved the flag.

Are you in pain, sad in your Heart, because of injustice in your relationships or because of the misery in the world?

First, be aware of the full worth of your life: only then can you place a first stone for a new, beautiful earth, born in love. Now, first allow yourself to born in yourself: no longer push this child away. Resolutely choose this ONE, happy path; no more crossroads!

Spontaneous joy; no "must" anymore.

HALLUCINATIONS

Fundamental anxieties because of an insufficient presence in yourself. You don't see clearly into yourself nor into your surroundings: you live too much in the spirit instead of with two feet on the ground, here and now.

You experience yourself as playing a piano with white and black keys: you mistrust the "black" as something negative in yourself; you are afraid of your own depths, of the "devilish" — you think you have to defend yourself against something "bad" inside you.

You take heavy burdens onto your shoulders; you do many things because you "force" yourself to do so, because you don't dare follow your spontaneous nature.

In this way you become ever more estranged from yourself. There's no more real contact with your deepest Core; you are afraid that one power or another might crush you; you believe in negative or black energies.

Illusions present themselves to you because you've suppressed a part of yourself, an important part of your emotions, of your longings: it was "dirty and bad" inside you — but now this repressed aspect is appearing again. The more you run away from it, the stronger it "pursues" you.

You think you deserve "punishment," that someone is pursuing you, that he will kill you, etc. — you are fleeing from yourself. You divide yourself into a good and a bad part: this split personality asks for a solution, especially because you begin to look upon this rejected aspect of yourself as an other, a devilish figure, someone who wants to harm you.

Possibly, you believe in this evil aspect of yourself in such a way that you begin to identify yourself with it, and you might apply force to, or manipulate, others: a consequence also of your own feelings of powerlessness and anxiety.

Allow your feelings to flow freely. You are not bad: change these negative convictions regarding yourself. Stop this self-condemnation; with clear eyes take a good look at yourself and your surroundings. Integrate completely your "negative" feelings, or, rather, that which you consider to be

negative: anger, hatred, revenge, sex, power, wrath, etc. Nothing is bad; everything is evolution.

Accept these emotions, work them out, don't run away from them. Calmly place all power in yourself; don't seize for power over others nor manipulate them. The more open and honest you dare to be toward yourself, the better you will get to know yourself, the stronger you can evolve. Trust in the goodness of your inner Self and stand solidly, self-aware, with both feet on the Ground. Place the authority in your Self!

HANDS
(See also Callus formation, Skin, Warts, etc.)

Psychological correspondence

Giving, leading, and being led; cherishing and caressing; the way we "undertake" our lives and our work. Holding on and letting go. The generous, heartfelt offering. From the hands radiates an enormous power if we live from out of our deepest Self; this radiation offers healing, love, recovery, softening.

If one "feels" with the hands, then one will "see" with the inner eye at a deeper level — as long as one opens oneself to the strong, beautiful Authority in oneself. The hands symbolize the "adoration" of an idol outside yourself or else they symbolize the thankful realization of the divine kingdom in your own being. . . .

The symbol of the balanced cooperation between the left and right poles (See Brain); a link to other people, striking or soothing; being open to others — but above all daring to accept and follow your personal direction without blinders.

Ailments, in general

Are you too hard on yourself, with iron discipline? Are you not open to gentleness, enjoyment, and joy? Do you only notice that which is sad and that which limits you? If so, then you are throwing away your life.

Do you force yourself in *one* certain direction, blindfolded? A path on which you don't take your true nature into account?

Are you constantly "thinking" instead of surrendering to your inner Self, to your intuition? Do you not see clearly with both eyes? Are you prejudiced? Do you close your eyes to the essential? Do you limit yourself to the rational or external, to image, status — in other words, do you not make yourself welcome in your totality?

Do you swear by God or by the devil, by one or another religion or sect, which brings you further away from yourself?

Do you lock yourself away in isolation? Do you have no real contact with others? Do you shun people? Then you will probably also shun yourself. What is it you push away in yourself? Your body? Your feelings? Or something else? Why not open yourself up fully to yourself, to others?

Completely accept your feelings; don't switch off one part of yourself; acknowledge the harmony of the female and the male in you. Take away all blinders and surrender to love for yourself, to your inner Authority. Don't be stingy with a laugh, dare to enjoy life; feel your higher powers, and handle them with mastery. Open yourself up completely to the abundance of life: don't push it away.

Hand blisters
(See also Hands, and Blisters, in general)

Emotional vulnerability, especially because you don't allow your higher energies to break through. Because you underestimate yourself and idealize people or things outside yourself. You'd sacrifice yourself, be too hard on yourself. You keep yourself too closed up, your larger energies are hardly allowed to develop themselves. You deprive yourself of this possibility because you think it has to be that way, because you think you

have no right to it — possibly there is a stubborn refusal after being hurt emotionally. But this also was a result of your self-restriction, your self-degradation. Held-in potential energies — until they burst! Underneath this lies a deep Anxiety of being yourself; you mistrust or look down on your content — you think there's something negative inside you, it threatens you, and that's why you don't break through. In this way, your nature is kept in an iron grip; anxiously you close up yourself and your spontaneous energies. This blocked self-realization can lead to sharp aggressiveness, to hard action: self-destruction.

Feel those strong life forces which grow inside you, and allow them to produce in a spontaneously active way. Calmly turn yourself inward: don't be afraid of your own depths, your natural aggression: build your life on a solid Basis with only your Self in the center. Be good to yourself, relax, don't hurt yourself, don't reject a part of yourself, allow all creativity to flow through freely, don't block any emotions. Are you angry? Then look at the causes for this (your powerlessness, your discontent with yourself, your self-degradation . . .), and express them. Come to an understanding, and change your opinion of yourself. Acknowledge your worth; don't bottle things up; turn outward in word and deed! Your nature is safe: listen to it. Follow your impulses, your intuition; don't be afraid of your emotions: no longer keep things in. Love for yourself chases fear away.

HEADACHE

Headache, in general

Anxiety. You insufficiently trust your Self. You try too hard to comprehend everything, with nervous brooding and thinking. Hesitation, self-doubt: shall I go on or not? Shall I choose this path? Stagnation because of anxiety and unsureness.

Life is a question mark to you. Emotions: sadness, pain, anger — a consequence of your hesitating conflict: "Shall I go back, or do I dare evolve onward?" An inner battle and resistance against transformation. This leads to confrontations with sad, ambiguous situations in your surroundings: a reflection of your not going on in a consistent, self-assured way. Inner friction because you are insufficiently aware of your Worth! Self-condemnation. You look at yourself through the critical eyes of others, and especially through the eyes of people for whom you have high regard. You place the center of your existence too much outside yourself. Am I doing it right? You don't dare to completely be yourself, experiencing your nature the way you are: you anxiously clasp and hold on to a lot of feelings. You think and control more than truly living from out of your true nature. Do you worry too much about others? About those for whom you feel responsible? Do you want to anxiously watch over them? Can't you let go of your partner? Does the thought of death unconsciously occupy your mind?

Go on! Change direction, completely trust your intuition, your deepest Self; don't ask yourself what others expect from you. Stop with self-criticism and acknowledge your worth now. Fret no longer, let go, and trust: there's no negative happening in your life that you haven't unconsciously called up yourself. Therefore, completely depend on the solid Basis in you, and achieve creative construction of your life. Without hesitation, create a joyful future. Stop trying to comprehend everything with your "thinking"; trust, relax. If your expectations regarding your life are no longer anxious ones, then sad situations will disappear out of your life. Give yourself freedom and oxygen; no longer oppress yourself. Nor hold back your feelings in a tense way. Allow your nature to

grow spontaneously. Dare to cut the knot and no longer look back at that which has passed. Direct all creative energies onward.

* * *

People who are often bothered by headaches also need to examine the following in themselves:

Energetically bottling up and suppressing (no spontaneous, honest, direct reaction or "expression of feelings," etc.). This goes together with a fundamental feeling of doubt regarding one's own "I," often feeling victimized ("I am not allowed to" or "I *have* to do it this way or that way.") A feeling of being the underdog or playing the "obedient one" toward the Authority that one places outside of oneself (while in the meantime one listens to one's own small, little ego-aspect, which is hard and severe and which is afraid because it's closed off from the Greater "I" being). "I have no choice, I *have* to swallow what 'they' are saying or doing to me," but, actually, one does it to oneself. In short, a denying of one's own Mastership, of True Inner Authority. In this way the person is not obliged to take life in his own hands, and he can constantly blame the "cause" of his problems, his pain or sadness, on Something or Someone OUTSIDE himself. Doing this, he doesn't at all help himself. On the contrary, he pulls the rug out from under himself. In the first place, he subjects himself to "laws" and "rules" to which he "has to listen" — instead of opening himself up to what his Life-Heart asks. Transformation is asked!

You collect energy inside; you pile up and suppress emotional energies and fertile seeds instead of allowing these fruitful life energies to flow in a spontaneous, self-assured way in one continuous motion; instead of resolutely swallowing certain things — as well as speaking, acting, putting your feelings into words or expressing your emotions in a straightforward way, acknowledging your true feeling and possibly making it known to others. But you'd sooner take a position of expectation toward the outside world . . . as if you have to be the "wronged victim" who has to swallow who knows what! Don't hide behind this . . . . show yourself as a Powerful male-female "I"! And express yourself, *be* yourself, don't stand still in a passive, bottled-up way, subsequently suppressing your so-called emotions (Oh, this lie; denying your mastership!). Behaving like an emotionally tortured "victim"! Go onward!

You hold back your spontaneous, creative, emotional, and fertile powers; you block them. As a result, an abundance of sexual energy can develop in *certain* people. This, however, is not the cause of headaches; instead, it's a result of "holding yourself back" in a broad, energetic field.

Don't play the role of "the underdog." Headaches call to you to take a position at the head of your life! Therefore, a fundamental solution is not to work this off — for instance getting rid of your frustrations in sexuality, or in one or another kind of sport, or in an outburst of fury or irritated reactions. But realize where the CAUSE lies that makes it necessary to spit out everything, to work it off or to lose yourself in certain things . . . it's because you "suppress" the "first" feelings, the "first" creative forces and spontaneous expressions that well up in you, because you don't immediately and spontaneously experience within and bring out your feelings, because again and again you wait and bottle things up instead of giving yourself the "free, natural outlet." A constant bottling-up and curbing yourself (in emotions, deeds and creativity), which can lead to the search for safety valves.

So, become yourself in a POWERFUL way, without doubt, so that aggression does not accumulate, nor frustration pile up. Feel sure of yourself from out of your honest feelings and spontaneously express yourself. Don't allow yourself to "be lived," don't live from below, don't bottle things up, not for

the eye of society nor for relations. JUST BE YOURSELF, in all honesty, without fear of losing something . . . when you are yourself (the approval of others, your image or whatever).

Are you constantly rushing yourself? Do you hurry, hurry, bringing your nerves under high pressure? For whom? Why? Are YOU not in the Center of your existence? Headaches will force you to listen first and foremost to yourself — not running ahead of yourself for the sake of society, "work," the job or someone else, rushing for them . . . at THE COST of yourself. Because this means "holding on"; "Let go" says life! When you hold on to this or that, to what this or that person might think of you, how "they" judge you, to what happens if you don't do this or that — all reasons to force yourself, hurt yourself — instead of calmly but resolutely BEING yourself! Do you like to force a certain behavior from others? Do you want them to approve of you? Do you prefer to remain in a victimized role while looking up to the Authority outside yourself? This Authority doesn't have to be a person; it can just as well be some idealized image you have and strive after for yourself, or some social pressure . . . an image, a job, a god (the god of Time and Structure for instance) — it's always about Something or Someone you place ABOVE yourself and above Life. This is easy: then you don't have to evolve, because then you don't take any responsibility for your TRUE SELF-EVOLUTION!

Therefore, no longer flee from yourself, no longer flee from your responsibility. Don't place yourself under something (for instance your work; achievements, etc.) or someone. Don't put on an act. SHOW YOURSELF in true form, the way you are. Don't place anything above Life! Express yourself and live life to the full, according to heart and soul, not according to desires (wanting something from others or wanting their approval for instance) but LET GO of others and *do what YOU feel you have to do, living from out of your HEART, from out of your BEING.*

*   *   *

Waiting, expectant — piling everything up inside you, holding on to emotions, a forced attitude, instead of swallowing everything right away; strongly reacting and going on, firmly, as "I," be it in a female-forceful or male-forceful way; you remain stuck, you hold back your fertile seed. Throat glands might swell because you try to save face before the eyes of the outer world, of others. You don't want to make your real feelings known.[1] Even when you feel emotionally or psychologically raped, as it were, you still keep these feelings to yourself. You have a need for swallowing the past, things that have gone by, getting a clear and bright insight in "why" you have attracted certain things and still do. There is anger, possibly bottled-up fury in your throat. It would do you good to spit every thing out for once . . . not by blaming someone, but just to free yourself from everything that has been bottled up. Finally, via this emotional expression, you can get "in touch" with yourself, with your body, with your "I"; to feel, to know, to realize that you as an "I" have the right to a "free" existence.

You have no reason at all to get angry with someone, even if it seems there's a reason. These are alibis behind which you hide so as not to become YOURSELF. Possibly, you have attracted many situations in the past, offensive and painful, as a result of the fact that you didn't step forward as "I," that you took a waiting position as an underdog or victim. This is "shutting yourself out." Therefore, don't blame others now, but resolve to break with holding yourself back, with this suppression, holding on to things or persons and denying your true Central "I." Instead, *STEP FIRMLY FORWARD AS "I" from within, from the heart, and allow your*

feelings, your energies, to flow freely and sincerely! Only you can free yourself; only you can make yourself completely free. In your emotional experience you will see how no one outside yourself really is the cause of your problem, of your headache, but how you have held on too much to your surroundings, perhaps cared about their judgment or their reaction, possibly were emotionally dependent on them or dependent on the approval of society, a group, etc. Don't blame them for it, but begin by living FROM OUT OF YOURSELF . . . from out of your inner basis of Authority, honestly listening to what you feel! No longer bottle things up; no longer keep things in to please others or to be considered good.

Feel that fundamental fire power inside, which is waiting for you to forge yourself into a human being of a Noble race. Now, allow that power-stream to flow honestly, and don't suppress yourself: just BE yourself, do what you feel you have to do at any moment of the day, without checking yourself, without bottling up, without passively waiting, on the fringe of yourself! Bring yourself completely in! Now, possibly, you blow everything out of yourself, as if fire and backed-up vomit flies out of your throat; for far too long you have held yourself back, and you were not really yourself. Now the moment has come that you enter firmly and in a concentrated way into yourself, into your body; that you no longer keep yourself silent and expectant, nor as a zombie, or dependent on a social sphere. Let the dragon spew, all that is bottled up possibly wants to come out, so that subsequently you can turn yourself restfully toward inner peaceful relaxation. As a divine, powerful, and at the same time a loving, bulldozer, you make yourself a way; Your Path that lies ahead of you, and nothing or no one can stop you here.

You have to realize *"yourself"*; not a job, not an "image," etc.! The heavens then will clear; you now enjoy life, Nature — you no longer worry about anything! You now learn to see true beauty, and you discover the pure values of Life. You now really live from out

---

[1] Read in this connection about the symbolism of the thyroid gland.

of the joy of your Heart, the happiness about your "being." You no longer hold on to anything or anybody! You go out like an adventurer with a knapsack in search of all that is beautiful in Nature, to the green meadows and the playing ducks, the singing blackbirds, and the bleating sheep. You really come home to the nature in yourself, among all that is beautiful, which only NOW you can see, because you no longer wait or take an expectant position for someone else to make you happy or give you relaxation, for someone else to stop hurting you. No, you know now that you have everything in your hands, and that, when you no longer hurt yourself, you will automatically meet other people on your path who share in this happiness. You now sing, as it were, along with the birds, you glow with health; your happiness cannot be broken anymore; ARRIVED HOME in yourself, *in the NATURE of your being, in your Center, your Sensations, your Body, your Great "I AM" from which you had strayed away so far.*

You no longer RUMINATE on things, thinking all the time, but immediately spit out the negative and enjoy the beautiful newly discovered delights! You no longer run after an "image" of yourself. You now live "according to truth" (see Part I). *You no longer inhibit yourself, no longer put a damper on yourself, on that spontaneous life stream, since you are living from out of your Heart, your deepest feeling, not dominated by desires, "seizing." Now there's no longer any question of doubt, nor of anxiously holding on or seizing/curbing things with your thoughts; only Trust dominates in a self-assured Going Onward!*

Cluster headaches
periods of severe one-sided pain
around the eye socket, mostly at night

You feel yourself to be *whipped up* from left to right, as it were, up and down; you don't very well know where is north or south. One time directed earthward, then again heavenward; you might become dizzy from it.

Nervously seeking outside yourself, deviating from your inner focus, from your deeper bottom, from your heart. Seeking and looking and moving toward everything outside yourself in an exaggerated fidgety nervous way, so that your head no longer knows where it is. IN THIS WAY, YOU DEVIATE FROM YOUR OWN CENTER! Therefore, come back to yourself and learn to let go of everything! To do this, of course, it is necessary that you BELIEVE in yourself, in the worthiness of your Center, your Content as a Worthy Human Being!

An inner feeling of chaos, not knowing very well how to proceed. You are searching . . . but you don't very well know where. And for what?! Therefore, take yourself to the deepest layers inside you . . . to the Plutonic treasure chamber inside yourself; which is REAL and authentic, and of the most noble gold. You may trust in this! You never have to ask someone else for "advice" — although you can open your ears once in a while or pick up something here or there; but only YOU can decide WHAT exactly is right for you, what is good for you at THIS moment; "I," here and now. Therefore, ask yourself: "*Where* is that deep Core?" In your own dearest Self, within the precious content of your being. Don't search further than *your HEART,* than *what you FEEL,* because there it all starts; there lives love, warm love for yourself; there lives self-appreciation, self-respect, and there begins an appreciation for that which is truly beautiful and pure in yourself and in the world around you!

So, *turn profoundly inward and liberate yourself from all feelings of guilt and anger, of powerlessness and penance, of all doubts! Place yourself at the head of your life and listen to the loving feeling very deep inside yourself. No longer lose yourself* in things and surroundings, your thoughts nervously looking here and there, up and down. Allow those nerves to calm down by turning yourself INWARD in a very pure way, by FEELING where you are, who you are. Let everything outside you go — come home to your content; no longer live with your brains going round and round in chaotic nervousness. *Stop that wild merry-go-around from turning and turn toward yourself in REST and AS-SURANCE.* DON'T RUN AWAY FROM YOURSELF. Trust that deep Content, that treasure chamber of gold. KNOW how life is put together: read Part I of this book; nothing just happens by "accident"! You have your life in hand; everything goes along beauti-fully and smoothly if only you let go more and know that everything falls into place . . . TRUST! You don't have to cling to every-thing from left to right, from earth to heaven; you don't have to move in such a busy way, throwing your thoughts all over the place. Always keep both feet on the ground and don't turn this matter upside down!

It might be necessary to build up clear, pure structures, and if you don't immediately see "clearly," then trust that everything will become clear without your having to imme-diately look/run all over the place. Know that everything falls into place at the right time, that everything will be all right as long as you have faith, as long as you connect yourself closer with your heart and know that YOU, as Master, stand at the head of your life. That there is NO chaos, that you just experience it that way sometimes; calm your-self; *don't fly from here to there with your eyes, your thoughts, your total being. LET GO of things; no longer hold on to them through your senses, through your thoughts! Now, STRICTLY turn toward the Center in yourself, very deep and calm inwardly; FEEL your heart and offer yourself love and appreciation . . . so that pains can disappear. You no longer LOOK for it AROUND you . . . you no longer move around in a dizzy way . . . you descend deep inside yourself and NO LONGER STRAY FROM THIS INNER CENTER. You establish yourself firmly on your own foundation.* You believe in this fundamental basic force in yourself, so that you no longer have to look outside yourself in an anxiously reaching nor nervously seeking way. NOTHING "IS A MUST"! No longer live according to the conviction that

you are "nothing" or just a "passing" little ego or a nervously turning brain with an at-tached body that is dependent on the outer world for its existence! No — your life is solely dependent on yourself, on your con-victions regarding yourself. Therefore let go of the negative conviction that you might just be a moving shadow, a madly turning head, an energy field searching and grabbing out-side itself. No, you are YOU as a Content in an earthly body: come to this realization. DESCEND into yourself: only there can you find rest, only there will you find that funda-mentally secure basis. Surrender to this! Listen, listen . . . very deeply to your content, to your feelings, to your intuition, to your heart, to the golden content of your abdomen, to your INNERMOST BEING. Here, you will find Fullness, Rest, and Silence; here, you will know yourself to be ESTAB-LISHED in a strong and stable way. Now, you will no longer look around WILDLY. Arrived at home, landed, full of self-confidence.

Migraine
See also Headache, in general

If one takes away the left side of the trium-phal Arch, then the entire structure collapses. If you, as a child of humanity, cut yourself off from that motherly, intuitive, emotional source in you, then migraine can manifest it-self.

Insufficient awareness of your own worth. You see yourself through the eyes of others. You condemn yourself according to the norms of your parents, according to people to whom you subordinate yourself. Paternal authority pushes away the gentle, peaceful feelings.

You don't at all live according to your spontaneous nature. Perhaps you give the impression that you are *authentic,* but you are misleading yourself.

Migraine now calls on you to be who you *are,* completely, in all rectitude, not to be the way you are "supposed to be," nor to appear a certain way in order to please to others, nor to try to satisfy the silent expectations of your parents — nor to satisfy that part of you which represents the authority of parents!

In this way, also, your emotional life — your spontaneous emotional flow — is being tied down. You have, for instance, the feeling of being stuck to the Authority of your father, your mother, your employer, etc., or you bow to another dominant "Eye" that constantly supervises you. But this severe eye really lives inside yourself: you constantly place yourself under control. The environment is just a reflection of this.

You are too dependent on what "people" think or say about you. You still always place Authority outside yourself, or in a voice inside you that isn't really a living voice.

You don't dare to really autonomously live from out of your true nature! This leads to inner conflict. Your emotional world battles to be free while you constantly suppress your nature. Migraine raises the white flag, asks for a cease fire! After all, the eye with which you supervise yourself really means thinking and fretting, lingering too much over problems; ruminating anxiously on your problems because you try too much to control everything with your "reason" and your senses, without daring at all to trust your intuition.

Moreover, you are experiencing your deep emotions, your rich emotional world, as threatening; you hold on to authority outside yourself. You scarcely dare to build upon your own deepest Core, your fundamentally strong Living Self.

Because of this, you fixate endless "thoughts" on certain small problems: you are afraid to fail or you think you aren't doing things right.

You don't trust in your intuitive, inner knowledge; you distance yourself from your feelings; you ignore an important part of yourself. Migraine, therefore, attacks mostly "one-sidedly" in the head.

However smoothly you function via your outer ego, your freedom is deceiving: it is not freedom, but imprisonment.

You don't *really* live from out of your total self, but habits cause you to not even know who you are anymore — who you are separate from your upbringing, separate from indoctrinating restrictive rules. It all has stuck to you like a second skin. (Don't reproach anybody: after all, you've attracted everything yourself, consciously or unconsciously.)

You feel like a victim who can be hurt.

Possibly, you've attracted in life a cold, dominating figure because you've also relegated your emotional life to the cold, the shadow.

Find rest in yourself, relax, allow your brain to cool off, surrender completely to a deep, restful maturity within.

Now acknowledge your Worth and build your existence in an autonomous, self-assured way; uncouple yourself from bindings or the Authoritarian Voice under which you have placed yourself, and because of which you can't spontaneously be yourself.

Become aware of the armor in which you suffocate yourself, throw out the nervous thinking-pattern, and live according to your nature, your intuition.

Don't live according to the expectations of others, but according to your personal nature. Don't be afraid that you're not good enough: if you live in harmony with yourself, if you don't deny your originality, then you can consider yourself honest, good, and pure. Dare to live from out of your deepest core! Stop self-curtailment; no longer look at yourself through the eyes of others. Don't desire to be like this or like that: be yourself!

You are asked to look at the wisdom that is inside you, not to look at someone else, not to point at things or people outside yourself . . .[2] but to expand the deeper, funda-

---

[2] Read about the symbolism of the forefinger and the middle finger.

mentally strong "1-Power" which lives inside you. Go on, go further, follow the signals on your path and don't get stuck, don't stand still! An extremely strong energy inside you asks you to come to the realization of your Content, your Power, your Central Worth.

This illness indicates that there are enormous Forces inside you, and only when you completely and totally appreciate your being (your physical, strong body of flesh and your treasure box with its rich content, as a Human Being), only then will your life-core stop sending you signals like "migraines." Again and again it's pointed out to you when you "deviate" from yourself — first of all by directing yourself too much toward others (via criticism, via "looking," instead of looking inside yourself for wisdom and true worthiness) or toward "minor" things in existence.

If you again start looking for it outside yourself because you remain stuck at the "superficial side" of your being, too little realizing your content-in-your-body, which is strong and full of wisdom, then you will be *called to order* (by your Living Self) with Saturnal severity! To make you conscious of the fact that you need to follow the HIGHWAY in yourself, and none other! IN ORDER FOR YOU TO SEIZE YOURSELF POWERFULLY WITH AUTHORITY, BECOMING AWARE OF THAT INNER WISDOM, THE DIVINE AUTHORITY WITHIN YOUR OWN BEING, and placing this content "honestly"[3] inside a SOLID, RICH PHYSICAL BODY! So that you no longer will go beyond your borders by deviating from yourself, outward: this can have to do with people, work, etc.

With migraines you call yourself severely and harshly to order! As long as you refuse to acknowledge in yourself your inner greatness, the central authority, you will possibly call up severe pointing fingers in your surroundings "as a result" of this — or do you have this feeling at least, for in reality this

doesn't have to be: this "for as long as needed" dictator lives then first of all within yourself. On the one hand, this calling to order of yourself, via migraines, bringing yourself home within your own circle of wisdom, is necessary. But, on the other hand, this happens rather "harshly" and painfully. Is this perhaps because otherwise you would not listen to this demand to "return" into yourself?

Punishing yourself, also, because unconsciously you know that you have denied or neglected yourself in your greatness. Come into yourself in LOVE and GENTLENESS; acknowledge that grand, broad power in your being, and stop punishing yourself now; stop directing yourself again and again toward minor things, things outside yourself. Now, resolve to place the Authority inside yourself, no longer placing the "priority" in things and people outside yourself. In this way your head will reach inner rest and at the same time sense that you, as a Worthy, Loving Master, are ready to navigate your ship of life!

It is also asked of you to realize how secure and protected you can feel inside yourself: you, in your divine, powerful being. That nothing or no one can take down that strong giant of a Human Being — who you are — as long as he attunes himself to his great Heart, to Life, to his powers and not to: "look at this!" or "how do others do it?" or trying to "force something through no matter what," "instinctively desiring," or sheer "sex without love," or "hard ambition," etc.

After all, this indicates only that you as a human being insufficiently realize and use your creative powers, that you still have to discover the greatness of your Human Nature! The chain has to come off your neck; you feel suffocated. It is you who keeps you suffocated — not one or another Jupiter, pedantic index finger from the outside! Detach yourself, feel free, and no longer take your breath away by acting like a tyrant toward

---

[3] Read about this in *Large, Beautiful, and Healthy.*

yourself, nor by deviating from the Highway of life.

Don't be "limp," "weak," halfhearted, changing with the wind; follow the solid Central Pillar inside yourself, the main line of Life! Develop that solid, central force in yourself, no matter if you are born as a man or a woman: place the solid Authority inside yourself. Raise yourself, firmly, from within your divine center. On the other hand: listen to the feeling of your Heart . . . but, then, as a masterful leader over your existence! If you live according to this inner Pillar of Authority and also develop love on a higher level inside you, emotions, energies will also flow out in a loving way. You no longer will look for a safety valve as an escape from the severity you experience, but the result is giving your energies very Conscious leadership; in your work, in your physical relation experience for instance, or in other dynamic activities in which you feel delightful and good. No more compulsive instincts which looked for a way out under the eyes of the tyrannical voice inside you, but a conscious, joyful, gentle — though at the same time forceful and strong — experiencing of your loving nature. Human according to soul and body.

It's indeed important here to realize that awareness-energies and physical body long to exist in "unified alliance." If someone keeps living on the instinctive level, then his body will ask for safety valves on this level; however, the human being who acknowledges the greatness of his being will experience the unifying alliance with his body, very consciously, in love toward himself and others. The flow of energies then happens FROM THE HEART, not from an exaggerated fixation on the surroundings via the head-brain-rationality-looking at . . . Wisdom is looked for within one's own "I." One no longer directs oneself instinctively outward, toward others; one doesn't gossip maliciously; one no longer looks for things greedily outside oneself.

The Person is now standing at the Head of his existence and follows that Highway from

out of his Heart, allowing his energies to flow freely, in love, soulwise and bodywise.

A healthy balance between "work" and "relaxation" accompanies this; one listens to the heart, to inner "knowing and feeling," which goes far beyond ordinary thinking and acting. The person lives according to truth, and does precisely that which he inwardly feels he should do from out of his Living Self (read Part I).

"HEARING VOICES"
without having an objective exterior cause

In this case, we're not talking about our "inner voice," nor about that which we intuitively perceive in ourselves as a "felt" indicator of a direction.

Here, it's definitely about perceived "voices," which can command you or give you messages — voices that are apparently separate from yourself. It's as if they penetrate your head from "the outside," as if they come from "someone" else.

We find this phenomenon in persons who suppress parts of themselves, who have called up in themselves a kind of "dividedness" in order to survive psychologically.

Taken by itself, this does no harm, especially not when one realizes that the "voice" represents a part of you that has been pushed to the side.

After all, one's complete unconscious content can be projected onto a separate part of the personality, and that content can then enter in the form of a voice. Instead of integrating all feelings, all unconscious powers, natural urges or impulses into one undivided personality, one divides oneself as it were. In this way, aggressive powers are being suppressed. One is afraid of them: the same powers can again come to the surface by expressing coercive commands; the part in you that you anxiously keep suppressed then will surface again, in a more forceful way, via a voice. You don't dare to speak up completely for your total Self, so therefore you (unconsciously) let "voices" speak.

You don't accept yourself the way you are; you feel stuck, frustrated, your true nature tied down, psychologically bound, powerless to be yourself.

You feel anxious, shadowed by evil, pursued by badness — but in fact this Anxiety, this paranoia, is only a reflection of your own fear of your deepest Self, of your true Nature. You distrust those strong powers that are very deep inside you; you think you have to arm yourself against them. You flee from yourself; voices call for integration: after all, you are being confronted with the result of fearful self-suppression! Also, pent-up aggression can find its path in this way. Were you taught to control yourself, never to let your nature go? To mistrust your feelings? Told again and again to live obediently and nicely, subjecting yourself to regulations? Do you strive after a projected ideal? Do you inwardly feel cramped because you can't answer to that ideal? Do you consider yourself, therefore, to be bad or devilish?

Intuitively follow your path! You don't need to perceive "clear" voices of "spirits" outside yourself: the wisdom is inside you! Direct yourself inwardly: everything is good here. Don't suppress part of yourself; integrate all parts of your nature into the Unity of your self. Tune in to that which is deepest in you, and listen to your Heart. Follow the path of love, and don't be afraid to let your enormous powers flow. You're allowed to erupt like a volcano, to flow like a waterfall — as long as you are yourself. In that way, you don't hurt anyone. Feel safe in that imperishable, fundamentally solid Basis, Your Living Self. Don't accept any other authority in your life than your own "I."

No longer close yourself up in a cramped way: let go of everything and let everything open up. Nothing or no one outside you

threatens you. They are the voices from out of your deepest Soul, voices which can manifest themselves in an exaggerated way because for too long you've suppressed the natural powers they represent! Therefore, don't build your life only on your "rational mind," nor on that with which "others" make you believe, nor on that part of you which does satisfy your projected ideals while you keep on suppressing that part of you which is rich in energy. Accept yourself completely; trust in that deep, beautiful power source in you; it is divine and made of gold.

Don't be afraid of your own powers, of your intuitive channels: allow them to circulate freely so that they don't have to seek side roads. You are only being "shadowed" by the Heart of love: don't look for "evil" where there's none at all. Your fears create voices, create devils, etc. In "reality," they don't exist.

Come home into yourself; know yourself to be safe; don't crawl into a corner of your house. Welcome the child in you, the female, the male, and don't suppress any of those aspects in yourself. Merge into unity.

THE HEART

Psychological correspondence

Left and right, the female and male aspect kept in balance within a balanced structure; in the middle functioning as a channel to allow life energies to flow through. Receiving and passing on within the light of "BEING."

A passage of energies, an opening-up of yourself to that which wants to come through and flow through in and via your body, your head, too, without fixing it or grasping it in any way. Continuously allowing it to pass, allowing life oxygen to flow through within the solid basic structure of your being, steadfast and strong.

You surrender to yourself, to the ever-flowing life energy inside yourself; you don't grasp anything; you don't stem the flow of life; you don't blockade with resistance, with thoughts, with desires. You receive and pass on, in absolute surrender to Life: this dynamic, therefore, is not being hampered anywhere.

You establish yourself strongly on left and right legs, balanced, *the spine solidly erected in the middle;* you open up your head, *with your higher consciousness,* to all kinds of forces, energies, and winds of life that want to flow through it. Not fixating with your thinking — on the contrary, rather a state of not-thinking, of letting-go of everything with the head — rather a letting-be, letting-pass; *a deep, restful experience of your "being," in surrender.* Nothing is being grasped or fixed. Allowing everything to be, *allowing yourself to be,* allowing that everything Life has to offer you in essence comes in and passes through you or inspires you. This gives a supreme feeling of rest, relaxation. Especially because you are solidly established in your unique structure, you can afford to let go of everything, allowing energies to flow through your being and cause a blissful feeling of relaxation. By *opening up,* by *letting go of everything, opening yourself, as if cherished in a blissful, warm wind of life.* Absolute blissfulness because of letting things pass and by just letting yourself "be."

A readiness, willingly saying "yes" to the really pure and beautiful that wants to offer itself in you; *flexibly bowing your head to the real pure gold that wants to flow into your body.* Not resisting the beautiful in life that wants to fertilize you. *No resistance, no stubbornness, no blockade or boycott of what life wants to reveal to you from within or from without.* It speaks for itself that you don't at all have to open yourself up to the negative that wants to force itself upon you. But this organ says: *tune yourself to the most supreme feeling in yourself, a combination of heart and consciousness, a higher knowing*

and feeling, so that only the beautiful will be able to come inside you. Believe in this; therefore surrender to that which is highest in you so that the divine light that is inside you can fructify you, so that only that which is purest in the outside world can visit and meet you.

Ailments, in general

You close yourself off, "hard," rejecting, not even allowing the most beautiful, loving flow to go through. Feelings and life energies are not allowed to come in, nor are they allowed to find a way out. No open, spontaneous, flexible communication with others, no passage. You keep yourself closed. You no longer open yourself at all for energies coming from the life-source that want to flow through your body and nourish it. Nor do you open yourself up to pleasant contacts and information or whatsoever from the outside. "Closed. Shut!" you say. Hard feelings, hard thoughts, tense structures, a refusal, perhaps anger — nothing is allowed to come in anymore, nothing is allowed to flow out anymore; tying yourself down, not flexibly being open toward Life.

You refuse to swallow anymore; you think too much has come toward you, that you now have to set the limit, and you spit out the excess as it were. "Stop," you say. And in this way you would spit out the baby with the bathwater. It's important to find a balance, on the one hand allowing things to come through from the outside world, in communication with others, and on the other hand to say "stop" (to an excess of something), in honesty with yourself. But still always opening yourself up to that which wants to let itself be known, coming from your deepest emotional source and inner center of truth: to that wind of life. Never say "no" to it. Allow it to come in from within yourself, those deep warm life-forces; allow it to become a blissful flow running through your living body, and enjoy it. Get in touch with yourself, warm and intimately merged, and don't say "no" to yourself, to that loving wind of life in yourself. Take yourself in completely into your body, and experience the relaxation of simple blissful being, as "I."

Things go wrong when you actually lock yourself up in a hard way, like a hard-boiled egg in its shell. Therefore, don't tie yourself down in fixed patterns, but break open and allow things to flow, allow yourself to live; allow life energies to flow through your complete being, don't paralyze any dynamics by holding on to things, by closing a door where life wants to come in and animate.

Don't feel frustrated; you are bursting with life forces; attune yourself to them. Don't clamp on to things or people in a feeling of inferiority, of doubt about your own ability or goodness; don't clamp on to "false values" because you deny your actual life value as "I."

Break through frustrations by allowing yourself to be who you are, the way you are, not thinking you have to "achieve, hold up an image, or satisfy . . . ." Come into loving, gentle communication with yourself and, as a result, also with others. Don't lock yourself up behind a frustrated shield of pent-up energies and immobilized feelings. Dare to be yourself, the way you are, the way you really feel it. Surrender . . . to Life, to the REAL self that you are. Be yourself from within; don't close yourself off in a rock-hard "manly" way, but open yourself completely in order to allow those "female" energies in your being. You are not at all silly or weak when you allow, let through, when you open yourself up in surrender to life in yourself. This is exactly your power; that this receptiveness, this allowing of energies to flow through in yourself, can go together with a fundamentally strong establishment upon your own foundations, a solid spine, your skeleton in balance. Allow, permit: not the unauthentic, not the false, not spurious values, but everything that represents "life."

This will give you blissful relaxation, a happy feeling.

Also read the text: *Blood, heart and blood vessels: psychological correspondence*

Adams-Stokes attack
sudden unconsciousness, caused by cardiac conduction defects (AV block) or arrhythmia

You have tried to overextend yourself and to embrace more than you can handle. You hold something in your grip, in your thoughts, which it would be better to let go of! Accumulation of emotions, nervous aggression, painful confusion of thoughts. Because you, in fact, feel powerless, you try to "seize" and hold on so that nothing (or no one?) will escape you. But what you are holding on to weighs so heavily that you can no longer carry it; you then no longer take external action. You finally retreat and let everything collapse in powerlessness.

Surrendering to your deepest intuitive self leads toward trust; don't try to oversee everything with your rational consciousness. This is a restricted way of life. Just get a grip on yourself. Wanting to maintain outward power indicates feelings of powerlessness. Your "I" is strong, mightily strong: don't disparage it. Radiate, radiate! Radiate outwardly from your deepest self instead of absorbing everything until you overflow. Letting go and self-trust, relaxation, discharging, and outwardly directed breakthrough.

Angina pectoris

You hold on to certain feelings or situations in such a way that you might explode! Your thoughts fixate on them. You perhaps want to hold two elements or people together (you and your friend?), which it might be better to let go. A relationship grows by itself: seizing or forcing is of no use. Let everyone freely be himself or herself: don't try to "change" anyone. On the contrary, let go; evolve yourself, liberate yourself inwardly. When you try to bring yourself into harmony and let go of all holds you have on others — and also let go of them in your thoughts — only then will you attract that which is good for you. Give freedom; you will liberate yourself through doing this. Or, you hope and think that "it" might still come to fulfillment: let go! In every respect, you carry a heavy load and don't quite know what direction to take, but you keep on holding on to everything. You fear that when you let your emotions flow freely, or when you let go of a person or a situation, then your life will be "lost," that you might fall into the abyss. You are for the most part silent about these deep feelings; you completely turn inward. Your heart can no longer relax and radiate freely, because you hurt your Self too much, and because you offer yourself insufficient attention and appreciation — no matter what others might give you.

Let go of everything and everyone: give, radiate, and don't accept anything in return. Offer real love to yourself and also to your relations — without expectations — and love will be given to you. Be faithful to yourself; speak, say what is in your heart. Free your emotions; express your feelings; work them out, and evolve. Enjoy your pure being! Lazily bask in your own sun-warmth. No one else can make you happy if you haven't first discovered the joy in yourself, joy because of yourself, thankfulness for life itself. Feel the earth beneath your feet, here and now, instead of projecting your thoughts ever further. Don't live in a dream castle; direct your eyes clearly to reality: in this case, the joy will stand or fall depending on whether or not you are content with yourself.

Arrhythmia, in general
abnormality of the rhythm of the heart

Unsure, indecisive, seeking in several directions at once.... Confused thoughts; you get many contradictory impressions: you are a slave of them, cannot handle them all. You

don't follow a straight line, don't take a clear stand. You cannot say farewell to something or someone even though the facts indicate you should let go and go on. You think and fret in a vicious circle because you don't have enough faith in your Self, in your intuition. You are stuck, as it were, with your head in something, in someone. You'd like to tear yourself loose, but your feeling of dependence and your lack of self-worth, the under-appreciation of yourself, cause you to suppress yourself: your feelings, your longings, your autonomous self-realization.

You cannot bet on two horses at the same time: first and foremost, you have to make choices that are for your own good and for the sake of your health. This dilemma — yourself or your surroundings? — is the consequence of unbalanced seeking for yourself. You want to do good for others, but also for yourself; you might do too much for others so that they would accept you, so that they would like you. Because of this, you are holding yourself back and don't live resolutely in *one* direction. You are being pulled in two directions; this tension is becoming too much for you.

It could equally as well be a dilemma of having to choose something involving your job, your relations — a nervous, insecure quest: yes/no/yes . . . jerking and jolting along.

Stay close to your feelings, your intuition, and don't fill your head with confused thoughts. Allow all emotions to flow freely, don't bottle them up, fret no longer, let go of that which causes inner collisions. Quietly take time for yourself; don't let yourself be rushed by others. Follow your true nature: trust this and go on your way, imperturbably, without paying heed to the opinions of others. Say farewell to certain views, or bring about changes in oppressive situations. First of all, achieve peaceful harmony in yourself and trust that your environment will be a reflection of this. Make a choice, determine your direction, and go on in a steady rhythm.

Heart attack

You don't really dare to show yourself as you are, for you consider yourself to be not good enough. You feel afraid, small, unsure, full of emotions and perhaps full of sadness, but you will not admit to this! You give the impression that you are harder, more stalwart, than you are. Lonely, in pain, but you will not let anyone enter your actual heart! For perhaps you want to keep up your pride, dignify your image as a strong man or woman. Or are you severe with yourself? Do gentleness and flexibility mean "weakness" to you?

Is it anxiety that prevents you from looking deeper, under the surface? Are you afraid that if you begin an honest confrontation with your feelings then you will totally drown in sorrow, in powerlessness? Are you anxiously keeping the lid shut? Why be so hard on yourself? Why this mask? Why this ostrich-like behavior? You take distance from your deepest Self, from your own warm heart, pushing away "the little one" within yourself. You don't want to know about any "weaknesses"; you push others away from you: "I don't need anyone; I can handle this." You sometimes take a sharp attitude toward others in order to keep anyone from entering into you. A self-protecting attitude, with which you hinder others from working themselves in. This can be a reaction to having repeatedly been hurt: "You won't get me anymore." This hard attitude has a destructive, even lethal effect. Realize here that it was the original self-rejection which attracted painful circumstances in life. The only solution is to resolve this basic cause: by true gentleness, by love for oneself, by becoming aware of one's self-worth.

You act as if nothing is the matter; you constantly direct the spotlight away from yourself. You think, perhaps, you will find respect and appreciation this way, for after all you don't appreciate yourself enough. You blind yourself and everyone else. There is no question anymore of joy coming from the depths of your heart: at most, only superficial happiness. You want to prove yourself; you cross a boundary — in your job, in a certain task, in an ideal for which you fight. You live too much in your head, in your thoughts; you don't really live in harmony with your nature, with your body, and with your heart, which asks for gentle attention to yourself.

Be yourself, in all honesty: "Now that is me." Drill down to the deepest well of your soul: look at the neglected sorrow there; allow your small aspects — your gentle feelings — to exist freely. No longer force things. Be loving toward yourself; totally open yourself up to self-searching and don't anxiously keep everything closed. Totally stretch out your soul in relaxation; dare to feel the joy of your existence and put no harsh requirements on yourself! If you simply dare to be yourself, without camouflage, and realize that you don't have to answer to a certain "image," a burden will fall from your heart. This can only happen if you now contentedly accept yourself the way you really are. Spontaneous joy, security in the depth of your Self.

Congenital heart disease

One does not realize the importance of, the use of, taking earthly life seriously. One prefers to joyfully dance and prance into life, though only superficially; one does not realize the depth of oneself nor the true value of life on earth. Limited to pleasure, to agreeable fairy-tale fantasies, to games and teasing, one does not reach the essence of Life nor the core of oneself. This psychological game seems to signify fleeing: it is playing hide-and-seek with oneself, with life; the playful child thinks, "Ah, that's not for me — I can't do it. I can just as well go back to where I came from."

He doesn't realize how, through experience in earthly life, he can reach awareness, intense joy, real growth and evolution. He is not aware of his depth, of his richness, nor of the richness of life on earth. The undervaluing of life, with a laugh of mockery sometimes, is a pathetic escape. One is afraid to look deeper; one does not find oneself; one clings to the surface; one twitters and chatters along; one bypasses one's values, one's gold. An *escape* from oneself. It is necessary that such people truly let themselves be born, that they intensely become part of earthly life, that a baby joyfully experiences its first steps, that it can feel present, here and now, through concrete contact with its surroundings. Experiencing the rich beauty of life, knowing that it is enjoyable to proceed onward into life itself and that one should not flee into a fairy tale sphere, into a superficial world, into a spiritual dream realm by which one will lose contact with the earth. Discovery of and appreciation of oneself. Feeling, intense sensual contact, discovering oneself as a physical and earthly being. Feet on the ground; discovering the sun, the wind, the sand, the rain. Enjoying a cookie, milk. Honest, open, profound contact with oneself, with one's parents; love and the realization of one's "I"-center, of one's powers. Coming to AWARENESS!

Such people are being born in order to cast off an incorrect conviction regarding life on earth; they very much underestimate their creative possibilities as earthly beings. They *play* with life: returning, or staying here on earth? One may point out to them the Value of Earthly life, the profundity in themselves.

Heart, enlarged, hypertrophy

In panic and anxiety, small and lost, you look further and further outside yourself for something to hold on to. You feel alone in the desert; it becomes wider and wider; you run away, further and further, from yourself: because of this, you don't get a grip on anything. You don't feel safe in yourself, not safe in whatever structure; you are search-

ing. . . . It is all so far away from you — this is, of course, because you refuse to acknowledge the fundamental, strong, trustworthy Basis-essence deep within yourself. You ignore your worth, your power, your divine self: you place all authority outside yourself. Come quietly to self-introspection: here lies your safety, your wisdom, the power over your life. Self-construct your life on this basis; don't let yourself "be lived"; don't float around; no longer seek outside yourself. Offer yourself gentleness and appreciation; in this way, you will attract pleasant situations into your life and will do so without having to "search" for them. Self-trust! Perhaps you try too much to grasp hold of others, using "power"; let go and grasp hold of yourself. Quietly realize yourself.

Heart failure

You don't believe enough in yourself: you doubt whether you can solve your problems, especially emotional ones (which are often the result of a primal trauma). You bring yourself into question: "Who am I now? Good or bad?" You hold yourself back, offering resistance to your most beautiful feelings. You carry on too stiffly, too tensely, too forcedly; your emotional flow is being blocked, and perhaps you have the impression that from the outside you are being held back, that you cannot go in the direction you wish to because if you did you would be stopped by "circumstances." But it is you who tie yourself down. Because you don't make yourself master over your nature, because you don't trust your nature, you don't feel able to go straight ahead. You deviate from your straight path: seeking something to hold on to, you are looking to people and things outside yourself, such as to your partner, your Image, your function at work, your accomplishments, possessions, etc. — you refuse to live from your heart, from what you truly Feel. You doubt the powers of life itself, thinking and brooding too much about worrisome things, about death and illness.

You are too hard on yourself. Despite the emotional burdens you carry, you will keep standing up straight and stiff for the sake of outer appearances, possibly not letting anyone notice anything. You present yourself as more stalwart than you inwardly feel. You don't feel completely good inside yourself, in your body; you look at life through glasses that are too dark because you don't believe in Life, because you don't see how you are the creator of your life. You withhold your spontaneity; you retain and hold on too much to things and people, out of fear of losing control over yourself.

You stand before an obstacle, and it seems as if you can't get over it: you refuse to let go of that which is not good for you, holding on in such a way that you feel confronted again and again with an unsolvable problem. You don't flexibly go along with your nature, with your longings; on the contrary, you think you have to fight against yourself, against life. Possibly, you care much for others, are always busy with others, or you fill up your life with your partner: instead of, firstly, filling it with yourself. Your Awareness is too absent from your body. You accumulate so much emotion and thoughts that your life can seem a nightmare.

In love, come to yourself!

Listen to your nature, to your intuition, to what you feel; don't force yourself any longer. Spontaneously be yourself; honestly show your feelings. You are master of your earthly existence: no longer look through dark glasses, but open yourself up to joy in your existence. In love, come to yourself; don't condemn yourself because of your inner nature or outer appearance. Just be faithful to your nature; a free, spontaneous flow of movement, without holding back, without tensely closing yourself. You are in the Center of your existence: put all Authority in yourself; make an end to all idols. Don't be afraid of emotions, but let them flow freely. Come to insight, work it out, and let go! Be convinced that you can solve

every fundamental trauma, every emotional problem, by looking at — among other things — the convictions you were born with regarding yourself, and by turning them all in a positive direction. You are strong, your heart is strong: as long as you believe it and don't block your emotional currents!

Myocarditis
inflammation of the heart muscle

Powerlessness and anger: you feel stuck, tied down, locked up; your head is spinning with thoughts that are trying to get a "grip" on.... Instead, you feel "gripped," like a martyr; inwardly you make a fist, but your thoughts stubbornly hold on to an idea, a person, the past. Your head is being driven by the motor of Anxiety: you don't dare go on, don't dare liberate yourself. All these are needless burdens, mostly created in your Thoughts: your mind dominates your emotional life and hinders higher consciousness-energy from coming through. You are, after all, angry with yourself because you don't dare let your "I" come through! You are sad because of your own powerlessness.

Be aware of your worth now; respect the spontaneous, joyful child in you and at last let your feelings flow freely. Say what you have to say; dare to handle your active powers with mastery; don't doubt yourself; allow healthy, aggressive creating energies to come through freely — let it all go; allow love and joy into your life. Place in yourself the power over your existence; don't cling to the mental, surrender to your intuition, to your feelings....

Heart pain

Holding on, you clutch to a person, a system, something that oppresses your existence, but you refuse to let go of it. In fact, this dependency destroys you: finally let go and free yourself! Because you lay your values aside and refuse to wear the crown of human divinity, you want to cling to something else — outside yourself. In this way, you smother yourself. . . . You pull things toward yourself instead of giving to yourself, giving to others. You might force things, absolutely wanting to take hold of a certain range of ideas, of a relationship, instead of going onward yourself: but you are full of sadness and uncertainties, not daring to trust your own Essence. You feel anxiety because you refuse contact with your own deepest soul, are afraid of death. In this state of insecurity, nervous tension is sometimes driven to the limit; you are on guard, easily startled, on edge, sometimes aggressive.

Nevertheless, you'd like to throw yourself open to a broad feeling of space and time, without limitations — you'd like to experience relationships with others in a warm and intense way, but this is not yet possible because you first must come close to yourself. Two royal children can come together only when they don't cling to each other out of necessity, but — as two autonomous beings — make a gentle, free choice, each being aware of his or her worth, and experiencing the joy of life and love within himself or herself.

Thus, place the center in yourself; live resolutely, going in your own direction, and in this be faithful to your nature. Let go of everything and go on! Don't hold yourself back by again and again reaching back. . . . Active energies want to come through: no longer direct them inward in a self-destructive way, but transform them into Joy and Creativity! Put on your crown, realize your worth, take up all your space — without asking yourself again and again, "What impression do I make? What will others . . .?" Don't fight against the truth, which you can find inside yourself. Then, out of love for yourself, and in honesty to others, go straight ahead. Fully enjoy life, here and now; don't tie yourself down. Love of yourself liberates you from all anxieties and brings you closer

to others. Let go of the sorrow from the past; create a happy future yourself now: with self-awareness, take the rudder in hand.

Heart palpitations: extrasystoles
Your heart skips.

Your legs, *tired* and walked on until they are bowed, as it were, dead-tired. You finally don't know anymore how far you have gone, *for how long you have been persevering in this direction* (literally or figuratively), but one thing is definite: it has been going on for a long time! But you keep on going on and on and on, so that that your legs might take on an O shape. You probably think *it all HAS TO BE that way,* just like the long distance runner or jogger who is totally convinced that this or that distance *must* be covered: *that it is supposed to be that way,* or for the sake of fitness, and in the meantime one doesn't realize that one causes oneself to grow older and shrink instead of becoming healthier, but one is convinced that it *is* okay, no matter how much effort it costs! Life itself doesn't ask for this. Why such fixed, crazy ideas? Why still live according to "oppressive laws" without questioning them? *Use YOUR INDIVIDUALITY, your highly unique thinking Ability, in order to place it all in question . . . and to see where you constantly FORCE, EXHAUST, push yourself, where you do things that are hard for you, where you absolutely keep it up and don't even question: "Is this LIFE; is this really good for me?" Then stand still . . . and think about this. See how you have allowed yourself to keep on walking in a tense way for too long, have acted or thought strenuously in this or that direction, in this or that hard way.* Now take away those blinders. Stop "following," doing what's "supposed to be done," what others, or society, norms, and rules tell you to do because it's good for you — FOLLOW YOUR HIGHLY UNIQUE PATH in a loving, but truly creative way.

After all you are not a monkey, not an imitator, not an idiot who runs in circles or does this or that every night because "someone" says that's how it's supposed to be . . . that's how it has to be . . . as if YOU are not allowed to exist as YOU! As if life asks you for strong efforts!

Time to change the rudder: you live from your inner Feeling, from your heart. It's okay for you to work and make efforts, build up thoughts, but as long as they don't hurt you, as long as they are not "pushed on you" by doctrines, habits, social norms or whatever. You do take responsibility for your existence, but you now begin to live from out of your creative "I"-thinking and your supervising brain!

Stop walking on in this way. Reconsider everything. Look at *where* you just do and follow what the rules and others and society have told you to do: realize then that LIFE doesn't ask that from you. *IN-DEPTH UNDERSTANDING is being asked; possibly seeing through certain indoctrinations which give importance to things of no importance.* Find a new source inside yourself and ask yourself what's GOOD for YOU personally.

An *example:* don't live automatically or think that sport is healthy because everyone says so; the same with dietetics. Eat what you are in the mood for, and know why you need this or that food product and why your body enjoys it, no matter if it's chocolate or pears. Know that nothing is unhealthy if the signal comes from out of your deepest self, from your soul-center upwards, and tells you to take this or that. But at the same time understand the cause of your liking this or that food product, and work at it. Don't make yourself believe that sport is necessary, that dieting is necessary. . . .[4] A human being is HEALTHY when he JOYFULLY experiences his own nature and eats what he likes and does what he feels he has to do, from out of his deepest self — not because it "has to be that way" or because that's "the way it's done."

BE . . . BECOME who you *really* are! Also regarding the exterior: don't allow yourself to be fooled into believing that skinny muscles are healthy, and fat might be unhealthy, that you have to be slim, and being heavy might be bad or unhealthy. FEEL what is good and healthy for you, and also see through the cult of the exterior: true beauty lies in the extension of truth, not in someone who creates a body made to manipulate with power, emptied inside and filling himself with things and/or people from the outside.

No longer ACHIEVE on any level, but just be yourself: live according to the truth, from your heart, in goodness, and *SEE THROUGH* things, look for *the ESSENCE,* for *the CONTENT* of life, no longer FORCING yourself in order to GET, *to want TO HAVE* this or that. *Let go! Arrive at the vibration of BEING instead of HAVING!* And this "having" doesn't have anything to do with material things (although this is also possible), but it can be about *"wanting to have a certain situation" that is not there (yet)* . . . and you WANT this to come to be! *LET GO! Don't force anything; and trust. Experience the joy of your "Being."*

Stop making it so hard for yourself, stop also FILLING yourself with the things you think to be IMPORTANT but which in fact in the view of Life itself are of no importance. Listen to that gentle but resolute voice of your inner heart and follow only that path. Don't live on the SURFACE, on the outside of your being, but live and act from out of your deepest source, according to what you feel deep inside. *It's necessary to look THROUGH things,* to realize thoroughly that everything has a reason. *DON'T JUST KEEP ON WALKING ON AND ON without coming to the realization of the fact that there lies something MUCH deeper under the surface and false layers* — search for that information of truth. This can be done by no longer thoughtlessly doing things the way you used to, by no longer keeping on going

---

[4] Read more about this subject in *The Horn of Plenty.*

in a direction you used to think you were supposed to go in. Now listen to your inner ear. WHAT does your heart really want? *What* does life ask? No longer make yourself so tense. No longer fill yourself with things, but EXPERIENCE YOURSELF in your own fullness; enjoy your being. Don't just be occupied with your work, or with just what you do or achieve, but *connect yourself with your INNER EMOTIONAL CORE, with your heart, and FEEL how it calls for a "stop," NOT KEEPING ON RUNNING the way you are at the moment . . . in thoughts and meditations or in deeds.*

Return to your deepest source, turn deeply inward, be good and gentle with yourself. Stop "filling" yourself, and now fulfill yourself completely with the love that will flow through your total being. *For a while stop living, thinking, working, organizing at the Surface . . . and listen to the deep, wonderful voice of your Feelings, of your heart.* No longer tire yourself; don't exhaust yourself in thoughts and deeds. No longer keep on walking on that way — but in a very loving way reflect on yourself and dig deeply for the ESSENCE of life, of yourself. You no longer live out of your *Head,* out of *Obligation,* but out of your total being, out of what you feel in your middle, out of your warm navel region, where life begins. You live out of your feelings, out of love, and you fill yourself with new life-energy — resting a bit — no longer running on the way you used to. Stay very close to yourself, to this heart of yours; *no longer concentrate on the outside of things, people, matter; nor linger by outer factors and material details.* But *essentially* turn toward that which will nourish you, and in such a way that instead of shrinking, wasting away and degenerating, you will constantly regenerate yourself: now you lovingly FEED your body. A warm glow, an energy full of love, flows through your entire body. Your cells continuously renew themselves. You warm and feed yourself. You no longer run past yourself. The life energy

comes from within . . . and you feel that now, and you now open yourself up to it. *You stop for a moment of reflection about yourself and don't rush yourself with your head, with indoctrinations, duties, norms, thoughts. . . . No, you now continuously STAY close to your heart; your thoughts/mind/spirit are not separate from your body. Your heart-energy now feeds every fiber of your body: doing good, giving rest; warming and giving health.* You feel yourself growing in this inner power and rest. Steadily, you do your tasks in life, no longer taking leave of your "I," your heart, your body. You are *One* — in the alliance with yourself, according to heart, soul, and body. You no longer skip yourself, the Essence of yourself . . . you no longer run along till you fall down exhausted. You live according to your inner being, and every chilly distancing from your body, your heart, your feelings, has disappeared.

You don't live in the tower of your thinking, but very intensely and connected with mother earth. *A delightful coziness in matter; very close to your inner "I," and never again will work, thoughts, details, the superficialities, etc., get the upper hand. You are gentle and full of love, one in unification with yourself, according to heart and soul.* You take the time to reflect on yourself. Whenever you do something, no matter what, you no longer "separate" yourself from yourself, you no longer just run on. You don't do ANYTHING — with your head, your thoughts, or just out of habit — without your HEART and your BODY being involved with it! *Only in this way will you FEEL when you are running away from Life, or whether you stay present in your Heart, your body, your total being while doing or thinking. You no longer skip the essence of yourself, of life . . . and your heart doesn't skip anymore either.*

YOU ARE . . . NOW. You no longer RUN just anywhere in the desire to obtain something or get somewhere — whether it has to do with insisting on finishing a work or reaching a finish line or running the kilometers "someone" tells you is healthy. You no longer want to get "somewhere," no longer want to "endure," from your head, from your programmed *fixed ideas,* from your acquired convictions, because this destroys life. *You no longer insist on getting something "done," fixated in your head in a hard way: you let go and you arrive now at the essence of yourself, in love and mildness.* You now question everything and arrive at your true Heart: you learn to feel what life asks of YOU. Nothing is a "must".... Except "listening to this essential feeling of life," listening to your heart, to what your heart tells you is good for you.

Don't dwell on unimportant external factors or details. Live according to the essence . . . and Be who you ARE; remain always present with this BEING and don't "force" yourself into anything. Goodness and love count — not achieving, shining or responding to false ideals. Live and experience yourself in love, from the Core of your "I." Don't demand things from yourself . . . but LIVE out of the joy of your total, unified essence. Come into deep contact with your heart, your body, your content of treasures. *You no longer force anything; you no longer want to obtain anything; therefore, you no longer get angry, in impatience or nervousness. You live out of goodness, in thankfulness for your being, looking at the Content, the Essence of things, people, life.*

Heart valve, problems

Prolapse

A feeling of powerlessness and aggression: you cannot free yourself from your sadness, from a situation which is suffocating you. You want to escape. . . . You have accumulated and held on to a sea of emotions: your life is being dominated by irritation and annoyance with yourself because you don't feel able, with your Conscious "I," to get a grip on your life, on your feelings. It is beyond you, and you refuse to let go, until things burst.

*When it comes to prevention, it is necessary to allow those burdensome emotions to come through freely, to work them out and leave them **behind**. Resolve, with self-aware power: "Now it has been enough!" Cut it off, go on, let it drop: your heart calls for gentleness and joy. Don't flee from life, break with self-destructive habits!*

Regurgitation (fails to close completely)

You are emotionally at rock-bottom, but you will not let others sense how heavily everything weighs upon you. . . . You force yourself, exert yourself to the limit, in order to still be able to "keep up," until you finally collapse and refuse to paddle on in this way any longer; you feel wrung out. It is all the same to you now; you are dead-tired of fighting. You feel empty. You no longer participate! Stop! You anchor yourself. Because burdens and sorrow are becoming too heavy, you don't want to go on anymore. You feel vacant, apathetic, no longer caring about anything. . . . This ailment calls for self-liberation, for joy and open space for yourself.

Stenosis — narrowing (opens too little)

You aren't doing what you want to do in life: you don't dare to Live to the fullest; you feel time going by, and you are already thinking about Death. You don't dare to let your feelings go; you protect yourself against. . . . You wrap yourself up, you tie yourself down, constantly putting limitations on yourself. You would, however, like to live and play spontaneously, like a child. But with an aggressive thought-pattern you put a damper on yourself. You are anxious, feeling threatened by others, by your emotions, by death or a devil. You are afraid, as if you might collapse or go up in flames.

Don't doubt your deepest Self; don't destroy yourself with unrealistic dark thoughts. Push out all your feelings, let them flow, and don't hinder yourself from Living. Open your feelings and thoughts to an optimistic horizon, to a life you can create yourself. Don't fool yourself with the thought that a "destiny" determines your life. Fatalism is foolish. Don't underestimate your possibilities any longer; surrender, without fear, to yourself, to your feelings, to your longings.

FEAR OF HEIGHTS

Fear of forces over which you don't have control; fear of pain, because you feel vulnerable. A shyness, a mistrust, a fear of being dragged along into anonymity. You don't believe that your deepest Self doesn't call up negative things if you don't wish it to. Afraid of "evil." Insufficient grounding; fantasy sometimes surpasses reality; in thought too much, in your body too little, with feet off the ground. You often escape in daydreams with your thoughts; you don't live enough in the here-and-now. It's necessary to use your common sense and to unmask the so-called threat or evil. Laugh about it. With your Conscious thinking capacity look at the relativity of it all. Make a distinction between fairy tales and reality. Follow your inner, wise advise.

Trust that you determine your own Life, without any question of a negative happening if you have not first longed for it or called it up.

HICCUPS
exaggerated

There's something that is beyond you; you don't have an immediate grip on it. This can have to do with a certain fact, a happening, or the words of an Authority above you (you feel yourself being pulled up by the hair by a master).

Possibly, you step back too much to make room for someone else, for an authority outside you.

Possibly, you can't completely grasp what you've seen; you are shocked; maybe it splits you in two.

There's something you can't comprehend or assimilate right away. You are startled; your structure seems to be temporarily absent. Where is your solid backbone? Hold on to that which belongs to you, and calmly open yourself up to that which is new, to others. You are not defenseless; take good care of yourself. Calmly assimilate. . . .

Are you afraid of something bigger than yourself, something you can't handle right away? Are you afraid of falling? Nothing has more power over you than you have over yourself: grow open and "rise" on your own. In this way you'll no longer have the feeling that others, or a situation, or a Something, are "beyond" you. Indeed, in this way the hiccups can be considered a symbol of "growth": small moments of crisis that one must rise above, again and again, on the path to more authority of your own, and toward a new stage!

HIPS

Psychological correspondence

They represent not only *the supporting power* of your being — preferably *in balance* — but at the same time, they represent the structure, the solid lines you set up, after which you *choose one* well-determined direction, in a resolute and self-aware way. Calmly standing still, considering yourself, in order to finally go onward with *Power* and Flexibility, without hesitation.

Here, the following problem is often being experienced: do I live from out of myself or for the sake of the eye of other people? This duality causes an imbalance.

Two safe points; within this structure, an enormous energy flows in a certain direction. Letting yourself go, without anxieties, in that direction in Life which you, yourself, have indicated. Going on, in balance, on the path of evolution.

Ailments, in general

In imbalance: you don't know what decision to make; you hesitate. A confrontation with at least two possibilities in which false motives can play a role.

Are you allowing yourself to be guided by motives such as "image," sex, compulsive urges — instead of determining your life in a self-aware way?

Duality: am I allowed to choose this path for my happiness, or shall I sacrifice myself for others? Or, do Anxieties hinder you from choosing your path? Why don't you dare go on? Love doesn't know any sacrifice: first, cherish yourself. You don't take action; your energies are being held back; you are twiddling your thumbs instead of truly *living* and coming into action.

Inwardly, you are filled to the top with energies, but you just think and fret; perhaps you constantly make yourself angry; you feel imprisoned. *"Doing!"* is the solution.

After all, frustration leads to aggression: free yourself from this. Do you force yourself by putting up structures that are too restrictive, too disciplined? Perhaps because of the urge for achievement or because you are being a "severe father" to yourself? Do you correct yourself in a harsh way? Break out of this and allow your spontaneous energies to flow freely. Or, conversely, do you not keep yourself to any structure? Do you not see any path? Do you have no ideal or goal to live toward?

Perhaps you refuse to go on: and one "I" says to go here, the other to go there — you

withdraw into yourself. You are standing still, without evolution! The basic structure of your Life comes out of your deepest Self: Don't stick any artificial, purely rational framework onto your life, but take your feelings into account.

Does it all weigh too heavily on you? Can you not decide?

Cut through the Gordian knot; trust your intuition and be faithful to your specific nature! Straight as an arrow, going that one Living Direction!

Arthritis of the hip joint
coxitis

You are sitting inside armor plating: you don't give yourself much room to move, but you are of the opinion that this feeling of "being stuck" has nothing to do with your psyche; you blame it all on others or on Destiny; you think you are a victim, including being a victim of illness. Afraid and shivering, you withdraw into yourself.

Like a lemon in a wheelbarrow, you allow yourself to be transported, dissatisfied and fatalistic.

You feel suffocated, seized by the neck, as it were; you can't go one way or the other; you experience anxiety, coldness, and darkness; you experience "cold" inside yourself.

You live too much toward others, toward the norms of society — mechanically, as it were — and live too little from out of the spontaneous longings inside yourself. You bind yourself up so tightly! You don't see any other future than the one that leads to death.

Powerless anger. Disillusioned and reproachful if others don't give you what you expect from them.

Don't be estranged from your longings, from your warm feelings, from love: offer yourself life, give yourself what you deserve, and warm yourself; don't expect from others that which you keep from yourself!

Dare to be completely who you are, and don't put yourself into armor. Listen in supple versatility to your nature, to your wishes: let yourself go, no longer blocking spontaneous energies. Determine, in a self-assured way, your life's path. Firmly seize the oars and go in one well-determined direction, which you and no one else indicates. Don't let yourself be diverted by others: go on, and allow pent-up energies to come free in action and creativity.

Enjoy your body, the nature around you, the things you like to do. No longer limit yourself; don't allow yourself to be limited. Throw away your crutches and Live!

Degeneration, decalcification, of the hip joint

Productive earthly powers are being suppressed. It is hard for you to embrace life, your emotions. You hinder your evolution by not building upon the wisdom of your inner self. You don't truly live from out of yourself. Possibly, you read a lot or listen to the "knowledge" of others, or you are content with the spiritual adoration of one religion or another outside yourself, or possibly you feel like you are the king in the land of the blind: all signs that you don't build your life on the basis of your Self, that you "immobilize" yourself in untrue or worthless systems, that you build your life on dogmatic or intellectual knowledge instead of on inner wisdom and the joy of life itself.

You don't take up your space; you pare down your existence; you suppress the most beautiful personal energies in yourself. Do you feel threatened? You hide yourself; you don't allow your true "I" to be born; you're afraid of those deep powers, of emotions in yourself. Still, you feel more and more like one who is being hanged, a prisoner of yourself. Possibly, you direct your life solely toward others: thusly, not to have to *become* yourself. Spiritual energies by far dominate the earthly concentration. Sometimes it all

becomes too much for you. You feel unable to be master of your existence; you are convinced that you have to "hide" yourself instead of realizing yourself. You establish yourself on the mountain of the past, without daring to make one step toward true evolution. You aren't working out the past; you're not opening a space for the future.

Going on, productivity, self-realization, a strong concentration of energies in your body; you are protected in the safe basis of your living Self; everyone at his own tempo: calm, powerful, self-assuredly going on in the direction which you, yourself, determine. Toward life, not toward dematerialization.

HODGKIN'S DISEASE

The absence of one's own Authority; one isn't really motivated to live from out of one's own goals and longings. On the contrary, one tries, left and right, to do good for others. One's own will remains absent: one is too obedient, too docile, not assertive enough, not yet truly born in oneself!

One tries to find oneself in achieving, or in doing good for others; one thinks to find love in "giving" to others, but this has nothing to do with love. . . . One doesn't find oneself; one searches desperately, hopelessly, without getting a grip on oneself.

One would "dress" in all kinds of guises, would present oneself in different roles, because out of fear one doesn't dare to feel one's own roots. "Who am I?" Changing like a chameleon — all authority is given up to the surroundings.

The origin of this life-attitude lies in doubting one's own Worth and in the fear of the powerful eye outside you, fear of others, of extermination by those who look at you: you feel so powerless. Because of all that you will do anything not to be destroyed, but to be accepted. So you no longer at all live according to your personal longings — you fly all over the place to be helpful to others. Do you think yourself so bad and untrustworthy? Your life, your emotions, your sadness, and your anxieties have been too heavy for you, convinced as you are that you are "weak": that's why you collapsed, that's why you pull the noose around your neck. In this way you remain just at the surface of life, possibly as the Santa Claus for the whole family.

Take the reins in hands yourself, fearlessly, and build your life on your own authority. Play the main character yourself in your own life! Action from out of yourself, not to please others. Come close to your emotional essence and love yourself the way you are: others will truly love you if you love yourself. No longer push yourself away. You aren't bad; you didn't do anything wrong — these are misleading convictions. It's only about a shortage of insight, about evolution. Don't fool yourself; begin to discover things deep inside you: search for your values, your talents, your wealth of feelings, and dare to exchange them honestly with others.

No longer run away from your Core, your Living Self, and no longer live for others, but first of all for yourself! Offer yourself life and joy. Straight ahead and unified; resolutely determine your direction, your point of view, your goal. Now bring yourself to realization.

HUNTINGTON'S DISEASE

hereditary, degenerative brain disorder with jerky involuntary movements ("chorea") and behavioral disturbances

A longing that can't be fulfilled — you feel so empty, so emotionally lonely; you aren't sure who you are, you look for yourself in an insecure way; you might greedily throw yourself upon things, people, all kinds of sources, in order to swallow up everything, to load yourself up with tons, with masses — desperate, distraught, because you can't reach yourself, because you are directed too much toward the outside instead of toward your deepest Source. You try to cling emotionally to relationships. You might drown yourself in a relationship because of exaggerated identification, which results in your filling yourself up with the other person. But it makes you desperate that this other person is only partly accessible to you, hidden, as it were, by a hazy mist. You want to get closer; you want your partner to come closer emotionally — but this isn't possible. Outwardly, you'll try to compensate for these feelings of empty powerlessness: perhaps in a formal attitude, or in beautiful clothing, or in a stiff role: if these things fall away, then you hardly feel yourself, so you cling to these outer structures. You expect very much of others, in proportion to that which you withhold from yourself. You ignore your content; you swim at the surface: therefore you will attract partners and friends who don't satisfy your longings. You want more and more — it's never enough. Finally, you become angry and resentful because others don't give you what you long for, because they behave completely differently from the way you wish them to. You might behave like a parasite because you deny your own roots. You try to get more of a grip on others instead of on yourself; you will direct things — until you get a scare from your deep, unconscious emotions, which all of a sudden make themselves known in an intense, nervous language! Your bladder also can suddenly release, because your deepest Self says, "Just let go, just let go!"

This language asks you to turn deeply inward, to bend your grasp for power toward a search for your Self. No longer exert yourself like this, trying to bend others to your longings. Become aware that the deepest cause lies in your powerlessness, your self-

negation. Anchor deep inside yourself: only there lies all hope. Free yourself of self-destroying emotions and no longer shun yourself. Give others freedom, and in that way free yourself. The true pillar of your life is not to be found in your partner or neighbor, but in your Self-awareness, an inner Power that you thus far have ignored. Free yourself from everything which in the past you've tried to hold on to, and make an end to it; say goodbye to the past. Open your hands now and give, in Love, to yourself, to others, without expectations. That which is good for you will then automatically come to you. Now calmly relax in yourself and take time to observe the little things in life; respect all this, treat things with gentleness: this is only possible if you first dare to stand still and observe yourself with respect, no longer fleeing, no longer greedy. A strong grounding — a balance between spirit and body — is necessary: now give concrete form to a powerful Human presence, instead of remaining in the mist like a vague shadow any longer. Establish yourself more strongly, independent of others, in earthly "matter," not in "spirit," because after all it was this Neptunian absence which made you grasp for exaggerated "earthly" compensation. Feel with your senses, here-and-now; put down roots in the earth, descend totally into your body. Get a good grip on yourself.

HYDROCEPHALUS
"water on the brain"

You are wearing a big hat, so to speak, to protect yourself, and you don't dare come out from under it.

You come into this earthly life with emotional burdens, anxieties, heart pains, feelings of guilt and shame, with a mountain of sad memories.

You'd prefer to keep dreaming in a fairy-tale world; you don't really dare look at reality.

Sadness of the heart fills your head: you are so afraid of your own feelings and of your strong intuition; you consider "Feelings" in a negative way. The harder you try to run away from them, however, the harder they will pursue you. It totally fills your head. You don't believe in your mastery over yourself: you feel afraid and not self-assured. Inner conflict in your emotional world: you don't really know which path to take now, do you? Back again to where you came from, *away* from the earthly spheres — or will you go on, after all, with your feet seeking for solid ground?

This physical situation is unconsciously being called up in order to come to complete acknowledgement of your rich emotional world, of your inner wisdom, which reaches beyond rational knowledge. So that now you will find self-assurance in your deepest Self; so that in yourself you will acknowledge the moon fully as a silver valuable, the emotional treasure.

Feelings and intuitive experiences are positive, not negative! Don't be so afraid of those deep sources in yourself: break with the past.

Clean out the sadness and the anxious experiences from the past, and now create your future in a well-aimed way. Acknowledge your worth, the Authority in yourself; don't hide your feelings behind an Image or under a big "hat." You may blindly trust your intuition; experience those radiant, beautiful emotional powers in yourself, and no longer run away from them. You have come here on earth not to develop a narrow rationality, but to finally offer yourself full space for your feelings in confrontation with the earth, with people. The salt of the earth lives, it is good; integrate it into yourself. Develop all your intuitive gifts; allow energies of consciousness to flow through freely.

No longer let your life be a flood of anxieties and sadness: don't pile things up; let everything go, and direct yourself, in self-confidence, toward Joy. Free yourself of fears!

Parents of children with Hydrocephalus sometimes need to solve similar problems in themselves: feel safe and protected in your Self; don't suppress any emotions; give all the space to intuition, feelings, and creativity; don't lock yourself up in a superficial, or one-sided, intellectual life; acknowledge that inner Worth of your Self, and allow transformation.

HYPERVENTILATION

Unsure; not knowing very well which direction to take; you doubt, but instead of listening to your inner voice, you open your ears to others. You run away from your Self! Shy, inwardly in conflict. "Shall I break with it or not?" You unconsciously refuse a solution: you hold back your evolution. You keep a tight hold on yourself; in fact, there's an abuse of power over yourself. You run away fast from the true solution — unconsciously, you prefer to remain in a position of so-called "powerlessness" instead of forcefully taking your life in your own hands and carrying all responsibilities! The fear of doing this paralyzes you. An anxious resistance to evolution, to a change for the better. A resistance to looking DEEP inside yourself for the solution; you are walking on tiptoe, anxious about your Self, tense and agitated, clinging to the surface.

"No!" A refusal, angry, closed-off. You don't want to go on this way. Hard and coercive, you hold yourself back. A stop. It's been enough now. You don't want to talk about it anymore; you would prefer to withdraw inside yourself, "alone." You close your ears, as it were; you close yourself off.

You have made your decision and no one can do anything about it anymore. You are no longer open to changes, to something new. "That's the limit," you say, and you close the door. They are allowed to come in, but they have to be silent. This attitude is because for too long you have made yourself dependent on others, on the outside world, and have much too little been "yourself" from within. An unconscious longing to step out of this prison-structure, but your first reaction can be one of anger toward the outside world. Know that the cause lies deep inside you. Now bring yourself one step further!

Blindness, not wanting to listen to that which is more elevated; hardness and willfulness. With this you only bring your evolution down. But hyperventilation now points out to you that the time has come to change direction.

You pull yourself down, and you close your ears completely to the new insights and information life wants to offer you. Because you are not "stuck": you only block yourself by not taking the steps you should take for your liberation!

A deep, suppressed fury/frustration can be present: because of feeling powerless to live on like this, powerless to liberate yourself completely from an old, established pattern in which you are not able to be "YOU." You might act as if it's all good for you (the smiling role you possibly play), but inwardly you are past the boiling point; a nervous kind of irony overpowers you. One more step and you will swipe all the glasses from the table. You can't and won't any more. For you it is finished!

Unconsciously, you want to start searching for your "true life," for your "self," for a life that completely connects with who you *really* are. Breaking with "play-acting," with a kind of showy behavior that you keep up, or "this is how I have to be/act toward others," an attitude, habits, in which you weren't yourself. Now masks fall off and you want to emerge, but you still suppress your forces: in a destructive way you direct them inwardly. You have the feeling of being suffocated by them. *Till — you make that step, let go, throw off your mask, become completely "yourself," allow all the forces to flow outward, your real feelings, no longer assuming an attitude, no longer play-acting. . . .*

Powerful energies, feelings, and creativity ask for a breakthrough: allow them to come through. Your safety lies deep inside yourself, not at the surface. Exhale calmly and deeply while you drain away your anxieties into the earth under your feet.

From out of your deepest Self — your basis of trust, which never leaves you as long as you dare to depend upon it — you then again calmly inhale powerful energies, which enable you to take your life resolutely in your own hands and to direct it in that way which is best for you. No longer allow yourself to "be lived," but choose, produce, enjoy — full of trust.

Go on and make the necessary adjustments, changes. No longer put yourself into a pressure cooker; lift the lid; don't be afraid of the freedom.

Transformation!

Make peace with yourself; live in honesty with yourself. Know and see how you have played a part, how you have placed a mask in front of your REAL self, have kept yourself hidden in a situation — behind a partner or who/whatever. Now you break through! Know now how you TRULY can be yourself and don't have to agree with an "attitude" or make compromises, showing yourself only partly, with your true "I" hidden behind a screen. Disarm yourself, unmask yourself. Come to peace; live in truth out of your deepest content, the core of your "I." Give to yourself and give to others, without lying to yourself, without going beyond a border there, where you hurt yourself, and have to place a mask before yourself in order to keep it up. An honest face? It is you who has to break with "false appearances" in order now to be "yourself in all honesty." That is the most beautiful thing that exists.

First, come home, deeply and calmly, to yourself; then manifest yourself out of these honest, inner depths, no longer immobilizing yourself in these forced patterns, no longer placing upon yourself a "role toward the outer world" — for instance just to respond to the desires of your partner, your parents or whomsoever. You now are "honestly" YOU! Liberated: in genuine peace with others because you now no longer fight against your true nature, because you now live in peace out of your TRUE essence. Love, gentleness and contentment with the free flow of life-energy, with the evolution you allow in yourself.

HYPOPHYSIS

Psychological correspondence

The consciousness that lies in/throughout/behind our earthly, material existence and is at the same time its driving Force — that consciousness we call our Living Self-Core, because it doesn't die, because it continuously feeds our body via energies — will grow into Self-awareness, thanks in part to the medium of our physical Body, and especially thanks to the receiving, processing, and transmitting qualities of our brain and glands. Here, together with the epiphysis, the hypophysis plays a very important role.

Energy impulses are being received and then translated physically into hormones, which are being produced via the glands. Here, the hypophysis is the most important regulating center. These energy impulses are, in fact, signals from our Consciousness on many levels.

When we receive sensory impressions from our surroundings, there is a direct reception by our Living Self via the brain, the nervous system. Epiphysis and hypophysis are delicate antennae that are open to impulses from the outer world as well as from our deepest inner Self. One can consider them as important pylons in the electric network — which ultimately will make it possible for us to grow and materialize our own future.

We are not victims of our brains, of our glands and hormones!

Deeply stored memories, unconscious regions, feelings and experiences from times long gone, perhaps not of this life, all information which has come to us consciously or unconsciously, lies or truth, the psychological web in which we are imprisoned, convictions regarding ourselves, old wisdom — the Hypophysis is an entrance gate which leads to a tunnel into other dimensions. This gland is open to stored information in the "old" parts of the brain and will react to this on the basis of our Content and of our convictions deep in ourselves. It will react to *all* parts of the brain, to all received impressions, and also to the light-energy impulses that emanate from the epiphysis (see Epiphysis). The hypophysis is a gathering place for a very complex Human existence; it produces hormones in a certain quality or quantity according to the extent to which it is being stimulated by the inner Self.

The more self-aware we become, the more we become Master over this gland and its workings; as long as we live "unconsciously," then we'll continue to lean upon its automatic functioning, but this will then mean that our traumas, our compulsive urges, our fearful memories, etc., will have such an influence on our brains, and therefore also on our hypophysis, that this gland will react by, for instance, over-producing hormones. Trust in our deepest Living self is beneficial; but the self-aware observation and experiencing of our selves is necessary so that we don't allow ourselves to "be lived," but instead create our lives ourselves. Therefore, on the one hand, we will have to use the hypophysis as a pass-through for our uncon-

scious Self, and, on the other hand, we need to direct our lives very Consciously and also to direct the hypophysis, by bringing in new information. No slavishly following programs or physical habits from the past: we can revise things (for instance, Menstruation). The brain and the hypophysis only react to our Awareness-content. We are not victims of our brains or of our glands!

Brain and Hypophysis obey the conscious or unconscious orders from our Self

The hypophysis is a contact point between the spiritual and the physical, between our inner Self and our physical existence, here and now. The gland gathers, holds, and functions as a funnel to our earthly existence. We lead this existence according to our convictions. Are we convinced we are worth nothing unless we achieve in an exaggerated way, sexually or in another area? If so, then our brain and hypophysis will react to these unconscious impulses and will call up certain reactions in the body via the nervous system, via hormones and blood. Perhaps we will produce an extraordinary amount of hormones, which in turn will influence our behavior, etc. This vicious circle can only be broken by our becoming conscious of deep-rooted programming in ourselves.

Therefore, we have to see the hypophysis as a source which transmits things to us, as a "suction magnet" which draws things from our deepest Self, as antennae which — in the form of spirals — go back to our origin. The hypophysis is like an arbitrator. On the one hand, it works on the basis of the many messages and experiences from the here-and-now, and on the other hand on the basis of knowledge and convictions from our inner world. All this causes the hypophysis to secrete certain hormones, to have a certain influence on other glands and organs, because of which we constantly feel ourselves changed psychologically and physically, more healthy or less healthy. On the basis of this externalization of our unconscious convictions, we can, if we want to, bring about changes, very Consciously, in the storage place, in the Content of our deepest Self. This changed inner condition will make us react differently to impulses, experiences, from the outer world: the hypophysis, the brain, react in a very specific way on the basis of your Consciousness-content. In this way, you can make yourself healthy and release yourself from compulsions or unpleasant characteristics which come to light in earthly existence.

The Will to Live is the motor behind the hypophysis. The gland functions by drawing from a content which is full of energy. Not with our brain or our glands, but with our Self-awareness do we ourselves have to force a new birth. We shouldn't wait until we are born once again out of a woman. We shouldn't "be lived" any longer by programmed cells, by a hypophysis which react to unconscious convictions, upon which we supposedly have no grip. In this way we make ourselves victims!

By Consciously Now discovering, by bringing in new information, by reprogramming, all the cells in our body will react, and the hypophysis will integrate in a new system. A human being doesn't really have to suffer and die before he can enter his earthly paradise. When we reprogram, bringing in new information, then our glands and brain will do the rest. Our body is constantly kept alive by our Consciousness: all glands are important antennae for the receiving of impulses from this deepest Self. The hypophysis is very important here, just like the Queen in a busy beehive: symbolic of the concentrated life-power source, which constantly determines which horse can be spurred on. . . . The enormous power which is being attracted here comes straight from our deepest Self.

Hypophysis and Epiphysis

We create our reality. The hypophysis is symbolic of the search for balance, when we receive new experiences, which then need to be digested and assimilated in the present content. A base which sends out and, by receiving new information, also will influence the genetic material; the arbitrator who decides what will or will not play a part. A retaining function, a gathering of information, while the epiphysis is more immediately radiating, like a flower which blossoms. Both glands represent the reception of Awareness-powers in an earthly body, as links, as reception bases, as pass-throughs, but each in its own way. The EPIPHYSIS can be considered as the window through which, from out of our inner Self, our Consciousness, we turn toward the earth. The immediate incarnation of our divine spirit. We experience this gland as an inner lamp, a strong energy-core in our head, of which we can easily make use to go through consciousness-experiences and relocations on many levels. We also use the epiphysis to produce and send out electrical particles, to materialize our inner intentions — in other words the epiphysis as a catalyst of consciousness-powers toward materialization. The epiphysis obeys, moreover, the conscious or unconscious convictions that stimulate the sending-out of electromagnetic radiations, which lie at the basis of physical circumstances that happen to us. A gland which constantly exchanges information with our warm, guardian angel, the thymus gland, and with our wise Old one, the hypophysis; and which places on our head the Crown of awakening on earth, here and now. The HYPOPHYSIS represents the following: a window which looks deep inside ourselves; an antenna to a storage bank of consciousness information, a gland which tells us clearly: "The richness, the heavenly, lies inside you, not in heaven high above your head." A gland which enables us to draw from old wisdom, but which also allows old programming to be bent toward new convictions, and which in turn transfers this to our deepest Self. This Self will, in its turn, give renewed commands to the hypophysis, which is in immediate contact with the epiphysis (and with the rest of the body), through which new outer circumstances will be created as a reaction.

The Key to Self-Liberation, Christiane Beerlandt © Beerlandt Publications

It is, therefore, necessary that we realize how we stimulate not only those two very important glands, but also our total body, to create circumstances around us in the physical world.

If we were only Consciousness, we would, (until now) not have any grip on matter. In which case we wouldn't materialize; it is thanks especially to these fine, material connecting channels, the glands, and thanks to the nervous system and the brain, that we are able to constantly influence, change, and create our world in a "material" way. When we become aware of this instead of allowing ourselves to drift upon mostly negative, unconscious convictions, then we not only will learn to fully develop these physical organs, but we will create a new beautiful world. Then, a stronger Unity between spirit and body will be experienced; then, a stronger penetration of consciousness into matter, and of body into consciousness, will take place — then Father and son become *one,* then matter has changed, then Consciousness has an immediate impact on form. In other words, a new human being, a new body, a new, immortal Individual develops.

The condition for this evolution to take place in a human being is: Heart and Insight, Love and Wisdom, going hand-in-hand. In the body as it is now, we can translate this as harmony between the glands of the head (epiphysis, hypophysis) and the heart (thymus). The other glands (adrenal glands, thyroid glands, sexual glands, etc.) will be lifted up, as it were, in their function and will be at the service of this higher union: Love-Wisdom. Left and right brain hemispheres, intuition and rationality — all will work together in unity, until the duality disappears, even on a physical level. This probable line of the future is open to us.

Conditions for a healthy and well-functioning hypophysis

Calmly, and full of trust, making contact with your deepest Self. Being open to powerful energies from unconscious regions, which are also experienced via the consciousness, via the stimulating epiphysis. Being open to the deepest dimensions in yourself and not simply living in a *part* of yourself.

Take up all your space; dare to break through, to intuitively sense things: do not allow yourself to be "indoctrinated" by others, but dare to dig deeply into your personal wisdom. Don't lower yourself, don't push yourself down, don't hurt yourself: allow life to flow in, and exploit your creative possibilities.

Self-manifestation, without beating about the bush. Place the sun-center inside your, not in an authority outside you. Don't refuse to cooperate with the building up of your existence. If you say to yourself, "I no longer participate; I close the books; I go on strike; life isn't worth anything to me anymore," then the physical counterpart, the hypophysis — as the central regulator — also will stop functioning! Dare to make the present count more strongly than the past; let everything that wants to be purified come through. Being open to your evolution, to growth toward your path, to truths about yourself — and working on this! A constant transformation of unconscious impulses and instincts into Awareness.

Hypophysis, diminished or absent activity or production

You feel like a beast of burden, stuck in your own unpleasantness (unnecessary emotional burdens, dark convictions from the past about yourself); you listen to what others have to say instead of listening to your own inner voice. Perhaps you position yourself like a servant of others. You live on a very small piece of ground, as it were: you don't take up the psychological space that is good for you; you allow yourself to suffocate, allow others to silence you, instead of standing up for yourself. You don't achieve creativity; you rather stagnate in passivity — protesting energies bubble to the surface!

Allow that life-energy from your Living Self to come in; experience those rising, eternal powers from your deepest Source, and draw from it. Now, create wonderful things and drop your burdens. A resolute intervention in your life instead of stamping yourself as a victim. Allow the motor to turn; fly like an eagle, with the power of your own wings; no longer fool yourself by thinking you are bad or "inferior"; no longer kneel; make life lighter for yourself. Be convinced of your profound possibilities for the development of a joyful existence. A stronger anchoring is necessary, a more solid intertwining of your physical self and the underlying deepest Self.

Tumor of the hypophysis

You anxiously hold on to certain things; you become completely "in the grip of —" You don't dare trust your deepest Self; nor, therefore, do you trust in the course of your life's further path; you feel as if others have seized you by the neck. Sadness; no longer seeing a way out, not being able, or wanting, to go on. You are, in fact, strangling yourself by bottling everything up and holding on to it; you are also distrustful of others and therefore don't talk about your deepest problems, although they are becoming too heavy for you. You imprison yourself. Life energies are no longer allowed to come through.

Let "it" all go — problems, people, past. In this way, free yourself! Feel how strongly you are positioned in your inner Living Self, that constantly propelling Awareness, and know that you can count completely on yourself. Healing will follow the conviction which you bring to yourself. Become Master over your own existence!
(Read the previous texts, Hypophysis.)

HYSTERIA

You have waited much too long to stand up for yourself and to honestly reveal what goes on inside you. You don't want to see what's really going on, although you get the impression that "they" are pushing in your eyes, that "they" are hurting you. You are afraid to be yourself. You've too much considered yourself inferior, as a slave of others. You withdraw into the background; your emotional world is being totally suppressed! You feel imprisoned; no one sees you anymore. Your feelings don't matter to others. . . .

With willpower and perseverance you can keep this artificial situation going for a long time, until you no longer even feel your emotions. You become distant from yourself, resigning yourself to the situation; you even have no tears left. The experience of "sadly feeling pushed aside" converts into hard aggression, into rebellious fury. . . . Ultimately, it becomes a force that stirs things up, a force with which you can't deal anymore: your unconscious, deep Powers — which for so long you've controlled, suppressed — now go beyond you. You are lifted up, as it were, into the air; your Will and Mind no longer have any say now, no matter how desperately you try to hold on. Until the last moment, you've said "No" to your emotional world, to those spontaneous energies, those creative possibilities in you that ask for your self-appreciation. You resist this inner breakthrough. A volcano will erupt. Your attitude automatically evokes certain behavior from your surroundings: they also will "suppress" or not understand you, or not appreciate you; but it is your self-denigrating convictions regarding yourself that are at the foundation of this. You don't pay attention to your worthy content, but you expect others to do so. You don't give yourself love; you treat yourself like a rag. Do you then expect appreciation and love from others? Of course, this isn't possible!

Because of your powerlessness, you burst out in a fury, but you direct it at others; in an exaggerated way you'd demand their attention because you're not giving that attention to yourself. An uprising of the Self, which for too long has been hidden; you'd force others to listen to you, as it were, but you don't listen to your own longings; because you refuse to acknowledge the power and force in yourself, you'd like to have the power to force others. A powerless, desperate cry for Attention and love from others: because you short-change yourself so. You feel small and unprotected. A call for Life from out of the deepest roots of your existence, because for too long you've tied yourself up, have made it so you can't breathe. Aggression now looms over you; you might spare no one. It is clear that hysteria will arise in people or groups who feel themselves discriminated against.

"Here I AM!" Allow your powerful energies to flow freely under the watching eye of a Self-aware "I." Trust in that natural flow of your emotions; don't bottle things up, but acknowledge your totality: your worth, your unique humanity, your creative possibilities. Don't expect others to make up for that which you withhold from yourself. Don't blame, don't criticize, don't hurl your anger at others: the cause really lies in your not acknowledging yourself, in self-humiliation — it lies in yourself. No longer buckle yourself up tight; allow spontaneous impulses to pass through freely, and follow your natural wishes. You are not powerless. If you accept the Authority in yourself, which is self-evident, you don't have to stand up for yourself in such an intense way.

Every human being has an inner, powerful Source, an immortal basis which is fundamentally solid and sends you signals when something goes wrong in your life: hysterical forces rise to the surface in order to make it clear to you that it's high time you, as an Autonomous being, take up your scepter so that you may enjoy and experience joy, just like everyone else. Transform your suppressed energies, your aggression, into energetic action, without hesitation, without feeling inferior to others. Express and fully experience your feelings, respect yourself: then others will approach you with respect.

I

IDIOCY

Instability regarding presence or absence on the earthly-dimensional level: one experiences complete incarnation as kind of threat; one doesn't dare to come down completely into the earthly spheres; one remains for the most part under the "bell glass" of a spiritual world. This flares up, as it were, and then goes out again. The channels to other dimensions are constantly open; the language of an idiot can bring to the fore wisdom from strange sources, as well as simple foolishness. But the idiot isn't Aware of this.

One can't "come outward," as it were; one remains too much in the "spirit." The strong spinning energies are often being turned inward in a suicidal way because they aren't directed by a Conscious "I," here-and-now — because they are restrained by fear and suspicion instead of being used in earthly creativity. One wants to absolutely achieve something, such as "earthly incarnation," but actually one is afraid of it: powerless. One is born with the conviction one is an outsider, not able to *truly* live, sometimes with a powerless feeling of aggression, with a feeling of being hurt, and "I have to protect myself from the threats surrounding me."

It is of importance that those kinds of people learn how to place trust and pride in themselves, that feelings of powerlessness are being replaced by the realization that one is master of one's life, in charge of "leaving or not" for unreal regions. Feet on the earth; an intense sensorial presence here-and-now, daring to take the steering-column into your own hands regarding certain tasks, so that awareness is being increased through energetic action and self-confidence. A defining of individuality, but no longer an anxious withdrawing. A complete coming out, a blossoming on this earth, and a closing down of the escape-route to elsewhere. However: don't close off the channels to inner wisdom.

There is a vacuum, as it were, which forms an impenetrable screen between their true deepest Self, their deep feelings on the one hand and on the other hand their outer "I" the way it functions toward the outer world. This duality needs to be solved by teaching them to trustfully bring out their deepest Self and their deep feelings (even the most primitive ones) in a direct and honest way.

Encouraging them in "love that gives." After all, they also sense, just like everyone else, that "grabbing" and "desiring" ultimately only bring with them anxiety and looking for escape. Whereas lovingly sharing and giving will help them find the path to true and complete Living on Earth in happiness.

IMMUNE DEFICIENCY DISEASES
insufficient formation of antibodies

You don't acknowledge your own autonomy, nor your own worth, nor your own capability, with the life powers from your deepest Self, to neutralize every "strange intruder." You're insufficiently present in yourself; insufficient faith in yourself, on the one hand,

The Key to Self-Liberation, Christiane Beerlandt © Beerlandt Publications

and on the other hand emotional tension that is too heavy — these make you vulnerable and susceptible to negativity. Belief in your immunity makes you immune: this also means that you are convinced that *true* immunity lies in Awareness and that physical immunity is the result. This can only exist on the level of goodness, of Living in truth.

Do you live only for others, rather hollowed out, instead of fully enjoying life, giving yourself love? Do you flee, instead of bringing yourself to realization? Do you perhaps force yourself constantly, carry needless burdens, constantly put prohibition signs up for yourself, allow yourself to be hurt by others, allow yourself to be used or misused? Or do you constantly try to get everything under control, without trusting the processes of life?

Transformation from an unconscious life to conscious insight into your Self leads to mastery over yourself: self-awareness that has faith in its deepest mechanisms, that doesn't shut its eyes to physical signals that are being sent out by the inner Self in order, via this feedback, finally to achieve a correction and a better balance. Immunity is about faith in your own loving divinity, about the knowledge of the power you have to self-create physical health. If you aren't convinced of this, then immunity will disappear. (See also the introductory chapters of this book and the category Infections.)

INCONTINENCE
involuntary loss of stool and/or urine

Incontinence of feces

Not realizing that you have your own "backbone," being unable to choose one's own direction. You feel like a baby, dependent on care, unable to direct your own life

yourself. You are not really aware of your worth as a human being. You allow yourself to be ruled by others. Sometimes, it is all about unconsciously asking for attention or you partially flee out of your body, all because of fear of being hurt as a grown-up. Therefore, you would rather be a baby, without having to take responsibility for yourself. Atmosphere of absence. Perhaps you appear to be perfect, but you are almost "not present in the here and now." A feeling of emptiness, of no "I"-being. Neptunian spheres. Roaming deep under ground, like an unborn one, not really knowing that you are, nor who you are. Every energy, the slightest Mars-Force, is being reduced to nothing; there's no noticeable active force toward self-manifestation. A standstill, a not going forward, a non-manifestation. Keeping yourself absolutely quiet, under water or behind the shades of life. You feel even smaller than a baby, like the head of a pin, because you, as YOU, is almost "nonexistent": you hold yourself back, you don't want to go on; something inside you says that it can't "go on," can't develop. No active participation in your "development"; on the contrary. You break down your own progress; you go backwards instead, you hide yourself in the great nothingness, in the indefinable primal womb, so that you are unreal, invisible (as "I") to the living world. An extreme of self-escape.

Be consciously born in yourself. Don't throw away your self and your production: words, actions, creativity — appreciate and cherish them. Be aware of your worth as a Human Being. Stand on your own feet. Build up your backbone in a firm way! Awareness of your own worth and self-love chase away all anxiety and feelings of insecurity.

Now, open yourself up, allow the human child inside you to be born on earth; push it out, give it every chance for existence; free yourself from what you've been walking around with for so long: your "I" is allowed to, and must, develop in full glory! Let go, release, allow the child to come out of your womb into the world. Give it a hand. Don't say "no" to letting go of that which lies behind you, or to going further in truly becoming your "I," no matter how difficult it seems: it will result in happiness, in true "life." Find that key to your feelings and dive into the water of life; don't be afraid; don't hold yourself back. No longer camouflage yourself. Reveal yourself completely as "I," the way you are. No longer shun life; don't withdraw; no longer remain anonymous or "retracted," but throw yourself with complete surrender into the sea of life: as wonderful "I"! Spread your arms and legs and dare make that leap into life; surrender, give yourself everything, give yourself Life! Anchor your heels deeply into the earth.

Incontinence of urine

You unconsciously protect yourself against your feelings; you resist; you reject that healthy flow of emotions. You lock yourself up in yourself, as it were, or you talk away your feelings. This can happen by placing the damper of your rational mind on top of things, but here it instead is about a Power-grip on yourself: an aggressive self-blockage. You are so anxious, you feel so small and powerless, that you don't dare let yourself go; you anxiously lock up your feelings inside yourself, offering resistance, with all your might, to emotions in general.

You are hard on yourself: you forbid the gentleness to come through, because you fear to be dragged along, as it were, by those feelings. Instead of living your life in a Self-aware way, you think you constantly have to protect yourself *against* life, *against* the power or the grip that others might get on you; but in fact it is you who are a *too* difficult, *too* hard, mother to yourself. You turn your back to life.

You keep your emotions in , you constrict yourself so anxiously, keeping yourself tightly shut. You experience yourself as a helpless child, vulnerable and unprotected. You offer resistance to a supple, free flow of

emotional energies. Your nature now calls for a correction; feelings find their outlet in the letting-go of urine. Because of this, you get even more a sense that you don't have the power to keep yourself and your feelings in hand, to remain master over your situation; as a result, you possibly close yourself off even more. Are you so anxious and tense because of the severe Authority above your head, no matter if it's a god, an idol or a parent?

Place the authority in Yourself, so that you live in a calm way, so that you don't have to be afraid.

Don't be afraid to surrender to your deepest Self, to your feelings; it will only strengthen you. No longer offer resistance to your emotions. No longer hinder yourself, but allow yourself to blossom. Don't flee from your feelings; they are a part of your Power to create your life yourself. Allow energies to flow freely; don't be afraid of the gentleness in you; this is only possible if — in a self-aware, more loving way — you become master over your life, if you feel safe and secure in yourself, if you don't experience the outer world as a threat. You control your existence in a self-assured way (The urine won't flow involuntarily anymore.) On the other hand you give all the needed space to your gentle, intuitive emotions, so that no outlet needs to be sought (discharge of urine). Harmony, peace, self-confidence, awareness of your personal worth. Being open to Life.

INDIGESTION
digestive disorders

A feeling of anxiety, threat — you try to surround yourself with a protective shield; you are spasmodically shooting a cannon, as it were, attacking and defending at the same time. You feel threatened in your emotional life. Fear of life, fear of death, of the future, of those who might threaten you, of the accident that might happen to you. In other words, you have insufficient knowledge of the Ability that every human being has to create his life, himself. Fear of the depths within you that you consider to be untrustworthy or dark: you flee from that which is most beautiful in you, from the motor of your existence: your creative Self. A flight away from your deepest Self to the outer ego, into all kinds of activities, into sport and games. But, in fact, you are running away from your Self; you push away your strong awareness power, your guiding spirit; cut off from your fundamental roots, you don't believe in your worth as a human being. You don't dare to fully live from out of your deepest core. You feel bound hand-and-foot, as it were, your piled up emotions looking for an escape valve. Your Conscious "I" no longer has a grip on deeply hidden unconscious emotions that now threaten to overwhelm you. . . .

For too long you've offered angular resistance to your spontaneous deep feelings instead of allowing a flexible flow. You've been holding on to things for too long (impressions, experiences, people, emotions); you've been trying to keep a "grip" on outer circumstances for too long; you anxiously draw things in, until you burst. Powerlessly, you try to get your feet on the ground; you can't reach your own basis, and this makes you aggressive and drastic!

Dare to glide into that which is deepest in yourself: nothing threatening lives inside you! Be good to yourself and others: come closer, don't be estranged from your deep core; dare to make contact with the warm, affectionate part in you and allow feelings to flow through, spontaneously and smoothly. Insight into your own trustworthy Life-core, and generous love toward yourself: that drives away all anxieties. No longer live like a metal puppet, forever on guard, inflexible and tenacious: build your life in a productive way, make yourself useful and fruitful, go along in a flexible way with the impulses

from your deepest Self and — let go without fear! Dare to look at your emotions, your anxieties, become aware of them. Come to Insight regarding your personal abilities, transform them.

INFECTION, GENERAL CAUSES
(See also Part I)

Infections manifest the ultimate climax of emotions, tensions, which have been suppressed for too long. For too long you've held on to somber thoughts, tense, heated energies: now, allow this psychological pus to escape, allow the volcano to erupt in order to come to rest afterwards, to calmly cool down.

You don't dare to fully come through; you suppress true self-realization because you don't really believe in the powers and security of your Self. Perhaps you anxiously hide yourself. Do you love yourself? Sometimes it's really about a feeling of powerlessness and anger, about helplessness and sadness. You might become angry with others because you feel unsure. For too long you've lived in stress, have suppressed feelings; sad or anxious. Now, these accumulated emotions and thoughts spurt to the surface as a discharge. A time for self-analysis and great purification!

Now, allow all thoughts and feelings to flow freely through you, in total surrender. Let go of everything, don't block anything anymore; look deep inside you for the true cause, and purify your feelings in self-confidence without holding on to negativity any longer.

In people with a VIRAL INFECTION, we find — along with the above-mentioned facts — the following causes:

You're almost Absent as an Authority in yourself. Where *are* you? Why don't you resolutely reveal who you really ARE? Why do you *let* yourself "be lived" instead of leading an existence that accords with your true disposition, your nature? When you deny the completeness of yourself, when you live according to the Authority of others, of a god outside you, then your deepest Self admonishes you. Stop! Come back into yourself. The virus pushes you with full force into yourself! Now, you are obliged to rest and come to self-contemplation. You've hurt yourself by not truly living in harmony with yourself. Perhaps you've held on to a lifestyle which doesn't really fit you. Have you lived too superficially or according to what others want you to do? Love doesn't ask for sacrifice. Healing means first and foremost being lovingly present in yourself and remaining faithful to your unique nature; only then can you do good for others. Do you think you are desperately struggling in the clutches of a virus? No. You are master over your own body. It's only a sign of the fact that, before the contamination, you were already stuck in the power-grip of an "unauthentic" life. The virus took place on your empty chair in order to make this clear to you. Now, truly accept your kingship; reign over your life with certainty and with a steady hand. Be faithful to your nature; no one can do this for you. Openly express yourself and stand up for yourself; don't force yourself. Truly being present in yourself, here and now: allow your creative energies and your feelings to flow freely, and find again the balance in yourself. Place the Authority INSIDE you, and allow yourself to heal.

Fungal infection

You feel stuck in a restrictive structure. You are inwardly angry because of being tied down, extremely irritated because of your powerlessness. It's your feeling that parents, guardians, or others exercise too strong an authority on you, and you'd like to break out of this with a glowing fist! But you don't dare; you are silent, or you lock yourself up in silent fury. A silent revolt. It goes against the grain for you to do what others ask of you; you'd like to run in the opposite direction from that in which you now have to go. In fact, we're dealing here with a minor form of self-destruction: you feel so powerless to be *yourself;* you feel anxiously so alone, standing on your own, that you crawl under some Authority to be safe. In this way, you refuse to develop the enormous energies of creativity and personal possibilities: you place them behind bars. This has a frustrating effect. You are an ostrich, and you deny your enormous potential energies, spiritually, as well as on the physical, creative plane. *That* is your imprisonment! Discontentedly, you do what others tell you to do. By accumulating angry, wrathful emotions you only worsen the fungus.

You offer yourself insufficient respect and genuine love: therefore, you don't give yourself what you deserve, namely the discovery and realization of your possibilities. Because you condemn yourself and really don't love yourself very much, you waste your life in useless activities, or perhaps in an ironic, ridiculous, clown-like attitude: mocking yourself and Life, itself. A breaking-down of life, destruction. That which you don't give to yourself, you expect it from your fellow man, from your friends; therefore, instead of *giving* to them, you expect too much from them. You will become jealous more quickly and will feel rejected, not realizing that it is you who's excluding yourself. You don't easily trust anyone anymore because, after all, you lie: you ARE NOT present; it's only a weak shadow of your true self that is there!

You transform into negative, self-destructive, angry energies all those beautiful energies that are ready to come through. Those energies then turn into fungus. Because you don't get a grip on yourself, it is possible that you place yourself under the authority of Institutions, Sects, Leaders — all of which, however, won't bring any satisfaction. You feel small and at the mercy of someone's grasp; you experience this as if someone were seizing hold of your most intimate sensibilities. You close yourself up as best as you can. Sadness, anger, and powerlessness seek a place to dump all this waste: fungus.

Be content with yourself, with LIFE, itself! Be happy with the task you can fulfill. Experience the power in yourself to be master over yourself. If you refuse to rely on your own Authority, you naturally will have the feeling that others exercise too much authority over you! Don't put the brakes on yourself, your energies; allow all creativity to flow through. Achieve Respect for the higher values in life. Place the value in yourself. Stop (self-) destruction, and begin building up! Stretch out to all sides; love yourself; be aware of the joy of being able to live every moment.

Self-confidence will drive away all anger. Don't get stuck in the material: freely develop all your talents.

LOCAL INFLAMMATION

Anxious, seeking thoughts — it might cause your head to be burning hot — often there is angry resistance to your personal frustrations, because of your being stuck, because of your limitations. You are looking for a way out; perhaps you can go two ways; because of this uncertainty you feel indecisive and at the same time aggressive. You are too hard on yourself; your life is too tight and too tense within certain structures, laws, or rational rules. Your emotional world and intuitive channels are clogged up; you are too removed from your nature because you force yourself. You hurt yourself! Perhaps you determinedly want to glue together two things which are impossible to join. You hold on to it, you insist, and you won't let go. In this way, the flame of your deepest Self ignites, and it says: "Let go, and trust in this

evolution, which now will unfold — what you want is not always what is best for you." Ask for the best solution for your problems, the most beautiful evolution, but then let go of these things and don't try to force the solution that now appears to be the best one. Call up the positive, let go, trust, and it will happen. Have you, in a state of insecurity and anxiety, tied yourself down in structures, in authority, in relationships? Did you look for support in situations which now are being experienced as oppressive? You want to get loose — you don't want to get loose; you are strong — you are weak. These are contradictions which ask for a solution. Which Gordian Knot in yourself do you need to untangle? What part of your body is inflamed? (See specific categories.)

Trust the inner authority — the healing powers within you if you transform your inner frustrations into Self-confidence! Experience the calmness, the peace within you, if you let go of that which you now so intensely hold on to. Give your feelings as much room as your thoughts: acknowledge that intuitive spontaneity within you and take yourself out of that vicious cycle of worrisome thoughts. Break through! Don't build upon authority outside you, because that only leads to an aggressive revolt in yourself. Be faithful to your nature; dare to be yourself, the way you are! In a free-flow of feelings and creativity, unload that which you've been holding on to for so long. Dare to proudly experience your autonomy; no longer block Joyful energies: they purify and make whole!

INSOMNIA, SLEEPLESSNESS

Anxious, needless fretting; you trust neither yourself nor life. You think that everything in life "just happens," that the human being has no say in the course of his life. You expect rescue from the outside; you are afraid that you can't handle it all. You don't create your existence in an aware way *yourself.* You see everything blacker than it really is because you don't believe in the possibility of directing your life yourself, because you don't believe that that which is good for you will happen if you open yourself to it in trust. You look for solutions; with a heavy heart, you await events. . . .

Free yourself! Come to Self-awareness and build up your existence yourself, without anxieties, with the knowledge that your Living Self will attract those occurrences which at this moment are best for you. Don't block up this faith-process; don't try to comprehend everything with your rational thinking; don't hinder your evolution with anxieties; trust your intuition, let go, stop fretting and brooding. Feel free! Nothing in life "just happens" by coincidence; surrender to your deepest Self and relax. Know that you can create your Happiness. Be convinced of this, do it, and be happy in this awareness! (Read Part I)

INTESTINES

Intestinal bleeding

The feeling that life has nothing nice to offer you anymore. You feel tired and old, seized by the neck, by "death"; unconsciously, you long to withdraw because you hurt and feel so much anxiety. . . .

You refuse to stand up straight, self-aware, and say, "I am here." In loneliness, you step back and let your energies drift away, unused.

Come to reconciliation with life; choose a radical route to joyful incarnation. Be born, finally, in your total Self. Become master over your life.

Intestinal cancer
(See also Cancer, in general)

Deep, vague anxieties. . . . You don't know where they come from, but you think you are sliding away into a deep, dark hole. You have the impression that you are at the mercy of a dizzying, turning Wheel, which you can't do anything about. You don't direct your life *yourself.* Fear of being gone, of being toppled, of losing all control — powerlessness.

You hold on to something, but at the same time you'd like to throw it away: "Help! My horse is bolting, and I can't get hold of the reins. . . ." Afraid of your deepest Self, of your emotions, of your natural feelings: you keep yourself hidden under a metal structure.

Take a good look into the depths: bring up your Plutonic emotions and observe them; don't be afraid of them. With your wisdom, look closely at your suppressed energies and let everything flow upwards; remove your anxieties and sadness at the surface. Let trust, warmth, and love circulate through your total heart and body; powerfully become Master over yourself and become aware of your divinity! Enter the daylight with your emotional wealth! (See Part I)

Intestinal catarrh, enteritis
inflammation of the intestinal mucous membrane

You run away from yourself because of fear, because you don't know who you are. A black, primal scream; the fear of disappearing, mortal fear.

You run away from your deepest Self: you are, after all, afraid of your deepest "I"; you don't trust it. You experience your depths as being black and unsafe to live in. The feeling of a sword hanging above your head; a feeling that certain people are hostile toward you because you experience yourself as being dark and hostile. Nevertheless, surging inside you are enormous energies which want to rush in all directions; a longing for freedom; a longing to go on and take up all possible space. Suppressed aggressive powers — but you remain in the same place; you don't really evolve, because you are so afraid.

Allow your healthy energies to flow freely; no longer block anything by needless anxieties. The deepest security and rest is to be found inside yourself! Place the center in yourself and make contact with your highest Awareness: calmly take in everything, observe the situation, and recover your balance. Acknowledge your mastery. (See Anxieties)

Colics, cramps, spastic colon

Anxiety. You'd like to crawl away; you feel like you don't belong. A sort of shyness regarding your surroundings. You run away from certain social contacts or from a certain relationship.

You feel weaker than the others. You feel pushed into the corner by a group or a person; a feeling of loneliness, desertion. For a long time you haven't *really* been in your body; you've been absent. You've lived like a shadow, expectant and afraid, a feeling of not totally being of the earth, human. Nevertheless, you want to live!

On the one hand, life is heavy upon you; you can't handle it anymore. Others irritate you — "Leave me alone!" On the other hand, there's the fear of being left alone. . . .

Confusion: because of the feeling of "not being human," insufficient grounding, too little concordance and self-assuredness. Only letting yourself and your life energies come through in fits and starts.

You cling stiffly, anxiously, like a small child to the hand of his father. You feel small and look for shelter outside yourself. Afraid to live as "I."

Comfort the little child in you; know yourself to be gentle and safe. Be aware of your unlimitedness, and integrate light-earth-water-fire in yourself: fully become a Human Being, self-aware in the here-and-now. Unlimited trust in your deepest "I." Allow your energies and emotions to flow freely, don't hold back, let go of everything. Dare to give yourself calmly to human contacts, without fear; don't place yourself off to the side with feelings of inferiority.

Rest, and trust in your Self.

Constipation, slow stool

In anxiety and unsureness, you hold on to *a lot:* you think you can't handle and digest such an amount of information and emotions. You remain stuck where you are, immovable like a rock, without evolving onward. Fear of letting go of an old situation.

You trust too little in your deepest Self; you direct yourself too much toward material things, your possessions (things, people. . .), or things that are of secondary importance in life. You do this without realizing that because of your anxious fixation on "possessions," you will at one point have to let go of these material things. If your life is built too much on material values, then you are a poor human being and don't allow true joy into your life. Transformation is impossible if you don't permit contact with your higher Consciousness.

Are you so on guard, anxious? Do you want to hold on to too much? Are you functioning like a mechanical robot without really allowing your personality to evolve toward a wise incarnation, becoming truly human? Do you, for instance, take in material nourishment but no spiritual nourishment? Or, is it because you put too little trust in this inner Basis in yourself? Do you feel threatened or caught in the act, seized by the neck? Do you experience yourself as a powerless being? Do you "hold on" to things, people, situations, instead of letting go and building your life upon your ESSENTIAL basis, your core, upon the essence of Life itself?

Or do you cut yourself off from your emotional world because you are afraid that the ground beneath you will disappear if you surrendered to your gentle side? Nevertheless, you are probably full of undigested emotions and experiences, which are waiting to be assimilated and let go of.

Do you cling to superseded values, old useless philosophies, to situations and ideas from the past?

No longer resist natural, healthy evolution; let yourself go, let go of your emotions and all needless burdens from the past. Dare to take a new look at everything and make room for renewing thoughts, experiences, impressions, in order to finally come to flexible digestion and integration. Stubbornly or anxiously refusing to let go of material things or of the past leads finally to decay and death. Trust in your deepest Self: a complete surrender to your natural impulses under the supervision of your Self-awareness leads to a "lighter" feeling, to joy for the new, for Life.

Crohn's Disease
chronic inflammatory disease
of the intestinal wall

To you, the world forms a threat; you find a system in order to survive. A constant escape-mechanism: you feel cold as ice and inwardly unsure; you hide behind a mask. Your outer image is intended to present a factitious picture of yourself — with a chic or seductive or sexually attractive appearance. Your life is built too much on pleasing others, on attracting partners or friends, preferably with magnetic drawing power: this is to compensate for your inner emptiness, so that they might tell you how worthy you are, how beautiful, etc. The game: power-powerlessness. Of course, this doesn't solve anything. In extreme cases, you dress in a fox pelt, as it were, the camouflage of a sly fox, who hides his truth, and who catches others with tricks.

As a tough body-builder, as a glittering dandy, as an enslaved puppet of the fashion world, etc., you are confronted again and again with your failure. You lose yourself more and more in this world of desires, sexual passions, superficial fantasies: an ice-cold road to death, cut off from the true, warm love for yourself and others; being dishonest with yourself, a lie to the outer world, you only utilize part of yourself, taking on a particular posture in order to camouflage your weak inner condition. . . .

In order to keep a power-grip on others (because you feel strong only like this), you don't at all reveal the person you really are! You become more and more estranged from yourself; you "fill" yourself with others because you anxiously run away from yourself. Slyly, you conceal yourself. You are afraid others might discover your true nature, especially that part of you which is unwholesome and bad (according to how you condemn yourself)!

Suffocated by this situation, you can't really evolve. Moreover, it makes you inwardly peevish and angry when you discover that the game isn't working nor giving you true satisfaction. It makes you sad, but cut off as you are from your powerful Self, you don't dare show this emotion either. You are afraid that if someone takes away your sham world, then nothing will be left, because to survive — so you think — you have to be the first to declare war, and your camouflage technique is an especially powerful weapon. You are on guard! Anxious. . . .

Lay down your weapons, become aware of the richness within you. Stop this self-demolition, this self-negation! True Nature doesn't form a threat. Seek contact with that which is Essentially important in yourself and in your environment. Dare to be small again, and look at this baby: allow it to grow slowly in you, this time with true love.

No longer flee out of yourself: fill yourself with attention and warmth. GIVE to yourself and your partner instead of attracting and expecting; give, and open yourself up to positive things which spontaneously offer themselves. Don't use yourself nor others, but LIVE freely, the way you feel. You are GOOD the way you are; you don't have to be afraid of energies, powers, or traits in yourself anymore. Neither your natural characteristics nor the outer world form a threat for you. Don't play-act. DARE to live in self-aware honesty and trust. Neither the outer world nor what others expect from you is of importance, but what matters is that which you truly feel — your inner essence. Know yourself to be safe in yourself! Reveal your true "I."

Diarrhea

In certain cases, diarrhea can mean a sigh of relief after a long period of tension and cramped retainment or holding on.

You forcefully push yourself away from something; you react against something or someone. You feel as if you are stuck or held down: you'd like to run, to run unrestrained, in an urge for freedom!

Or do you fear, beforehand, landing in a situation of imprisonment? You'd like to live your nature in total freedom: you show your teeth to everyone who, according to you, is seizing you by the hair.

You are anxious that something or someone might get a grip on you or power over you: this is really a result of being insufficiently rooted, with a basis that is too uncertain, too weak, — it is all going beyond you. You run away. You look at everything too much from below up, not from out of your higher Self-awareness, but hesitatingly, with a feeling of inability. You'd prefer to flee instead of confronting yourself because you "won't be able to do it" anyway. . . .

Feelings of anxiety and nervousness hinder you from manifesting yourself the way you'd really like to. Or, possibly, you are so overwhelmed by certain things that, as a reaction, your body offers a fast passage and outlet to whatever is overwhelming. Or do you refuse to take in the psychological sustenance? Do you flee?

Feel your strong basis, and in a self-assured way take up more space for yourself. Your anxieties are based on insufficient trust in your deepest "I"; no one can hold you back; you can calmly be yourself the way you are. Be born in yourself; no longer run away from impressions, people, or experiences that you think you can't handle: select and determine, yourself, from which sources you want to draw and which information you will pass by. You determine your life, your encounters: don't let anything get pushed upon you. Don't be disturbed by the comments of others; feel solidly established in yourself; manifest yourself, and take hold of your boat's rudder! Know yourself to be safe in yourself; nothing or no one can threaten you if you become aware of your unique being, of your worth, your inner Mastery. Look at everything calmly and achieve gentle, peaceful production inside yourself. Dare to develop your creativity in a calm tempo of growth; don't slow yourself down, nor flee from it!

Diverticula
the presence of abnormal blind tubes or sacs, mostly in the large intestine

Extreme fear, mortal fear, as if at any moment an earthly disaster will take place. You don't trust life at all; you are constantly on guard. You feel as if you are taken up in a gray-black sphere, as it were, one in which you no longer really hear or see, feel or know. You anxiously cling to things: your emotions, experiences, thoughts; you don't dare to acknowledge your healthy aggressive powers and emotional energies, nor do you dare to use them in fruitful productivity. You are afraid of self-realization! Emotions from your childhood as well as spontaneous feelings — you keep them all covered under a black mantle. You hide your true nature, not daring to show the way you feel inwardly. You mistrust your nature; you constrict yourself; you don't dare to let go because you feel so unsafe in yourself. You peek out at others — peeking through your fingers, so to speak — without really stepping into the stream of life yourself.

Look clearly: there's no black threat. Let it all be born; allow your emotions and creative energies to flow freely; break the chains with which you have imprisoned yourself. Don't cling to things or people; cut that knot which for so long needed to be cut. You are your own guardian angel; know yourself to be protected in yourself and trustingly create your life yourself, so that anxieties will disappear. Don't tensely close yourself up; come toward open contact with others; don't put the brakes on yourself and your feelings. Discover those nice, peaceful, gentle energies in yourself; life is safe if only you become aware of the creative possibilities in yourself. Allow those powers to come through and free yourself! Discover the enjoyment and the joy of life. Dare to immerse yourself completely in life; there's no reason for mistrust.
(See also Anxiety.)

Intestinal gas, flatulence

Anxiously, you hold on to so much. You'd like to embrace it all, lift it up or solve it — including your worries for others, a feeling of responsibility, but it's too much for you. A partner or possessions, old sorrow, accumulated thoughts and emotions: you are afraid to let go. You fear that something or someone might get a grip on you, and that you won't be able to control yourself anymore: that's why you hold yourself back, don't express everything: you try to keep the lid on the pot. You're afraid that suppressed contents will come to the top: you anxiously cover it up, beneath the surface.

A balance between earthly responsibility and spiritual Awareness is necessary. Calmly take the time to build up structures in your life that mean unburdening to you. Think clearly and methodically, and plan methodically, with a clear overview — not brooding, holding on to certain things or people. Trust and let go. . . . Don't cling; that which is good for you will automatically come to you if you freely surrender to your deepest Self. Your deepest emotions don't form a threat for you; allow them to flow freely; finally, sadness transforms into joy if you don't block your feelings!
Live enjoyably in "your body" and don't get caught up in worrisome thoughts too much or in a head full of emotions, anxiously holding things in.

Malabsorption
bad absorption of nutrients in the small intestine

Putting your life in the hands of others, listening to guidelines and norms that don't at all come from you. Too little grounding, too little earthly resoluteness; outwardly, you take care of your ego, directed toward the outer world, but inwardly you don't acquire power or a grip on yourself; you place all power over you outside yourself. Instead of being aware of those divine, creative powers inside you, you kneel before an ideal, a religion, or a guru outside yourself. Indoctrination, feelings of guilt; obedience and loyalty to restrictive systems: you don't really live from out of yourself. Instead of standing on your own feet, you slouch; you ignore the powers inside yourself. Healthy fire-forces aren't being used; you lead an existence that is unauthentic or too "spiritual." Your consciousness seems to be separate from your body.

Be aware of your unique worth! Place inside yourself the Authority over you, and allow intuitive emotional powers to unite with your

Self-aware assertiveness. A unity between fire-force and emotion. Take your life resolutely in your hands, and in full consciousness take in all experiences. Don't let yourself be led. Don't give others power over your life, but place this power completely within you: with your Conscious "I," direct your energies, your body, your life. Absorb vital powers into your body by believing in your genuine worth as a human being. Live from the inside out; feel that fullness and don't degrade yourself any longer into such a state of emptiness that you have to compensate for it by absorbing matter or people from the outside world.

Intestinal polyps

You feel stuck, seized hold of by others; you have the feeling you have no say about your life, that they do what they want with you. You let others drive you; you even have the feeling that others cut you off, that someone constantly hinders you in your life. But, in fact, it's you who hinders yourself! You live in a position of dependency and often even of submissiveness, because of need, because you don't think you are able to stand on your own feet.

And still you would like to get out from under this; wanting to feel separate and free, because you feel to be without breath. You barely find room in your life to move.

Depend on your individual Self; think for yourself and don't build your life on the philosophies of others! Be conscious of your own worth: live under the authority of your own mind and no longer follow others. No one can block your way: now, realize yourself. Free yourself, no longer allowing yourself to be belittled or hurt. Stand solidly on your own legs; become aware of all your possibilities. You, yourself, also need to let go — of everything and everyone — and create a free passage for yourself, your Content!

Obstruction, intestinal blockage

You have been very hard on yourself; you've broken through something; you've gone beyond your limits, and now you are bearing the consequences.

Even if you *can't* do it anymore and should urgently stop (or let go of something), you go on, offering enormous resistance. An inner battle; you'd like to resolutely break with something, you put pressure on your nature, perhaps you force your body. Consciously or unconsciously you'd like to break off something. You act like a severe, merciless judge toward yourself! Perhaps it was a matter of an inner shock, an extremely harsh gesture toward you or a harsh happening involving you, attracted by your harsh attitude, of course.

You feel pushed, as it were, into a tight spot, into a corner, and you can't get away. You'd like to run away, but it looks as if you no longer can find an escape — a way out. Time to realize that "confrontation" is necessary. Turn yourself around, look straight in the eyes of that (or the person) from which you are fleeing, and you will see there is no real danger (that you've created this for yourself, in thoughts and feelings); you will see that fears will ebb away: because now you stay IN yourself, no longer do you flee, but you seek a definite solution for your problem.

Do you experience on all sides that which is negative? Do you see that which is devilish, that which is frightful? Is your imagination going wild, and do you now have the tendency to see things ever darker?

Filled to the brim with pumpkin forces[1] in your being, but instead of developing them in a constructive, conscious way — doing something with your feelings, your potential, in a creative way — you'd rather instinc-

---

[1] Read more about the symbolism of the Pumpkin in *The Horn of Plenty.*

tively take flight, like a mouse escaping into its hole. You don't really trust life; you consider certain things as being too dark.

Transformation is asked for! Go onward and bring all your powers and emotional potential into action. Now, no longer think of things that are long gone; revise certain things, make your decision and know that YOU have your life in your hands. Straighten yourself up as "I AM," as master over your life. . . . Be honest with yourself; confrontation with your "I." Don't run away from yourself; don't try to "bite," to conquer facts or people (reflection of your inner struggle); just solve that doubt in yourself, that anxiety, to become/be yourself completely. Acknowledge the true golden content you are, and no longer avoid it.

*Now, make yourself inwardly peaceful again; open the roof above your head; no longer "strap" yourself — suffocated with thoughts, convictions — in forced habits or duties that you think "this is how it **has to** be," but feel FREE in that blue atmosphere of life.*

There is not a speck in the sky. It's only you who has created it. Communicate on a higher, purer level with yourself, and also with others: if necessary talk certain things over in a very open, honest way. Arrive at that feeling of inner freedom. There no longer exists any pressure, nor a tendency to instinctively escape instead of coming to a conscious, resolute confrontation and solution. . . .

Just hang your armor on the hook, bend reverently at the knee, and flexibly follow your nature! Calmly determine your limits, mark off your territory, say to others, "This far, and no further." Respect yourself. Make it easier for yourself. . . . Let go!

Become nicer and gentler with yourself.

Full of trust in your "being," your "I," allow life to flow through you, free and unhindered. Peacefully agreeing with your Nature, with what your Living Self longs for, without offering resistance.

Intestinal yeasting

Emotions ferment; you feel stuck; you allow anger to yeast in your intestines; you hold yourself back in order not to come to an aggressive outburst — you withdraw. Perhaps you will put on a mask to the outer world, friendly, but you feel so powerless inwardly; you bottle everything up; you look for revenge, or with confused thoughts you look how you can get a "grip" on something or someone. You are tense, restless.

This inner, nervous dynamic asks to be allowed to open up, asks for liberation, but you feel suppressed or you suppress yourself. Instead of letting go of everything and everyone, you wish to arrange everything, to organize, to control, you intensely hold on to everything, but outwardly your mouth is rather locked up. If things don't go well, if you feel hurt, then you will remain silent, red, and angry.

Suppressed action; ostrich-attitude. You don't *really* see what's going wrong in yourself. Certain experiences or thoughts are hard for you to accept and digest — this leaves you anything but unmoved; this makes you anxious. . . .

Show yourself the way you are, the way you feel; don't hide it; in dialogue you will grow. In fact you are boiling with Powerlessness: you close yourself off from your strong basis. Stand with both feet on the ground and come to peace. Don't reach outside yourself, but come close to yourself. Know that you are good and safe within a certain structure, but allow your spontaneous emotions and energies to be free! Become more concentrated in yourself, crawl close to your core, handle your fruitful energies with mastery: in activity, in creativity; don't turn yourself toward details, and no longer poison yourself with dark feelings. Spread your wings wide and cast your seed on the earth: digest, let go, and be productive. Let it all be — loosen your grip.

DUODENUM

Psychological correspondence

Experiences, ideas, impressions, confrontations — new information is being assimilated: the stomach refuses or accepts, and it gives its content to the duodenum. The duodenum represents further sensing and digestion. "Do I dare to leave it all to my deepest 'I,' to my 'unconsciousness'? Shall I let myself go? Can I trust myself?"

You are on the verge of totally surrendering to your Self, and of counting on your strong "I." This trust in your deep Self leads to activity and the production of energies. You have the secure feeling that, "Here, I'll always be taken care of by myself." In your relationship with others, this means being ready to do a service, helpfulness, lending aid, taking care — not with the intention to show off, but rather with a feeling of "you can always count on me," and with the awareness of solidarity and cooperation among people. Also, the feeling that by performing your daily tasks — your job and other activities — you are contributing to something greater and more beautiful. Life, itself, moves on. You radiate trust and joy, unselfishly: you, as well as others, experience these energies, which are not visible to the eye but which propel life onward. You participate gratefully. On the one hand, watchful, active participation with others in Life, and on the other hand a surrender to unconscious processes: trusting the positive result of the digestion of new information that has been received from your surroundings; and then the use of that information.

Ailments, in general

You give up and refuse to make use of new information that enters. You withdraw into yourself, like a hermit, no longer wanting any contact with the outer world and closed off from your deepest inner Self. Objection to new impressions or ideas, which seem to you as being heavy burdens; you refuse to participate any longer in certain things. Passivity or revolt: energies can't freely develop themselves now. Perhaps even animosity toward certain fellow men. Because you don't permit those deep streams of joy that come from your divine Self, because you have black feelings about yourself and others, you go on strike.

First of all, lead your life: trust in your intuition, in your deepest Source; first come into quiet contact with yourself. Only then will you appreciate living together with other people.

If you don't sufficiently trust your own Powers, if you mistrust yourself, then you can't really communicate with others. Your deepest Content is good. Be open to renewing impulses.

Duodenal ulcers
This condition is sometimes erroneously named "Stomach Ulcer."

You feel like a child, dominated or led by something or someone much bigger than you. You feel propelled onward, as it were, by a thrusting, unconscious power that is much stronger than you. You are afraid. You think you are at the mercy of so many emotions and impressions that you can't handle, impressions you hold off and would like to push away from you. Reality seems hard to you; you would prefer to escape it in dreams or fairy tales and not really participate in life. You mistrust others, and you suspect certain people of having a grudge against you — indeed, that they would push over your pedestal if they could: that's how unsure and mistrustful you feel.

You feel too weak to truly participate in life with others. You think, "I don't fit in; I'm an outsider, a strange being." All the more so because you often would escape into other-worldly dream-images. The physical, the fleshly, the earthly, sometimes appear to you as a threat: you prefer to play the Lady and the Unicorn.

And, still: you do belong. Feel safe and warm in your nest. Fill yourself with that cozy, peaceful atmosphere just like "twelve apostles of Life" sitting around a table exchanging new information in an genial way, freeing new energies and trusting in further life processes.

("Duodenum", a portion of the Small Intestine, is so named because of its length: "duodenum" means "twelve fingers' breadth.")

SMALL INTESTINE

Psychological correspondence

The small intestine stands for synthesis of passive receiving, on the one hand, and active digestion, on the other hand. An optimal functioning of the small intestine asks for a balance between giving-and-taking, between the self-aware, active digestion of received impressions, on the one hand, and ,on the other hand, the surrendering to unconscious processes that you dare to trust. This demands a strong awareness of your Sun-center, and also that you dare to trust in your own solid Basis as well as that you know how to move lightly via the navigation-power of your higher Consciousness. This demands complete surrender to your Living Self, to your intuition. If you don't do so, then oppressive thoughts or emotions full of mistrust will disturb the digestive processes.

Then you are afraid of the future: a defective, hesitating movement of the intestines. Or do you retain your feelings? Do you hold on to the past? Can't you let go of experiences? Do you unconsciously cling to old things? Intestinal sluggishness or putrefaction are the result of this. Carrying needless burdens.

Do you dare to fully open your brains, your senses, to higher energies? Do you walk forward on your own legs, powerful and self-aware? Are you productively making use of new information, new feelings, and do you thankfully assimilate these new

experiences into your present content? Then, as efficiently as possible, the required nourishment will be taken up in your blood. Harmonious digestion in your digestive center corresponds with a balance: taking up and sending on of digested experiences: a constant process of enrichment, renewal, transformation.

Ailments, in general

Directly opposite to trust in your unconscious processes, in your Self-Center, is Anxiety. You make life difficult and "sour" for yourself by blocking your own lighter energies, by ignoring the central "I." You again and again look for support from others instead of trusting your own solid Basis. Just to secure the attention or support of others, you'd even be too good, or would make compromises that go against your true nature. Without hope, you feel drowned in experiences from your past, undigested emotions; you neglect yourself; perhaps you've lived for a long time under the heavy dominant pressure of others, and now you are holding on to this cold pattern. In other words, you are too hard on yourself. Digest, now, those experiences from the past; look at those traditional habits or influences and allow the negative to remove itself. . . . For every circumstance you have attracted in your life was already a consequence of / a mirror of your own inner condition. Don't reproach others.

Healthy digestion of emotions leads to transformation; this process, this rebirth in yourself, can only happen if you trust in the Authority of your Conscious spirit. You decide, digest, and let go: the intestines react with joy to the command of the Master. Let the Conscious human being pull his life out of unconscious sleep and solve underlying problems.

If you ignore this mastery, if you anxiously run away from yourself, then the intestines will break adrift. So, calmly and fully, take in all experiences; observe the emotional obstacles that suddenly arise and digest them. You are not empty of content, but are worthy: manifest yourself in self-assuredness! Your experiences and feelings all come from *one* source — your deepest Self: allow this deepest "I" to grow by assimilation, digestion, and passing through.

Ileitis
small intestine inflammation
(If necessary, see also Crohn's Disease)

You anxiously hold back from letting yourself go, from experiencing yourself emotionally. . . .The burdens from the past weigh heavily on you: often, as a reaction to an experience of life which was too strict and too authoritarian, one develops a hardened behavior.

You hold on to your emotions; inwardly you feel so soft and hurt, but around all that you've built a hard coconut. You'd like to give yourself completely, to open yourself up totally, but unconsciously you hold yourself back: "That is mine and no one will touch it!" You hold on to everything; you would even adopt a false posture so as not to expose your deep core. You do not in the least trust your solid basis. With suppressed aggression, you are ready to defend yourself against a threatening environment. You experience yourself as like a child full of "bad" characteristics. Because of these negative convictions regarding yourself, you attract unpleasant situations. The burdens become heavier. . . .

You are safe in yourself! Allow your emotions to flow freely and sadness to work itself out: feel free, throw off the burden from the past! Nothing can hurt you anymore if you acknowledge and appreciate your strong, deep Self: it isn't the world around you that forms a threat, but it is your self-negation, your self-betrayal, and your anxieties that hinder you from taking up renewing, joyful experiences. Make yourself welcome in your safe Sun-center, and let go, now, of all stressful sadness.

APPENDIX, BLIND GUT

Psychological correspondence

The function of the appendix, as well as its psychological symbolism as a mirror, are strongly underestimated. The appendix is like a Guardian at the threshold, offering you a choice: Do you choose life or death? *A fork in the road:* do you choose the living path of liberation or do you keep going on a path that doesn't offer you any living prospects at all? Do you choose the "dead-end street"? Do you refuse to persevere and evolve? Or do you flexibly turn toward true Life? Here, we find ourselves in an active meeting room, where — after brief digestion and without hesitation — progress ultimately is chosen: a choice made under the impulse of trust in our deepest Self. With the force of a catapult, this decision stimulates advancement in Life. However, inner resistance, or standing-still for too long with heavy, burdensome emotions or happenings from the past; or, unconscious resistance to resolutely going on in life — all this can cause an illness in the appendix (Yes, in earlier times, also death). It is of the utmost importance that we understand the alarm-signal of the appendix: now, *choose* life, evolution, and no longer allow your emotions, anxieties, and tensions to ferment.

The appendix is located on the lower right of the large intestine, where the small intestine becomes the large intestine. After initial digestion and integration of information in the small intestine, passed on by the Guardian to the large intestine, where the highest energies are released, witnessing the transformation of emotions and matter into Awareness and liberation. To arrive at this final phase of the ultimate liberation of needless burdens (and daring to surrender to your deepest Self so that renewing energies will be able to be released), you constantly have to CHOOSE — saying "yes" or "no" to this very profound process of transformation. This process will be carried out to the utmost in the large intestine: the appendix represents *this* moment in the digestion process of assimilated experiences, ideas, emotions — the choice.

If in "blind" faith one chooses Life, then the appendix is an intense, broiling little place which energetically radiates and stimulates like a fragrant flower. The appendix represents "yes" or "no" at the effervescent, joyful feeling of conquering the world like a child. And it represents the celebration and enjoyment of things in life, without having anxieties, unhampered by emotional or material burdens. In active surrender, throwing off everything that hinders you on the way to enrichment, and triumphantly absorbing everything that leads you to higher wisdom and to more intense joy in yourself. A healthy appendix, therefore, asks you to choose your own evolution without *too much* hesitation. If immobile, the appendix wilts. From clear insight and trust, draw a straight line, without resisting, toward a higher awareness-level, toward self-liberation from hindering tensions, anxieties, uncertainties. . .

Being alert with your "I"; being open to liberating insights. Come to a clear decision and act accordingly: the appendix, as a guardian, doesn't allow *any* going back, allows no anxiously standing still in yourself. Let go and go on.

Ailments, in general
(See also the above-mentioned correspondences)

Don't you dare to choose the path of your own liberation? Do you keep hurting yourself by holding on to old pain? To needless anxieties? To an Authority above your head? So that it's impossible for you to grow any further from out of your own soul-core? Do you see everything as being so dark? Don't you come to a clarification, and can't you resolutely make a decision? As a result, is the threshold now overburdened? In this situation, you will burn on the spot: it is be-

coming too warm at your feet. You feel: "I have to get away from here!" Don't stand still any longer! (At a job, a love-relationship, a teacher-pupil relationship, etc.)

We're often dealing here with inner conflict, a choice that has to be made between two possibilities.

Or do you, with a flag in the air, shout like a fanatic for an ideal, a guru, etc. — because you feel yourself to be so powerless and refuse to evolve toward inner wisdom? Then the appendix also will become deformed. Do you drown in anxieties, in piled-up tensions? And do you now pray to a superior Savior instead of seizing your life with both hands? If so, then this beautiful flower — the appendix, which sees its purpose fail — will decay. For, the goal of the appendix is to send experiences and burdensome emotions in a transforming direction (the large intestine) and to be a link in this process toward joy, security, and higher knowledge.

Appendicitis
inflammation of the appendix
(Also read the above text)

Appendicitis places the human being before a fork in the road. He will have to choose, to make a decision.

A psychological battle of Life or Death: attack, or stop fighting? Knowing better, but still fighting on with sword upraised until you collapse and can't go on: appendicitis, or the end of a path of sorrow. A conflict, a constant overburdening: you will now have to choose! Deep anxiety and insufficient faith in yourself: because of this you cling to someone or something outside yourself. You escape into your work, for instance, into your achievements. You allow your life to be directed by that which is prescribed by others, by society, or by a guru; you follow guidelines that force you and don't at all come from within you. You don't trust in your deepest Self, nor do you trust your intuitive, gentle emotional side. You think you have to keep on; you exert yourself again and again; you climb further and further away from yourself — until the appendix says, "Stop!" Now, you are being forced to reflect upon yourself; now, you are being directed at your Center: now, follow your own Authority, your own rule, and no longer live for the sake of the eye or authority of others. Now, choose — in favor of yourself. Anxious about and mistrustful of yourself, you hold the torch, the ideal, high in the air; you fight for it, but — it lies outside yourself and only serves as a compensation for your under-valuing yourself. You fight on, against your better judgment. You are fixated on some-thing outside yourself; you blind yourself concentrating on it — you desperately try to get something into your grip, into your power. In fact, it's all about anxiety because you can't find the power over yourself. In this way, you cling to things or to situations; you become a prisoner of your "blindness"; you drag a ball and chain. . . . You can't handle it anymore. Finally, something unex-pected happens, as a last straw, and that does it: the appendix calls you to attention and begs you now to place the Center of your life inside yourself in order to allow for true joy and relaxation. No longer keep on running in place, but go on and cut through the knot. In thankfulness, choose Life, say goodbye to that false path that leads to death.

You needlessly reach too high and take on burdens that are too heavy: anxieties tell you to choose another path and way of life. When you again feel the sun shining in your heart in peace and relaxation, then you know you are taking the right path, and the appen-dix will heal quickly. One can't serve both the divine, authentic Self and the interests of the False or Unauthentic.

Introspection, love for yourself, and faith in your feelings; no longer doing that which you are expected to do, but living, very sin-cerely, from out of yourself, and choosing in favor of your own Life.

LARGE INTESTINE

Psychological correspondence

Even more strongly than does the small in-testine, the large intestine indicates the con-version of basic instincts into consciousness under the mastery of our Self-aware "I." If we have Love and Trust in our Self, then op-timal assimilation and removal will take place in a healthy large intestine.

Here, the final digestive processes take place: a final breakdown of substances, through which certain important nutritional elements and fluids end up in the blood. Unusable waste products are then transported to the rectum, the anus.

This is the ultimate place of transforma-tion of matter into energy. Under the author-ity of our inner wisdom, our Self, we let go of old things in order to make room for that which is new. Here, a complete surrender to your Self is demanded, a letting-go of need-less burdens.

Here dwells a very powerful dynamic, an extreme energy, the top of a pyramid, where earth (matter) and consciousness (energy) reign in peace and balance.

Here it is determined: *"This* is my Terri-tory, my Content; I represent *these* values; I trust in the Power of my 'I'; I feel safe; I am Master of these energies, these ever-growing possibilities, my qualities. I stand in the Center of myself and now let go of old, di-gested emotions; nothing or no one can threaten me. I won't poison myself with anxieties, with old sorrow, or with any power-grip on others, nor will others get me in a power-grip and hurt me. This is because this Super-powerful energy, which is re-leased by complete trust in my loving 'I,' makes the release-and-transformation process taking place in an optimal way. This allows me to become ever more Aware, self-assured, and powerful and gives me a feeling of being completely protected and safe."

If we flexibly surrender to experiences, if we don't cling to material or emotional things, if we dare to accept the fullness of ourselves and let go of all the old, then the large intestine will function smoothly.

The symbol of resolving deep-seated emotional conflicts so that you can arrive at peace within yourself: there is no more fighting, and the new situation is *better* than before the start of the battle.

Large intestine: the Power of a human being lies in his Content, his Worth, the Love of himself. If he gives this power, this mastery over himself, to others, then he will become an anxious, powerless being at the mercy of others, and one who feels threatened. If he seizes Power over others, then this misled energy stream will hurt him and others; if he doesn't become aware of the power — of the mastery over himself and his unconscious instincts, impulses, or urge to possess — then he is an unhappy slave.

The large intestine is symbolic of the building of Wisdom by accepting and processing new information and eliminating that which is unusable. Wisdom grows by being open, without prejudice, to impressions from the outer world as well as to the unconscious content of ourselves, our experiences and knowledge from the past: a flowing-together of both channels leads to trust in our Leadership and is reflected in the peaceful, healthy functioning of the large intestine.

The way a butterfly, renewed and transformed, leaves its cocoon, so does the stool of a human being mingle itself with the Earth: the human being renews himself and transforms.

Conclusion:

The large intestine is like the great Sphinx: its content symbolizes wisdom and Power, its form has the shape of a well-defined structure, with a lion's paw to the left and right — just like the ascending and descending parts of the large intestine — as guardians of our safety. Transformed matter under the

Authority of our individual Mastery. Being aware of our royal worth and content. Quiet Power over ourselves through deep faith in our own divinity and our love for eternal life. Here, within this fixed structure, it is best to take your time and become fully aware of the wealth of your Self and your Existence (calm digestion and transformation).

The fundamental feeling of warmth and security deep inside you. The stronger is this trust and awareness regarding your worthy content, and the less attached you are to material things — being able to take in everything and to let go of it all again — the healthier your large intestine will be. The large intestine represents the most profound, fundamental necessity for Autonomy of the human being who succeeds in transforming desires and emotions (such as anxieties) into a growing Mastery over oneself.

Ailments of the large intestine, in general

You feel anxious, threatened by something you are facing powerlessly. Your Self has no authority over certain compulsive emotions or actions. . . . You allow yourself to be hurt by others; you insufficiently trust your strong, safe Basis. Perhaps you've heard some shocking news, felt like a blow against your stomach: aren't you digesting it? Do you have anxieties (spasms)? Do you quickly run away instead of confronting yourself with your deepest Self? (See also Diarrhea) Do you deny your worth, and do you pour out despised contents, like a poison? Or do you, on the contrary, realize very well the value of your productivity? Do you pass your stool fast and in a hurry because you feel so empty?

Or do you, in a cramped way, hold on to everything? Is the resistance in you so strong that you can't let go of the old? (See Constipation) Do you refuse to transform?

Reprogram your convictions regarding yourself: consciously become master over your content, and be fully aware of the worth of yourself so that you experience a safe and

warm feeling in order to achieve calm diges-
tion of food and to have a healthy stool.
Mark off your territory in self-assuredness.
(See also psychological correspondence)

Ascending part of the large intestine, ailments

You keep running in a circle without really going onward and upward: your powers are deep, but you refuse to let them fully come through. You insufficiently manifest your-self. It is as if you were on a flying carpet, sitting tensely, full of anxieties, not trusting the navigation of your superior "I," nor trusting the unconscious processes. You are looking for happiness, but you are holding on to the past: the shining energies of your Con-sciousness are there, but you only direct yourself to dark remembrances or to the black, emotional aspects of your life. In this way, transformation can't happen. You are "bound" into a structure that is too oppres-sive, too static: you can't get away anymore; "Help!"

Aggression turns inward, emotions some-times overflow. You have no power, no grip on your existence, and you try compulsively to force it. The same goes for your projec-tion to the outer world.

Free yourself, and liberate yourself from this
prison! In fact, you are not bound to any-
thing or anyone: it's only emotions that bind
you; so be yourself, know yourself to be safe
in your deepest Self; go along flexibly. No
longer resist true evolution; don't cling to
things, people, situations, possessions —
find, only in yourself, the divine power.
Firmly seize only your life and direct it to-
ward a joyful future.

Descending part of the large intestine, ailments

Do you allow your "I" to sag completely? Do you consider yourself a poor victim, powerlessly pushed in the corner? "Am I not allowed to exist, then?" You experience your surroundings as being crushing and dominating, or perhaps it is you who are so severe with yourself. Do you feel agitated? Do you anxiously cling to things? Are you not able to make your binding to material things subordinate to your higher conscious-ness and your Heart?

Do you knock yourself into the ground in total self-destruction? Perhaps you think you always have to make room for someone else; you feel uncomfortable and anxious, cold, pushed to the side.

Just calmly take the time to observe your
worth and to polish up your diamond! Allow
your energy field to radiate in warmth and
joy from your deepest sun-center. Take care
of yourself securely: you need first of all to
be accepted and loved by yourself. Now, ac-
knowledge this worthy content, this enor-
mous Consciousness-power; you don't need
anything more in order to create a produc-
tive, rich future. So, calmly let go of that
which is superfluous; give full trust to your
powerful Self.

Colitis
inflammation of the large intestine

You allow your life to be too dependent on others: you remain in an attitude of waiting or expecting. "I can't, I don't dare go on alone. . . ." You blame the fact that you are not really making progress on resistance from outside. Possibly, you have the feeling that a strict, dominating environment hinders you from having a free existence. But it is you who nips your life in the bud: you hold on to happenings or experiences from the past, to people or things from the present. You hold on so tightly in the conviction that you are powerless. An inner, accumulated, creative energy; all these restrained powers and anx-ious doubts lead to frustration and inner re-sistance!

Now, stop this self-destruction and give
warmth, love, and trust to Yourself. Free
yourself, open up your parachute and jump!

Dare to experience your personal autonomy, separate from your environment; come close to yourself. No one can give you that certainty — only you.

(See Large Intestine, in general)

Ulcerative colitis
chronic inflammatory disease
of the large intestine, with ulcer formation

Duality, communication problems: from pure powerlessness you outwardly show yourself as different from how you inwardly feel. In a manner of speaking, you bend your head like a submissive servant, but inwardly you spit venom and fire — from powerlessness. You allow yourself to be turned round and round like a little bird on a perch because you think it has to be that way. Possibly, you amuse others in your harlequin suit, but inwardly you cultivate dark thoughts. Or do you seduce, do you make love, out of powerlessness and sorrow because you think you have to please others — or sacrifice yourself? The latter also goes for the kitchen slave. ("I am so good, obedient, or holy.") You do what you have to do in an exemplary way, but meanwhile inside you there's a turmoil of aggression, powerlessness, sadness, anger. The victim can't, or dares not, take up his or her true place. The victim feels to be in the power of.... Finally, you collapse under burdens that are physically or emotionally too heavy.

Because you experience yourself as empty and cold, you try to fill your life with a partner or family or material possessions, etc., to which you hold on. It seems, then, that all happiness is slipping away from you: because you don't direct yourself toward your Self, because you refuse to acknowledge the fullness of yourself.

Stop offering yourself to one or another person or god. Get rid of death, and come to joy in life! Resolutely take your life in hand. Quit being a slave! Develop those powers in yourself: unfold yourself in love, and come to

open communication with others. Stand up for yourself; dare to sound the gong. A healthy mental capacity: you don't have to expiate any guilt or "karma." Free yourself, and now stand in the center of your existence in a Self-aware way. Let the past be a closed book where necessary: bring about the needed changes in your life and create your life yourself.

Mucous colon
mucous deposit in the large intestine

For a long time you have felt "empty"; you don't know very well which direction to take; your body is a compilation of gathered emotions and experiences, so to speak, but they are unmanageable. You feel anxious, unable to get a perspective on your experiences or to control the course of events in your life. Your heart is constricted in a tight straitjacket: you string your bow too tightly. You've built up restrictive structures in your life, and you think that therein lies the solution for your inner labyrinth of emotional impressions: contradictory impulses are being picked up, but they are neither being looked at nor digested. This anxious confusion piles up. Unconsciously, you possibly attract a strong, dominant authority outside of you in order to compensate for your feeling of emptiness; or you constantly put a damper on your natural, spontaneous, relaxed emotional life: afraid of falling into a deep hell because of your dark emotions. You constrict yourself, which doesn't hinder you from functioning flexibly toward the outside in these falsely secure structures. Inwardly, the despair gnaws.

Your feelings can be experienced in full surrender, without self-curtailment, if they are under the supervision of your Self-aware I.

Don't be afraid of an endless or uncontrollable sea of feelings or impressions: your Self is extremely able to let all experiences come through and be digested, in full openness, within certain structures of time and space. Have no fear of your spontaneous experiences, nor of intense experiences from the past; your true seed can slowly grow via harmonious cooperation between your gentle openness toward emotions and your resolute, active digesting Powers. Open your lungs wide, take up all your space, PLAY your individual role in your life, free yourself from a false role.

Ulcers of the large intestine

A suffocating feeling, resistance to letting go; you retain and hold on to so much. In devilish anger you push yourself away from the past in which you are imprisoned with your emotions. Fury, powerlessness.

So, free yourself from this burden, spur your horse like a knight — noble to yourself, to others — and let go of everything. A self-aware choice to build up a healthy future. (See Large Intestine).

RECTUM

Psychological correspondence and Ailments, in general

We are not spirits, but instead are warm-hearted earth-beings directed by a powerful Awareness. Symbolic of grounding, extreme shelteredness in yourself, knowing yourself to be safe in the power of love for yourself. Balance in work, labor, and relaxation (rest).

You feel strong: your emotions are being carried by the secure, trustworthy Basis, which you offer — the absolute trust in your Self. Daring to show your naked content, the way you are, and not hiding these values — not from yourself, nor from others. You mustn't hide yourself. Reveal yourself!

Calmly trust the play of cooperation between rational, healthy thinking, on the one hand, and the unconscious intuitive processes on the other.

Take good and gentle care of yourself the way a mother treats her baby.

Ailments are caused by the inner denial of the above-mentioned certainties. One feels shut off from one's own basis. Do you have to go through some kind of experience, perhaps make a decision, choose this or that way, and do you keep on hesitating indecisively at the fork in the road? You don't dare. You withdraw. Now, determine your path *yourself* — one-pointedly directed, and go on. Don't be too hard on yourself, don't hurt yourself, be faithful to your Nature!

Anorectal bleeding
blood in the stool

Anxiety. You feel threatened, pushed into a corner. You stiffly hold on to patterns from the past. You don't break away from them; this hinders your evolution.

Fear of looking ahead.

The frustration of being unable to be yourself makes you angry. Still, you keep on stagnating: you don't dare to trust your nature, and you don't accept certain characteristic features in yourself. Afraid of not being good enough, not meeting the expectations of others. Like an ostrich, angry, with his head in the sand, you will not or cannot experience the NOW, separated from the past. You are inclined to "blame" the past for your present powerlessness. But it is you who denies your Worth, your Heart. That is why you have attracted experiences in your life which have confronted you with this lack of appreciation of yourself.

Also, in relationships or in sexual encounters you can feel fear of being "crushed." Or, do you also have an aversion to your body? Not realizing that you block yourself, you might be angry with those who (supposedly) "hinder" you.

Trust your nature, experience love of yourself instead of being angry. You are good the way you are. Take the veil away from your face, be honest and open with others. Don't try to keep your balance on unstable foundations from the past, on the norms preached by your mentors or those who brought you up — norms that absolutely don't fit your true nature.

Experience yourself the way you are and thereby get rid of your frustrations. The world around you is friendly toward you if you no longer dislike yourself, your body, your own flesh and blood.

IODINE
Deficiency, insufficient assimilation of

Loneliness, anxiety. You step aside; you hang your head; you stay under the authority of those who raise you or your partner; you refuse to acknowledge your own mastery. Unconsciously, you live toward death. This psychological self-negation leads to degeneration; you write yourself off. . .

Refusing to become an adult; making yourself small, like a helpless baby. You cling to cold structures.

It is necessary that you become aware of your inner greatness and translate it into action! Allow yourself to blossom instead of pushing yourself down. Creativity, talents, independence in relationships with others, daring to demand your space, no longer allowing yourself to be classified as "subordinate" or as a wallflower. Discover the warmth and security in your deepest Self.

IRON
Deficiency, insufficient assimilation of

You don't live from out of *one* central power center. On the contrary, you *let* yourself "be lived," you allow others to treat you the way they want; you are perceived as "disintegrating"; your borders are open, without limita-

tions, without self-protection, shoreless — you don't know where you can go, since you don't feel safe, since anxiety makes you flee instead of coming closer to yourself.

Flexible, anxious, chaotic, without direction or incentive; you experience yourself as cold and aimless.

Discover that safe, calm feeling in the father aspect that also lives in your soul: don't expect that cozy homey warmth from others — it lies inside yourself; inner warmth, produced by feelings of thankfulness and love for yourself. Life is a goal by itself. Inner secure love: offer it to yourself, look for security in your deepest core. Love for yourself without self-criticism, self-degradation or self-condemnation, will fill your life; this warmth toward yourself will be the motor behind the direction, the goal, in your life, by which anxieties will disappear.

ITCH

In general

Energies well up now and burn on your skin: it asks for a complete breakthrough of your Self. Do you have too little self-confidence? You have already felt it for some time: you search, but don't seem to find the solution, or you neglect the true solution. Something has to change here, but perhaps you don't achieve clear insight? It irritates you; you might jump out of your skin, be beside yourself, because of it; your patience is exhausted: "How do I get out of this situation?" Energies have been piled up, bottled up, for too long. Perhaps you blame your partner or your colleagues; you experience unhappiness with your life's present situation. If you keep yourself blocked, you don't have to get angry with others. They only seem to be the cause of your discontentment: in fact it's you who doesn't take up his or her full space, who keeps himself or herself imprisoned in a structure that is too narrow and limited. All your possibilities, also your higher spiritual energies — your talents, your complete Self — ask to finally be allowed to exist freely. Instead of bringing yourself to realization, you develop negative feelings of indignation, anger, anxieties, etc. You don't trust yourself enough to come to true development.

You walk in frustration. You, *yourself,* would hold on too much to others, but you think others restrict you. You look for a way out.

Self-confidence! Let go of others and free yourself! Break through structures that are too limiting: give yourself a large living space so that you'll also do the more annoying chores of life with pleasure. Try not to want to have a clear view of everything at once, but start with building your life, step-by-step. You are only imprisoned, only irritated, if you allow yourself to be restricted by others. Experience your life as reaching very far; develop your creativity in several directions, then your life will become lighter.

A child will perform "annoying" tasks with pleasure if it believes in its own Worth, is aware of its responsibility, and also can develop a wide range of possibilities regarding creativity.

If he doubts his great worth as a human being, he'll only look for "pleasures" to fill up his life and will neglect his "tasks." It's therefore necessary that both parents are aware of their worthiness and also develop their talents, making use of their energies in a creative way, so that the child, who is strongly influenced psychologically by the parents, has this example in mind.

Strong belief in your Worth and Possibilities as a human being will free all energies that now want to be born — the itch disappears. Give yourself time; have patience; don't condemn yourself!

Go onward in faith!

If necessary, see also: Anal itch; itching of female genitals.

Itch on the scalp

Confused, you think and search. Because of the presence of contradicting elements — because you don't trust enough in your deepest Self — you don't clearly see the sense of things. You think you have to figure out and solve everything with your rationality. Energies, active decisive action, and aggression are being held in: you don't know which direction to choose. Desperately, you look for a solution; you keep running in place, making no headway. Nervousness; you are impatient and angry, discontent, because certain things are not going the way you want them to go. You would like to force things, to bring about change. You live too much in your head, too little with your whole body.

Your deepest Self "knows" it already; trust and let go; try not to force, to grab with your thoughts, that which should follow its own course. No longer fret. Make a choice, leave others free, express your energies outward, don't stand still. In the contentment of the Present, you are allowed to expect everything that is good for you in the future. Trust banishes nervousness.

J

JAWS, JAWBONE, TEMPOROMANDIBULAR JOINT

Psychological correspondence

Symbolic of the ability to "divide," to allow impressions to come through in such a way that you can handle it all emotionally. The controlling mechanism in you that closes or opens up to others, to new information.

The power in you to choose — without forcing, without resistance — certain situations in your life. The will to be open, yourself, to meet your own needs and longings, and then to brush away that which you no longer need.

The protecting, secure structure in you; the will power to push yourself through, on the one hand, and on the other hand the co-operation and exchange with other people, in reconciliation.

Being able to trust your basic structure, calmly experiencing yourself in balance; building up your own house, sheltered in your personal, protected territory, and freeing yourself of, or removing, all pain and sorrow.

You hit the nail on the head, if necessary. Fighting for the truth, standing up for yourself, showing your teeth. Being aware of the full extent of your life; intuitive, emotional, rational, creative — the awareness of the scope of your existence itself.

Symbolic of the Power of your inner Authority; manifesting oneself in a resolute, active way in earthly life; self- liberating and bringing freedom. You are not being "swallowed up" by a system or a person. You allow others to be free; you don't "swallow up" others.

A primitive, fundamental power needs to be directed by the Conscious "I."

Ailments, in general

Do you consume yourself in fury, in vengefulness, because everything is not answering to your "narrow" rules or expectations?

You live only partially; you ignore your rich emotional world, or you live only according to primitive needs. You deny the large space of your existence; you live in a way that is too restrictive.

Anxieties block you: you dare not be open to your personal powers and possibilities, nor to what others bring to you. Your self-negation can lead to the worship of a golden calf, to fanaticism; you put all authority outside yourself. Are you perhaps being drawn in by a sect, a religion — and just like them you want to burn an effigy?

Possibly, the feeling of responsibility for yourself has disappeared. Where is the will-power, the self-manifestation? You are not yourself (any longer). Do you succumb to the adoration of false values?

This situation, in powerlessness, ultimately leads to aggression, perhaps to enormous fury, to a revolt! Also, if you've placed yourself in subordination to others instead of building upon your own Authority, then your life will become "twisted," and you don't know how to get out of it. But you'd rather suppress everything, clenching your teeth. Your anger, your resentment, are being inwardly experienced. You'd like to knock someone down, but you can't. You feel so incapable that you might collapse. Jealous or resentful thoughts can make your head spin! But, in the end, you prefer to let everything ferment in silence and not really stand up for yourself.

Your worries will resolve themselves if you become Aware of the deepest powers in your Self, if you acknowledge all power and authority in yourself and no longer flee from that calm, safe Basis which lies at the origin of your existence. When you find peace in yourself, then you will be able to be open to others, in a peaceful, loving way. Dare to fully experience your feelings; don't close yourself off from them! Replace anger with active self-realization; let go of the past and see how you've attracted all these sad happenings because of narrow convictions regarding yourself. Now, open yourself up to new, Conscious choices and don't cling to that which is not beneficial for your evolution. Trust! Don't put the "other" on the flaming pyre; know that it's your own inner fire, your very personal energy, that you aim destructively at others; look into your own heart and make it free of hardness; fight only for truth in your life. "Bite" into life with joy, in love; participate fully in it! Relax....

Abscess of the jaw
(See also Abscess, in general)

You enclose yourself too much in a cocoon; your feelings, your anger, can't be experienced freely. Full of anxiety, you live on a shaky, insecure basis. The emotional burden weighs very heavily. Afraid of your deep emotions, of death. You don't trust your deepest Self; you place all authority outside yourself, in a religion, a structure, or a philosophy, but you are unconsciously so afraid that this world might not be the true one. In this uncertainty regarding your own Basis, you cling anxiously to things, to people, so as not to fall — energies are asking for a breakthrough!

Find yourself quiet, sure, and safe in your deepest Self: no deeper value or guarantee of safety than your ever-living Self. Stand fast upon your own Basis: the burdens you carry are needless. Replace anxiety with love and trust. Don't be afraid of emotions, nor of powers from your unconscious which raise their heads and call for recognition! Don't push them aside any longer! Let the volcanic, divine energy in you break through! Don't be afraid of your anger: don't bottle it up; express it; come to confrontation until you've gained Insight, until you realize that the anger and anxiety grew out of your unsureness.

Cysts of the jaw
(See also Cysts, in general)

You open yourself so much to everything and everyone that this costs you somewhat: you perhaps mother, coddle or dominate others. Or you cover others with patronizing attention. You fill your Content with others instead of first and foremost Growing *yourself!* Large and full of sensitivities, sympathizing or meddlesome, you take everything in, like a gathering mother Crab (zodiacal sign Cancer). Emotions, sadness, melancholy — including about others — after all, these others "fill" you up in the first place. With your head, with your thoughts, you are constantly "away" from yourself; you take in sorrows and problems. You don't "forget" problems from the past.... You "collect" everything.

Jump into life yourself instead of giving life to a cyst; create in a balanced way, "give-and-take"; allow energies to flow out instead of holding on to everything and everyone. Keep your mind on yourself; the other person doesn't profit if you dive into his pool of water; resolutely stay to the side. First of all, strongly build your own foundations and realize yourself; only then can you open yourself up to others. Be present in yourself, with your feet on your own piece of Earth, here-and-now! Also, let go of problems from the past.

Fractures of the jaw

Frantic, because of powerless aggression. Desperate: you don't know what to do anymore. You feel hurt in your most intimate sensitivities. . . . Sadness! This leads to thoughts of vengeance and sarcasm. You might force things now! You are jumpy from insane fury because of happening(s), because of pain from the past; you feel so hurt, you can't digest it. You feel like someone who's been decapitated, like a slaughtered chicken — which can lead to biting self-mockery. It can also lead to a furious reaction against people who have "hurt" you. You don't see that your Self-denigration and self-negation were the cause of the sad or troubling happenings that occurred in your life.

Now, go your own way so that your life no longer stands or falls on that which you expect from others. Leave it behind and go on! Full liberation from black thoughts about yourself and others. Despair, aggression, powerlessness, and resistance resolve themselves when you attack the true cause: therefore, now come to an autonomous, self-aware realization of life and no longer hitch yourself to others. Be convinced of your powers and possibilities! No longer diminish your life-space by fixating on others.

Lockjaw

A feeling of being unable to express yourself the way you really are — unable to go on. You don't dare; you withdraw into yourself.

Sadness is inside you, but you don't dare to come out with it. As unsure as you feel, you constantly question whether you can handle a "task" or expressing yourself outwardly.

Inwardly hesitating and emotional, but outwardly cold and distant: instead of occupying yourself with your personal growth, you direct your attention at others as a diversion.

Outwardly, you'd place yourself "above" them, like a teacher or a horse tamer; you would hide your doubts behind a whip!

But, actually, you look at the world from below upward, like someone who's inferior: "Is it alright if I do that?" This uncertainty oppresses you and inevitably leads to frustration and anger! Just to feel the slightest bit worthy, you'd climb a step higher.

Give yourself the place you deserve and realize yourself, full of self-trust.

Come into contact with your deepest feelings; no longer close yourself off from them!

Place your personal worth higher, direct your attention inward instead of outward, and no longer doubt your unique Being.

Let the ice water melt in the warmth of love; accept yourself — don't reject yourself. Place all power inside yourself instead of wanting to keep a grip on others. Discover the peaceful, relaxed core in yourself. You don't "have to," but instead you "may"; don't resist life, don't resist your feelings, and allow them to flow freely.

Ailments of the temporomandibular joint
a tendency to dislocation

Do you show yourself outwardly the way you feel inside? Or do you wear a protective mask, as it were? Possibly, you wear a friendly, polite costume, but inwardly the battle rages. From undercover, you fire aggressive arrows, but you won't say anything; you keep your aggression inside your mouth. Possibly, you feel like a victim on a cross because you don't succeed in expressing your point of view, which goes directly against that which your fellow man proclaims. Or, you don't succeed in resolutely transforming your healthy, aggressive powers into energetic self-realization. You smile, and you wear a beautiful bow tie, but inwardly you feel black and suffocated with emotions.

You doggedly fasten your teeth on something; you can't get it out of your head; you are angry and unrelenting, but you experience it all Underground. You have pain and sadness, but upon it you build up a fury, rancor: a stone-hard inner reaction. You push yourself away. You swallow up and swallow up experiences; outwardly, it appears that nothing is going on. You harden yourself. You learn how to live with this disunity, with this play-acting. After a period of artificial suppression, primitive powers break through.

Don't bottle things up; reveal yourself the way you inwardly feel; express your anger, dare to be yourself. Always be faithful to what you feel, to your nature. Don't harden yourself, but arrive at insight into situations. Why did you attract this or that situation? Solve your emotional pains by looking thoroughly at yourself and becoming Aware of the fact that your powerlessness begins with suppressing your Self.

JOINTS

Psychological correspondence

The joints immediately reflect to what degree you listen to the inner Authority of the master inside you, or whether you balk at this and would sooner obey an Authority outside you. To what degree are you stuck in the system of sacrificing because of Reverence for? . . . Because you undervalue yourself? You bend completely. . . . You feel like a martyr, guilty, the burden-carrier for others. Perhaps you think you are bad and inferior; you allow yourself to completely sag; you blow with the wind.

Denying the power in yourself, you'll perhaps get irritated easily, especially when you even slightly sense that someone is going to tell you something — stubborn, resistant as you are.

In this way, the joints symbolize the ease or the difficulty with which a human being dares to trust his inner Self and dares to surrender to the stream of life. Does he refuse evolution and change? Does he cling to old values in his life? Does he listen to false gods? Does he live in a flexible, supple way, or is he instead recalcitrant and stiff? His joints will tell that.

Ailments, in general

Do you trust too little in your Self? Are you anxiously fleeing from your emotions, and are you making a wrong leap? Are you looking for everything outside yourself? In books? In that which has previously been taught to you? And are you afraid to deviate from this? Are you digging in your heels?

Do you force yourself? Do you tie the girdles too tight? Or, do you hurt yourself? Why don't you flexibly and joyfully surrender to love for yourself and for others? Are you afraid of being hurt, or do you walk on tiptoe? Are you suspicious? This unsureness only hinders your own smooth evolution.

Therefore, consciously put things into order where necessary, but for the rest trust your living Self, which automatically regulates everything for you without you having to constantly monitor it.

Allow higher energies to come through. Don't cling to the material or superficial. Feel supported by yourself; don't strain yourself, but in life be open without prejudice so that you can make the necessary turns without problems.

Arthralgia
pain in the joints without objective physical anomalies being necessarily present

You fight against your own nature, and you fit everything too tightly within a structure: this is because you consider yourself too weak, and as a result you imprison yourself.

You attach yourself to exterior things, to structures, to form, to details and trivialities — you do things "because that's how it's supposed to be" according to the rules that you, society, or the system of which you consider yourself a part, place upon you.

You don't build your life on your own foundations. You barely stand with your feet on the ground; your shoulders become stiff and angular in this unauthentic life with needless burdens.

You remain superficial. You are not straightforward because you don't trust yourself, your own nature. After all, a human being can't possibly be "good," can he?

As a result, you'll also point a finger at others. Because of discontentment with yourself, you'll also soil others, will look at them distrustfully, criticize them; you gossip. You are on the alert for. . . .

Stop fighting and offering resistance to your own gentle, beautiful nature! Allow all feelings to flow smoothly. Learn to relax; direct yourself to the Core of your life, not to the appearance of others: content is what counts. Bring that warm, friendly Teddy bear home, into yourself.

Arthritis
inflammation of one or more joints

You feel like a martyr. You are the eternal victim. But by playing this role, you do get the attention you so badly "need." Sometimes, you appear to be a clown who weeps inwardly, but the clown, at least, gets attention from his audience. You criticize or gossip; this is but a camouflage for inner powerlessness. Anger, because of this powerlessness! But perhaps you blame it all on another, or on this or that situation, on an illness, etc. You might writhe and twist, almost breaking your neck like a real acrobat, in order to receive attention and love from others. Doing this, you force yourself, and when you realize that all this is not working and you continue feeling powerless, you become sad and reproachful.

Perhaps you appear to others as being arrogant, conspicuous, or sometimes dictatorial, and you constantly take the contrary position. But, actually, you are hurting yourself, condemning and suppressing your deepest, gentlest parts. You long just for love. Why be so hard? Are you afraid of your gentle characteristics? You will project this onto your surroundings. Here, we can speak of a certain suppression and duality in yourself. Possibly, you hang out the dirty wash of others because you find yourself "dirty," or you shun yourself.

*The cause of your sadness lies in your expectations from life: were you of the opinion that you were a victim? Then you have attracted situations toward yourself (and also this illness), which confirm this. Are you convinced that you deserve to be healthy and happy? Then your healing will begin. Your criticism of others is self-projection. Experience now your good and gentle side. You deserve love and attention from yourself; this can never be compensated for by attention or love given by others. When you respect yourself as being worthy and place the power inside yourself instead of thinking yourself to be powerless, only then will others give you what makes you feel good. Your surroundings reflect your inner vision of yourself! Look deep inside yourself and attack the problem at its foundation. You can only change **yourself**. Become master of your own life and give value to yourself. Are you treated as an inferior? Then this means that you don't appreciate yourself! Change your convictions! Those who don't wish to acknowledge you will then disappear out of your life.*

If necessary, also see the text Arthritic Fingers.

Charcot joint
neuropathic joint disease
total degeneration of the joint

You take life away from yourself: slowly, you flee into the spirit. You withdraw from the earthly; you would isolate yourself from the rest of the world — a pulling back.

Your earthly energies are not really allowed to come through; your Mars-power is being suppressed; you push yourself away in self-condemnation or like a "lowly servant" who is not worthy of building his own self-aware, powerful existence.

You place high demands upon yourself: emotionally, you keep yourself shut, tightly wound. . . .

You hurt yourself. Why don't you allow yourself to really live? Why don't you give yourself the right to exist? Don't you love your body, or do you look down upon earthly life?

You live only in your head, not really in your body: energies flow away. . . .

Confront yourself in the mirror: come to gentle, warm, proud acknowledgment of your personality. You belong. Accept your totality, your body. Concentrate your energies in your body and call up your powers under the authority of your Conscious "I."

No longer push yourself away: acknowledge your worth as a human being of flesh and blood.

Dislocation

You feel stuck in a certain pattern, structure, or under an Authority; possibly you feel squeezed between the columns of an organization, a religion, a school, etc., but you refuse to carry burdens any longer. You wish to withdraw; you wish to cut a tie.

In the past — because you were insufficiently grounded in yourself, weren't really sure of yourself, felt vulnerable — you were too much "drawn" into a system or an Authority outside yourself, into which you allowed yourself to be taken up. It all comes down to self-doubt, to the powerlessness to manifest your Self in a strong and autonomous way. You now resist it; for too long you've lived tensely, alert, on guard, aggressive, in a defensive posture. Your natural feelings were suppressed in a tension-bow of thoughts. You don't really feel comfortable with your emotions; you don't really dare to take up your space. Unexpected aggressive

reactions — unconscious reflexes for self-liberation, as it were — can suddenly happen. But you'd sooner slide away instead of bringing yourself forward in open dialogue or in honest behavior.

Relaxation, trust; daring to look at your deepest feelings; knowing yourself to be protected in yourself; offering no resistance to the smooth flow of your own feelings; strongly establishing your "I," knowing yourself to be secure in yourself, so that you can build your own life independent of whatever authority. Calm self-confidence, not forcing your nature. Transforming aggressive powers into active self-realization. Peace in yourself.

Hypermobility syndrome
abnormal, exaggerated
mobility of the joints

Like an infant, you are at the mercy of. . . .

Your self-awareness seems to be absent. Your life is being directed by anxieties, by your unconscious emotional world, by others — you are so afraid of your own depths. You want to grasp for things or people outside yourself because you don't take hold of yourself.

Initially, the feeling of "I can't get away, I feel locked up in a dark cell," makes you pull and tug violently; but you can't detach yourself from it, nor can you detach yourself from your own emotions, nor from others who think they can tell you what to do.

At last, this leads to: "It's all useless. . . ." You then let yourself droop completely; anyone can walk over you; you then can only position yourself defensively instead of (as previously) offensively — you give up. A feeling of Aimlessness.

BECOME AWARE OF THE FACT THAT YOU DON'T HAVE TO MAKE YOURSELF MASTER OF, OR OVERTHROW, ANYTHING OUTSIDE YOURSELF. TAKE POWER OVER YOURSELF. Joy of life of-

fers solidity! Grounding, self-assuredness, enthusiasm, action, trust. Lead your emotions in a self-aware way, direct your life yourself! Acquire power from joy. Joy because of yourself!

Ruptured, torn ligaments

You fixate on *one* point in *one* direction. You hold on to it. . . . You refuse to listen to your own inner Authority! A demand for change.

You too little follow a "personal" direction; your self-awareness seems to be absent; you follow a certain path like a ball that rolls and rolls, without really consciously choosing!

You think a lot; you feel like you are stuck somewhere in a run-down street, but you don't do anything about it. You remain sitting, stagnating in the old situation. You go on living in a certain pattern because it supposedly has to be that way, or because you refuse to take responsibility for positively building up your life.

Like someone who doubts, or like a robot, you automatically follow a direction that doesn't really suit you. There can be many reasons for you to cling to a job, a relationship, etc. — anxiety and unsureness lie at the bottom of this. You insufficiently believe in your Self; in certain matters, you are too pliable, too compliant. Your own "I" isn't really present in everything you do. This leads to an inner rift because suppressed powers and potentials rage inside you!

A tear or rupture indicates that it is necessary you change your direction, choose a new path: surely a direction that is inspired by your own longings and insights.

Higher, new energies wish to come through: don't limit yourself to superficialities or materialistic outer goals.

*No longer live like a train without a locomotive: you are in a good position when your life is impelled from within and can evolve under the supervision of your inner Author-*ity. *Birth in yourself. Now, direct yourself toward your ideals and wishes; be productive. Leave the dead-end track; leave the paths that don't really suit you; leave the job that you are only doing because of money, etc.*

Now, quit the battle against your deepest Self and flexibly follow the signals you feel. Joy doesn't come from security built on the basis of the outer image, but from a profoundly experienced self-confidence.

Allow higher awareness-energies to flow freely.

Osteoarthritis

You feel hurt and alone in your sadness. You are like a martyr who drops his shoulders ever lower. You allow yourself inwardly to be swept along with your feelings. You demolish yourself by developing negative energies (thoughts, emotions). You hold on to a painful memory, to a pessimistic life-philosophy — "I was born just to experience sorrow." — to a disbelief in life without burdens, to thoughts of death, etc. Your warm sun-center and feelings of self-appreciation are being disconnected. This holding on to self-degrading feelings leads, indeed, to a distorted life-consciousness and goes chronically from bad to worse. You hide the suffering deep inside yourself, sometimes being totally unaware of it; often, you are an ostrich hiding its emotions in the sand. You don't want to, or cannot, see true reality any more, sucked along as you are by your own sad thoughts and convictions. Negative thoughts burn up your body like a candle. Are you trying to prove to yourself that you *are* good, and do you live like a saint, perhaps out of fear of ending up in "hell"? Do you not dare to fully enjoy life? Are you doing too much for others? Do you try in such a way to fit in that you strain yourself and are in pain? Do you neglect yourself? Do you force yourself to serve others? Out of feelings of guilt, out of fear, because of a lack of self-esteem?

Open your eyes wide: dare to see the truth. Life is joy! Give love and radiate in gushing enthusiasm. Don't extinguish the fire inside you, but give yourself warmth instead of deadly, icy cold. It doesn't benefit anyone when you, like a martyr, are doing good for others. In this case, the motives behind your actions are not pure, and they will not get you anywhere. Live from out of a feeling of self-esteem; respect yourself. If you don't love yourself, then you don't truly act out of love for others. Sorrow and anxiety are the lies of our world (see Anxiety). Give your warmth to others, and then you will fill yourself with magnetizing, healing energies. Allow yourself to enjoy. Don't mope. Resolute Action! Completely integrate all your energies. Don't get stuck in the past; draw a line and create, Now, life as you would like it to be for yourself! Change your negative expectations of life, and the results will not fail to come. Become conscious of this potentiality!

Rheumatism of the joints
(See also Rheumatism, in general)

An inner urge to break through all boundaries, to begin fighting for absolute freedom!

You'd like to push over all structures; nothing or no one can contain you any longer! You revolt against all those whom you accuse of placing limits on your life! You might get angry and begin hurling criticism! An intense longing to open up. . . .

A desperate search for one's own depths and distances. . . .

For too long you've undervalued yourself and have put yourself into a straitjacket. You've attracted oppressive situations (unconsciously); now you long for all the freedom of movement.

Therefore, listen to your inner authority; don't blame others for what you have unconsciously permitted for such a long time. Now, walk other paths, follow your impulses, but don't give others the "blame" for your not acknowledging yourself! Dare to enjoy; allow all feelings to flow freely. Don't break down any doors, but throw open all possibilities for yourself — also those doors that you used to fearfully keep closed. No one else curtails your freedom: you have "immobilized" yourself for such a long time.

Structure, form, rules — these automatically arise from the blossoming of your content, your talents, your possibilities: a structure which leads and regulates, but which no longer curtails. A structure which gives you all the freedom of movement without your having to hurt yourself or others. Step out of your armor; no longer allow yourself to be drawn along by others, by an authority, gods, or a philosophy — free yourself!

If you no longer grumble at yourself and limit yourself, then you'll no longer reproach others.

Be gentle to yourself.

K

VITAMIN K
Deficiency, insufficient assimilation of

You build your life on the Authority of *others*, too much within oppressing structures, because you don't trust your own foundations enough.

You "oblige" yourself to satisfy certain requirements in order to guarantee your safety, but these are only unstable requirements. Actually, this suffocates you; your suppressed spontaneous aggression wants to break out!

Resistance! You feel tied down, not at all free; you'd like to run away as it were, to go beyond your limits, like blood that gushes out of its veins, in order to free yourself from the situation in which you feel trapped.

A suffocating situation — also because of the fact that you consider yourself to be weak and, therefore, dependent on others; you allow yourself to be ruled by others, you feel seized by the neck, you experience yourself as being a powerless victim who is not able to live an autonomous life.

Your thoughts, boiling with anger because of this powerlessness, are seeking a solution. Then again, you are dropping your head in sadness. . . .

Become aware of your independent, autonomous worth and rely on the security of your deepest Self. Gradually build your life in pride.

A balance between structure and spontaneity, between feelings and form; don't force yourself to live in a straitjacket or in the grip of others.

You are no victim; it's this negative conviction regarding yourself which makes you crawl and makes you sad.

Transform these thoughts into joyful consciousness. Discover your worth and enjoy your emotional wealth; don't suppress yourself, but dare to live your life to the full, in an unconstrained way!

There's nothing you 'must' do, you are allowed to live happily and peacefully.

Determine, yourself, your definite Limits!

KAPOSI'S SARCOMA
a kind of cancer, mostly originating in the blood vessels of the skin

You can't really reach your feelings: you feel like a victim, deep inside a pit of anxiety. Possibly you've allowed yourself to be dominated, or you've lived for too long according to the standards of others, instead of accommodating your own personal wishes. In every way you start to revolt with a powerless fury! You'd like to get out of this oppressing situation; energies from within push in all directions and ask for your breakthrough, but you are frantically searching with an inner nervousness, without really getting anywhere. An aggressive powerlessness, a frustrated fury — finally you say: "It all leads to nothing. . . ."

In fact, you are pushing yourself away from your poor, sorry Self (at least that's how you see yourself): free yourself from this vicious circle. Make yourself warmly welcome, be your own father and your own mother. Place all power in yourself instead of expecting shelter outside yourself. Every human being has a beautiful, good Core within himself. In the first place, make Peace with your deepest Self: you are not powerless. Experience yourself as an autonomous, creative individual who's able to heal his body, simply by Lovingly Accepting himself, the way he is, without condemnation, without turning away from himself. Pamper your body like a child and be happy for life itself; don't put any conditions on it. From out of this self-contentment in the here-and-now, you will attract joyful circumstances. Reconciliation in your heart, no more discord. Freedom instead of suffocation. A happy CONTACT with your Self: the love toward yourself will get you out of the abyss. Decisiveness and action instead of fury and frustration. Self-confidence!

KLEPTOMANIA
irresistible urge to steal

The cause really lies in a combination of different factors. Because of the inner feeling of imprisonment, one would attract a "prison cell": you feel as if your nature isn't allowed to exist freely — you "forbid" yourself to lead a free, natural, spontaneous existence.

You smother yourself; also, your upbringing has *possibly* added to this. You suppress many beautiful and creative energies in yourself; emotionally you keep yourself too tight, too closed. A self-imposed imprisonment; you'd peek out of the corner of your eye for the right moment to break out of this!

Suppression of longings leads to exaggeration. Because you have the feeling that it's others who block you or limit you, you'll act in a way that represents an escape out of this world-imposed prison.

On the other hand, there's a deep anxiety here and a compulsive "collecting" of products, as an expression of the primal instinct of mankind to survive.

Seeking, sniffing with the nose forward, taking in. . . .

Anxiety, which is a result of not having real contact with one's own deepest Core, and which is the result of one's self-negation, of the negation of natural, intuitive, sensual longings; ultimately you feel not only imprisoned in yourself, but also so empty. Because of this, an urge develops to constantly "fill up" this emptiness with elements outside you. This happens on a very earthly plane, since it's particularly your earthly nature upon which you look with an angry eye — and refuse to fully acknowledge.

Kleptomania is looked for as a way out of this inner schism: compensation for that which is "missing" or is pushed aside within you.

After all, this schism leads to stress, to a hard anxious tension, which apparently will only disappear when one can fill one's own emptiness: by theft.

This collecting instinct, in fact, leads to actual psychological survival, although it doesn't offer the *true* solution to the inner problem that lies at the foundation. Here, it's about a revolt of the prisoner.

Another aspect is the undervaluation of one's worth and one's possibilities.

You anxiously cling to everything and everyone in order to find a feeling of safety.

You don't at all believe in your own mastery; you are convinced that unconscious powers direct your life, that your hands lead your head, that you're not at all able to take your life in your own "hands" and aren't able to build your life into a joyful, satisfying existence.

This frustration, this dividedness in yourself can be solved by completely opening yourself up to all the qualities or aspects of yourself: accept your intuition, your nature, your instincts, and don't close yourself off from natural, sensual feelings!

Don't mistrust your Nature, allow it all to come through freely; otherwise it will look for its way out in exaggerated manifestations such as sleep-walking, kleptomania, etc. . . . Unconscious powers that surface shouldn't be ignored, but should be integrated — that means: accept them, look at them, deal with them, under the supervising eye of your Conscious "I."

When you no longer consider yourself a threatened being; when you're no longer on guard against your own nature, but fully surrender to yourself; when you push your worth, your talents, your physical longings outward, also in relation to friends — then you will begin to experience your fullness in "giving," and no longer in "taking" in order to fill yourself. Experience that fullness in yourself; don't be ashamed, don't feel guilty about your feelings or your dreams, but fully experience it and no longer push yourself away!

Then get a good hold of yourself and know that the Self-aware "I" fulfills a superior role Now in regard to that which is compulsive: if you are convinced that unconscious powers follow the Guidance of your Order, and if you no longer put your feelings under a glass bell, then you'll no longer be bothered by kleptomania. Instincts will be transformed into Conscious creativity: you can at any moment start this transformation. When you carry through this liberation, you are Master over yourself.

KNEE

Psychological correspondence

Symbol of the power of inner perseverance, of the proud "I"; of placing yourself in the Center, in a strong and compelling way.

Symbol of the willingness to flexibly bend in life; of surrendering to your deepest Self without resistance; of willingly allowing yourself to glide on the path of true evolution; of being Proud about yourself without stubbornly holding on to false or external values, which might block inner evolution.

The power to stand up for yourself, not just allowing others to bend you; the central power in you which radiates outward full of self-confidence.

Kneeling before your deepest worth as a divine creative being; reverence and respect for yourself and for others; a flexible openness toward the world, not being stubbornly closed up.

Ailments of the knee, in general

Anxiety, not trusting your Self, your intuition; being on guard, bracing yourself, being on the defensive. You doubt your worth, your possibilities.

Hard and inflexible, stubborn, indomitable, arrogant, proud in a exaggerated way: thus you immobilize yourself completely and are displeasing to others.

This attitude simply follows from an insufficient trust in your deepest "I" and the resultant anxieties. You dig in your heels; you won't give in, stubborn, because you feel threatened. Energies turn inward instead of outward.

Sometimes an exaggeratedly dominant attitude, an abuse of power — because of powerlessness.

Working against the flow, despite knowing better; you don't allow gentleness, love, to enter your heart. Do you love yourself so little? Do you despise certain things in yourself? Don't you allow yourself to enjoy that which is beautiful? Do you hinder the happiness of yourself and your fellow men? Afraid that if you give in the cannibals might eat you? In other words: that others might get power over you. You stick to a point of view that isn't sound. Perhaps you resist people you think are seizing or suppressing you. Angry resistance, also to those whom you suspect want to push you into a certain direction, while you don't want this at all.

Possibly, you think that deep inside you there's a little devil, something very bad; perhaps you think you have to suppress your feelings and your nature: your knee protests. Resistance to that which is new, to evolution; holding on to old patterns.

When you trust your nature, your emotional world, your intuition, your deepest divine Core — when you arrive at Insight into yourself and others — then you'll understand and will have the ability to love. Then you'll allow yourself to flexibly transform all your talents into creativity, to handle with mastery all your energies. Look deep inside yourself and let go of all that is superfluous; don't burden yourself with proud, stubborn thoughts, but for once dare to be good and gentle with yourself. If you collide with your own "I," with your own nature, then you will also collide with others. If your attitude is sharply aggressive, then you'll attract aggression. When you become aware of that Fundamentally strong, safe Basis in yourself, then from here on you will create your life yourself and will take on a flexible attitude regarding everything that is new on your path. A tense defensive attitude is no longer necessary if you only become aware of your potentialities, of your true worth. Placing authority within yourself means self-protection.

Obstinacy and Powerlessness disappear when you acknowledge all forces in yourself: bring your Self to realization, instead of blocking and wasting energies in exaggerated aggression toward others or by putting on a puffed-up Image.

Calmly go deep inside yourself; discover here that which is good, and radiate this goodness. Stop considering your disposition, your Nature, as something grayish or threatening: after all, because of this you have considered the whole world to be hostile and have taken a position against this. Deep in his core, every human being is good. Be open to that gentleness inside you. . . .

Swelling and pain in the knee
(See also Ailments, in general)

An enormous energy, often aggression, is being suppressed, and it asks for a breakthrough.

Outwardly you might appear self-possessed and Big, but inwardly you feel unsure, anxious.

Your emotional world has hardened because you put yourself into armor: you no longer allow yourself any gentleness. Inflexible and stubborn.

Enormous, stubborn anger — extreme resistance to something or someone — often lie at the basis of a swollen knee, but you keep these feelings inside! New energies, creativity, and longings want to flow, but are being stopped.

Often, an enormous potential of possibilities, but again and again they are being suppressed. . . .

Allow these enormous forces to come through: no longer resist the spontaneous, flexible flow of your feelings. When you are angry with someone, it only indicates your own powerlessness to bring yourself to realization.

Allow that natural aggression to escape; confront yourself with the cause of your aggression; Speak with your fellow men, no longer stubbornly bottle things up! Be open to your inner wisdom; feel the leadership in yourself; acknowledge your powers, your intuition, and live freely, without anxieties. Transform piled-up energies into Action, into creativity! Allow yourself to enjoy; no longer be so hard on yourself.

Meniscus
Ailments, deterioration, tears
(See also Knee, in general)

Possibly, you appear to the outer world as a dancing, foolish clown. Possibly, you puff out your chest to show who you are, but inwardly you are not aware enough of your own worth, and you unsurely bring yourself into question. This duality leads to an inner tension, sometimes to a sharp nervousness, but also to grimly holding on to certain things or people outside yourself (possibly to a partner) of which you don't want to let go under any circumstances. You place in others the power and the authority over your being because you don't acknowledge the authority in yourself as an independent value. Sometimes you'd punch, fight, and force yourself into all kind of twists, psychologically and physically, so that you hurt yourself! On the one hand, to please; on the other hand, to revolt against your own dependency. Your feelings and movements are influenced by your nervousness; too angular and too hurried, too sharp and tense; you no longer make any smooth, flowing movements, you are becoming too hard with yourself. One could compare these inner and outer movements to a saw, which, because it has sharp teeth, doesn't relent, and constantly makes the same movement, cuts at last through the piece of wood. In the same way you constantly suppress, or fold, your aggressive powers into the "demanded" direction in order to satisfy the expectations of the outer world, so that you destroy your own nature. Because of a lack of confidence in yourself ("Am I good, am I doing it right?") your inner sharp hurriedness leads to a chronic "sawing" in the knee. You are not at all flexible toward your nature anymore; you force things. Your knee only works smoothly if you "grease" it with relaxation, with flexibility toward yourself; if you, independent of the opinions of others, are faithful to your nature, in self-assurance, no longer doubting yourself.

If you get angry, then this is a result of doubt about yourself, of your feelings of powerlessness, of insufficient presence as a strong "I."

Do you live too much according to others? According to an audience? Do you let your "being good" and your "happiness" depend on the approval, or not, of the outer world? Do you experience yourself just superficially, without knowing your Content?

The Meniscus asks you to live from out of your Self, flexibly and with self-confidence, not for the eye of others. Discover your inner wealth and don't try to obtain confirmation or approval from others by forcing things or forcing yourself. Be faithful to your unique nature! Open yourself up in a relaxed way and give yourself freedom; surrender to your nature without resistance. Transform grimness and anger into the realization of your own wishes, without asking yourself what "they" might think of you. Don't live for the spotlights: listen to what you feel.

One can't "force" anything or anyone: let go. Just be yourself. The people who are in harmony with you will appear on your path if you don't block it by tensely wanting to hold on to something or someone. Trust will make you create your existence and attract in your life those things that are good for you; don't force anything.

KORSAKOFF'S SYNDROME

serious amnesia, often fabricating stories in order to hide this; mostly caused by Vitamin B₁ deficiency in alcoholics

You're not really present in yourself; you have no contact with your deepest Self; you have taken distance from yourself in a cold way. You don't know very well who you are; you don't really live Consciously.

You do play your external role in the world; you identify yourself strongly with this external part of yourself; perhaps you play your act in an authoritarian way (One has to do what you order one to do!); you might in a tough way forcefully push yourself outward, but in this way you become more and more estranged from yourself, from your own authority.

Your attitude is cool and supercilious — toward yourself. You might transmit that same coolness to others.

Here, we're actually dealing with a dividedness: you play a certain role because if you'd be yourself you'd feel totally lost, seized as you are by your emotional world and not at all able to get the least grip on it.

"I am the big one; you do what I say." This is the role in which you feel best, because you no longer know who you are anyway; you are like a zero who then takes on a strong role as compensation for his inner emptiness.

Sometimes, it's about anger, aggression toward yourself, and you identify yourself unconsciously with the attitude of a cold person from your environment. This person is only a reflection of yourself.

Make a few steps backward; don't push yourself further away from yourself; look closely in the mirror, into your heart: "Who am I?" Now come back, become one with your soul, with your gentle feelings.

Get a hold of the Core of your being; turn yourself toward your central feelings; dare to go very deep inside yourself; arrive at respect for your inner Mastery, and be honest with yourself!

Look for the true worth and characteristics of yourself, and stay very close to your core, without coolness, but with love.

Don't be angry with yourself, don't be supercilious toward yourself: you are unique and good the way you are now.

Now be flexible with yourself and others: you don't have to be Napoleon in order to be accepted! Bend toward yourself, with openheartedness.

L

LAUGHTER, CONVULSIVE, UNCONTROLLABLE

A relief valve for accumulated tensions, nervousness, energies, emotions.

A grateful and friendly backing; you fall back on this because you don't yet dare to really show or express yourself the way you feel inside.

You feel too much "tied down"; you have to curtail your energies and your nerves, especially when you are in the company of people who can somehow "tie you down or admonish you"! Emotional tension, a secret pleasure that has been held in for too long, an outlet for overcharged nerve tensions. A form of being unbalanced: you don't really manifest yourself, on the one hand, and when, on the other hand, this suppression becomes too much for you you perform a circus act. Also, when you don't know what to do anymore or when you look somewhere for "rescue," you let it all go. You don't get a hold anymore, because your Self-aware "I" isn't yet developed enough.

This can be a camouflage for inner feelings which are not at all cheerful, but in this way you still can manifest yourself strongly. You put on a show, and in that way you get attention from others, without having to expose yourself.

But most of the time it is just an expression of accumulated tensions, which are the consequence of not yet daring to really be yourself. A vivid imagination, which is not being kept under control by the "I," makes it worse.

Healthy self-realization, self-acceptance, releasing energies, calmly showing your nature, the way you feel, not piling up tensions and creative energies, not being secretive, but open; rest and calm inside yourself. Balance and self-confidence.

LEGS

Psychological correspondence

The ability, the power, to leave the past behind and to evolve ever onward, to go on to a new future which we create in a self-aware way. We don't allow ourselves to *be* carried; we know we are being carried by our living Self: that's why we endure adversity without difficulty, that's why we have no fear, that's why we dare to leave behind the needless emotional burdens from the past. The creative process of life is all movement; we joyfully take part in this, without resistance or standing still. We resolutely go on in life.

THIGHS

Psychological correspondence

Energies!!! Potential possibilities of power-development in yourself. The thighs represent primal power. Strong self-manifestation! Broadly, take up your space. There, where one's own fundamental energies —

creativity, productivity, personal "pressure-power," proud potentiality — are reflected. Symbolic of the ability to stretch — elasticity of the psyche: what do you and what don't you allow "to be" in your life?

Do you dare be intimate with yourself, with others, or do you shut out your deepest and most sensitive self? A loving embrace of the Power and the gentle Child in you.

The reflection of accumulated energies, of emotions from the past, or — Now, making use of your own energies.

Ailments, in general

An accumulation of unused energies! Do you suppress your wide range of creative and productive possibilities? Do you want "to jump into" something, to start something in Action, but don't see where and how? On the one hand, you are filled to the brim with potential powers and are very strong. Perhaps you might express this all verbally! But inwardly you feel "unable" and don't know *how* to express and use your energies. Suppression can lead to aggression, to powerless sadness. Did someone (or some system) determine your life with a lot of pressure? Did you suppress your energies for too long? In passiveness, in obedience, in self-doubt? The deeper cause always lies in yourself!

Possibly, you lived for a long time under a dominant system (or a structure, a person, etc.). Now, you want "to jump out," but you still hold on to that which is old, because you don't yet have a clear view on that which is new. But, inwardly, resistance grows: "I want to get out of here! I want to feel and experience MY powers."

Do you "narrow" your life, are you looking at the world with "blinders" on?

Attack! Bite into life with all your energies! ENLARGE YOUR SPACE; self-liberation.

Your energies turn, turn, turn — direct them according to your longings! Use them; handle them with mastery; direct them; don't hold on to them, but radiate them without hesitation and deal with your longings in an intuitive and active way. Nothing "has to be

done"; you are allowed to be productive in all the areas that you have kept dormant, in the spiritual as well as the physical sphere. If you wish to put your powers into singing, then sing; if into writing, then write; if into sexuality, then experience your body and your creative powers; if into bicycling, then bicycle, etc.

Acknowledge the Sun in yourself: your center of self-confidence and radiating warmth. Crawl deep into your most intimate Self, into your warm feelings, and feel safe there. Your power center is always there, even if you don't always realize it, and it constantly sends out enormous energy streams with which you can very powerfully Create your life in a Conscious way. Do it, and don't remain sitting, down-heartedly. Enlarge your space! Broad-mindedness, without prejudice.

Thighbone

Psychological correspondence

Solid, secure basic structure in your deepest Self. Solidity, and at the same time the flexibility to accommodate your own space: open-closed. Regulating your space: allowing, not allowing; this far and no further. . . . Are you well and solidly situated? Then you can go on. You can always count on your inner mechanism, which intuitively indicates how far you can go. Powerfully taking up your life-space, feeling protected in this security. Establishing yourself in life, manifesting.

Ailments, in general

With an exaggerated urge for self-manifestation, you go too far, in an aggressive way: "This is mine! Don't touch." This mostly happens when one experiences insufficient security in one's own Basis. Or, conversely, when there is suppression of one's own "I." Not knowing anymore. "How can I be self-reliant?" You feel inadequate, unsafe. You don't take up your space; you allow yourself to be pushed to the side by others. In this way, you are too much directed to outer values: "How do I appear?" Instead of basing yourself upon inner Power. Revolt against being "pushed away." Revolution!

You can depend completely on this deepest, inner basic power in yourself, this basic structure; it demands space for you, gives you solidity, and protects you. Calmly take up the space that belongs to you; don't get angry about it.

LOWER LEG, SHINBONE

Psychological correspondence

The ability to go on in life in a rhythmic way. With joy, you bear the fruits of your life: first of all, your body; or do you bear yourself like a burden?

Symbolic of mobility, maneuverability, of choosing your own path and then changing it again: this can mean your salvation. Wanting to achieve something, ambition, and taking the necessary steps toward this. Walking on your own! Or do you allow others to direct your life? Do you follow others? You can break through! Step over obstacles. Sustain efforts.

Symbolic of going on to more beautiful, more profound life-motivations. Overhastily going on or standing still in your development. You follow *this* way, which you decide in self-assuredness to take; kicking away, hurting others, or feeling hurt, attacked. Powerful pillars.

Ailments, in general

Do you feel seized by the neck, attacked? Do you allow yourself to be hurt? Do you not allow yourself supple movements? Do you lock yourself up in a space that is too small, literally and psychologically? Rest rusts! Are you standing still? Do you refuse to evolve or to let go of the past so you can grow toward a new future? Possibly, you carry enormous burdens, needlessly. Perhaps you direct yourself too much toward achievements or toward material things, and

you are not truly advancing toward spiritual enrichment. You don't feel stable: "I'm only made out of wood. . . . I'm afraid of others, and I don't trust my own supporting basis." You experience your sunny "I-center" as a threat; you hide behind others and refuse to powerfully stand up Straight yourself. You withdraw into yourself and don't dare manifest yourself.

Desperately doubting: "Which way shall I go?" Resistance against authority: "Go away! I will determine my own path!" In the meantime, you're not so sure. . . . Aggressive attack upon others, because of fear, of feelings of being threatened; frustration.

Push back your frontiers; dare to explore space, in all directions — the cosmos! "I AM": then you don't have to defend yourself. No one will attack you or can hurt you if you are aware of your strength, of the fact that you are always protected in your Self. Calmly building up your future at your own tempo. Don't suppress your longings and ambitions. Follow your intuition, trust your deepest Self, be faithful to that which is in harmony with your true nature! Be straightforward, in positive anticipation. Don't let yourself be distracted from your path by futilities. Don't attack others; realize yourself powerfully! It's not outer authority that hinders you from truly living, but it's your denial of your inner Possibilities. Bear life joyfully and throw off the needless burden of the past.

Calf muscle
(See also Muscles, in general)

Ailments, in general

You are rigid, and you look too much in *one* direction: whether it's about fixation on a material or an emotional problem, on a job or an ambition. In unmovable stubbornness, you refuse to listen to your inner voice, to your nature. You don't truly evolve; you stay in the same place. You force yourself; you cling to something; the happiness of life doesn't seem to exist for you anymore because you hold on tensely to. . . . You should be joyfully walking and jumping, dancing and singing; you should be rolling around in the grass and playing, like the eternal, spontaneous child in you — but you don't allow joy into your life, no supple evolution. You feel overburdened, sad. Sometimes, you can go so far that you become blocked by biting irony, hardness, or bitterness. You don't allow supple transformation in yourself; you make your joy depend on facts and people outside you, instead of autonomously moving on in a direction of ever greater happiness about life itself. You hinder yourself from truly enjoying. Do you believe so little in yourself, in Life? Do you direct yourself toward anxiety and death, mistrusting your nature? Do you live with prejudices, with blinders on, so that you hinder yourself from truly going onward in life? Are you demanding too much from yourself?

Direct yourself, without prejudice, in all directions; don't limit yourself in life. Softening. Come to a supple versatility; unburden yourself of sorrow and tensions! Live freely, and in a self-aware way create your optimistic future: don't stand still. Don't sink your teeth into sad things: it's your sad convictions about life that cause this sorrow. Let go of everything and everyone. Resolutely choose a new, happy life-course. Don't allow your life to be dominated by false values and false sadness (materialism, achievements). Don't force your nature, neither to satisfy others. Open your heart: let go of all the hardness aimed at yourself, aimed at life.

LEPROSY

You withdraw from life; you refuse to exist any longer in these circumstances.

You Don't want to be; you degenerate. You simply don't let life come through anymore.

A feeling of being a victim of circumstances and unable to change anything about it.

You become "spiritualized"; you withdraw into a more spiritual state of being instead of being present, physically, here and now, with your feet on the ground.

You don't see life as being worthwhile; condemning yourself as a worthless being, powerless. "We poor people — confronting an overwhelming fate, or one or another god or idol." By your negative, fatalistic convictions, you've already put a noose around your neck: you already feel doomed to become ill.

"We're not able to Live and be resistant to contamination": a strong belief in one's own powerlessness, but also in your "Body's inferiority in the flesh."

Come to loving acknowledgment of your body: in "matter."

No one is "just" born somewhere by coincidence: environment and circumstances are a reflection of the unconscious dominating convictions in every human being. Via confrontation with this mirror, it is possible to become aware of this.

This becoming aware is the only way to positive evolution of all of mankind. The world grows from within, from out of the hidden dimension, the world soul, the soul of mankind: we can influence this growth in a positive way if we look inside ourselves and from here reprogram ourselves and the world. Physical reality will change when we change our convictions, our philosophies, our thoughts. After all, we create our world with our Awareness-powers. There's no god who will rescue the world: we'll have to take on this responsibility ourselves. This can only happen if we acknowledge the divine, creative powers in ourselves, if we dare to acknowledge the Worth of our existence in a Self-aware way.

A break with rooted philosophies which consider sorrow and illness in the world an unavoidable drama!

A radical change by which we acknowledge life thankfully: we cast away the idea that we might be powerless and victims.

It is necessary that we acknowledge the value of our Awareness AND of our Body: the power of the spirit directs the body. Our body is not "just" there: it offers us the possibility of growing in interaction with the propelling power of our deepest Self, developing an ever-stronger creative power. The world is asleep and in the grip of false and Neptunian theories that are unworthy of humans: this is the insanity which reigns in mankind. It's the fact that the Human Being neglects his possibilities and keeps on solving SYMPTOMS instead of pulling out the roots, instead of attacking the causes, in order to arrive at a definitive solution. The conviction that ruin will come leads to ruin.

Belief in one's own worth and in the possibility of (from now on) "deserving" positive evolution will reward you. Illness that is being experienced by the masses asks for reprogramming of the masses.

(See also Part I: Infection, Contamination.)

LEUKEMIA

You are estranged from your own nature. What are you hiding behind? Behind your father or your mother? Behind a limited part of yourself in which you function very well? You don't take up any responsibility for your life.

Just like a "marriage of convenience," made because of social class or religion, you live in an understanding with yourself: Where is that originality of yours? Why do you hide behind dark glasses? Now, take a good look at your Self.

You degrade yourself to being only a Part: you keep yourself squeezed in a pair of pliers, so to speak.

Your creativity! Your original impulses! Your spontaneous natural power! Where did this go? Why don't you live life to the fullest? Cut off from your deepest basis, from your Living Self! A false situation, a factitious, unauthentic, unreal situation; perhaps you also live with a certain person in such a "relationship of convenience," or with a certain religion, or authority.

Artificial, like a little dog that has been fashionably trimmed: you allow yourself to "be lived" instead of, from moment to moment, choosing in favor of your breath-of-life.

There is a blank spot, as it were, in your life — a large hole. Because of passiveness? Or do you think Life and your being are not Worth living? You lower yourself; perhaps you live like a machine, and you look upon life as all "possessing or having," and the rest doesn't interest you.

Deeper contact with your true nature is gone. What sense does life have anymore if you're not involved in it?

Come close to yourself, to your original nature: there lies joy. Come out of the shadow, MANIFEST YOURSELF: you!

A break with falsehood, with appearances, with facade, and with having only half a life.

A total break with the past: throw out what you are hiding behind. Distance yourself from those with whom you, for some reason, have an unnatural psychological tie. Heed your Natural disposition, your spontaneous ideas and longings: live according to them!

Return to nature in every way; be born, now, in your Self and take distance from indoctrination by your mentors. Lifelines that are not created by yourself lead to estrangement from yourself, so that at last your spontaneous life-urge will also disappear. Don't live off others, nor live on only a small part of yourself, but break through! Burn up that lifeless personage from the past and grow now, from your own roots, independent, and ready to accept happiness.

In all honesty, confront yourself with your own deepest core: dare to manifest yourself the way YOU ARE, one hundred per cent.

It is possible that regarding children with leukemia, the parents, too, need to solve the above-mentioned psychological problems in themselves. Radically choose true, ORIGINAL life.

LIPS

Ailments, in general, symbolism

Do you close yourself off from others, or do you cordially open yourself up to them? Do you close yourself off from your intuition, from your natural feelings, or do you actually allow yourself to be dominated by the sensual, by unconscious anxieties?

Are you stubborn, willful, obstinately closed, too critical — or do you actually feel weak, limp, and unsure? Do you close yourself off from natural gentleness, or do you sink into weakness?

Unconscious, primitive emotions (anxieties, aggression, etc.) are reflected in this sensory organ: Do you insufficiently trust in your intuitive channels, and are you constantly on guard, alert, testing, with your ears up like a guard dog?

Do you not dare to say all the things you feel or think? Do you press your lips together? Are you angry but don't dare to speak? Refusal? Revolt? Anger? Either you swallow your criticism of others, or you throw kisses and compliments in all possible directions — passing yourself over. Where are you? Do you just chatter away to others instead of *doing* things yourself, evolving yourself? Do you not dare trust in your own feelings? Do you think they form a threat to you? Are you afraid of sensuality? Or do you fix yourself — by means of a suction power, as it were — into affection, into the

flesh, into others, without wanting to live independently any longer, without letting go because you insufficiently believe in yourself?

Investigative, alert, critical behavior is good as long as it does not degenerate into mistrust.

Know yourself to be safe in yourself; don't separate yourself critically or stubbornly from others: this only indicates unsureness. Don't spread yourself too thin: concentrate in yourself. First bring order to your private domain; protect yourself. Trust in your deepest Self and dare to reveal your true nature; say what you have to say; don't keep your mouth tightly closed.

Offer your love, your affection, without forcing. Achieve autonomy and, without putting up obstacles, allow your feelings to flow freely. Self-awarely and intuitively explore your path!

Offer with your heart; speak from out of your heart and don't GIVE as compensation for a lack of Self-love. Dare to trust your feelings and go adventuring; be open to new things in your life.

Be honest: let words and deeds merge.

Don't be silent when you feel you have to speak. But know that the cause of anger lies in yourself! You can speak out, but expect nothing, demand nothing, from others.

Be faithful to your nature; don't suppress your feelings.

Cracked lips, chapping

There's a crack in you, as it were, a split: on the one hand, experiencing the here-and-now and, on the other hand, your thought world in which you hide. Thoughts, imaginations, fantasies, reveries about the past, daydreams — instead of actual creativity. You develop an enormous amount of energy, also aggressive powers, but you don't do anything with them; energies flit past your brain too much; you don't really live with your soul and body in the here-and-now. It seems as if you are outside your body, as if you are observing your own body from out of your high thinking-tower. You hide in this tower, because you are on your guard against others, who can hurt you.

You don't really trust life, you think that others are about to hurt you; you are ready, in a defensive posture, with a knife under your pillow. You don't really dare to come forward in life, here-and-now. You feel too weak, too distrustful, to step into life with deeds, with your body. Either you hide in romantic, dreamy, nostalgic thoughts, or you blow up the negativity in your thoughts — thoughts that have to do with sorrow, with illness and death — as if in this way you can keep the "darkness" out of your life. An illusory life in an unreal world. In the meantime, aggressive powers are asking for a breakthrough, but you check yourself, which can lead to hardness, to aggressiveness that is too sharp ("Watch out or I shoot!"), to angry nervous thoughts, to nervousness because of the inability to realize yourself. When you are unsatisfied with yourself, or when you think yourself ugly, then you can create in your imagination a more ideal reality, but this only leads to frustration when you land again with your feet on the ground.

Accept yourself, love yourself as an unique being with unique characteristics; don't measure yourself according to the norms of others, but just be yourself, here-and-now. A balance between the spiritual and the earthly is necessary: become one with yourself. Create your dream world for yourself in reality. Don't flee from yourself; allow aggressive, creative powers to flow through, and handle them with mastery.

Express yourself, say what you have to say, don't hide, even if you are angry; resolve the distrust in yourself. Don't dream about the sensual, but enjoy, in reality.

Come with both feet on the ground and don't live in the future, nor in the past. Don't dream about Love, but develop it in actuality in yourself and toward others.

Cherish your body, don't run away from it. Seek peaceful contact with others, so that you don't have to look for it only in dreams. No longer push yourself away; in this way you will no longer be on your guard with others. Close the gap in yourself; then you will be closer to others.

LIPOMAS
benign tumors of fatty tissue

Fundamental anxieties and feelings of insecurity lie at the basis here. You think you have to safeguard and protect yourself against a supposed danger. Often, the growth of a lipoma comes to be after an emotional shock is received. You feel hurt; inside you it brews and ferments with emotional experiences that you can't let go of. Emotionally, you are knotted up with yourself, and you are afraid that at any moment you will be overpowered by something or someone outside you: anxiously, you lock yourself up inside yourself. You don't really live in reality, here-and-now: you live too much in thoughts, in "spirit." You don't trust the ground beneath your feet; you don't trust the life-processes, so as a result you try to force certain things or try to keep them straight — things it would have been better to let go. Possibly, you cling to an outer affirmation, to matter; but here, also, you are afraid of being pushed off your pedestal or of coming out as a loser. You are most afraid of the emotional powers in yourself, because you don't really use them in original creativity, because you prefer to keep the lid on this jar.

Place yourself in the center of your existence! Let go, feel open and free: unburden yourself in trust. You are protected by Nature unless you convince yourself of the contrary. You don't have to safeguard yourself at all; give yourself over to the now-moment, to those spontaneous powers in yourself. Anxieties block joyful existence. (See further under the subject Anxiety)

THE LIVER

Psychological correspondence

The liver stands for the Power of a human being who becomes Master over his unconscious content, over his emotions, by trusting the transformation processes. *Actively building a peaceful existence.*

The liver stands for *Faith* and *Trust* in our Self, for our *critical digestion of our experiences.* This Faith, this security in the living Self, drives away all anxieties, all destructive aggression.

The liver receives and purifies the blood; it has a detoxifying function.

In the metabolism process, nutritive substances are transformed into useful elements for the body. Absorption, digestion and breakdown, purification and excretion.

The liver represents, therefore, the constant psychological transformation process: the transformation and digestion of new experiences and emotions toward Growth, toward spiritual Evolution, on the basis of the already present unconscious content.

The blood — symbolic of light, joyful, divine warmth — changes constantly under the influence of our psyche. The liver shows us to what degree, under the authority of our deepest Self, we smoothly digest and *purify* our primitive emotions and burdensome feelings — *employing them as new building stones in order to restore harmony in the house of our Self, and to place it in the light of joy.*

A symbol for the *illumination and observation* (on the basis of unconscious convictions that dwell inside us) of our experiences. In accord with these convictions, received impressions either will or will not be assimilated in us in a relaxed way. Arriving at insight will then lead *to understanding and to letting go.*

Symbolic of: *giving yourself the chance to grow toward joy, peace, and cheerfulness.* For this, it is necessary to be psychologically open, to have trust in your Self, and to "let go." Joyful labor in life; *"burning" to unselfishly build up something beautiful for yourself and for others. In the awareness of your worth and possibilities, taking care of your tasks with pleasure.* Seeing to it that everything will go beautifully and smoothly, with love. *Utilizing energies in productivity;* calmly *letting go* of things that had better play no part in your life anymore because they would slow you down in your growth!

Powerful, dynamic energy-production: don't put a check on your energy flow!

Ailments, in general

You suppress your powers, your emotions, your productive energies.

Deep anxieties, anger, because of your feeling of incapability, of standing still. Black thoughts. Possibly, you flee into unreal spheres that are too "spiritual" (See also Alcoholism; Epiphysis, working too strongly). You don't trust in your own light, divine source, and as a result you "hold on" to certain people and situations. In this way, anxiously despairing about life, you cut yourself off from your deepest Self. These anxieties are a signal from your living Self, indicating that you are on the wrong track; turn away from death and come to life.

You retain emotions. Fury, hatred, vengeance. You don't come to terms with the past — so much so that you are poisoning yourself. You suffocate in your own stool.

You seem unable to get a grip on compulsive actions, thoughts, or feelings; you want to get out, but you can't as long as you don't trust yourself, your nature, as long as you don't self-assuredly become master over your unconscious content.

Pent-up aggression; approaching others with an angry and threatening look; in this way, you try to get rid of your feeling of imprisonment. Possibly, Content that has been smoldering for too long explodes in fury from time to time. Or do you keep bottling everything up inside?

Softening, trust. Come into action, creativity, into dynamic self-development instead of bottling up all your energies and emotions. Criticism of others only hinders you from truly evolving yourself. Transform everything in your life into something beautiful and peaceful; enjoy that which is natural, the sun, life. Look at everything in a much lighter way, from out of your deepest Self; actively build a new life, with joyful, optimistic energies. Release, let go. You've unconsciously called up all happenings in your life. Now allow evolution and go on! You can permit a new turn in your life. This is not possible if you don't first of all let go of the old, of the feelings in which you have immobilized yourself. Now, direct yourself deeply inward, not outward, and look at your anxieties, your anger. Which destructive convictions lie here at the basis? You are not powerless. You are not "in the grip of—" Become master over yourself, grow in gentleness, in love and peace, toward yourself.

Abscess of the liver

Emotional overburdening: mortal fear, pain, anger. Here, suffering leads to aggression.

You daydream; you aren't "really" here and now. Your thoughts are heavy and dark: you are full of mental worries, your head burns from it. You don't take any Action! You don't digest the past, you're not really going forward because you absolutely want to maintain something, to hold on to something; you refuse to go on. Cramped, tense, tied down. . . . Anxiously, you cling to something because you feel unable to do it on your own. . . . Too much "spirit," too little Here.

Self-destruction: you allow unpleasant and unconscious spheres to dominate you.

Come to clear Insight: look closely at where you will go. Stop brooding and daydreaming: self-aware Action! Fight for your ideals of life and don't occupy yourself with death. Work out your sadness and live in the moment of now, in a joyful, intense way; create your own future now; no longer allow yourself to be carried along by unconscious negative convictions. Transform yourself into a powerful fighter for Life, autonomous, master of your emotional world. Unhesitatingly, let go of dark, painful memories from the past by understanding how you, yourself, have attracted these happenings because you considered yourself powerless. Replace this self-poisoning with love and gentleness.

Cancer of the liver
(See also Cancer, in general)

Despondent; you don't see a way out. You can't handle it anymore, you give up.

Sadness, fundamental anxieties.

You cling to something or someone because of fear of losing.

You have too much directed your attention, your criticism, at others; you have filled your life with others instead of actually realizing your life yourself! You don't feel very worthy; you lean on others because you think that without them you can't live. In order to not have to realize yourself, you'd even "worm your way in" into other people's lives, would meddle, would make yourself angry at them — while you, yourself, are burning because you refuse to evolve.

Here, cancer asks for a total transformation, but you resist changing! Rather die than change — or not?

Because you don't realize your own worth, because you don't allow yourself to grow and create, in joy, you'll unconsciously attract people who are a reflection of these negative thoughts regarding yourself: they will cause you the sadness you asked for. Don't blame them, but change your life!

Review everything — come toward honest, open Insight into yourself, into the (above mentioned) causes of your illness. Put your helm over; become aware of your Worth as a human being; allow new life energies ,which also will destroy cancer. Self-respect, love, joy, humor, and putting things in perspective!

Cirrhosis of the liver

Words are being kept in, a natural spontaneity being suppressed: you put a damper on your life. Joy and enthusiasm are being strangled by Prohibition or routine, by Commandments and Rules that you place upon yourself.

Anxiety and belief in death, mistrust regarding your own nature; you feel so unsafe because you insufficiently believe in your own solid Basis.

You experience yourself as an insignificant pawn in the mass-happening; you don't stand up for your rights and your space as an individual. "What meaning does my existence have?" You let yourself droop.

You forbid yourself from living powerfully and inventively! You don't allow Love into your life! Why are you so hard, perhaps even embittered and angry? You have a difficult time letting go of sad occurrences from the past. You don't allow yourself to enjoy all earthly things: suppression of a part of yourself can lead to exaggeration — for example, to alcohol abuse. You're not enough aware of your Worth and possibilities. You feel the earth shaking, as it were, under your feet: anxiety and lack of self-acknowledgment give way to alcohol (possibly). You'd like to hide: because of fear and unsureness, you don't really dare to reveal the way you feel. You allow yourself to be sadly sucked into a dark hole.

You shut yourself out! You refuse to let cheerful life energies flow; you flee — passivity, disintegration of the "I," not believing in yourself. You become more "spirit" than human.

Burst out of your house, which is too closed up, and accentuate your freedom and your Worth! A radical turnabout: acknowledging your "I," pushing back your frontiers, manifesting yourself. Action! Break through with your very personal nature and give to yourself what you deserve: all Love, attention, and a large living-space. Free yourself from the habits of the past, and say goodbye to the useless emotional burdens that hinder you from truly living, enjoying. Give yourself all individual rights; sit solidly upon the basis of your deepest Self; trust in this fundamentally strong creative Source in yourself, and take your life in your hands in a self-aware way. Anxieties disappear if you realize how you can create your life yourself, and also realize that death as a destiny doesn't exist. Bulldoze your old, sad, fatalistic lifestyle, and begin your life Anew! Your body and your liver will regenerate via the magnetic powers that are ignited in your Self by the influence of the positive impulse of feelings such as Love, Joy, and by faith in yourself!

Hepatitis A

Something weighs on you enormously: it keeps haunting you. Piled-up emotions now overflow. . . .

Anxiety, sadness, anger — now you flee from an unbearable situation. In fact, you are fleeing from yourself; you can't handle certain things anymore; instead of bringing about Changes, you refuse to listen anymore! Were you once sharp, aggressive, fully convinced of masculine self-manifestation? And do you still feel those powerful, turning energies inside you? But — Are the brakes now being put on you, and do you feel overcome by feelings of guilt? "Did I do it right?" Is it a matter of a sort of contradiction in yourself? "Was I a sly fox with shady behavior, or am I a good human being?" You are afraid that "they" will also point it out to you because you already have condemned yourself. Inner shame.

Did you ignite a fire, and do you run away from it now? You experience yourself as being stuck in a certain pattern, seized by a person or a structure, and you want to get out of it.

You'd like to roar like a proud lion, but you are not sure if you are on the "right" track: "Who AM "I" really?" Sadness, doubts, feelings of helplessness, sometimes a feeling of being irretrievably lost, the victim of. . . . Suppressed aggressive powers.

You would run away from yourself, from the past; you begin to see reality only through "limited" glasses. Everything seems too heavy to you; you can't put things in perspective anymore!

You blow small details up into feelings of guilt and into self-doubt. Ultimately, everything weighs too heavily on you; now you feel small and alone, at the mercy of. . . .

Your previous aggressive courage transforms itself into sadness and powerlessness. All you feel is that you are like a butterfly caught in a net.

Too much tension piles up — especially your unresolved feelings — and forces you now to isolate yourself, to rest, and to reach self-contemplation. This is just what you need so badly.

You are confused and you can't get a clear picture of the truth; imprisoned in the grasp of self-doubt, self-condemnation, frustration, and detrimental self-questioning about your person.

The rational aspect is being too much influenced by your feelings. Possibly, you are ashamed about certain things from the past; you'd now like to withdraw. Yellow shame (feelings of guilt).

Translate your aggression into resolute action, into transformation: bring about change where necessary. Reap the harvest you have sown: resolve things, and don't keep walking around with unresolved problems.

Pick up the pitchfork and take hold of the straw! Never condemn your experiences from the past as "bad": consider every phase of the past as a necessary step in your evolution and let go of everything.

Give yourself the blessing of beginning with new courage: do good; give love to yourself and to others. All sadness, anger, and feelings of guilt can disappear.

For once, illuminate everything clearly, from the right direction, and arrive at a perspective; make your decisions and direct your energies onward in full force, no longer standing still in the past.

Everyone learns from his lessons; now build a plan or structure in a balanced way and come out of your confusion. Make a clean sweep and go onward in full force! Joy and optimism about the future.

Look at yourself as a positive, creative human being, no matter how others or the small voice inside you have deluded you. No longer allow yourself to be "stuck." Free yourself. At last, by letting go of your emotional burdens, arrive at Rest in yourself: confront yourself with this; resolutely bring about the needed changes. Don't flee.

Hepatitis B

Anger, because of your own powerlessness, because of being stuck, because of your own inability to evolve. Deep anxieties, often amplified by the anxieties you've sucked in with your mentor; you still are reacting to experiences and influences from your childhood years, or from the recent past. Hatred and fury because of your own attachment, because of not being able to be "yourself." You'd like to blast yourself loose with the aggression of a cannon shot; you might shoot someone dead. . . . Twisted, self-poisoning feelings. The virus lives instead of YOU, yourself.

Anxieties, threatening clouds above your head, will smother you — you shiver, and you bend yourself into all possible angles, but you don't *really* live from out of yourself. You don't get a grip on these anxieties. You carry a heavy load of emotions, memories, influences from the past: your own identity now must grow up; strange anxieties and emotions from the past need to be worked out and purified so that you'll know who YOU are, so that this body becomes your body. No longer be the personification of anxiety-sadness-anger from the past: release yourself from that which is false and arrive at your pure "I."

Angry and shut off: in this way you can't get a clear perspective on yourself.

Do you perhaps cling to "earthly treasures," to material things, to money, or to outer status? In this way, you won't find yourself. A requirement to come to complete transformation: higher awareness-energies wish to come through; your deepest Self asks for self-contemplation and acknowledgment, but you anxiously hold on to the old; you refuse to let go and explore your own deep "I." You flee outside yourself.

The virus and the symptoms it causes, form an extremely essential escape valve for your deadly emotions: in this way, you now can survive. Listen to this language of your deepest Self, and don't hold back change; your snail-pace, sticky and slow, may transform itself into powerful progress! Be faithful to your divine Self. Don't sink your teeth into false values. Dare to observe your feelings of anxiety, hatred, and powerlessness; work them out, let go. Stay within your limits, build a safe structure, yourself, and pay attention to the gentleness in you: open your smallest veins up wide, and breathe in freedom. Detach yourself from oppressing thoughts and emotions; let go of whatever or whomever does not fit your true nature. Come to life! Allow joy to propel your blood in a direction where there's room for Love; look closely at your SELF, feel the powers in you, and self-create your life — lighter!

Know *that you, yourself, have attracted every situation in the past, be it unconsciously, because your Living Self-Core wants you to arrive at the insight that there are dark emotions dwelling inside you which ask for a definitive cleansing. Don't angrily*

blame anything on someone else, but always ask yourself the question: "Why" do I again attract this? ***What*** *do I need to change, to solve in myself, so that my life becomes complete joy and light, so that I only encounter happy situations? Let go, in thankfulness! Turn yourself deeply inward. Believe in your goodness, your power — and go on without demands, desires, resentment, etc. A light, happy existence!*

LUMBAGO

Insufficient faith in yourself; an absence, a *No:* you don't really take up your full space. A refusal to acknowledge yourself completely; a refusal to be.

Enormous energies, beautiful powers, natural feelings — all are pushing to the fore and asking for a breakthrough; you are holding yourself back.

You force yourself, absolutely wanting to look in another direction; you are violating your nature: you are carrying enormous, useless burdens because you aren't actively manifesting yourself from out of your own self-assuredness.

You insufficiently concentrate yourself within yourself; you allow yourself to be overpowered by emotions instead of resolutely taking hold of your energies and using them.

You dream, and perhaps fly far away with your thoughts, but inwardly an unsureness gnaws at you. Beautiful consciousness-energies, creative powers, like pure organ tones, push ever harder and ask for liberation. It is as if you refuse to allow fruits to grow.

Do you so much doubt your own worth? Do you feel so unsafe in your own nature? Do you think you have to be a victim? You refuse to accept your beauty, and rather than acknowledging your feelings and possibilities you put them under a glass cover.

You sag under these energy burdens, under this self-doubt.

You tensely force yourself to keep on standing; you tighten up yourself in anxious insecurity, with no more flexibility left. You might aggressively defend yourself — against everyone who attacks you, or against supposed danger, because you feel threatened. You don't feel really protected in your deepest Self. Because you feel so small, you exist chiefly insofar as others notice you.

You are like a child who asks for attention. You want to please others, to be noticed or acknowledged; you cling so much because you ignore your own autonomous worth. In your feeling of powerlessness, your outer image plays a role: after all, you don't really live from out of your heart, from out of your spontaneous emotional world, but you would rather observe the reaction of others to you. In this way, you begin to force yourself and start doing things that are too taxing on you — an estrangement from yourself.

By demanding attention, or by your provocative attitude, you can manipulate others, "seizing" them, and placing them in your power.

Acknowledge your self-worth, come to self-respect! Lift yourself up in self-assuredness, and build your life on your own solid Basis. Without worrying any longer about what others think of you: discover your powers, look at your feelings and let them flow through freely; feel your masculine solidity, your fruitful productivity. Place in yourself all power over your life. Be faithful to your nature, live in harmony with yourself, don't force yourself — so that you don't carry needless burdens. Active self-realization without hesitation! Don't let yourself be overwhelmed by feelings and powers, but seize them, realize yourself here and now. Don't flee. Concentrate yourself in sureness. Feel safe and protected within your deepest Self, independent of others. Self-create your life and know that nothing "just happens" by accident.

LUPUS ERYTHEMATOSUS, SLE

autoimmune disease with a great variability of symptoms from person to person (possibly involving the skin, joints, muscles, kidneys, nervous system)

You wish to die because of the fear of having to live. You can't handle it all anymore; you feel full of sadness.

Fear of pain, fear that others might skin you, torture you! Frantic, a plea to others: "Please leave me alone, don't hurt me!" In fact, behind this hides the fear of death: a feeling of not being safe anywhere, not in death, and not in life.

Powerless aggression demands a well-determined attitude from others. Unconsciously, you even think you don't have the right to a peaceful life: you feel guilty, although you don't really know why. You deny your worth as a human being.

As long as you remain convinced that you are bad or guilty, that you deserve punishment or will be tortured by others, you'll call up situations in your surroundings which will, indeed, correspond to your convictions.

Look at that small baby deep inside you: no longer push it away, integrate it in yourself, look at it. "Why is it crying?" Don't flee from this sadness, but bring it to the surface. Dare to look at your own nakedness, allow your feelings to come free; don't run away from yourself, don't run away from life: death doesn't offer a solution. Here and now, through honest confrontation with your deepest feelings, you will ultimately end up at your inner wisdom, and you will look at everything in a different way. You will discover that fundamentally strong Basis of your deepest Self, that immortal guarantee, the possibility to *self*-create your life: change your expectations of life in a positive way, and you will discover that joyful power of life in yourself and will lead a totally different life. In love and freedom, self-aware and joyful.

Acknowledge your unique Worth. It is you who condemns your body of flesh and blood: welcome it lovingly!

LYMPHATIC SYSTEM

Ailments, in general; causes

The deepest cause of a dislocated lymphatic system lies in not acknowledging oneself as a Unity: spiritual awareness-body. Several possibilities here:

Unbalanced in the "spiritual" area — you live in unreal spiritual realms, in a mist, with your head in the clouds, allowing yourself to be taken up by Neptunian spheres, by unconscious influences.

Thus, you lose all sense of reality here-and-now; you insufficiently feel the ground beneath your feet. You lose contact with the earth; you live in other dimensions. You are insufficiently present in your body in a conscious way: you consider memories more important; you float in the barrel of your unconscious being; you are "being lived" by associative emotional processes; you float.

Perhaps you do yoga and think you possess wisdom, but you are so fragile and transparent that one could walk right over you. You don't have a "grip" on life.

You go beyond all limits; all individual demarcations and every awareness of structure, of time-and-space, have disappeared.

Anxiety, doubts, mistrust. You don't believe in your health: you might keep yourself ill because of your negative thoughts, because of imaginary nonsense, because of hallucinatory self-deception. You are constantly in a defensive posture without reason.

Suspicion and mistrust: you'd sooner see the bad in everything, even in things that are very good. Your interpretations rest upon the

negativity that you experience in yourself: you don't have both feet on the ground; you don't know anymore what's true or untrue — all because you don't have a perspective on your Self! You live too "spiritually," too much estranged from the earth, from your body. You mistrust your own Nature! You are not sufficiently a Human Being of flesh and blood; you don't really assume your earthly task and your responsibility because you make your thoughts sick! As if you reverse the story of the Creation of yourself: you go back to your source of existence, to your original state of awareness instead of evolving toward a greater Individuality — an autonomous "I."

The reverse is also possible: an imbalance in the area of the physical. An exaggerated life of sexual passion, tense and unexpressed; strong desires, bunched-up lusts. Unsatisfied, wanting to possess ever more. The cause of this is insufficient awareness of one's own Worth as a human being, an imbalance in the relationship of conscious-unconscious, male-female. This is because you insufficiently believe in the power of your creative "I"-awareness; because you leave these enormous creative energies lying blank; because you don't allow yourself to transform in the Light of your Heart and your Self-aware spirit.

Solution of ailments and the psychological meaning of the Lymphatic System

Bring structure into every level: pure, beautiful straight structure, under the Authority of spiritual Awareness.

Get a grip on yourself through Insight; shape your existence into a concrete form. This also means: making your life *whole,* bringing it again to Unity, specifically the soul and the body not being separate from each other; a body nourished by the spirit; your Consciousness governing every cell of your body; a beautiful merging of heaven and earth, of your earthly dimension and your original spiritual womb, your deepest Self.

Be a unified, straightforward human being; don't cut yourself into pieces. Get everything under control, lead everything along good lines, bring everything to its rightful place, finish it off, round it off — and dispose of the excess.

Here, the psychological symbolism of the lymphatic system becomes clear; a balance is reached in every human being who, on the one hand, allows himself to be guided by the Authority of his Conscious spirit, but on the other hand stands solidly with his feet on the Earth. Immunity of the earthly body by being completely tuned in to our deepest Self. Calmly stand in the middle, between heaven and earth, as it were, and in this Center of your Self be aware of your worth, of your divine Power. This awareness of autonomy is Immunity, Itself.

Superfluous emotions will be worked out and disposed of; we don't have to brace ourselves anxiously in order to defend ourselves: Faith, Knowledge of this divine nature of the human being form an impenetrable protective shield.

The lymphatic system demands that we be open to our Awareness, to the signals of the Living Self. If, however, we don't trust our deepest nature, the lymphatic system will become overburdened, even will refuse to function. If we close ourselves off from the Consciousness that directs our lymph, if we're exclusively directed at material things, superficiality, or loveless sex — at possessing instead of giving — if we ignore our true worth, then the lymphatic system will become overburdened. Anxiety blocks healthy drainage, needlessly burdens the defense mechanism.

Love and trust in our deepest Core stimulate a smooth digestion and excretion of metabolic waste matter (of emotional experiences) via the lymph system; also, antibodies are formed in a calm way in the lymph to protect the body against foreign intruders.

Thus, if we live too strongly in the spirit and not enough with our feet on the earth, if we allow our lives to be dominated by inauthentic spheres or by dream realms — with anxiety and mistrust as the consequence — then the lymph reacts to "false" signals from our head. There's nothing at all to be defended; this has to do with anxious self-delusion, a battle against ghosts! But the lymph will react to this situation in an extremely intense way by overworking or else by a work-stoppage. . . .

Healthy functioning of the lymph requires that we be close to our nature, that we produce earthly fruits via creativity, that we cultivate grape vines so that later we can pick the grapes from them: balanced growth of our life, the unity of body and Consciousness in incarnation.

Just as the lymphatic system controls and regulates, cleans and critically defends, so should we acquire a clear perspective on ourselves, not dwelling on the sadness of yesterday, but believing in a fruitful future.

Transforming via the processing of our emotional experiences. Feeling yourself taken up lovingly and warmly in the midst of your vineyard and, if necessary: REORGANIZE all your ideas, your framework, your way of life, your functioning. RECONSIDER your life; a tabula rasa, in order to be born again. Inner worth and earthly joy harmoniously converging.

Lymph node swellings, in general
(See also Armpit, Groin, Neck)

Emotionally holding on to things; you don't digest things; you refuse to direct your life in a Self-aware way and to trust your intuition. . . . You stand still. . . .

You don't make any progress, no matter how hard you try, because you are emotionally stuck.

You are being blocked by inner contradictory feelings; you think and fret a lot, but you float in the air; you try to get a grip on a situation, but by doing this you smother yourself. You don't give yourself any room to breathe anymore! You fixate on something; you Want absolutely *that* in just that way: let it go! Energies wish to come through, aggressive powers are being suppressed.

Your stomach no longer digests your emotions, you feel uncomfortably stuck.

Let go of your anxieties, no longer fix your thoughts always on the same problems, surrender in Trust to your deepest, intuitive inner Self, and let go now of everything unto your utmost depths! If you completely surrender to your Self, everything will be arranged for you; express your longings, but don't fixate on something that, perhaps, is not at all good for you now. Everything at the right moment — your deepest Self knows this. Don't be afraid, trust in this inner, divine mechanism that enables you to create your life yourself, but which at the same time protects you from missteps that later on could cause you sadness. Solidly stand with both feet on the ground and go on in a self-aware way, allow your emotions to flow freely, work out the past, and give your future every chance.

You float, away from the earth. "Spiritual energies" turn strongly but don't find a way to materialize in the body. You are like a Shadow, a Silhouette: you're too absent from your earthly Self. Too spiritualized; not enough present, here-and-now, on Earth. Your head's high up in the clouds; imagination, thoughts, spirituality, nervous thoughts, etc. — all this is not at all integrated into your physicality.

The cause of this non-integration (spiritual awareness-body): the earth appears just cold to you; you don't believe in your divine worth as a human being; you refuse to wear your crown and take up your responsibility as a human being in the earthly realm.

You are so afraid of the emotional, of those earthly feelings, of confrontation with your own body, of confrontation with the sensual or the sexual in a relationship. You feel threatened by certain contacts. But you don't really see very well how to realize yourself on earth on the emotional level. You *think* too much; you insufficiently trust your emotional wealth and your intuition.

You don't dare surrender to yourself, to your natural feelings; for these reasons, you might experience difficulties in the exchange of emotional and physical contacts with others. Because of unconscious fear, you cut yourself off from your feelings and from your body: an escape for the sake of self-defense. Nevertheless, you are filled to the brim with feelings and emotional powers; but the active Mars energy runs out in an exaggerated life of the mind, in the spiritual.

Concentrate all spiritual energies in your earthly body so that you are solidly anchored in your earthly self. In love for yourself build up the framework of your life.

Come down; you are safe here. Transformation; power over your emotions, yet still a free flow of feelings and creative energies. Heaven and earth in balance. Lofty thinking-power and rich spirituality are only justified insofar as you are solidly grounded, with your feet on the earth, and insofar as you are in harmonious contact with your earthly Nature, with your body, with your feelings. Live from out of your deepest Core so that trust and love of yourself blow away all anxieties and alienation.

Enjoy the senses, your nature, your power-development. You are safe in yourself; you shouldn't flee above or outside yourself. You are always established in your eternal, fundamentally strong Self. You don't have to shield your nature, because you are naturally protected in yourself.

Don't flee into unearthly spheres; take part in the hearty celebration of the earthly realms, in sensorial joy.

Lymphangitis
inflammation of lymph vessels

Suppressed aggression, piled-up energies that are not allowed to come through; you live in a way that is too stylized, too structured, too controlled — and now you'd like to burst out because of pent-up tension. Your emotions ask for a breakthrough, an outlet valve.

You feel locked up in yourself; you feel as if you are suffocating in a situation you've held on to for too long: you want to get out now.

You become nervous, overstressed; people or things that have been tied too strongly to you are now experienced as "clinging" and irritating. You now want to run away from this. You look for Freedom. Sometimes, you'd like to push everything and everyone away from you, with full force, but in fact it would be better if you opened the cell door of your prison because it's this self-curtailment that takes your breath away. It's your own thoughts and emotions that rob you of your freedom. . . .

Dare to realize yourself without the accumulation of energies, of healthy aggressive powers; produce, and no longer hold yourself back: allow your nature to exist freely; don't put yourself into a framework that is too narrow; don't deny your body and your sensory enjoyments. Dare to spontaneously experience your feelings; don't stress yourself so, don't wait until you explode. Trust your natural disposition and also dare to express your anger; come to the point that you work out those burdensome feelings. Don't silently hide away. Allow everything to evolve smoothly. Don't smother yourself with frustrating thoughts. Feel safe in your deepest Self, and dare now to blossom.

Lymphedema
swelling caused by accumulation of lymphatic fluid

You are looking for rescue, for hope, and for a grip outside yourself, because you feel unsafe here-and-now.

You "hold fast" to earthly things without really participating in earthly life in a self-assured and joyful way. You allow yourself to turn with the rhythm of the earth, but you anxiously cling, because you really feel defenseless. Afraid of stepping into real life; denying the joyful muscle-power, the flesh and the blood: you allow your inner fire to burn away without making use of it in an emotionally creative way. You don't push your Mars powers through; you don't allow yourself to truly "become." You feel you are in the grip of anxiety; you float in dreams, in thoughts, or in fretting — your feet are too far above the ground. You find it very difficult "to descend." You are at a distance from your earthly body; possibly, you look at yourself and others from such a distance that it seems as if you are living on a higher plane, desiring prestige and outer glitter. It seems, then, as if you have an inflated ego, as if you are above everything. But this is only a posture, necessary to survive. Actually, you feel afraid of being "seized" by something threatening, because the authority upon which you base your life is untrue (religion, an authoritarian leader or parent, etc.) because you don't at all feel safe in yourself. You run away, as it were, from the divine power and love in yourself. You don't trust in your intuition, your inner knowledge, your living Self. On the contrary: you think you have to protect yourself with drawn sword against the enemy. You're on guard. If others consider you to be dominating, then it's only because of your attempt to look at things from above, to control and oversee them because you are mistrustful. The head, the spiritual, the thinking, "masculine aggressiveness," are too strongly present compared to the soft, earthly, emotional, peaceful aspects.

Emotions are being directed by anxiety and by mistrust in your own divine creative power, so that precious energies are being wasted in self-combustion. You don't very well know what direction to take because you don't listen to your deepest Self; confusion, hesitation, and holding on in a tense way are the consequence.

Feel yourself safe and confident in your Nature: follow your intuition; build on that fundamentally solid Basis of your immortal self and construct a clear, strong framework. Depend only on your own fundaments, with both feet on the ground. Allow your body to warm itself comfortably in the sun of your Center; fully participate in earthly life and enjoy the beautiful, the sensorial.

Descend to earth and allow those "feminine" energies to flow, without resistance; experience your emotions, your creativity, and use all energies in constructive activities. A balance between a solid frame work, on the one hand, and the experiencing of earthly content on the other. Let go of everything; no longer cling, but allow those feelings to flow freely. Try to purify your thoughts. If you trust in your intuition and translate the signals from your surroundings, then you will definitely know: "That is the direction I have to take." Anxieties are needless; take up all your space, without self-suffocation. Allow nature to speak for itself; listen to that language of your body, of the earth. Experience those powers in yourself; root yourself solidly in the ground and develop your talents. On earth, here-and-now, you can create your life the way you think is right: take hold of this with both hands. Life will only become lighter if you don't cut yourself off from the earthly, joyful blood-circulation, from your heart.

M

MAGNESIUM
Deficiency, insufficient assimilation of

Anxiety, a crushing, suffocating feeling: you don't live in a self-aware way out of your own sun center. You'd sooner cling to other Authority (for instance, children to their parents), but you feel like a little dog who's master keeps its leash too tight. You feel in a grip, in a trap. You hunger for space for yourself. Because you don't really live from out of your deepest Self, you are afraid that that upon which your existence is built might collapse.

Mortal fears; many anxieties and emotions ferment inside you; you inflate yourself by drawing everything in, by attracting everything, but this suffocates you. Your heart contracts painfully, because you offer insufficient love to yourself, because you walk around with death instead of joyfully surrendering to life. You bottle up your emotional problems; you live in anxious "expectations" of — Tensely retaining and holding on to things, emotionally defensive against whomever or whatever might hurt you; you experience life as an unsafe fairy tale that might have a bad ending you can't do anything about. You don't even dare to stand on your own feet — that's how unsure you feel. You live too much "under" an authority or "at the service" of others: your deepest Self reacts to this and calls for its own free existence! Your beautiful energies, your creative possibilities, are being suppressed; you don't live in an authentic way; the sunlight of others can burn you, because you don't acknowledge yourself as being the Center.

Feel your Power, Consciously concentrate yourself in your body, pull your energies together and become that strong, loving RADIATING human-being! Instead of letting everything anxiously ferment inside you. Tear yourself loose from the grip that oppresses you, from the hand that beats you, by freeing yourself from your feelings of powerlessness or inferiority, by becoming aware of your fundamentally strong Self, your safe basis. Build up your existence in rest and peace, from out of your personal Sun center, and no longer doubt your worth, your possibilities of creating your life yourself, according to your longings.

No longer suppress those piled-up energies: transform them into action, dare to LIVE! Trust in that divine creative power, the love in yourself; don't allow yourself to "be lived." Dare to FEEL, to enjoy, to cherish that which is beautiful; a warm earth under the sun.

MALARIA

You experience yourself to be like a "victim," who in this life has a heavy cross to bear, from which there is no escape. Too much "spirit," too little "earthly" joy.

You feel desperately stuck in an oppressive situation: you'd like to tear away, to free yourself; you look for solutions, but in vain.

You look at everything from the dark side, from below, like a small man who doesn't believe in the fact that via our negative (unconscious) expectations we, *our-*

The Key to Self-Liberation, Christiane Beerlandt © Beerlandt Publications

selves, call up our circumstances in life. You believe in Fate; you think that death, a mosquito, and misfortune can be inflicted on you "just like that." You root yourself in death; you don't really live from out of your conscious "I"-center.

Look at everything from above: with your Self-awareness, from out of a powerful concentrated Center in yourself. Become conscious of your creative possibilities; know how, by your unconscious convictions, you program and attract a negativity, yes even death, into your life. Acknowledge your divinity, achieve Love in yourself: this rest, this balance, your gentleness, mean Immunity (See Infections). Experience the joy in that which is earthly — the natural, the sensorial, under the authority of a proud Self.

Be honest with yourself and stay faithful to your Nature: don't allow yourself to "be lived," not by others, nor by existing "impersonally." Take up the total space of your Being.

MANGANESE
Deficiency, insufficient assimilation of

Inner rift: your spiritual consciousness seems to be running away from your physical body. You'd like to run away from yourself: you feel so imprisoned!

Anxiety. "I don't want to." A refusal, especially regarding Love.

You feel emotionally so weak, you experience yourself as an incapable human being, cut off from your natural powers, from your body, from your instincts, from earthly contacts. Possibly, you are afraid of sexual contacts, of physical caresses.

It's as if a great authoritarian Eye constantly forbids you to become involved in a loving exchange with a partner. Mars and Venus separated. An inner conflict, perhaps running away from a partner, but in fact it's

about the inability to achieve unity in yourself: you push away the intuitive, the emotional experience, the earthly enjoyment! Do you live like an Image, artificially?

You want to get away! You are allergic to yourself: do you think yourself to be so bad? Were you taught to avoid everything that has to do with your body? Or are you so dissatisfied with yourself, inwardly and outwardly? Why flee like that from life? You would even run away from your own "brain influence," from your own thoughts? You don't even try to give safe shelter to your inner emotional core (which you consider to be so inadequate) in your clear-thinking Self-aware "I."

No longer run away from your own Nature: allow those feelings — your unconscious intuitive powers, earthly enjoyment, your body —to exist freely. Now, achieve love in yourself and give yourself room to exist: dare to enjoy the physical, the sensorial; be generous to yourself. Integrate body and soul, the "male" and the "female" in you. Trust in your deepest Self, no longer split yourself.

No longer condemn yourself or one aspect of yourself: dare to LIVE from out of your spontaneous Nature; surrender to your feelings. Become master over your Self: your brains, your glands, your body all are waiting for your instructions.

MANIC-DEPRESSIVE ILLNESS

You are convinced that deep inside you, in unconscious regions, there's something bad, something dark, which can appear at any moment like a little devil, and that you can't do anything about it.

You don't *really* trust in your deepest Self, in your solid foundations: you are afraid of a part of yourself; you suppress the "female" aspect, that which is rich in emotion, the intuitive, that which is gentle and supple!

You are afraid of your powerful, emotional energies, and you become too hard, even aggressive, toward yourself. You are not allowed to exist freely and spontaneously; on the one hand, you stay anxiously "within" your shell, longing for warm gentleness and loving shelter, for devoted sharing in relationships.

On the other hand, you push away these emotional longings; you would manifest yourself with a powerful, aggressive punch: "I don't need anyone; I'm not afraid; I'm big —" Again and again you plunge an aspect of yourself under water. This has a boomerang effect: that which you suppress will come up again after some time. Swinging back and forth from "big" to "small," from "powerlessness" to "power," from "hard, proud 'I'," to "falling back into uncertainty," from the suppression of emotions to an outlet of these emotions, from hope and optimism to despairing pessimism. There's an imbalance, a changeability from one extreme to the other, because again and again you Fight against a part of yourself. Two opposite energies that are complementary and ever seeking a balance.

Don't suppress your deepest emotions; allow them to flow freely. No longer fight against yourself: one emotion flows into another so that at last you "work things out" instead of suppressing them. To do this, however, it is necessary that you achieve Insight into Yourself; knowing that your "I" lies strongly and dependably in the Center of your existence; knowing that you don't have to be afraid of anything inside yourself, and that you will live more balanced in proportion to how open you are to that gentle, supple, sensitive female part of yourself (moon). This female aspect can constantly make itself a place within the strong Framework — the structure of your being, your male, proud aspect. Neither male nor female aspects will be neglected anymore: come to a communion in

yourself, feel that fundamentally strong Basis, your eternal, deepest Self, and hold on firmly to these central foundations.

Trust in that which is deepest in yourself. In self-certainty, arrive at decisive action, but surrender to your feelings, allow Sun and Moon to exist in constant harmony: find rest and satisfaction in a life that you build in a self-assured way. Integrate your emotional world — and physical enjoyments also — in a Self-aware existence; allow power and gentleness to meld inside you. Nothing in you is bad. No longer push away those elements which your mentors have condemned in their own lives. Be newly born in yourself: dare to allow harmony into your life.

(Read Part I.)

MASOCHISM

A false image of yourself: showing a pliable weakness in order to have someone else in your power. In this way you get others in your grip.

The reason why you want to get others in your grip is because you feel so powerless, like an "absent" puppet, like a servant for others; you are convinced that you can only come into your own by being a victim. Convinced, also, that "enjoyment" can be experienced through "pain": this kind of "enjoyment" is not a fraction of "Truly Enjoying" in Love without pain. Masochism *can never* lead to true Happiness. On the other hand enjoyment in (self-) love can!!

Suppressed self-esteem, bottled-up aggressive energies, extreme nervousness, a suppression of your "I" power, of Mars energy, out of which there actually grows a desire to *fight*. Outwardly, you can appear big, tough and strong, like a Superman, but inwardly you feel small and soft, powerless.

Emotionally, you feel hurt, stuck, at the mercy of others; because of your masochism you get, on the one hand, the needed Liberation from bottled-up energies, and on the other hand the needed attention from people (through the attitude of others whom you will attract as if they were your "torturers").

Masochism and sex
See also Sexuality, exaggerated sexual urge

Because of refusing to acknowledge yourself as a worthy Human Being, you will give much room to the "animalistic," the primitive, the instinctive and sexual powers in yourself. Your bottled-up, unused creative energies lead to a nervous, frustrated "explosive danger": in sexual masochistic games one can vent this steam. The emptiness to which you doom your human existence is being filled with pleasure and sexual excitement.

*Brainwashing. Acknowledge your worth, your inner wisdom. Allow your powerful, creative energies to come through under the authority of your Self-aware "I"; no longer frustrate yourself. Produce. Integrate your emotions and your longings into an energetic, active existence: instead of provoking active Mars powers in others, you need to push through your energies yourself! Don't hesitate to bring yourself to realization; don't allow your life to be at the mercy of someone else or of Fate. No one is a victim. Create your life yourself the way you want it; transform pure instincts and powers into conscious creativity; achieve **real** Joy. Masochistic enjoyment has nothing to do with the True Intense Enjoyment within a **true** love relationship. This Enjoyment belongs to Happiness. On the other hand, masochistic enjoyment leads you further and further down the abyss.*

Realization of your golden worth as a human being will lead to a changed composition of your blood, of every cell in your body; the glands will change the hormonal picture, which then again will influence your behavior. In other words, your convictions

*and your opinion about yourself immediately influence the chemical composition of your body. A relaxed and joyful existence of soul and body will come to be, if you are convinced that you deserve happiness and rest. And that enjoyment does **not** have to go hand in hand with "pain"; on the contrary!*

MEGALOMANIA
inflated self-esteem or grandiosity

There's a rift: on the one side, your deep Core, and on the other side, how you present yourself to the world; a dislocated "I."

Your deepest "I" lies hidden, is anxious, and feels wretched. You keep this supposed garbage can closed, afraid as you are of yourself. Doubts and unsureness.

You are afraid that others might see your so-called "badness," afraid that you might fall into the (power) grip of others. . . . You anxiously hide your feelings.

Fleeing from yourself, you might seek to make contact with the entire world: you are looking for self-affirmation. In an exaggerated way, you compensate for your self-negation — for your self-underestimation — by emphatically manifesting yourself outwardly. You stick out your chest. The world is at your feet. In this way you feel good, because it fills the enormous gap that you have created in yourself.

Possibly, as a consequence of your self-image, you have been deeply hurt and have been severely dominated by a powerful authority above you. This powerlessness, this pain, seeks refuge in megalomania, but it is blindness, false glitter.

Thus, now be aware of your true inner Worth. Feel your deep undercurrents, your very Core, and allow your feelings to blossom freely from out of this Self-core. Experience your personal fundamental tone, and no longer judge your value by the others, by the outer world. The gold lies inside yourself; don't doubt it. Don't fool yourself, don't hide behind self-delusion; honestly come to yourself and discover your rich emotional world, where there's nothing bad or threatening. Replace megalomania with true self-confidence.

There is an incredible grandeur in every human being; therefore, it's not necessary to puff yourself up with far-away dreams.

Achieve unity in yourself.

MEMORY LOSS

You feel incapable, unable to build only upon yourself: you look to others for support, for an arm to lean on.

You let yourself go; you sag. Nevertheless, you still experience your potential. You'd like to — But you are too sad; you think you can't handle it all, alone.

You no longer concentrate in the here-and-now; you no longer live really consciously; you no longer believe in the meaning or the power of your life here. Actually, you flee to a less-concentrated consciousness-level, to being less present in life.

Fear and (perhaps especially) fear of death at the end of the tunnel. Unconsciously, you prepare yourself for this other state of consciousness.

Sadness — you call up this problem in order to push painful experiences as far away as you can. In order to keep life bearable by, in this way, eliminating certain things from your life.

Experience the power of your Consciousness in every fiber of your body; from out of your deepest core, focus on the intense Life. Being present in a concentrated way, here-and-now, instead of taking flight toward death. Create your life yourself the way it makes you happy, and banish death. Be aware of your possibilities! (Read Part I)

MÉNIÈRE'S DISEASE
increasing hardness of hearing, buzzing in the ears, attacks of dizziness and queasiness

It seems as if the Structure, the Form, no longer can "carry" the Content, as if everything is becoming too much. The person has had to swallow too much, has had to bear too much, has had to assimilate too much — and this might have to do with Work, Tasks, or with the material he has to read or study, or with emotional information that he has difficulty assimilating. He might become nauseous because of this, his stomach reacting with all its defenses to that which now presents itself as being "too much." He can't look at it anymore, doesn't want to hear about it anymore. He closes himself off from it, closes his ears.

That which "in the past" he has "swallowed" too much — mostly without resisting — he will now vomit with all his powers, like a garbage can that all of a sudden empties itself. It has all been too much for him. It's enough now. The pot overflows!

For too long, one has violated one's own Structure. Yes, has bent it toward another or others, often in a cramped, tense way.

This person is not yet really standing in the "full daylight" of Life, of himself: he continues to live "hidden," as it were, "under the earth, in his hole" — and he will "bring" everything into his hidden hole, but he, himself, won't really come out into Life with his total personality. One could psychologically describe this situation as a "self-chosen imprisonment" of the "I": one looks out from behind prison bars at a beautiful Sun out there, and one can also enjoy it in this way, enjoy life there — but one does not truly participate in it. No matter what one does, whatever work one undertakes, one doesn't dare to fully "participate" in actual Life. One keeps oneself in the background of Life.

The deepest Self-core of this human being and his life-powers ask for a "breakthrough," for complete existence. One can compare this situation with a mole that digs its tunnels under the earth in order to slowly, very slowly, build a hill of soil. . . . Suppressed life-powers push the hill up ever higher, but this human being still holds back his energies, so to speak — No matter how strongly inner powers are calling for liberation, he still doesn't lift his head above the hill until the life-energies impel themselves upward with Coercive Power and overwhelm him (possibly in the form of queasiness, or as dizziness, etc.). It has all become too much for him. At first sight, it can seem as if it's the world around him, or work, or the task that he has taken upon himself, or the confrontation with emotional issues in his surroundings, etc. — any of which weigh too heavily upon him. This can certainly be so! Yet, this is only a Consequence of the underlying cause: suppression of one's own spontaneous, natural, powerful life-energies.

Because of the fact that he suppresses Life in himself, he'll regularly receive "signals" from his deepest soul-core — namely bodily malfunctions, which are necessary in order to prod him to stop neglecting these life-powers! If he keeps ignoring this call, however, and remains stagnating in this phase, then the soul-core will send him ever-stronger signals. In other words, ever more-disturbing bodily signals, until at last the lid could fly off the pot. (By vomiting, for instance: he vomits because of himself, because of his own "immobility," because of the unconscious refusal to evolve: read "Queasiness — Vomiting") Until, at last, the mole hill is forcefully being broken open, with volcanic power: the inner Self of this person now forcefully compels him to enter into true life!

If he still keeps suppressing his life powers — if he still doesn't "listen" to the signals his soul core has been sending him for quite some time — then his "hearing" will diminish. Then the ear (or ears) will reflect the fact that he doesn't listen to the message from his deepest "I"; the ear will indicate that

he bottles up the "water of life," retaining it instead of letting it flow freely and abundantly.

Possibly, this person has attracted others who will make clear that "There's something not right in your existence; you need to make changes!" But he doesn't listen, stubbornly closing his ears to it. Possibly, he prefers to keep living with the same old habits, obligations, traditions, rules — while he doesn't realize that a New Step needs to be taken. He really has but *one* Duty, which comes before everything, and that is to LIVE from out of *your* own Powerful Core, as "I." He now needs to get in touch with his own inner soul-core; he now needs to place himself in the Center of his existence and no longer stand on the side of the road, where he bows before an Authority outside himself.

His brain becomes overburdened, overheated, with "thinking," with "information." He "immobilizes" himself with thoughts. He can no longer "bottle" things up in his head; he needs to come out with his energies, with his thoughts, with his feelings of anger or sadness. He has to speak. He needs to step into life in a more assertive, decisive way! He'll live from out of his Intuition, no longer keeping everything in a "grip" with his narrow rationality. He has to trust what he *feels* and deal with this in an honest way. He no longer does anything "because that is how it has to be," but he listens to his Heart. In this way he will no longer overburden himself.

A feeling of Powerlessness — "I can no longer handle it all" — indicates that he pays too much attention to things it would be better for him to let go of; that he insufficiently believes in his possibilities of looking at life in a different way and beginning to organize it thusly. He needs to mark off his Limits! He's not allowed to "let himself be lived," like a robot or a zombie that can be "switched on" by others. He now needs to CHOOSE life: this means to "listen" to his living self-core, which tells him what is good. He will make sure not to place

ABOVE LIFE itself those values which are of secondary importance in life: money, material things, external things, status, "so-called" duties, etc. If, in spite of it all, he still does this, then that will mean the same as "killing" life. He now will have to look at the ESSENCE of life, of himself, and begin to live toward it. He will not be permitted to be "afraid" to take new steps; he will not be permitted to be afraid TO LIVE.

He has to get rid of the inner conviction that life is a "stressful" business; he will have to adopt the conviction that life is there in order to be happy, to enjoy. He therefore will listen to the signals from his deepest Self and will bring about changes where necessary: habit-patterns will then change; the method of work will go differently, or a change of job might present itself. He no longer "bows" to Authority outside himself, to duties and rules that make his life a Burden. He now needs to live from out of his own Authority.

This person should "let go" of certain things, but he offers resistance. He has a difficult time because he doesn't listen to the voice of Life, but listens instead to other (false) motives.

In a cramped and tense way, he holds on to old superseded habits, and in this way puts himself under pressure. He constantly "immobilizes" himself and needs to free himself from this. As long as he doesn't listen to his inner voice, he'll look and listen too much to people (or books, etc.), to elements outside himself— all of which might make him Dizzy!

He needs to come to inner rest by responding only to that which Life asks of him.

Suppressed energies are seeking their course; they ask for a "conversion" in action, in creativity, for a Transformation.

The powerful energy inside this person asks to be used in a creative way. He shouldn't "constrict" himself and push his energies into a "framework."

He first and foremost needs to come home, deep inside himself, in order to live from out of himself without suppressing the "red life-forces." He shouldn't cling to others, but he especially needs to live, solidly, from out of his own autonomy. He needs to throw certain "burdens" from his back. . . .

He will now resolutely stake out his territory and push away certain things, which previously he allowed to be forced upon him.

He now turns his energies Outward — like an Archer, he shoots his arrows — instead of "storing" everything inside. He expresses himself; he speaks; he lets go. . . . He no longer turns things over and over again in his mind; he now knows that you can't be good to everyone. He realizes now that he just has to live in Harmony with himself. Out of this honesty, out of this Self-love, he will automatically act in a way that is good for other people in his surroundings, even if it doesn't immediately seem that way. This person needs to honestly manifest himself, and he will no longer go on living in a "suppressed" way.

Does he live from out of himself, or does he live according to the norms of the family, of a society, of a religion or a race?. . . . Undoubtedly, he then drifts off his Own, individual Path: this can't be good. No one "possesses" the truth, but the human being always needs to live "according to the truth." This means in honesty with himself, with his heart, independent of whatever laws. He only needs to listen to the Authority IN himself. Then, he will no longer hold in his life's powers! Like a productive water spring he will spontaneously learn to let himself "come through," without putting a BRAKE on it, without fear, without feelings of guilt.

A person who knows that it's he, himself, who determines the direction of his life, knows that no Fate nor God has any say over it: he takes the reins of his life in hand, full of confidence. He's the only one who determines the way his life will go. (Read PART I about this.) In this knowledge, in this confidence, he knows that everything will go fine

— and the RESPONSIBILITY for certain things no longer WEIGHS so heavily! Living on the basis of positive convictions, he knows that ultimately everything that is Good for him will appear on his path. But he does need to listen to the signals that his living Self-core sends him in order to bring about the necessary changes.

Life is now being experienced in a relaxed way, and lighter.

In resoluteness and self-assuredness he has now become master over his life. He now knows that nothing "just" happens, that everything has its reasons for being, and that his life won't know any misery or sadness if he Directs it from a standpoint of positive expectations.

He no longer confuses love and helpfulness with "doing everything the employer, his friend, etc." ask of him: he no longer makes compromises with his own "I"; he now follows his true Nature. He isn't that "good soul," who hurts himself, violates himself. He doesn't expect anything from others, but resolutely lives from out of himself now. He knows that his body is undermined when he doesn't first and foremost listen, in Self-love, to the needs of his "I" — separate from desires. He will have to push the essence of his "I" even more strongly to the fore and will have to let go of certain things. He will look at the ESSENCE, at that which is Most Important in Life, and let go of that which is superfluous. He won't be sidetracked by needless burdens. Very often this illness is seen in good people, who keep going in a certain track — for instance, in the track of another person. They think that it has to be that way, but actually they are hiding behind this attitude in order to avoid HAVING TO ARRIVE AT LIFE THEMSELVES.

This person will have to step out of his customary behavior and habit-pattern: possibly, he does his Tasks and Duties just the way his father would do them, while this is totally against his highly individual nature. He will now have to become HIMSELF in a very individual way; he will need to build up a Solid Framework in himself and learn to say "No" to the information that is forced on him from the outside, and to certain people. . . . Nor will he allow certain things to trouble his conscience: "If you don't give me this, then I feel sad because of your behavior!" But he will need to take the necessary steps, after which he will feel "liberated." He now takes responsibility for himself according to the "essence." By freeing himself from the former exaggerated duty-pattern, by stepping out of exaggerated, oppressive frameworks and structures, out of self-oppressive spheres. By manifesting himself more strongly as "I," he will in turn force his fellow man, his friend, his partner, to become themselves in a stronger way. You never can be happy with a partner or in a relationship if you aren't first happy with YOURSELF. You can never change THE OTHER; you can never blame the other: you can only CHANGE YOURSELF. If you free yourself from inner tensions and take the necessary steps that bring you closer to your inner harmony, then the result will be that certain things in your surroundings will automatically change in a positive way.

So, no longer close your ears to real changes in yourself, in your way of living! Break with every indoctrination from the past and look at everything from a new point of view now. Step forward with your true "I"; don't suppress your powers and your feelings! No longer allow yourself to be overpowered and/or influenced by all sorts of things from the outside. Turn deeply inward and listen to the voice in yourself that says life is Joy. Everyone leads his life according to his own convictions. If you are convinced that life is burdensome, is something you can't do much about, then it will seem that everything "just happens" to you! Then anxieties and uncertainty will torment you. But Life, itself, is not built on these kinds of fatalistic foundations!

Once you realize that a person creates his own life on the basis of his own convictions, then you will no longer hesitate to live on the basis of the following conviction: "I know I have my life in my own hands, that I have my healing in my hands, and that everything that is good for me will appear upon my path." You then need to listen to the Signals, to the signs you receive in your life — signs that tell you which changes you need to bring about in your life. It's not enough to Trust; you need to add Action. This means beginning to act upon the signals that your deepest soul-core has sent you so that you may become a happier person than you were before. In this case the signal is an illness: Ménière's Disease. It disappears out of your life once and for all when you have "understood" what your deepest self-core asks of you, and when you then bring about the necessary changes in your life.

MENTAL DEFICIENCY

There are several reasons why a being is "attracted" by an environment in which it will be born mentally handicapped to a more or lesser degree. Here, there's never a question of "guilt": parents and children serve each other's evolution.

Here, we're often dealing with an outer manifestation of the conviction: "I'm only a wooden puppet." One experiences oneself as a "machine." Perhaps one was even afraid of that which is deeper: anxiety seeks a mask. One looks at the world in a superficial, one-sided way; an escape. In this way, one doesn't have to go deeper. In this way, one avoids responsibilities. The anxiety is very deeply hidden.

Many are stuck, however, in not wanting to look any further than the primitive, the sexual, the animalistic, the material: they have dulled themselves. Take their masks off and show them that there are things which go beyond the most primitive, the instinctive. . . . The Heart, *true* love. . . .

Ultimately, many of those who are in an extreme state of mental deficiency wish to be free, unencumbered by external laws, so that, without inhibition and in complete foolishness, they are able to discover themselves. In order to express their feelings, primitive instincts, intuition — unrestrained childishness. Feelings of inferiority, and a rebelliousness against humiliating experiences; the longing to learn to experience the world beyond the rational or intellectual.

In any case, they will have to be taught that "giving love" — not "desiring" — is the most important thing in life; giving Love, living honestly — the first steps toward a higher evolution of the human being.

It is possible that a mentally deficient person is born in an intellectual environment. This kind of situation is unconsciously evoked (by all involved) in order to break open, as it were, the life of parents and family and so achieve a "complete" life. The genes are directed by the consciousness that lies behind them. If one looks at heredity or at "spontaneous genetic changes" as a purely physical affair, then one ignores the power and the meanings of human consciousness. (See also "Congenital physical defects; genetic determination: no.")

MOLYBDENUM
Deficiency, insufficient assimilation of

You constantly hurt yourself; the inclination to self-destruction. You are burning because of pent-up aggression. Extreme powerlessness. Powerful energies are being turned inward and becoming self-destroying attacks.

Allow that masterful power from out of your deepest Self to give form to your life, to your body. Be aware of your worth and come to productivity; be fruitful, break through, in a positive, constructive way! Create! Use unconscious powers in creativity and elevate them to Consciousness. No longer break yourself down: find love, and transform negative convictions regarding yourself.

MOUTH

Symbolism and Ailments, in general

Symbolic of either being open to, or else refusing, new ideas or experiences.

Symbolic of "bringing into being," of allowing something new to be born out of you. Radiating your volcanic consciousness-powers outward or holding them back.

Represents whether or not you harmoniously pass things on in communication with others. You, as an individual, in confrontation with mankind.

Also represents the manner in which you handle this: Honest and open? Or hypocritically deceitful? Do you enter into straightforward contact, or do you play the role of a saint? Every bird sings according to its nature, literally and figuratively. Do you give expression to your true feelings, or do you play a comedy? Perhaps you take a critical and condemnatory stand regarding yourself. Or are you shortsightedly critical toward others? Skeptically distrustful. Reprimanding. Keeping things hidden, or revealing things.

Juggling, or honest interchange.

Being a unified person, undivided, straightforward, with deeds that are in accord with one's words.

Daring to calmly stand up for yourself, not walking around with heavy burdens: giving expression to your emotions. Or is there a question of powerless aggression?

To what do you close yourself off? To the physical-earthly, or in particular to the spiritual-intuitive? Powerless aggression: are you sinking your teeth into something? Do you grab?

Get a grip on yourself and stay within your limits. Don't project onto others that which you suppress yourself.

Corners of the mouth, cracked

The cause of this lies in an inner conflict. On the one hand you feel sheltered, protected, and safe under an Authority (parent, partner, etc.), and you wish to remain bound to this because you don't get enough of a grip on yourself and on your feelings; because you can't *really* reach your feelings. Hesitation, uncertainty — yes/no/yes — confused fretting, resistance.

On the other hand, this situation leads to frustration; you want to get *away!* You fight for *more* space; you might collide with others in a sharp, hard, aggressive way because of this duality inside you. A tense forcing, an inner aggression, but in fact you don't get anywhere with this.

Allow gentle feelings, the female aspect, to exist freely, in harmony with the self-aware, resolute male aspect. Don't be too harsh; bend flexibly, acknowledge the loving aspect, the gentleness, in you; but feel strong on the Basis of your deepest Self so that you feel protected in yourself. So that you don't think you have to defend yourself in an aggressive way. Your frustrations will disappear thanks to your unhesitating self-realization. Calmly trust in your nature, your intuition. Don't paralyze yourself with harsh thoughts of powerlessness. Inside yourself, you find more space — not by forcing open to the outside. Open yourself wide with all your possibilities.

Dry mouth

Fleeing from life; anxiety, fear of pain, of hurtful experiences.

Too spiritual, not really completely present on earth here and now.

You control your natural energies, your feelings; you hold the reins of the "horse" too tight — a way of "killing." You live at a distance from your body.

"I AM here." Become master over yourself and allow your Nature to exist in all freedom. Trust!

Don't flee from life; don't be afraid of pain: take all responsibility for your life and create it yourself! Trust your feelings, your intuitive urge for creativity, your liking for joy and enjoyment. Feel your powers, and give yourself all opportunity to live without a harness! Anxieties disappear when you Consciously take hold of the reins! You see everything as being too black: allow your personal Creative powers to break through!

Palate, ulceration

You want to say it all and let it all come through, but you think you can't do it.

The past, emotional energies, words, aggressive powers are being swallowed. You are silent, you resist a spontaneous outlet. You release nothing, so that ultimately you also feel emotionally "compressed." You don't really believe in yourself. You are afraid of a total breakthrough of yourself. You bind and close yourself tightly, because you fear you will be completely crushed by something overpowering: you don't trust your nature. Your consciousness powers, your spontaneous energies, are being tied down by your "thinking."

In the first place, there's a communication-disturbance regarding yourself; you cut yourself off from your feelings; you carry needless heavy burdens; sadness and anger are being retained, as if you don't allow yourself to live Freely and think Broadly or manifest yourself outwardly. This of course leads to communication problems with others; but don't blame *them*, for your pushing *yourself* down. You are too absent, a stranger to yourself, because you are afraid of those pure emotional and physical energies, of that fire inside you. You show your teeth, but that's as far as you go.

Trust your deepest Self, your body, your inner powers, and allow yourself to go freely.

Say what you have to say and allow the fog to lift: make yourself clear to others and create clearness for yourself. Know who you are by surrendering to your nature, to your intuition, to your feelings, and just use your common sense. Push through what needs to be pushed through. Confront yourself with hidden feelings and be open and honest in relationships. Chase away the sadness and anger in yourself by building up your life in a self-aware way and by listening to your heart and your wishes. Say it, put it in words, without hesitation. Self-manifestation; let go. Respect your Self!

Thrush
fungal infection of the mucous membrane of the mouth
(See also Infection, fungal)

Imprisoned in your own powerlessness, you blame others because you don't get a grip on yourself. With aggression, sometimes with enormous anger, you'd like to seize others in your power-grip because you have the feeling that you are at their mercy. They bind you fast, you think, but it's you who are stuck to others, to your emotions, to your emotional, confused train of thought!

You don't see the right direction; you can't make a clear decision for yourself; you feel like you are "suspended," disabled, powerless; you don't feel able to consistently push through into a well-directed future. Doubts and anxieties.

Powerless to evolve onward. Still, you develop many energies that are waiting for your active breakthrough, but you don't feel able to resolutely make decisions. This frustrates you. This makes you furious.

You feel like a Giant, as it were, full of enormous energies, but you can't direct them, or you direct them totally wrongly (for instance, by staying stuck in the past, wanting power over others, exhibiting exaggerated machoism, etc.). Actually, you just keep running in place, without making any progress.

You don't really live in this world, as it were. "Where am I?" "Who am I?" With thoughts and dreams you try to get a perspective on yourself, but you don't know how. You stand far away from your nature; you don't live here-and-now, not really in this earthly space; you confuse past, present, and future. Extreme identity-confusion, including in the area of "female" and "male". At one moment you feel as if you are wearing the trousers, with aggression, with proud and stubborn thoughts, and then again you experience yourself as rather small, gentle, handicapped, oversensitive, and overflowing with emotionalism. At one moment you experience yourself as being in charge, and then again as incapable. Book-knowledge or inner wisdom; rational or intuitive; foolish or wise?

Stop blaming, criticizing, or finding fault with others. Observe yourself and become aware of your own worth and possibilities! Dare to externalize. Dare, from out of your deepest Self, to express yourself; allow your powers to come through in a self-aware way. Productivity. Trust in one's own solid structure; develop yourself without hesitation; become master over yourself, over your emotions. Don't suppress your emotions, but allow them to flow smoothly. Don't feel inferior; feel the power in yourself and let go of the power you want to have over others. Dare to transform all your potential energies into realizations! Make decisions intuitively; no longer feel threatened, trust in your deepest Self and go on, without scrambling back! Let your mouth be purified by the production of beautiful fruits, by not washing one's dirty linen in public, but by purifying yourself of black thoughts.

A loving relationship with yourself, with others.

Wake up from your dream and descend, with both feet, onto our planet "Earth." A sense of reality; the union of body-spirit. Come very close to your nature; dare to harmoniously experience the "male" and "female"

aspects in you: accept every part of yourself. Don't flee from the earthly. Become master over your unconscious spheres and dreams in a self-aware way. Accept active decisiveness in Yourself; dare to express the way you inwardly feel. Dare to think things through; act on your Insights. Especially don't stifle powerful energies: live your life to the fullest in the here-and-now. Transform anger, stubborn aggression, into Action!

MUCOUS MEMBRANES

Psychological correspondence

The ease with which you slide through Life; flexibly and trustingly, you let yourself be carried by your Living Self, by your purest nature core.

You allow your feelings to flow freely; you don't block your joy. You enjoy, and you take part in, the happy celebration of life; you dare to enjoy the exuberant feast of life with a wealth of music, dance, and delicacies (like in a painting by Bruegel)! You flexibly go on toward your life goals, without hesitation, without anxiety.

You don't make it too difficult for yourself: you don't tie yourself down too much by too many "duties" and too little "indulgences."

Thankful and reverent openness to life, to feelings, to that which is beautiful in life. A thankful, happy diffusion of energies which well up out of your deepest Self. Humor, laughter: "Go ahead!" Benevolent, full of trust, knowing that everything will be all right; trustfully shooting your arrows. Daring to experience your life without hesitantly questioning it; daring to completely scatter life to the winds, letting yourself go without sadness, without pain. The mucous membranes also represent the Protection of yourself: feeling yourself to be protected.

Proudly, and in self-awareness, acknowledging and conserving your inner treasures; through creativity, through beautiful, divine emotional experiences, giving your strong awareness-energies freedom to grow. Being able to build up a crystal-clear structure in your life because your life is being illuminated by the inner Source, the Living Self. Being open to that which is within, to those beautiful, creative energies in your deepest Self, which ask for honest, pure development, like rock-crystal.

Ailments, in general

Perhaps you swim in many waters; you do much, but in fact you don't touch the essence of the matter, of life. You remain stuck at the surface of existence.

Perhaps you see it all as *very* important, but you are like someone who constantly keeps filling a jar that has no bottom — senseless activities, fillers of emptiness. You don't feel protected in yourself because you don't make contact with your Living Self. Inwardly, you feel anxious and powerless, so that you might strive for power. Possibly, you waste time in thoughts of sex, of death, of black magic (wanting power over others), and losing yourself in decadence. Do you perhaps throw away your life or your body in sex or in perversities because you have to fill your inner Emptiness somehow, because you don't value your life sufficiently, because you ignore your beautiful Awareness-content?

You feel without love, cold, sad, naked, or "seized" by others. You don't accept your own Mastery; perhaps you make yourself angry with others, but that is only a sign of powerlessness. You pile up your beautiful energies; feelings can't flow through; you restrict your life!

When you throw a bomb at others (dark thoughts), then it will end up on your own head. Speak! Express your true feelings in all honesty.

Don't put on an act, because by doing so you hinder evolution. Discover the diamond in you, your worth, your most beautiful feelings. Feel protected in your Self; you don't have to build a protective shield. Don't use the sexual, the tasks in your life, as a compensation for emptiness, but discover your own fullness, and in true Love come to yourself, to the other one.

Don't throw away your life, but discover it in all its spaciousness, much further than the purely physical or material. Don't remain at the surface. Feel the joy of life itself. Trust your nature; allow healthy mind and feelings to merge in harmony: build a pure structure in your life but don't imprison yourself by so doing. A structure in which feelings and creativity are permitted to freely grow in the light of thankfulness and love. No more pulling yourself down: Self-respect! Joy!

(See "Psychological correspondence.")

MULTIPLE SCLEROSIS
MS

Unrelentingly and harshly, you scream "NO" to yourself!

You feel so cold in your being; you lean toward death, because you refuse to acknowledge your "I," your NUCLEAR POWERS, the solidity in you.

In "absence" you could waste away; you don't become master over yourself. You don't believe in your own foundations and possibilities.

You push yourself away; you'd even push away people who lead you by the nose to point out your powers and positive characteristics or your Self-healing energies.

Sharp resistance to self-acknowledgement, to love for yourself. . . .

Someone has hurt and underestimated you because you were born with these denigrating, self-destructive, bitter thoughts regarding your own worth! Perhaps these negative convictions regarding yourself have attracted to you humiliating situations or a physically self-destructive illness. This is to confront you with your thoughts — with your convictions — regarding yourself! Your body reacts to conscious and unconscious impulses. If constantly you break yourself down inwardly, then your body will break down. If you think you're only a cold, worthless rag, then you will no longer feel the warmth of love and the flow of blood.

If you are stone-hard with regard to yourself or happenings from the past, then certain parts of your body will harden: Have you developed a false ego toward the outer world, a self-willed, stubborn attitude in order to hide your gentleness, your anxieties, your injuries — all because you fear being hurt even more? ("They won't push me down anymore!") Inner anger toward yourself because of your own powerlessness, because of rejection of yourself by yourself and by others. Your body now begs for acknowledgment! Your total being is tired of being condemned! Let go of others. You live first and foremost for yourself: it's up to you to allow yourself to LIVE. You will receive appreciation and love from others if first you come to yourself in UNIFICATION. Don't ask for confirmation from outside, but at last give that confirmation to yourself. Don't cry out for acknowledgment from others: come to yourself! You experience your personality as being "imperfect": therefore, you will be physically limited. Stop this process and turn it around. Feel your body in all its fibers, feel your total being, as a beautiful piece of divine nature. Accept Life itself in thankfulness.

Experience yourself as being good, very good, and worthy — forget the indoctrinations or condemnation of your mentors or your parents, because these were only expressions of their frustrations, and had nothing in fact to do with your unique being. Don't expect that others will see or admire your worth, not even people who are older than you. Only accept the authority of your "I"; come to calm self-assuredness, independent from others. Lovingly descend into your body; learn how to feel every fiber.... Purify yourself from piled-up negativity: express your anger, show your teeth for once, allow that dirty smoke that blocks your brain to escape! Firstly, come "thoroughly" to insight into your emotions, and don't run away from them; look at your anger, your self-rejection, self-delusion: "I'm not worth anything and I can't do anything." See that the cause of this lies in self-rejection. Now turn warmly toward yourself and cherish that small, poor, deserted little child within you. How long will you let it cry without gentleness and love? Is the little child inside you not allowed to exist? Do you take away all joy from yourself, the way a mother punishes her child by not allowing it to have an ice cream for an entire year? Do you place hard demands upon yourself? Do you follow senseless, severe diets? Why not build upon your self-healing energies?

Energies are freed but then are immediately stabbed down; your healthy mind is made subordinate to limited knowledge, to that which you have been taught, to traditional habits.... There's ENORMOUS resistance, an obstinate, clinging Willfulness, a stubbornness. No matter how uncertain and anxious you might feel inwardly, what counts to the outside is your tough, hard Image through which no one can penetrate — or your superficial, cheerful clown suit — but there is no *true* JOY FOR YOU, for your life! You'd rather try to satisfy the norms of your parents or the needs of others; perhaps there's a lot of talking, but little is actually *said* from out of your ESSENCE, your core. Perhaps you give much pleasure to others, but in the meantime you *deny* your Self. You look through the eyes of others, too little from out of yourself. This dualistic attitude, which makes you finally disappear completely in the background, ultimately leads to hard, STEEL nerves. You have great long-ings, but you begin to float in the clouds in-stead of standing with your feet on the ground, here-and-now, and realizing certain plans, step by step. You nip enormous ener-gies in the bud. Surrender to your deepest Self, relax, allow yourself to slowly blossom.

Look very closely at your buried emo-tions, at the dark aspects, at death; dare to confront yourself with your deeper reality. Your world is different from the worlds of your mentors. Don't be a parrot, but open yourself up to wisdom, which you can only feel deep inside yourself. No longer brace yourself behind a bunker, but gently come into yourself, in complete surrender. Allow yourself to be happy; give yourself freedom; feel safe on earth. Now unwind your wound-up defenses; unfold yourself in a butterfly dance: transform yourself and recover.

MUSCLES

Psychological correspondence

Muscles symbolize energies revolving around a central structure; muscles symbolize growth, evolution, truly going onward in life, vitality, joyful awareness-powers.

Constant transformation: old values you treasured in the past — don't tensely hold on to them, don't restrict yourself, but allow your energies to freely go onward and climb upward! Allow the new to be born, and don't feel imprisoned in an old structure.

Muscles: supple, free space to move in; you go where ever you want. Or do you im-mobilize yourself? Do you just live within limiting structures? A human being is *more* than just a Skeleton. Without muscles and tendons we would fall apart.

Do you pay attention only to the sober, businesslike or material side of life? Then you neglect your muscle-system. Your deep

feelings of warmth and love for yourself and others; a volcanic fire force, warmth, emo-tional development.

Without muscles we wouldn't be able to stand solidly: they have a connecting, stabi-lizing, regulating value.

With common sense *alone* you aren't solid in life: give your trust to your deepest inner Self, your core, your soul, your eternal pow-erful "I" (use whatever term you wish), in which are found love and wisdom, an inex-haustible source of information. Don't resist this inner power, and allow true wisdom, in-tuition, and true feelings of warmth to come through. This divine core in you is the solid basis of your existence.

We are in contact with our guiding "I" through our feelings, our experiences, our intuition. With our mind we can reason and can build up theories, formulate hypotheses; these will fall in the water, when they go against our inner Knowing, against what we "feel" inwardly.

Muscles will relax or restore themselves when you calmly surrender, offering your trust to this deep Self, which will give you that which is best for you.

Let go of everything instead of forcefully holding on, don't keep yourself imprisoned! Nothing "just" happens in life: *every* situa-tion has been unconsciously attracted by your Self. A friend calls off an appointment? Be sure that your Self knows very well *why* this happens! At any given time trust in what happens; adjust only your negative convic-tions.

Therefore, don't try to absolutely force something: that which you want isn't always what's best for you. Let go, and open your-self up to your inner guide, who will lead you on a path to peace and happiness.

Muscles are ready to "receive" informa-tion from outside and from inside: sensitivity. Your muscles will hurt when you are too hard on yourself, when you don't open your-self up to love or to intuitive information — when you are cold and emotionally tense.

Ailments, in general

Anxieties: Where am I going? Thusly, you don't trust your inner "I" as a trustworthy guide. You try to encompass everything in a rational way. This isn't possible of course.

Unsureness: you deny your true inner authority. You've listened too much to the authority of others (or to society, to scientific requirements, to what OTHERS say, etc.). Inner resistance: perhaps you have let others walk over you for too long; you haven't stood up for yourself. Do you now feel yourself to be in a straitjacket without room to move? Suppressed emotions come to the surface, your vulnerability, your anxieties: "Where do I have to go?" You don't see clearly anymore.

Was your psychological sense of freedom being suppressed by dominating rules? Have you not dared to trust in your own strong inner Authority? The child inside you resists: It wishes to live in freedom! To go in another direction!

You no longer trust it all. You are tense, in stress, on guard, nervous, sad. Too strict with yourself.

Love yourself, be flexible and gentle with yourself; allow feelings to exist freely, don't retain them or hold on to them. Direct your life in self-awareness; build on your solid inner basis — an energy field of power and creativity. Go in the direction that you intuitively know you have to go in.

Don't withhold joy and pleasure from yourself! Enjoy. . . .

Trust; let go of old values.

Coordination; the cooperation of intuition, feelings and mind.

Enjoy your body, allow your heart muscle to be solidly directed by feelings of joy and love because of yourself. Open up your receptive antennae to beautiful happenings.

Integration of all your feelings; no more confusion, achieve rest and relaxation. Unburden yourself.

Muscular atrophy
shriveling, wasting away of the muscles

You don't take up your place: you limit your life too much to structures and duties, to carrying burdens and emotionally bottling things up. You are self-destructive: you don't allow yourself to really be born. Do you live dutifully according to a system, a religion, or a partner? Do you not dare to fully breathe, to broadly take up your space, to enjoy? You are a prisoner, full of frustrations. You feel unsure, but this feeling of insecurity irritates you. You look for a hold outside yourself. You crawl onward, as it were, instead of discovering the joy of life. You feel like a victim: you would sacrifice yourself, perhaps, for one or another god outside you. You are convinced that life contains much sadness, and that one patiently has to bear those burdens. You don't really *live*. You probably show yourself to the outside world as the strong bearer of the Fate that has met you. You become the personification of the Burden. You ignore that which is beautiful in yourself, in life. You experience yourself as being small, foolish, full of ineptitude. You are too strict, too hard, too cold with yourself.

Come to self-awareness! Realize your longings. No longer allow yourself to waste away. You, yourself, are the cause of your symptoms: in a positive way change your opinion, your philosophy about life, and your health will improve. Stop this self-destruction: no god outside you asks for it. Don't doom yourself to being a Beast of Burden, but take up your full space! Breathe deeply, enjoy all the beautiful things in life, discover the beauty in yourself, and awaken yourself to life in a loving approach to yourself.

Cherish yourself in warmth and partake in a hearty meeting with the earth, with your body, with others. You are not a victim, but the creator of your life: create new, joyful circumstances in your life.

Muscle cramps, calf cramps

Nervous tension.

Spirit and body separate themselves a little, as it were, because you burden your head too much with worrisome thoughts. You fret, think anxiously: "What will happen now?" You look for support somewhere, but you don't find it: you have to manage it all *yourself;* you anxiously cramp up, nervously looking for solutions to your questions, your sorrow, your uncertainty. You brace yourself, fortifying or defending yourself in a tense way; in your thoughts you seek intensely; you "claw" onto certain thoughts, perhaps imagining all kinds of things. By doing this you hurt yourself and block the flexible flow of energies in your body, in your muscles. You are very busy in your head with planning things, organizing or providing for yourself — not totally sure you will succeed. Anxious tension, by which your spirit is so concentrated on certain concerns that it becomes "separate" from your body. A cramp calls you completely back into yourself.

Let that steam go out of your head. A safe landing on your secure Basis, your deepest Self.

An injection of self-assurance and rest. Not allowing yourself to be rushed by anything or anyone. Know yourself to be supported in yourself. Come to complete relaxation; trust, and let go of thoughts. Everything in your life goes the way it has to, the way it is best for you, if you trustfully call up the positive. But don't pin yourself to the urge for achievement, or to exterior values. Be flexible toward yourself and feel how awareness powers nourish your body if you are present with your thoughts, here-and-now — not keeping your head in tense concentration upon one point. Stay here, with your body, Now. Don't run out of your body with your Consciousness!

Duchenne's muscular dystrophy

"hereditary" illness, with muscles dying off one by one, and at the same time enlarging

You enter life with negative expectations. You look at life as: "Everyone carries his own number, everyone has his task, everyone is tied to his little space, imprisoned and limited." You are afraid to truly live; you are filled to the brim with sadness; you shield yourself from the misery around you; you'd like to flee out of life. You consider yourself ugly and bad; perhaps you very much sympathize with your mother (or with the person with whom you have the strongest tie), and you make her ideas yours: "I'm ugly, unable to experience joy, etc."

You feel weak and hurt. You are convinced that others can constantly hurt you. As a result, of course, you will call up painful situations.

You feel at the mercy of others, helpless. "Which direction shall I take?" You don't know. You feel squeezed in a structure; you don't give yourself free living space! You submerge yourself in sadness and despair.

You don't dare to fully enjoy life. You don't trust your own Basis, your deepest Self. You don't really go onward; ear-flaps are covering your ears; you refuse to go on. Your way of existence is too "functional"; possibly too materialistic, or you wish to classify everything in life without really appreciating the essence of life. You keep yourself outside true natural existence, in deep anxiety and distrust regarding life: That's why in this life you have attracted these genetic conditions, which fit your inner convictions.

Self-awareness is always able to influence, to change, genetic codes. Put both feet on the ground, take up your large space, harmoniously integrate the elements — fire-air-water-earth — into your existence, and withdraw from the mousetrap which you have called up yourself! Don't strain yourself within a certain Structure; free yourself. Detach yourself, and enjoy the beautiful things in yourself, around you in nature. Offer yourself life; come to a clear perspective in your emotional life and don't close off your eyes or ears from Life: see how you have your life, your health, in your own hands. Don't allow yourself to "be lived"; become Master over your life. The cells of your body react to the instructions of your Self-aware "I."

Feel that powerful light-source in yourself; welcome yourself, in love, and come to a worthy Incarnation. Say farewell to detrimental convictions from the past! Drink in everything that makes you happy and that allows you to respect yourself. Life is not sinister and frightening unless you condemn it to be so.

Resolutely choose your path of life, and stand at the rudder of your ship.

Myopathy, muscle illness

Anxiety, bottled-up aggression: you are angry with life. A powerless flight.

You don't really believe in your self-aware "I"-power. You just feel like a cold skeleton, unable to experience true joy. Inwardly, you make yourself angry because of this powerlessness; you try to get everything and everyone into your "grip"; in a tense way you anxiously cling to material values because you don't succeed in building up your life *yourself* and working out your emotions. You feel bleak, filled to the top with emotions. You revolt against this feeling of powerlessness; you show your teeth instead of trustfully making yourself Master over your life and allowing actual evolution to take place. Your disbelief in yourself blocks you. You hinder growth in awareness; you don't allow your heart to lovingly radiate powers that would warm your body. You clench your fists, but you don't stand on your own feet.

Surrender now to the warm sun-center, to your Living Self. Feel that deep joy inside you, that possibility of creating your life YOURSELF. If you just believe in the negative, in your "powerlessness," then you are self-destructive. It's not someone else, but you who are able to call up your awareness powers and to make every fiber of your body vibrate with life-power, joy, and longing. Take up your full space; feel that warmth of the heart; make yourself welcome. Don't direct yourself toward others, but come to self-contemplation and discover that fundamentally solid, imperishable Basis in yourself.

Allow your emotions to flow freely, and don't bottle them up; don't be too hard on yourself. Arrive at self-assuredness; feel strong and loving; enjoy life to the utmost. Transform powerless aggression into energetic self-realization.

Don't delude yourself any longer with the conviction that you are unable to guide your body and your life in the direction that will make you happy. Open your heart, open your lungs wide, and allow yourself to truly Live — standing on your own feet!

Muscular pain
(See also Legs, calf muscle)

You've been too hard on yourself, or others have been too hard on you; in this case, however, you've unconsciously asked for it. An unconscious urge for transformation, change. Perhaps you now have to resolve some hard knocks: this is to wake you up. Bring about changes.

Sadness: you can't handle it anymore. It's too much for you.

For too long, you've held on to a function, a habit in life, customs from childhood — or you have held on to a role you play, but which doesn't *really* come out of you.

Or you have obeyed authority, have suffered pain because of others — but, in fact, you are doing this to yourself. Have you, in a cramped and tense way, held on to something for a long time? Now, you let yourself droop, in pain. There's no use for it anymore! A feeling of limpness, weakness, unsureness.

Your suppressed feelings now ask for a breakthrough. Your muscles no longer allow you to resist your own virtuous emotional energies — warmth, love, and mobility in all directions! It's a plea, from your deepest Self, to finally acknowledge your deepest "I," giving it the attention it deserves, no longer leaning on systems or authority outside yourself. A revolt against your own weakness in the past: having always done what others ordered you to do.

Feelings now wish to be acknowledged. Your inner "I," your Authority, now wishes to guide you.

Do you look sadly at the past? Let go, and choose a new direction.

What in your life asks for flexible adaptation? Changes? Allow yourself to flow with the current of life, without resistance: your deepest Self will bring you to the place where your evolution lies. Let go of the old and transform. Joy, thankfulness for Life! Surrender to virtuous life-energy; experience the comforting feeling of love inside you. No longer be hard on yourself! If you allow your emotions to flow freely, without blockades being thrown up, then these emotions will bring you further — also via communication with others.

Are you cold toward yourself? If so, then others will approach you coldly.

If you deprive yourself of love, then others will not be able to give you love.

Do you hold on to a limited structure? Or to narrow ways of life without true inspiration from your heart? Do you only do what you "have" to do according to belief-systems outside yourself, and do you not truly live from out of your deep longings? Then, your body, your muscles, also will restrict you.

Life is joy. You can only feel this when you allow yourself to experience all emotions, and when you place the Center in your

Self — not outside you, such as in systems, books, or authorities. That which is good for you, only you can feel.

Muscular rheumatism
(See also Rheumatism)

You are on the wrong track: you experience yourself as a victim who is not able to build up his own life. Sadness, repressed anger, disappointment, sometimes embittered. You feel cast out, written-off and "bound": you are silent; you feel treated unfairly; you don't really stand up for yourself; powerless.

You walk on the crutches of: "I can't." You don't get a grip on your life. You blame it all on others or on circumstances, but it is you, yourself, who are at the origin of your pains. Because you don't give yourself warm love; because you consider yourself to be inept; because you are stuck in sad occurrences from the past; because you don't build up your life Yourself, but you put your life in the hands of Fate, of a god or of your fellow men, because you deny your inner divine Power. Because you think life is a burden — that's why you will attract circumstances in your surroundings as well as in your body (rheumatism) which will give you a reflection of your sad convictions. Time to bring about changes!

You would sometimes beg desperately for a solution; for it you would cling to others, but this is of no use, of course, because the solution can only be found in yourself. You hope for happiness, but you feel too sad to still believe in this.

You wait instead of bringing about actual changes.

You duck away; your aggressive forces strike inward. You don't assume your leadership. You feel like a wagon on unstable wheels. You have no perspective on yourself, nor on the situation.

Your feelings become tight and stiff; you can't arrive at a free emotional exchange. You allow yourself to sag. Resistance to transformation. You hinder your growth by tightening yourself emotionally, immobilizing yourself in sadness.

Brake, and change tracks! Don't resist inner transformation. Discover the inexhaustible wealth in yourself; dig deeply and discover that fundamental source, your Living self. Grab hold of your life and create your life yourself with optimistic convictions. Don't fixate yourself on the negative, on sadness, because in this way you will attract more sad happenings. Know that a joyful, renewed life is awaiting you if you open your arms lovingly toward life itself. Take up all your space. Gather your powers. Dare to LIVE! Cut through what you have to cut through! Bite into life, stand up for yourself. Treat yourself and your body in a loving way; don't let yourself stand in the cold. SAY what you have to say. Get rid of those black emotions, your dark thoughts, and discover the sun in your Self. Feel your solid backbone; realize yourself! Don't stay stuck, don't weep. No longer restrict your life. Allow that stiffness, that resistance, to flow away from you, and experience your feelings in a flexible way. Don't immobilize yourself completely in angry powerlessness, despair or sadness: free yourself and open yourself! Allow that warmth in yourself; allow those enormous creative powers to flow through, and in a self-aware way take a new direction in life: the one that leads to Joy and enjoyment. Direct your life yourself; don't just stay where you are; don't let yourself "be lived" by religions, by the past, by the authority of others. Live from out of your Heart.

Strained muscle

"Where *are* you?" Do you flee from your true "I"?! You don't really live from out of yourself, but rather as a function of another person. You force yourself; you want to span something (like a bridge) in order to satisfy the expectations of your environment. You ignore your true nature; you hide your sadness and your inner anger. You feel you're not exactly going in the right direction: you probably follow the laws of the outer world too much, following that which you think

"has to be like that." Or do you outwardly, with your chest stuck out and head held high, present a proud demeanor as a mask? You feel stuck in a self-made prison. You too much allow yourself to "be lived" because you don't really feel secure in your Basis, in your deepest Self. Perhaps you feel hurt or not supported emotionally by others, but actually it is you who undervalue yourself! Because of anxiety arising from mistrust of your own nature, anxiety about the reactions of those around you, you don't really dare to reveal your deeper nature. You'd rather bottle up tensions and sadness than honestly manifest your nature.

Outwardly, you might show yourself to be tough and strong, but you don't really live in a Self-aware way. You're not in the center of your existence: your energies go around and around, as it were, in worrisome thoughts. You aren't flexible with yourself; you are too cold and hard on yourself. You act like this because you want to hide, to screen, your inner sensitivity and unsureness from the outer world. Do you consider yourself bad, guilty? Are you afraid you will not be appreciated if you show yourself the way you really are behind your mask of toughness? Why don't you pay attention to your inner Self? Why don't you love yourself? Do you play sports? Do you dance? Do you live only "for the eyes of others"? Do you feel inwardly so small, anxious, and unsure, that you seek affirmation in applause for your tricks? Self-betrayal. You hurt yourself! Why don't you reveal your true feelings? Do you go along with this condition of imprisonment? Don't you really care about your life? You demolish yourself. You carry a load of burdens and sorrow, but you shouldn't blame others for it, because the reason lies in fleeing *away* from *yourself!*

Your muscle asks for acknowledgment of your true "I," asks for Joy in your life.

Allow your feelings to flow freely: be yourself! Express yourself; speak, and come to life from out of your heart, your deep emotional core. Why withdraw so behind a screen? You are good the way you are; be spontaneous and never force yourself. Joy can only exist if one is satisfied with oneself. Be honest with yourself and do the deeds that you intuitively feel you have to do. Don't hold back. In a self-aware way express your opinion, your longings, and don't do things that go against your true nature.

Allow your energies to strongly circulate around your sun-center. Let go of sadness; don't trouble yourself with the outer world, with Image. Be faithful to your Nature! Feel the contact with your deepest Self and spontaneously give expression to your creativity. Allow all energies to pass through smoothly, in relaxation. Don't allow any discrepancy to develop between your outer and your inner Ego. Dare to manifest yourself the way you inwardly feel. Don't bottle up any anger or sadness: achieve open communication. Feel your strong Basis. Don't doubt the goodness of your nature, and honestly give in to your wishes. Come in love and warmth to yourself, and know yourself to be securely supported in yourself. You can truly make yourself and others happy only when you live in harmony and honesty with yourself. If you live rigidly, hidden behind a tough shield, then you can't really come in contact with others — then your fellow man can't be happy either, because you are not truly with them. Don't force yourself in public display: put things in perspective!

Torn muscle

Inner emotional conflict. Stop! It can't go on like this anymore. You suppress your own warm energies. Suppression of your true being, of your "I." You live too much according to the standards of others or of the outer world. Sadness, confusion. Revolt: you fight with your elbows, you squeeze yourself into a straight-jacket which is too tight, into a structure put upon you by a sports trainer or a yoga teacher, or by your partner or parents. Thus you don't really live "naturally" from out of your heart. You feel

vulnerable, like a martyr; you feel cold because you don't dare to experience yourself from within. You wriggle yourself into all kinds of turns; you sag with an enormous emotional flexibility because you make your life dependent on the approval of others. How do you feel inwardly? How do you want to be perceived? How do you adjust yourself? A "tearing" conflict, which asks for a solution. Do you consider yourself not good enough to live spontaneously the way you *are?* You make yourself subordinate to a society, to others.

You *allow* yourself to "be lived" by the outer world, by the sadness of not being able to be yourself. You feel threatened; you are afraid of being rejected or condemned. That's why you force yourself so. But your true soul-powers can't come through: you block your true self-realization. You crawl too much; you want to lean too much on others, as a child leans on the shoulder of his father, instead of discovering the Power in your inner Self. You don't listen to the voice of your heart; you tighten Yourself, you hurt yourself, you put duties and rules upon yourself just to "satisfy."

Are you afraid that the public, your partner, your father or trainer might lynch you, if you don't satisfy their expectations? Fear of criticism. Your feelings are kept in tightly. You think you have to carry a cross; you are of the opinion that life means exertion and pain rather than joy. You would call forth all your Mars powers, your aggressive energies, in an exaggerated way just to prove yourself, while inside you feel sad and small. You ignore the gentle beauty in your nature.

You Want to, but you Can't anymore: an inner collision which cries for acknowledgement of your "I" separate from the outside world. Lean powerfully on your Self, don't look for affirmation, but feel that warmth in your own being. Make yourself warmly welcome, and don't first expect this from others. Live from out of your heart, in self-assuredness. It's not the achievement, but how you feel, that counts. Put foolish thoughts out of your head and look at how your world might be built too much on a facade — at how you have paid too little attention to deeper values, to your emotional wealth, to your creative possibilities in a broad scope, to love toward yourself and others. You THINK too much, you worry needlessly. Dare to let yourself be born, and now live only out of your conscious "I." You are good the way you are, without forcing yourself. Now acknowledge your true nature and don't run ahead of yourself. If you live in harmony with your living Self, then you will notice how there is joy, relaxation, and peace at the origin of every human life. No longer leave yourself out in the cold. Rely on your fundamentally strong Basis.

MYELITIS

inflammation of the spinal marrow

Anxiety, insecurity, powerless anger, frustration, black thoughts.

All the things you have been accumulating for far too long — energies, feelings such as pain and aggression — now come to the surface; you burst open in revolt. No longer wanting anything; you are sick of living this way; strongly suppressed feelings that are piled up in the unconscious spheres spout to the surface. Time for a big cleaning, for thorough changes! You have stowed away your valuable diamond for too long; your deepest Self asks that you dig for that diamond. Dare to confront yourself with your feelings of Powerlessness; with the inability to be yourself.

You have not really been yourself; thus far you have carried a false scepter, have lived a life that goes against your worthy nature. You have built your life on foundations that are too unstable, that aren't really based on your own roots.

These symptoms ask that you call your self-destruction to a halt. Your feelings have too long been restrained. Again and again you have pent up your dark, bad thoughts, feeling imprisoned in a structure that doesn't suit your nature. You feel hurt. With impotent anger you only break down yourself and your body, but you don't dare to trust your intuition; you are not firmly standing on your feet. You cling grimly to the surface because you don't trust the depths within yourself. You consider your deepest Self to be rotten and untrustworthy. You have absolutely no perspective on your feelings anymore; your life is becoming unmanageable.

You are now flooded with emotions; you no longer can handle it, you push everything and everyone away from you; a longing for complete liberation.

You'd like to realize yourself, but you feel handicapped; you don't dare to build on your own solid basis.

Transformation! Let all powers and feelings now freely escape. Dare to let yourself rest upon your own deepest Self; the basis upon which you have built your life until now has been too fragile. Let yourself go now, let go of everything and come into harmony with yourself: be proud of your worth, dare to experience your feelings and your intuition. Fly freely and peacefully in your nature and discover that you are the creator of your existence! Self-respect. Take pleasure in your being. Now develop your new structures on the basis of your nature. Turn anger into action! Communicate with others, voice your opinion, don't play diplomat, live from out of your heart, dare to be honest with yourself, with others.

Don't blame others for your feelings of powerlessness: resolutely grab hold of your life, let go of the past, be solid in yourself.

N

NAILS

Psychological correspondence

Symbolic of the faith in your natural Growth from the inside out, in the structure which grows from out of your deepest core, your divine Self, outward. Faith in these inner Powers which form your body, which you can use in the creation of your existence.

Allow your wheel of life to go on in flexibility. Don't hold back change and renovation. Resilience; faith that everything will come your way: give, and you will get everything that is good for you. Don't try to force or seize too much.

On the one hand, symbol of the Power and Support which we experience in our deepest Self; if we trust our Self, then there is always a guarantee of Protection and Support. You will always be rescued by this eternal Living part of yourself, even if you sometimes fall deep.

The supporting powers in yourself. Symbol of Protection, of nourishing yourself from the inner source, with joy, power, and wisdom.

Taking good care of yourself; taking in things or experiences you need from the outside world and assimilating them; spiritual and material nourishment.

Arriving at where you have to be: propelling on toward your objectives. Going straight ahead for the goal. Going to the core of things, without detours.

Being one-pointed of purpose, ending up where you have to be: with the fire of your inner Self, you Consciously forge a life with well-determined goals and objectives which you try to accomplish; resolutely striving toward them.

On the other hand, the nails also symbolize the ability to be supple, flexible, and tolerant; to be open to changes, without anxiety or resistance.

Turning, in a limber way; taking your curves in a supple way, giving your steering wheel a totally different direction if need be: listening to your inner voice.

Ailments, in general

Anxiously clutching something or someone: afraid to let go.

A feeling of emotional threat, because of which you will begin in an exaggerated way to protect or hide yourself behind a thick impenetrable shield; but by doing this you totally immobilize yourself, and your feelings will be confined in a prison. You "arm" yourself against danger. You cover yourself up; you feel anything but protected in your Self because you don't have faith in your deepest Consciousness Core. You don't dare let go; you keep running in place; you're almost "immobile," your life becomes rigid; swollen, hardened, bloated.

You anxiously provide for yourself; you make sure everything is super-safe: you might take too much, swallow greedily, Wanting too much. . . .

Feelings of anxiety and uncertainty lead to aggression, to clawing at others, to self-destruction.

You can build up a dazzling defensive shield, a radiating outer image behind which you safely hide and which will keep others at a distance from your inner core.

A flower grows out of its root; white petals group around a center like a crown: this way we also will trust in the natural growth of ourselves. It doesn't do any good to reach too far, or for too much: letting go and bending flexibly with the rhythm of our heart, of our deepest Self. Working on ourselves, trusting in this inner power, without a feeling of threat; no forcing; not holding back changes. Being faithful to our deepest nature. Taking care of ourselves by evolving, without resistance, into a Self-aware life-realization, built upon powerful fundamental energies of which we gratefully make use, without hurting others. We know ourselves to be Safe and Protected.

Nail-biting

Anxiety, nervousness. Burdensome thoughts: your thinking-mill is turning nervously and tensely. You are not yet really yourself. Unconsciously you fear *"not-being."* You cringe in fear that others — your parents, your mentors — might "seize," punish or squeeze you: anxieties. But these negative expectations regarding life, with which you were born, can indeed be the cause of your having attracted people of whom you are afraid, against whom you are on guard, with whom you are angry. Insufficiently grounded in your own being, you don't dare allow your powerful energies to blossom: you insufficiently bring your possibilities outward; you hold back; you are insufficiently aware of your worth. You are afraid that others might grab you by the hair. You stifle your talents, frustrated. You don't always dare to be honest!

Feel calm, secure, relaxed in your Self. Discover your worth and be proud of your unique being. Allow all creative energies to open up freely; become aware of your deep powers, of your possibilities; externalize instead of eating up those beautiful inner energies. Reveal your thoughts, your feelings;

establish yourself strongly as an individual, no matter how young you are. Get a good hold on yourself; don't be afraid of anyone, and then no one will harm you. Step outward with your rich content; don't bottle things up; don't put talents into the ground. Place your faith in your divine, deepest Self.

Honest confrontation; resolute externalization of that which dwells in you; in this way, you allow yourself and others to evolve.

Crumbling, breaking, weak nails

You are insufficiently open to the powers, the sounds, from your deepest Self.

An inability or refusal to live in a self-aware way as "I"; you too much allow yourself to "be lived" by your parents (as a child), by an authority outside yourself, by the masses — you're too "anonymous"; you allow yourself to lie back like a baby at its mother's breast; you don't feed yourself.

You are too little aware of your genuine worth as an individual; you feel too small, too dependent on others.

You behave as if you have no backbone, too limp, too weak, too flexible; you feel in the grip of someone else. Emotions overpower your existence. Emotionally being stuck, bound to others. Sometimes you can't handle certain things anymore, can't digest them anymore; you close your ears to it, because you don't build on your powerful "I"-Consciousness.

Become conscious of your Self, of your Worth, and build a solid structure; mark off your own terrain, feel yourself protected within yourself. Under the supervision of a Self-aware "I," allow all powerful energies — your sounds, your possibilities, your creative power — to grow. Look deep inside yourself; don't sleep, but work; be open to those potential powers in your inner center. A solid, independent, resolute growth.

Ingrown nail
(See also Nails, in general)

You are filled to the brim with longings and ambitions to go forward, but you don't really dare to come out of your shell. With aggressive intentions, you'd like to overreach and get to the top, or grasp for a goal, but these feelings stay secretively hidden.

When it comes to realizing yourself, you feel so powerless and handicapped; you'd so much like to break through, even to seize for power, to perform stunts — You would attract people, would draw situations to you, would force things with an inner aggressive urge, but you feel so guilty about this aggressiveness, about these ambitions and longings.

The more you suppress your spontaneous powers, the more this leads to increasing frustration.

You feel anxious, guilty, powerless: you don't trust your inner wisdom. You think you have to find confirmation of yourself in the outer world; your ambitions and longings lie outside you; you think you have to prove yourself by external action. That's why you feel guilty; that's why you don't really break through — because you don't build on your inner powers and possibilities, on your consciousness energies. If you place the Worth in yourself, then the heated urge for outward self-affirmation will disappear.

You are afraid that if you live from out of your intuitive deepest Self, from out of your spontaneous longings — your natural disposition — you won't be good enough. That's why you search and struggle in your Thoughts. Stubbornly, you fixate on certain situations that you absolutely want to make turn out a certain way! Your thinking world is aggressive and clawing; you think you have to prepare certain things; you *think* and fret — but you are at such a distance from your inner Self.

In order to fill up your emptiness you cling to something — sucking on the world outside you, so to speak. But, estranged from yourself, you also have communication problems with others.

You are afraid of being hurt: you encapsulate yourself.

You sink your teeth into something: stubbornly, you remain where you are; with a so-called valid reason, you think you are not allowed to go on, but you don't in fact Want to, and don't Dare to, because of fear.

You hinder yourself from Being, perhaps from speaking, from showing yourself the way you *are* — afraid of being hurt.

Cast outward — with centrifugal force — your talents, your powers, and all your energies: dare to live from out of your deepest Self; build your life on inner wisdom, without hesitation. Come out with your feelings and possibilities; dare to freely communicate with people you attract on your life's path. Free yourself; let go of frustrating thoughts, and become active and creative. Anger is just the result of your standing still when inner powers are seeking freedom. Dare to be yourself, without shame or guilt.

Loosening of nail bed

You live according to certain rules or structures which are put upon you by the outer world, via your upbringing, via a system, a partner. You can't keep this up; you will have to "let go" of such an unauthentic life or your nail will loosen!

You absolutely want to do, to force, certain things which are actually not good for you, which go against your true nature. Mostly, you do things in order "to do good."

Wanting the impossible; you think you will fly far, but you are stuck.

You needlessly carry heavy burdens, especially emotionally. Your self-aware "I" is too absent; feelings are flooding you; you allow yourself to "be lived" by others, also — and perhaps especially — by those who mean well by you, but in fact are hindering your evolution.

An inner conflict can tear you apart: you flexibly allow yourself to "be lived" by others, but on the other hand you *do* want to live *yourself.*

You think you are attacking, but you, *yourself,* are being attacked by your anxious unsureness and your wanting to force things. You think you are going your way more independently, but your doubts are calling up a contrary reaction from your partner (Who, for instance, gets a hold of you). Being stuck; wanting to get away — a frustrating feeling. Are you looking for appreciation, for confirmation from outside? Don't you really dare to be who you are? Are you trying to satisfy the expectations of others? Where are you?

No longer undervalue yourself! Break the padlock and free yourself from bogged-down situations. Dare to experience your being, to show yourself the way you really are.

Don't look for acknowledgement of your outer ego, but live spontaneously from out of your deepest Self.

Go on: no longer remain stuck in oppressive situations, discover yourself in action and in creativity; don't let yourself be influenced by others. Show Yourself, not others, what you are worth. Protect your feelings, feel safe, and be a Father to yourself — don't expect this from others. Don't be afraid of your feelings; don't go against the current; don't always do what others tell you to do: follow the spontaneous flow which emanates from your heart and deepest inner soul. Dive into your deepest core; feel the earth, the confidence in yourself; allow yourself to blossom on your own basis.

Extremely thick, calcified nails

You put on armor because you feel threatened in your emotional core.

"Forbidden to enter," emotional blockage, impotently running in place, even though you might explode from pent-up aggression.

Because you doubt yourself so much, because inwardly you feel foolish or inferior, because you don't know how to deal with your emotional vulnerability — because of all this, you possibly put on a proud mask to the outer world, or you build up an image or an achievement-oriented job. In this case, inner unsureness leads to lion-like, proud behavior. Because you feel so limp and weak, you think you absolutely *have* to do certain things in order to stand up to others, to the outer world.

Possibly, an aggressive urge to fight just to be able to feel yourself.

You fixate on a certain something or someone; you hold on, you force things, although it goes completely against your true nature; here, it's about a natural outward growth-process from within you.

The world outside you appears threatening because you insufficiently depend upon your own secure Basis: you, therefore, will strongly push yourself away — with angry claws if need be — from those who, or that which, threatens to suppress you. But, in fact, it is you who suppresses your own natural powers. Sometimes impotent fury.

Softening, feeling peaceful in yourself. Opening yourself up to your inner Self; knowing yourself to be secure in this inner Authority. Do only that which you feel from within you should do, and don't compromise. Find yourself, build up your structure, allow those creative energies to run their course spontaneously; trust your own feelings, open yourself up to gentleness and love, welcome yourself and others. Self-protection is deep inside you; don't be afraid. Break down your shield. You are good the way you are; don't try to satisfy the expectations of others, but live according to your longings; dare to be yourself completely. Grounding! Self-assuredness! Action! Hold back no longer, don't hide; allow yourself to flow along supply on the waves of your Self. No longer be so hard, stubborn, recalcitrant, and aggressive — which has caused you to hurt others as well as yourself. At last, offer love and appreciation to yourself, the way you deserve it, and stop considering yourself weak or inferior: these are complexes which you can let go of! Discover the Power in yourself and become master over it!

White spots in the nails

Like a child, you lose yourself too much in others. You (unconsciously) allow yourself to be taken up into something or someone; you insufficiently affirm your individuality.

The strong urge to express yourself, to bring things outward, creativity — but you dream, think, fantasize, float, "think" or "plan" too much instead of arriving at *actual* self-realization. You are not getting a complete grip on your life; suppressed feelings weigh heavily on you. You are good and helpful, but are on guard because of your unsureness, which might cause you to aggressively bite when threatened.

Suppressed activity leads to pent-up aggression. But, actually, you are a dependent little sheep, afraid and expectant. You fixate your thoughts too strongly on certain things; emotionally, you have a hard time digesting certain things.

You allow yourself to be restricted, pushed into a certain direction (upbringing, influences).

It is good to do a lot for others as long as you don't lose yourself in doing so, as long as you don't do it only for self-affirmation, as long as these are your own longings and free choice. Come to complete incarnation; allow your energies to flow freely. Don't allow yourself to be restricted by others. Struggle free and become independent so that you first of all arrive at love for yourself. Make yourself welcome, as a child, but give yourself all opportunity to grow up in self-awareness: get a grip on your feelings, on unconscious powers, by living YOURSELF, on your own feet, autonomously, aware of your worth, trusting in your deepest Self. Not dreaming. Being present, here-and-now, on earth; enjoying

with your senses, resolutely building up your life; free navigation, without limitations.

NARCOLEPSY
always falling asleep

You pass over the essence of yourself, of life. You run out of breath: because you don't draw your energies from your powerful "I"-center. You pull yourself down. You don't really live from out of your true Self, from out of your heart. You lose powers by playing a Role, by wearing a mask. Perhaps you wear yourself out in order to satisfy the expectations of others, of the outer world: "Am I doing it right? What impression do I make?"

You suppress your gentle, supple sensitivity in order to manifest yourself outwardly as tough and manly, like a Lion who can handle everything or who directs and organizes things. In this way, you lose your powers in order to "satisfy."

You live too superficially; your true talents are unable to come to the fore; you are afraid of being yourself. You don't really *live;* you close yourself off from your power-source. You worry instead of trusting in your deepest "I"; you waste your thoughts on needless things. Emotional burdens weigh too heavily because you don't listen to your inner voice. Finally, you take the mask away because you are becoming so tired of this game, and you can't handle it anymore.

Possibly, you hold on to a situation which it would be better to let go of. You feel stuck to something or someone, and you'd like to flee from it! You defend yourself in a "manly," powerful way, but inwardly you feel anxious and unsure. You don't dare show your sensitive heart.

Do you put so much energy into outer values? Into your image? Or do you waste your life in futilities? Do you think you won't be accepted otherwise?

Be yourself; discover your deepest Self and draw from this bottomless cistern. Integrate all your feelings; dare to show your gentleness, your flexibility, your "female" aspects. Don't be too tough and hard. You are good the way you are. Don't be afraid to let go of things; don't force yourself to achieve something. Slowly, but surely, follow that route which you intuitively sense as being the one linked most closely to your nature. It's not the outer Image, but the way you feel inside that is important.

Take up your scepter, enjoy life; arrive at a clear perspective on your situation. Cut through a knot if necessary. Don't flee; get a hold of your life with both hands. Live joyfully from out of your deepest inner Center. Solve your emotional problems: confront yourself with them! Feel safe and sheltered in your warm sun-center, in the Living Self. Honesty, openness.

You will find your true life-motivation deep inside you, not in the outer world.

THE NECK

Psychological correspondence

The neck symbolizes relaxation and rest in ourselves if we trustfully open ourselves up to our inner wisdom. By doing so we will also be able to open ourselves up in a flexible way to others, to impressions from the outer world.

Being able to look at everything from above (with your Conscious "I"); daring to look in all directions without self-limitation. Daring to look at all aspects of a problem. Feeling free, casting yourself out of oppressive situations. Pride, inner self-assurance, but in service to, and gently inclined toward, others.

With prudence, you know how to keep to the golden center: "I or the others?"

Ailments, in general

Exaggerated pride: because of outer or false values, a result of being cut off from your inner Self; tensions, anxieties, and unsureness. Showing off your feathers so to seek conformation of yourself because you doubt your worth. You, yourself, are too absent; your life is built on having a Hold outside yourself, on image or on a function in, for instance, the religious, social, or political world.

Obstinately, stubbornly, holding on to a prejudgment, refusing to see the deeper truth; resisting. . . . Refusing to evolve further in life in a supple way on the waves of your flexible nature.

Holding on to obsolete values aggressively, critically, narrow-mindedly — because you are still ignoring your true worth. You resist that which others tell you; you cling to material, outer, or other less-important things because you deny the Power of your deepest Self. You block a supple flow to your body from out of your consciousness-Core. You unconsciously rebel against the request — from your inner Self — of acknowledging your large space, of beginning to look at things in a broader way, without blinders.

You cling to something, by which you hurt yourself: an inner feeling of being stuck, imprisoned. You'd like to radiate outwardly, but feel inwardly confined. You are too hard and too stiff, first of all, with yourself. Do you want to please others in a gracious way? In this way, you immobilize yourself!

Only do what you feel you have to do from out of your own nature; flexibly open yourself up to the longings of your inner Self; lovingly and self-assuredly open yourself up to the message from others. Free yourself of tensions; no longer cling to things or persons; arrive at gentleness, flexibility, openness. Be proud of true values, of your content, not of tinsel. Dare to open yourself up to the opinion of others, without feeling threatened: you are safe in yourself; you are allowed to calmly turn your head in all directions, flexibly attuning yourself to others without having to leave the Center of yourself. Inner solidity allows you to be flexible.

Lymph node swelling in the neck

The way the arms of a windmill turn and turn, although its foundations on the earth be weak and fragile, so are you with your head far above your body, so to speak. You think and dream, escape into your thoughts, away from the earthly here-and-now, although this doesn't stop you from appearing clownish, a proud Image, a joker, as if nothing's the matter. Inwardly, you don't feel totally safe in earthly nature; you experience as hard work that which is earthly, that which is natural, physical contacts with others, fully integrating your feelings. On the one hand, you would fearfully cling to others, but on the other hand you would flee out of life. You don't very well know what to do with your emotions; sometimes, you would defend yourself in an aggressive, nervous way, protecting yourself against the pain that others might inflict upon you; you are so vulnerable in your love relationships that you might flee into a vague thought-world. You want to protect yourself against evil, against those who want to hurt you. You build a protective fortress in your emotional world, but the cannons you aim to keep the supposed danger at a distance direct themselves inwardly so that you swell up. You hold in your powers too much; you don't allow your "I" to achieve true self-realization; you'd sooner lock yourself up in a high, unreachable spiritual island-sphere where no one can get to you. You don't really participate in life: in this way, creative and emotional energies are being blocked! You live too tensely. You are like a safety pin that pricks itself.

You are afraid of "the child inside you," of those original, spontaneous feelings, be-

cause you don't trust your own nature, because you degrade yourself to being less than human. Being stuck in the past, unable to go onward, because you don't really live in the Now.

"Help! I drown in my emotions, and I don't see how to integrate them into life." Mars powers are being suppressed.

Solution: see the category Lymph node swellings, in general.

Spinal fracture in the neck

The cause here lies in the feeling of powerlessness about the situation in which you are stuck. For too long you've suppressed your feelings, your natural powers: selfdestruction, which asks for a radical turnaround, a transformation.

It couldn't go on in this way — you don't really live from out of your self. Perhaps, outwardly, you have always seemed distinguished or polite, when in fact you inwardly were swimming in unresolved emotions. For a long time, spontaneous and creative energies have been suppressed: you do what's expected of you, but you are living like a wooden puppet by so doing. You can't keep on pushing away all those feelings, those energies; to do so is a form of suicide. Why aren't you really living from out of yourself? Anxieties? Are you clinging to false (external, material) values?

Fear of going on, of evolving.

An aggressive power-grip on your life. A nervous, desperate situation: an inner conflict. Going on or standing still? Evolution means Life, refusal means death. You oppress your heart, your soul, your life. You pile up worries, anxieties, and sadness: these seek a way out.

As long as you live here, you can free yourself: fly with your own wings and don't let yourself be held back. Listen to your inner authority, not to others; don't cling to worthless pillars. Surrender flexibly to your heart's desire.

Stop being so hard on yourself! Unburden yourself! Produce, create, express yourself, radiate love and warmth to yourself, to others, without anxieties. Trust in your deepest eternal Self; break the lock and follow the path of your longings, of your intuition, of joyful life. If you long for, and expect, rest and happiness, then it will come to you: no longer resist a positive, totally new path!

Stiffness in the neck, pain

Anxious stiffening: a feeling of inadequacy; you cannot or dare not completely "reach" things. You only look left or right, not daring to look in a wider scope. You feel "stuck," especially with regard to emotions. Your outer life-circumstances, the situations or things to which you stubbornly cling, are only a reflection of your inner anxiety and unsureness.

Too stubborn, but especially too Afraid of "hearing" or "seeing": you flee.

You feel too small to take full responsibility; you feel you're not able to speak Straightforwardly, to be completely honest with yourself. Too afraid to bend; you flee from the truth regarding yourself.

You won't be able to position yourself in a flexible and open way because you don't really trust your inner Self. In a cramped way you hold on for support or security to elements outside yourself. You ignore your own authority.

Intense resistance, aggressive and stiff-necked behavior, a reaction to your inner powerlessness: this is how you demolish yourself, not allowing yourself to evolve flexibly. Obstinately holding fast to your point of view without listening to facts that might mean enrichment for you: Do you feel so threatened? You close yourself off from your inner emotional core, from your nature; you hold on to needless tensions. You are too inflexible with yourself.

Build your life on the guidance of your inner Authority and feel powerful in your Self. No longer flee from your inner wisdom and from the message that others have for you: flexibly, and in a loving way, open yourself to others. Listen to your feelings, to your nature: don't force things, throw off needless burdens, let go of everything that oppresses you.

In a self-assured way, determine your direction; direct yourself in a flexible way at the path you intuitively feel is best, not allowing yourself to be slowed down by suffocating, conservative thoughts that hinder your evolution.

(See also Neck, in general.)

Whiplash injury
damage to the neck or spine
in a driver whose automobile
has been hit from behind or from the side

You have the longing to arrange everything, to hold sway over others, to keep control over your surroundings by overseeing everything in a dominant way. This inner urge awakens an enormous amount of energies, calls up a lot of electrical forces, but these energies remain ultimately within the closed circuit of yourself. This energy is not being exploited in self-realization; it charges itself more and more in accord with your wanting to embrace more and more. The causes of this injury are not only anxieties and an urge to dominate, but also feelings of responsibility and caring for others — and also an urge to achieve, to be loved and accepted by others, wanting to have a tough appearance, being hard and severe with yourself, doing too much for your fellow man: you put yourself in second place.

This closed circuit sometimes leads to a short-circuit: especially because you often hesitate — yes-no-yes — concerning the letting-through of energies that are ready to be unfolded by *yourself*. Energy, feelings, are being blocked.

In powerless fury you inwardly direct your aggression toward others because you feel that your grip or your Authority no longer work, because you feel that the role of authority or the game of being a stalwart attention-attractor no longer has the effect you had in mind.

Now you need to throw off your mask, or tough role. But then who are you anymore? In this way, you anxiously doubt yourself. "They floored me: I am stuck and can't do anything anymore" — powerlessness.

You blame the cause of your misery on others, but it lies inside yourself.

Integrate the gentle "femininity" in yourself, the receptiveness. Let go! Now turn completely toward yourself; make your Self and your powers emerge. Be a human being among human beings; neither place yourself at the top nor at the bottom. Be flexible and good with yourself. Anxiously holding on is not necessary; you can trust that fundamentally safe Basis of your deepest Self. Place yourself in the center of your existence so that you no longer have the need to stand in someone else's center. Be yourself; allow inner energies and emotions to freely flow outward. Don't block yourself.

NERVOUS BREAKDOWN

You can no longer handle things; you now ask others for attention regarding your situation. Your deepest Self now cries for Room for yourself, for acknowledgement of your worthy Self, because in the past you haven't given yourself the acknowledgement, the appreciation, everyone needs; because you have allowed yourself to be swallowed up by society, by family, by a partner, a group, a job, a function, an ideal — and you have given too little space and privacy to your highly personal "I." Possibly, you have constantly lived "the way you're supposed to"; perhaps you have even sacrificed yourself: this was an escape from your own "I," from your spontaneous nature, from your deepest feelings. In the past, you've clung too much to duties or to people. You just do, you just give, you work for others, until you run your head against a wall, because you are really running away from yourself. You have done too much now; you must go back: the path to yourself. You have done everything for others, because of a need for attention, affection, and appreciation, which you haven't given yourself. But nothing has been solved by this; now you are "stuck" in this self-sought pattern and you want to get out of it.

Everything went smoothly as long as you got appreciation and attention from your surroundings — because you were so decent, so good, so holy, so generous, etc.; because you were so much at the service of others. Until you became a victim of this role you played and which got out of hand. Emotionally and physically, things are becoming too heavy for you.

Now you are stuck in a situation, in a relationship, in a task, and it can't go on this way any longer. The true cause lies in the fact that you never really accepted yourself, unless it was under strict conditions: firstly having to prove that you are a good housewife or a model husband, etc. You don't unconditionally accept yourself. You don't really trust your deepest Self; you aren't really aware of the golden treasure hidden inside everyone; you want others to approve of you for self-affirmation. You feel oppressed now; you are no longer Free; you feel as if there's a noose around your neck. You no longer have rest and relaxation; you desperately long for your own space, to be free and left alone.

On the other hand, you can't be without others, because you don't lovingly and warmly welcome yourself the way you are, without "having" to fulfill this or that.

Powerlessness, aggressive feelings; fear of being yourself; inferiority; attaching more importance to outer or social norms and expectations than to your own Nature and its needs.

Despair: not being able to reach yourself; self-underestimation; being cut off from your intuition, from your deepest Core. Desperation, because you aren't living from out of your deepest Self. A feeling of suffocation because you allow too many people to penetrate into your personal terrain. Too little faith in your Individual powers and in the right to make your own decisions. Ultimately you feel Pain; you are hurt. As long as you don't consider yourself to be the true Center of your existence, as long as you wish your outer Ego to be acknowledged by your surroundings, others will hurt you. You claw at others, sometimes with power, because you experience yourself as powerless. In this way you again call up situations in which you are being seized (for instance, by medicines).

Deal with others in a free, relaxed, friendly way, while maintaining your personality and freedom. Determine your own limits, without losing yourself in a task, an image, in a group, in an ideal. In the first place take good care of yourself: this is "My terrain."

You feel secure and full of trust in your deepest Self; you don't rush for anyone. You follow the demand of your Nature; in the first place you offer yourself the love and appreciation, the rest and relaxation, which you need so much; only when you no longer Need to dedicate yourself to the cause of others will you be able to help others in an ideal way, without hurting yourself, without ignoring your "I." The pride of yourself, of your inner worth, is very good. You no longer drown yourself in others; no longer allow others to be parasites on you. You don't Seize powerfully for others; you no longer claw onto things or people because you undervalue yourself: now, you let go of everything and everyone and come very close to yourself.

A total confrontation with yourself is beneficial: your Self offers the guarantee of safe and immortal existence; you have only to tune into this, in surrender, and that which is best for you will automatically happen. Life is not a coincidence, but a happening that we ourselves determine and create. Anxieties are useless, since nothing negative can happen to you without your first having called it up.

Now, discover the silence in your Self.

NERVOUS SYSTEM

Psychological correspondence

In Freedom and Trust, being open to ourselves, to others.

The Light of our Awareness finds its way to a new dimension: the nervous system functions as an important system for receiving, transmitting, and communicating. Nerve cells react immediately to changes within the conscious or unconscious world of experience. Communication with our deepest Self, communication with others, through all matter and distances. Nerve channels transport messages.

Via feedback , via pain signals in our body, we understand what we have to "change" in our body.

Becoming aware is a very important process; our brain nerves immediately let us know when we are on the wrong track, when we are concentrating only on rationality and switching off our intuitive channels; we will become anxiously and nervously tense.

In order to live a calm and joyful life, it is necessary to have a healthy exchange between, on the one hand, the rational and logical, and, on the other hand, the intuitive and emotional. If we trustfully open ourselves up to our inner self, then anxieties will disappear.

You have harmonious contact with yourself, with your body: you enjoy sensorial impulses and pleasures, caressing gentleness.

A gentle, peaceful atmosphere, a fundamental trust in your deepest Self and in life: your nervous system receives these Consciousness Experiences and transmits them in all possible directions. You radiate light: to others, to every fiber of your body. Electromagnetic forces move strongly through nerve channels; you transmit, you receive. With your Self-awareness, you guide the functioning of your nerves. In order to have good health it is necessary to have a balance in the relationship between the Conscious "I," here-and-now, and your inner source of feelings, so that you feel stable, safe and sheltered in yourself, so that you won't cling to others, to things outside yourself.

If you don't trust in your Self, then your nerves will ultimately break down; if you aren't open to those light energies in yourself, then you will feel constricted, anxious, and dark.

The nervous system immediately translates just how much you are Free and full of trust in the Living Light of your immortal Self, or to what degree you close yourself off from this inner light, so that you can't really feel free and relaxed: you hurt yourself. If you refuse to acknowledge the mastery over yourself, then you can make yourself crazy, become Insane, paranoid, full of panicky anxieties.

Pent-up emotions, mistrust, disbelief, self-destruction — all these "weigh down" and "slow down" the light vibrations of your nerves: signals of sadness reach all parts of your body, until at last the negativity can settle somewhere in the form of an ailment or tumor.

In order to have healthy nerves it is also necessary that you don't allow yourself, via your head, to be "drained" up there into higher, thinner spheres so that you might lose all contact with the earth, with your body.

Stay here, within certain earthly structures; don't flee too much into dreams and thoughts. But don't tie down your intuition, your receptive channels; free yourself, and open yourself up to the most beautiful experiences.

Feeling safe, in surrender to life, aware of your worth. You know, you feel, what you have to do at every moment if you just listen to those stimuli and those signals in yourself. A fundamental trust in this inner clock. You don't close your ears to those messages; you don't close your eyes. You are completely open; you are aware of your unlimited possibilities with regard to "communication," sending-power, and radiation powers.

(Read Part I.)

NEURALGIA
shooting pain

You feel like a gull with clipped wings: you'd like to fly, but you are stuck. Aggressive powerlessness.

You hold back natural aggressive powers; you place yourself in stiff armor.

Your frustration — this bottling-up of energies, of impulsive forces, perhaps of talents — this blocking of natural emotional flow ultimately oppresses you so much that you break out in nervous arrows! Inner resistance to "being stuck," resistance to a life situation that strangles you.

You'd like to break with something, with a habit or an overly oppressive way of life, but you don't dare to — insufficient trust in your deepest Self. Possibly, instead of living honestly and spontaneously from out of your own longings, you attach too much importance to what others say about you.

You live in a herky-jerky way: your energies come through by fits and starts in your body because you don't allow yourself to flow spontaneously, to smoothly let your natural powers come through: you constantly block yourself.

You hurt yourself. This anxious self-suppression leads to enormous tensions, stress, anger.

You don't have to start "flying": the prison lies in yourself. Free yourself from the harness of norms, etiquette, "this is how it has to be," or "this is what others expect from me": liberate your nature and don't remain stuck to outer norms with which fashion or society tie you down. What counts in life are love and joy; dare to experience yourself to the fullest, from out of your spontaneity. For once, dare to express your aggression; don't be afraid of your powers, of your emotions. Speak out and stand up for yourself; no longer keep yourself so tight and tense. Give yourself all the space to be, in order to joyfully and creatively express that which really lives in your soul, in your heart. Say what you have to say; live in harmony with your nature; don't kill yourself by "politeness" or by artificial behavior.

Mark off your space and dare to allow yourself to blossom flexibly, without resistance, without inner objections or critical thoughts that consider only structure or matter to be important. Free your energies and dare to Live! Let go of anxieties and tensions: in all joy, demand life for yourself.

NICOTINE ADDICTION

You live anxiously hidden behind a cloud of smoke. Inner conflict: pushing yourself through as an "I," or remaining hidden? Behind an outer appearance of assuredness lies an inner question. "Who am I?" You don't trust yourself, nor the world.

You have the feeling that you can't really reach yourself; you are afraid of a part of yourself, don't really dare to trust your intuition, your energies, your feelings. You stay hidden; you push away this aspect of yourself.

You refuse transformation: *a complete break-through of your total Self, with all your massed powers and possibilities!* You lead a frustrated life; you too little acknowledge your worth; you let yourself "be lived" by your thoughts and feelings instead of resolutely taking your life in hands in a self-aware way and in all openness toward yourself.

You think you have to protect yourself because you feel insufficiently supported by your own Core; you don't trust enough in the intuitive part of yourself. You live *too* strongly in your head, in the spirit: thoughts, plans, anxious feelings — you can't digest it all; nervousness because your life is not built enough on your fundamentally strong basis.

Your reasoning ability and intuition are insufficiently connected with each other; you think you have to control everything with your mind; no question of surrendering smoothly to your intuition, your feelings, because *you experience the woman or mother in yourself as being too cold, distant, mysterious, too unreachable, absent.* The "man" in you — in the grip of this "dead," indrawing "woman" and her suction-power — is as if paralyzed (psychologically impotent).

Because you doubt your own worth, you build a screen around yourself within which you hope to find yourself, behind which you might feel secure. A *flight,* instinctively.

You don't dare to totally experience yourself. You hide, you think others can floor you or put restrictions on you, but you only *restrict* yourself. You are too *cold* toward yourself

Don't be afraid of your deepest feelings, your longings, your intuition; allow your energies to flow freely. Discover the warm-hearted, loving mother in yourself. Stand up as unified power! Destroy Doubt! *No longer flee from yourself; discover your powerful "I"-*

center, and from here allow your feelings and your energies to radiate outward. Dare to *fully experience* all your feelings and forces, separate from whatever prohibition. Surrender to yourself; don't hide; become aware of your deep worth; offer yourself trust and love. Know yourself to be safe and sheltered in yourself without needing support from outside yourself. Free yourself from dependency. Let go of anxieties, feel relaxed in your deepest core via absolute trust in that central power-source in yourself. Transform uncertainty into Self-awareness. Don't numb yourself, don't withdraw, don't push your feelings away, but experience them to the fullest; loving appreciation of yourself will destroy anxieties.

Openness, honesty, self-respect, active energies that turn outward; intimate contact with every part of yourself, *a melting together with all parts of yourself.* Bring upward that which is deepest in yourself; as a result, you experience honest communication with others. Confrontation leads to liberation; no longer flee. *A powerful breakthrough of yourself in your body: on a solid earthly Basis!*

If you have the feeling that you know too little love, then the cause lies deep inside yourself: you were born with fear toward yourself, with the feeling of not being worthy of love, with a *deep self-doubt.* Now, discover the worth and beauty in yourself: you don't have to hide. You are good the way you are. If you are convinced that your deepest content is mysterious and untrustworthy, then you will start to protect yourself and be anything but *honest and open;* then, indeed, you will attract people who aren't really honest with you, who don't give you the love you long for. So *emerge* from behind your curtain, break through in total self-realization. *Draw upward, OUT OF YOURSELF, that which is deepest, and GIVE . . . Let it all be born out of you!*

You don't get sick from smoking, in and of itself, but possibly from the psychological problem which lies hidden behind the addic-

tion. You can easily enjoy a cigar, without being addicted, without getting sick. But the need to smoke will diminish in accord with your taking yourself, in totality, into life. *Completely free, unobstructed flow of feelings, life forces!*

(Regarding the solution to this, read the very appropriate symbolism of *Red Cabbage* and *Yogurt* in *The Horn of Plenty*.)

NIGHTMARES, DREAMS

Unconsciously, you look for rescue from your anxieties: in your dreams. On a much lower consciousness level than a state of wakefulness, intense deep feelings will no longer be supervised or controlled by the attention of your consciousness and rationality.

Problems which are being accentuated symbolically or clearly in your dream indicate that which occupies you unconsciously or consciously in your state of wakefulness. The most suppressed things, the most deepseated emotional problems with which you really don't know what to do — precisely on those are the spotlights directed. Your deepest Self longs for growth and enrichment, seeks solutions to problems: a dream is the translation, mostly symbolic, of that which occupies you in your deepest Self. Working out fear can lead to a nightmare, especially if in your daily life you aren't really looking for a solution and would rather flee from it. In this way, a dream offers an outlet for tensions and emotions that have not been worked out.

If one flees into sleep from a hard, hurting world full of pain, anxieties, and sadness, then a nightmare will represent the cause of this flight.

Looking into this mirror one can begin to better understand certain problems, comprehending the dream language and its symbolism.

We need, however, to look at this from a broader and more beneficial point of view.

CONSCIOUS confrontation with yourself, here and now; consciously opening yourself up to your emotional world in THE STATE OF WAKEFULNESS will offer a real solution to those things from which you flee. In this way you will achieve rest and harmony with yourself. Then your dreams will only be stories, rich in images, like a symbolic representation of healthy spiritual evolution. Are you, in a state of wakefulness, joyfully directed toward life with your Consciousness? And do you, with a positive attitude, unmask your problems, your anxieties, death, without fleeing from them? If so, then your dreams will be peaceful. Then you can make dreams part of your conscious program; then, in the evening, before you fall asleep, you can for instance ask your deepest Self a question in order, via the dream language, to "realize" the answer when you wake up.

Another phase toward which we can evolve is *no* longer falling back into such a dream state in which we can no longer get a grip with our Conscious "I." Staying *consciously* present in your sleep, albeit on a different wavelength.

You rest very deeply, you totally relax, but you maintain control of your dreams.

In the dream itself, you decide and determine which way you go, or with what you experiment. You let go of the reins or dismount. You become master over your dreams and place them at the service of beautiful goals in your evolutionary process on Earth.

Via sleep and dreams, people slide back into a state that reminds them of the period(s) when they were physically dead. A fundamental anxiety of no longer being able to consciously live on earth, here-and-now, sometimes leads to a fear of sleep and of dreams.

So, the less we daydream (instead, separating ourselves very strongly from death), and the more intensely we live here-and-now, the more intensely we enjoy earthly bliss and sensory presence, and the more intensely we develop Self-awareness — the more will we evolve toward a condition in which we not only become master over our existence, but also unmask physical death as being the past.

Creating our reality in a self-aware way, acknowledging Life, and making an end to death. Making an end to unconscious situations upon which our Conscious "I" has no grip. Becoming aware beyond the borders of sleep or physical death: then there's no more death, no anxiety, no nightmares. Only a Life in Joy, day and night.

THE NOSE
THE OLFACTORY ORGAN

Psychological correspondence

The nose symbolizes that which is instinctive in a human being; spontaneous, natural growth, without having to be involved in it in a conscious way.

Intuitively following your nature, your nose, your inner Self, without having to think it all over.

Acknowledging the Power and the Mastery in yourself by trusting in those original powers, in your intuitive reaction-pattern.

As director of your life, take the rudder in hand in a self-aware way.

Symbol also of self-manifestation, of the determination with which you grasp something. The concentrated power of your awareness in your body: Do you have everything under control? If so, then the nose symbolizes the result of this mastery over yourself; a calm, powerful, relaxed, protected feeling.

A powerful "I"; the freedom to be your Self, without obstacles; being able to move freely in your emotional world, without frustration.

The courage for daring to be yourself, making your way and resolutely clearing up all obstacles, without paying attention to what others think or say about you.

Symbol of the rooted survival-instinct of a human being: thanks to the olfactory organ he found food, could smell trouble, could distinguish sexual facts. With a critical and keen nose he protected himself and the human race, guarded himself from danger.

In a human being, the instinctive force to reproduce. Symbol of the Human Being who is master over these instincts.

Self-manifestation, outer ego, full of self-confidence. In a negative sense: attaching exaggerated importance to how one "appears" to others; a behavior that is too self-willed, or aggressive, or vain.

Ailments, in general

You force something; you absolutely Want and Will push something through, instead of listening to your inner Self; you insufficiently trust in your intuition.

You feel hurt by others; insufficient self-protection and self-trust. Unsure, cut off from your inner powers, you might attach more importance to your outer appearance than to your true Self or to your feelings: this makes you extremely vulnerable. Hesitating, afraid, frustrated, hidden, not aware of your worth, not standing on your own feet, dependent on others. Sometimes this can completely turn around: over-confident, exaggeratedly proud, arrogant, liable to (sexual) instincts, intuitively going on and on — without using your brains; aggressive, stubborn, combative. "Did you see me?" I, the tough fellow. Don't cut yourself off from your inner Self, from your intuitive wisdom: build your life on your true values. You don't have to prove yourself to the outer world; you are allowed to give yourself all the love

and attention. You are allowed to realize your ambitions and longings as long as they don't go against the true well-being of yourself and others. Proudly dare to reveal your true content, evolve without hesitation, know yourself to be safe and protected in your powerful Self. Don't hold back your creative energies: action! Don't stick your nose into other people's business, but consciously live from out of yourself.

Don't allow the primitive-want-instinct (money, material things) to dominate; this is only a result of anxieties and unsureness. Love and Wisdom transform instincts into awareness: love yourself and gain insight into your Self.

Nosebleeds

You are too dependent on others for the balance in yourself: you feel like a victim, suffering, milked or misused, shut out — but *you shut **yourself** out*: because you feel as if you are nothing, or you think you are inferior, bad or not good enough. You look at yourself as being a rag doll or a little devil who should be shunned or at least who is not worthy of love. You feel like a harlequin on a thread: the thread being in the hands of others. Because you feel so empty and absent, you are too little aware of your individual worth and beauty, so that there comes to be a need in you to compensate, with more attention from others, for this estrangement from yourself: your nose bleeds — "Now look at me!"

You feel so cold, lonely sometimes, sad, uncertain; and you long for warmth and love.

You are at odds with your emotional life; you don't really know who you are: you now ring the bells so others might notice you somewhat and pay attention to you. But you push yourself, as well as others, away from yourself. . . .

No longer shut yourself out! Don't expect others to offer you that which you don't offer to yourself: love and attention. Come close to yourself; know yourself to be safe and warmly sheltered in your deepest Self.

Now confront yourself with the negative thoughts you have about yourself: Do you think yourself bad or ugly? This negative conviction will call up reactions from your surroundings which seem to be a confirmation of your opinion.

Change this detrimental outlook on yourself so that not only can you come very close to yourself, but you will also be able to attract people who can respond to your love.

Discover your specific possibilities, your worth, and come to self-manifestation. Know yourself to be accepted by others, not as someone inferior, but as an unique individual. Trust your nature and, in joyful spontaneity, surrender to life.

Make yourself heartily welcome; only then will you feel accepted in a heartfelt way by others. Don't put yourself out in the cold!

Don't live too much in your "head," denying and shutting out your body.

Nose picking, exaggerated

Nervous unsureness. Instead of resolutely going onward in life, you hide. You question yourself too much : "What do others think of me"? Sometimes you hide behind a nonchalant posture, but actually you are constantly looking left and right to catch the reaction of others.

You don't get a grip on your inner Sun, on your "I"-worth: you hide this powerlessness behind an outer ego, behind a certain outward behavior.

You are still so sensitive and vulnerable; you dare only cautiously to come out of your hiding place with your feelings; you hide your shyness behind a posture. Ashamed of your feelings.

Action! Direct your energies outward, go on without hesitation. What you feel yourself counts, not how you appear to others. No false ego: show your true "I," discover your powers — your possibilities, your rich feelings — and transform them into creativity.

You don't have to feel like a mouse in a trap: dare to openly and honestly voice your opinion to others without going around it. Stand self-assuredly with both feet on the ground; become master over your feelings in a self-aware way and don't feel at all inferior to others: every human being is unique and irreplaceable.

Accept your feelings and be honest about them.

Post-nasal drip
mucus of the nose that runs to the throat

You swallow your aggression and your sadness. You allow little *feeling and decisiveness* to flow outward; hurt and sad, you'd prefer to hide. Pain, having to do with relationships with others. If the ailment is chronic, then this often indicates very deep, buried pain; deep suppressed aggression. It seems as if you sometimes don't know yourself the reason for this sadness and this *withdrawal.* You'd rather let yourself sink into the ground with your emotions than come out with them. Consciously or unconsciously, you remain stuck in happenings from the past. *You don't dare to powerfully manifest your "I"; you hold back emotions and energies: you live with an extreme preponderance of piled-up spiritual or thought-energies* in proportion to the earthly, physical, sensorial, sensual experience. Possibly, your outer ego was hurt and you no longer dare to come out.

Sometimes, you don't really seem to stand with your feet on the ground, or you flee on a flying tapestry toward higher regions (thoughts, fantasies, dreams, etc.). A too-weak, limp-female, abstract or spiritualized atmosphere. You feel cold; sometimes it seems as if you'd allow yourself to be overrun by your emotions; emotions grow and seem to rise above you, without your really getting a hold on them. *Natural energies ask for a breakthrough;* you put the brakes on yourself and your evolution. You refuse to enjoy that which is earthly without sadness and tensions being involved.

Break through; take up your full space. Here "I" am! Integrate that which is earthly — the sensual, the enjoyment of tastes, odors and colors in your existence. Feel safe and at ease in that fundamentally strong basis of yourself and listen to what you feel. Dare to enjoy your body, the sensual, and the exchange of love with others; don't close yourself off, don't hold on to painful memories from the past.

Conscious concentration of your "I"; go onward, don't hold back energies and *healthy aggressive powers.* Feel good, calm, and peaceful in yourself; bring an end to the Neptunian in yourself and firmly establish the male pillar in the ground. *Allow the power of movement to flow through, from out of yourself; open communication; express your feelings; don't hide yourself; don't flee into your thought-world.* Grounding. Make an end to the garbage from the *past,* to that which hinders you from resolutely and Joyfully being yourself.

Running nose
(See also Colds)

You feel cold, and you long for warmth from others, because you short-change yourself. Inner sadness; you long to be hugged; you long for affection, for attention from others; you cling to someone. You are insufficiently aware of your own worth; you live too cut off from your own nature, from your inner power source: you look for affirmation outside yourself.

Outwardly, you can appear strong and stalwart, attacking your work with determination, but inwardly there's that gentle sensitivity. You were too hard on yourself; you have hidden your feelings behind a mask of irony, humor or puppet show, but inner tears now work their way out. Because of exaggerated accentuation of that which is "masculine" in you — like a mask — the "female" now rises up, or better yet: you are now looking for shelter in the great Mother, the gentleness, the sensitivity, in You.

There's a conflict in you: the way you outwardly behave — and how you feel inwardly. An anxious, small boy carries enormous burdens: outwardly, he's cheerful, a big strong man, but inwardly he feels sadness, and his heart is vulnerable and afraid. Perhaps you feel cast out by others?

You are afraid to be yourself, to show yourself the way you are! Don't hide your true nature; dare to experience your feelings freely; don't put on an act.

Mark off your terrain, and first of all feel in harmony with yourself: offer yourself the motherly love you deserve, so that you aren't dependent on others. Be aware of your worth, your greatness, and allow your Nature to exist freely! Don't "run" for others, but choose YOUR path in a self-aware and intuitive way.

You feel cold and, perhaps, cast out by others because you leave yourself in the cold. Offer yourself warmth and love, make your nature welcome and be faithful to your true disposition. You are good and worthy the way you are; you don't have to behave differently than you feel. Dare to be yourself; feel strong and free, go onward in self-assuredness! In Joy, build your life on that solid fundamental ground of your Self.

Sneezing, exaggerated

A refusal, a "no" to yourself: you don't really want to express your content and your possibilities. You are allergic to yourself. You withdraw. Resistance.

You doubt yourself, your worth; you are afraid of truly being yourself. Rejection. Still an unconscious urge for self-liberation. Rejection regarding something or someone outside you is just a reflection of not being able to manifest yourself frankly the way you feel inside.

A feeling of inferiority. You place yourself very low and in the back of the hall. You think you have no right to fully "exist."

You feel powerless; you hide in an anonymous mass in order to flee from your individuality.

No longer identify yourself but with the "little one" inside yourself: make it welcome, be good, don't reject it, but allow it to grow up. Discover the warmth and coziness in yourself; feel safe and protected in your deepest Self. Allow your energies to flexibly come through, keep them turning and no longer bottle them up because of feelings of inferiority: acknowledge your specific worth and your possibilities; no longer hide. Look in all directions, give yourself all the room you need: now acknowledge the leadership in yourself. Manifest yourself, produce, believe in your power, in your creative possibilities. Show yourself! Don't reject your Content or your Body. Mark off your limits in self-confidence.

Arrive at self-assuredness and ground yourself; no longer keep yourself so tight; allow your natural feelings to exist freely. Dare to be yourself without holding back.

BEING on earth: living in a self-aware way from out of your central source; not letting yourself "be lived." Work out excess emotions and let them flow away. Don't block creative energies. Spontaneously live from out of your intuitive, spontaneous "I," without constantly wondering what others think of you. You are like a closed-up flower bud: dare to reveal your unique being in the light of your sun. You, yourself, as the central worthiness, in a loving and productive existence. Now allow your feelings and creative energies to freely blossom.

No longer keep the bud closed up.

Stuffy nose
(See also Colds)

Frustration, holding back energy. Too closed-up in yourself; an inner demand to allow your energy core to burst open. Enormous powers are being suppressed; aggressive energies are constantly being smothered. Too little self-confidence, no confidence in the intuitive powers.

A bird that doesn't dare to sing its tune, that strangles its nature, that doubts its worth. Feelings are being suppressed; natural spontaneity is being hindered. Your own "I" doesn't get enough room to exist. Anger because of frustration. Inwardly, something calls: "It's enough now!" You'd like to turn everything around, to change it. There's a "power station" in you, which asks for a breakthrough! An urge for freedom.

A demand from the inner Self for transformation: for allowing your feelings, your powers, your energies to flow through freely, for acknowledging yourself in worthiness, and finally rooting yourself into the earth.

NUMBNESS

You don't really live from out of your heart, from out of your deepest Self. Your "I" lives in a suppressed way.

Possibly, you have unconsciously evoked a "whack" in order to awaken you; in this situation of numbness you will now begin to search for yourself. Do you feel that you are so foolish and worthless? You don't really "live." Because you don't have power over your feelings, over your existence, you will reach for power over others. The claw of someone who feels empty. Resistance, possibly revulsion, regarding yourself, regarding the past.

You hold on to others, including in your thoughts; inner powers are being suppressed.

Are you afraid of your deeper emotions? Of those powerful unconscious energies in yourself? Possibly, you are disdainful with yourself, or you experience yourself as an insignificant, small, loveless child; life becomes useless and boring when you can't really feel Joy and Gratitude for being, for the Now. You don't really concentrate yourself in the now-experience because anxieties hinder you. Anxieties are only there as long as you link life with death, as long as you don't really love yourself, as long as you don't trust in the immortal, Living Self.

Let go, let others go, no longer cling to something or someone outside you. Experience your own powerful, warm sun-center: fall back completely on yourself in order to discover that your deepest Self is solid and trustworthy, that you, yourself, can create your life.

Look for your direction and sail on in full force! Let go of that grip, and surrender to your feelings: if you no longer mistrust and suppress yourself and your emotional powers, then anxieties will disappear. Wake up now and come lovingly toward yourself: don't be afraid to fully engage yourself emotionally in life. The future will bring you joy, warmth, and happiness when, in a self-aware way, you steer your life in that direction. Grab for all power over yourself; solidly stand on your own feet; trust those creative powers in yourself and unfold them in self-realization. Don't allow yourself to "be lived."

O

OBSESSIONS
ideas or images that repeatedly
and persistently intrude on your mind

The cause of obsessive thoughts lies in Resistance to going *onward;* inner conflict. Out of Fear you hold on with your thoughts to a certain thing. Here, it's about unconscious anxiety-patterns that only will disappear if you arrive at Conscious and clear Insight in yourself, if you trust your Nature — and if you GO ONWARD!

You can't go one way or the other; you feel oppressed; you concentrate mostly on your own smallness and on your limitations as you experience them NOW.

You are hard, severe, and condemning toward yourself; you are afraid to trust your own nature, to listen to your intuition. You try to control everything with your mind. You hold on to things, although it would be better if, for your own good, you let this all go; anxious resistance.

You pile up anxious obsessive thoughts because of the suppression of your powerful energies, and *because you don't dare enough to acknowledge your own "I" and manifest it outward. Now look at yourself from above;* crawl out of that straitjacket: see that your anxieties are unreal and often concern imaginings directed toward the future and which are so non existent here-and-now.

Stand on your own feet in self-assurance and know that your obsession will only force itself on you as long as you refuse to *take your life in hand in a self-aware way:* with the power of the Conscious "I," every human being can get rid of obsessions. Make an end to suppression and frustrations: *dare to fully experience your Nature and to live according to it; you don't "have" to do anything — you are allowed to be joyful and spontaneous!*

By assuming the leadership over yourself, you will give yourself all opportunity to truly Live. *Don't get stuck at the thinking pole only!* Don't feel obliged; don't feel like you are a target for others — especially acknowledge your worth and don't allow yourself to be influenced too much by the words of others. Liberation! *Now allow your creativity, your energies, to flow freely!* Observe that which you keep suppressed; no longer hold on to that which prevents your evolution. Let go of that strictness; don't fight against your nature, against your self. Arrive at love and gentleness toward your self. Trust in your deepest Self, in your intuition, your inner wisdom.

OBSESSIVE-COMPULSIVE NEUROSIS, COMPULSIVE ACTS

You cut yourself off from your feelings; you no longer allow anything spontaneous in your life; you don't dare to live life to the fullest or enjoy the beauty, the earthly, everything which is natural; you have put yourself in an unnatural straitjacket. This calls up an intense counter-reaction! Alone, lonely, like a child who suddenly loses its parents, its hold — that is how you feel, standing in the cold; anxious and lost like a stray dog.

You don't feel your own backbone; they might drag you away.... "Why should I walk on my own legs?" You don't have faith or trust in your deepest Self; you don't have real contact with your essence. You are even afraid of yourself, fleeing from your emotions, your anxieties, and your sadness. You experience yourself only as empty, without substance, without worth. Eventually, you don't even *feel* anymore. Afraid to truly live, afraid of death, having a negative attitude toward your body or toward your deeper, healthy feelings of longing for intimacy, for good food or for another desired object, and as a result you completely oppress yourself, experiencing yourself as "bad" or "depraved" because of these longings. You don't love yourself; you condemn yourself or part of yourself as being devilish.

This suppression evokes opposition: a compulsive neurosis.

A constant battle, a resistance that is ready again and again to suppress the "natural," which wants to break through; this battle results in exaggerated "outlets," the compulsive acts.

Allow your feelings, your longings, your natural being, to exist fully and freely.

Don't be afraid of yourself: every human being is good and unique just the way he or she is. There is no question of "black" aspects to the Self: only when you suppress your Natural feelings for too long will the result be a "compulsive" reaction.

Come toward love, toward understanding in yourself, and surrender to your deepest emotional life; fight no longer against yourself. Dare to enjoy fully that which is earthly! Deep inside you lies the eternal, burning Light, immortal and powerful: turn yourself toward this Soul-essence; appreciate your personality, accept yourself in your totality and unconditionally. Be fully aware of your possibilities of action and creativity; no

longer block yourself, no longer frustrate yourself. Live in freedom and allow yourself at last to truly live. Allow the little child that lives inside you to grow up gradually, and offer it the love and understanding which, for such a long time, it had to do without. Independent of others, be your own father and your own mother, and cherish the child within yourself.

OPISTHOTONOS

contraction of the back muscles, producing an arched back and neck, as in tetanus, meningitis

---

Emotional confusion, nervous tension, looking for a way out of your inner collision: wanting to flee from life, from yourself and from your feelings, or then again seizing life in Anger! Fleeing or aggression. There seems to be no happy medium.

This original anger toward yourself and life can also be reflected in anger with your partner, with your father, etc.

Pushing yourself down: not really wanting to live. Sometimes, you are completely indifferent toward life; nothing matters to you anymore. You condemn yourself.

You feel "imprisoned" in life, in a situation. You feel like a ship anchored in a harbor: you want to get away, you want to stay.... You are afraid of death; you curse life.

You are afraid of the great Authority above your head: your father, a god, or commandment, Structures, etc.

You are too fearful to dare live from out of your inner divine Self: you don't allow the sun, the heart in yourself, to radiate. Dark, threatening emotions, anxieties, and coldness. You hide your true "I": you don't really dare to manifest yourself, and you remain in a haven that is not really your home.

You feel hurt; you don't see the sense of it anymore: Stay there or go away from the situation? From life?

You push life away, and then again you are afraid to be dragged into dark depths. Your life is directed by emotions, not by self-aware powers.

You make the sun go down, although you have such a need for warmth.

No longer resist the warmth of your Heart, the sun-center in you: discover your unique worth, and arrive at a gentle, friendly inter action with others. Warm your feelings; experience the peaceful, hearty, safe feeling in your deepest Self. Make yourself welcome in yourself and listen only to your inner authority. Be your own father and mother; know yourself to be protected in yourself. Enjoy all that is beautiful; dare to unfold your creativity. No longer collide with yourself, with others. Dare to express your love; don't place yourself at a distance. Bend flexibly to your fellow man; open yourself to a new course of life. Don't resist the life inside you.

P

PAGET'S DISEASE
osteitis deformans:
bones become larger and more fragile

Deep anxieties; you are in a dead-end dark tunnel. Despondency, distraught with mortal fear, loneliness, sadness. You don't feel supported by your own structure, by a solid Basis; you have wanted to cling to others, but all you are left with are heartaches.

You feel enormously threatened, but you have no foundations to stand on; you feel seized by others in a way that is not too respectable. You'd like to get hold of them, too, but you are too flexible; you don't really believe in your power; your resistance breaks down; you no longer have the courage to open your mouth or to keep standing; powerlessly you bend through your knees.

You think that others would rather put you in a grave, but actually it is you who ignores your worth and your strong backbone; you don't give yourself the love you deserve; you are destroying yourself with your negative convictions regarding yourself. You totally break yourself down: others will only react to these negative thoughts!

Develop that dignified, fatherly, male aspect in yourself, which every man and woman carries within: feel yourself supported by this powerful, secure part of yourself and no longer ignore it! Feel those sound, reliable foundations of your deepest Self, that central part in you which never dies.

Your body's cells are being formed by your consciousness: therefore choose in a self-aware way to creatively build up your existence.

Allow negative convictions to transform into joyful knowing: that you may be proud of your unique being; that you may come to self-manifestation and awareness of your worth.

Allow powerful energies to come through; unfold all your talents; don't withdraw from life, but with open eyes build up a solid structure: there's nothing threatening that will crush you.

Discover true joy and turn, in love and trust, toward your deepest Self.

Self-expression, humor, regeneration!

PAIN, IN GENERAL

You hurt yourself, unconsciously or consciously. Why? Your deepest Self calls up pain as a signal to bring about change in yourself. Pain is not necessary; it is not a necessary evil; it is not a must; without suffering and pain, one can evolve just as well. Transform. Don't wait until your pain forces you to. Becoming conscious without pain, freely and willingly, is beautiful.

We really don't need to endure any pain in order to be able to evolve. . . .

Deeply engraved in humanity is the conviction, the philosophy, that we people are nothing but poor sinners — that we have to pay penance and to suffer for our mistakes. This mass feeling of guilt, be it unconscious, which is portrayed in many myths — in the original sin, etc. — is a sign of ignorance, of

The Key to Self-Liberation, Christiane Beerlandt © Beerlandt Publications

a lack of insight, of the rejection of the divinity of the human being.

A person who's convinced of his goodness, who is full of love toward himself and others, will harm neither himself nor others. The primal conviction that the human being is sinful, bad, and guilty makes a person constantly doubt his own goodness and worth. He unconsciously calls up punishment because he is convinced he deserves it. Feelings of guilt and self-punishment.

More individually considered, we often choose this pain as feedback, as a signal: "Now I'm wrong; here I need to adjust my way of life." However, signals from our deepest Self can be received via our inner senses; we don't have to suffer. If we take our life in hand and direct it in a more individual and autonomous way, separate from the mass spirit; if we choose life instead of walking our Calvary of death; when we make an end to this mass-hypnosis, and every one of us listens in our personal way only to our inner wisdom; if we confirm ourselves in a solid, impenetrable energy and live in harmony with ourselves, full of trust in our inner self; if our outer behavior and our inner being say the same thing — then in this oneness we'll no longer feel pain. Contentment with yourself; don't live for the eye of others; joyfully experience your unique being.

PANCREAS

Psychological correspondence

The pancreas produces enzymes which help to digest the food; it also produces insulin and glucagon, two hormones which play a role in the regulation of the sugar level in the blood.

The pancreas symbolizes the sweet, loving presence in yourself.

Trust in your deepest self, in your inner Authority, which will constantly supply you with food: the "manna," the divine love. A deep trust in nature's powers of creation, in the endless supply of fuel (consciousness, love) that again and again helps new life to be born and that brings about new growth in your life.

You trust in the goodness of your divine essence, of the vivifying energies in the All; you nestle yourself securely in the womb of your warm nature.

Blindly, you surrender to your inner wisdom, to unconscious powers which push upward and transform themselves. Daring to give presents to yourself and to your friends, like a good-hearted Santa Claus. Daring to enjoy all that is beautiful in life!
Spontaneously dealing with and digesting emotions: spitting them out or swallowing them, not sorrowing and becoming immobilized by them. Confronting yourself; if necessary putting the knife at your throat in order not to drown in your emotions! Preferably dealing more flexibly with your feelings; resolutely taking a hold of life, trusting your nature. Giving your total self a chance to calm down, to allow your emotional life to sleep in the arms of your warm heart.

Balance in work and rest, between spirit and matter, intuition and rationality.

Fully trusting the adventure of life and not wanting to plan everything beforehand. Taking it well when you meet setbacks in your life and keeping them in perspective.

The divine love which flows from your deepest Self into this earthly dimension, into your bodily forms, is being translated into earthly terms: enjoying via the senses or allowing yourself to feel wonderful things, to eat delicious food, to admire with your ears or your eyes; the enjoyment of a love relationship between two people; the transformation of sadness into joy; working out sad memories from the past. Transforming warmth into loving participation in earthly life; actively dealing with unconscious negative feelings, in order to triumphantly go a step further in the awareness-process.

Ailments of the pancreas, in general

If you are convinced that you're not allowed to enjoy things, that sugar is bad for you, that you have to forbid yourself a lot, then you don't really love yourself.

Sugar only becomes poison when your thoughts condemn it to being poison! Do you sacrifice yourself instead of allowing love and happiness into your life; do you think that life needs to be "suffered?"

Do you have no confidence in the authority of your inner Self, and are you drowning in emotional problems? Do you not succeed in digesting them? Do you despise your body or that which is sensual? Do you think there will never be joy for you, and do you allow yourself to be washed over by despair and sorrow? You don't really believe in the power of your "I," of your mastery; you ignore your worth; you reject yourself: "My god, why have you deserted me?" You don't realize that you leave yourself out in the cold.

Come close to yourself: allow your Consciousness to warmly radiate through your body in every cell; fully integrate spirit into body. Realize yourself and feel yourself securely taken up in the warm hands of your divine Self. Trust earthly life and create your life in a self-aware way. Don't let yourself droop, don't let yourself be dragged along by feelings of powerlessness, by worries; and trust in the elasticity, the digestive ability of your consciousness. Don't allow yourself to burn away, but resolutely direct the creative fire toward new perspectives.

Love never asks for sacrifice. You have the right to happiness. Stop self-destruction!

(See also Diabetes. In *The Horn of Plenty,* read Sweets - Sugars.)

P.S.: Switching your eating habits and eliminating medications should not be done suddenly, but gradually: in direct proportion to psychological growth.

Pancreatitis

And now? Desperate, dark thoughts. Frustrated irritability. Angry and powerless. Extreme nervous tension; you can't handle it any longer; you no longer feel able to deal with an enormous mountain of emotions and burdens.

You now refuse to go on: you blindfold yourself so that you'll no longer see it all. You are completely stuck, imprisoned in situations.

Hopeless, you don't see any sense in it anymore; instead of looking for a solution, you completely sag. You are not on the right track.

Your common sense seems to collapse under an overburdening of emotions. You feel at the mercy of circumstances; you have pain and sadness; you feel powerless to stand up for yourself.

Uncertainties, anxieties; you shudder at the thought of the future. You become too feeble, too docile, too pliable; your will to live disappears. You feel so small and unable to face a future which you don't really trust.

Throw off all worries and problems and resolutely choose life; don't hesitate. Become aware of your powerful "I," of your total brain-content, of the relativity of your problems. Get your feet on the earth; wake up out of your nervous sleep; believe in your common sense; get a clear perspective on everything and see how your negative thoughts lead your life. Don't allow emotions to govern your existence: arrive at a solution on the basis of that to which your Heart inspires you. Don't pay attention to the external, to the fleeting values of life, and now offer yourself the love and warmth you deserve. Stop allowing yourself to "be lived"; create it yourself!

Joyful expectation will bring you happiness. No longer block your flexible emo-

tional flow by anger and self-destructive despair. Trust your intuition, your natural spontaneity. Feel yourself backed up by your fundamentally strong deepest Self; you are as strong as you want to be. Your life can take a radically different direction if you so choose. Bring about changes and Quit "things" or "business" that no longer suit you. . . .

Pancreas stones

Emotional burdens, feelings of guilt, self-condemnation, considering yourself to be bad or worthless. You'd like to get away, to sink into the ground; you are ashamed of yourself; you don't believe in your goodness because you feel a lot of aggression, anger, bubble up inside you! You never really dared to be yourself; anxiety has made you friendly and diplomatic with people with whom you sometimes would have preferred to voice your harsh opinion! You see everything too much in black and white; sometimes you don't know yourself anymore, because you don't really manifest yourself the way you are. Outwardly laughing, inwardly crying. Hiding your deepest emotions, until it all becomes too much for you. Now you feel the ties becoming too tight, and you'd like to escape out of your armor; inner resistance to your self-suppression. For too long you have forced yourself, adjusted yourself, inside a framework, a system or a relationship, without really spontaneously daring to be yourself. For far too long you have carried enormous burdens: for you, life isn't a carefree game, and at the moment you don't see any change in it. Don't be so hard on yourself: allow your nature to blossom freely, don't clip your wings; trust your deepest feelings, and no longer be afraid. Feel safe and calm in your deepest "I"; feel welcome among people and don't hide your true nature. You are good and worthy; don't put your true feelings and thoughts, your natural creativity, under the ground. Arrive at gentleness and love toward yourself, and transform! Change

that nervous self-suppression into an optimistic choice to be yourself, the way you really feel inside.

Don't hide your tears behind a smile, but work out your sadness and throw all needless burdens off your back. Don't fight against life, but enjoy: you have the right to joy and happiness. Don't punish yourself. Now look at life with balanced judgment, no longer in contrasts. Replace inner impatience and nervousness with healthy action, no longer jerkily, but flowing in a straight line.

Pancreas tumor

Powerless anger, deep anxiety about what has yet to come, not trusting in your deepest, secure Self. You might get furious with the small, gentle, powerless child inside you. Desperate situation; you have no more hope for the future concerning certain things. Help, help! Nervousness, overburdening of emotions; inwardly, you feel so unstable and unsure, you are cut off from your deepest Self, but outwardly you try to stay standing, with toughness. You cling to elements in life that it would be better to let go of, but anxieties block your evolution. You take a black view of things! Pain and sorrow ravage your total Self; you are no longer able to direct your life yourself; suppressed aggression, no more trust in life. Anxiety about failing, about collapsing.

Be good and gentle with yourself, feel safe and calm. Take care of the smallest child in your being and offer it shelter, warmth, affection, because only this love will bring peace, will chase away anxieties. No longer allow yourself to be overpowered by your feelings, but consciously get a hold of yourself. Trust the guidance of your deepest Self and transform aggression into consciously directed action. Let go of that which isn't really good for you; try not to cling to that which will drag you along to a fall. You forget that life means happiness and enjoyment.

Reorganize; change your life's direction: now build your life on inner wisdom, on true insights, not on outer or material values. Don't try to assert yourself with achievements or outer manifestation, but feel your heart, which begs for attention. Don't bottle up any feelings; allow them all to flow freely; don't feel obliged, don't be too severe, but arrive at inner peace.

PARALYSIS

If you are convinced that you are just a helpless, inadequate person, a victim, unable to create your life in a joyful way yourself, then you paralyze yourself.

Your nature, your feelings, your deeper emotions, live confined in a heavy, iron structure, like an airplane, which would rather take flight anyway, *away* from yourself, *away* from the earth, *away* from the Poison in yourself, because you are disgusted with your own "I." You put yourself in a glass bottle as it were; you hinder yourself from living cheerfully and naturally, from evolving: you pin yourself down. There's a kind of poverty in contact with your own heart, your deepest soul. You are hard on yourself! You turn inward, blindfolded; you refuse to go on; you go around in your own little vicious circle. You feel bound to the past, and you offer enormous resistance to breaking with this. You remain in your eggshell, instead of being born and solidly standing on your own feet. You prefer to retain negative influences from the past: was one of your mentors, for instance, an example of self-destruction, contempt, pessimism, fanaticism, fatalism? Or were you pushed away into a corner as an insignificant, inferior, cold being? In these cases, also, these life circumstances are but a reflection of your inner convictions regarding yourself and life in general.

For how long will you keep living in this eclipse of the sun — the denial of your own joyful, sunny, powerful "I"? Deep anxieties hinder you from breaking out of your eggshell, from standing in the happy light of earthly life. You paralyze, numb, yourself in order not to have to feel this anxiety, but this doesn't offer you a solution, because this sadness means only postponement in your endless life course, because life is Joy and Life will keep on calling up these kinds of situations for you, until you find this Joy and acknowledge it.

No longer flee from yourself: you are not bad, sinister or insignificant. No longer offer resistance to the Love and appreciation of your Self. No longer cut yourself off from your true nature: dare to be yourself, no matter how crazy; dance and sing; express yourself spontaneously, without limits, without yet again questioning whether you are allowed to, or what others might think of it. That powerful, dynamic dancing force wells up from your depths: participate in life, not from behind the bushes as an observer, but as the main character in your existence.

Push your self through; don't flee, but clean up all hindrances and cut the tie with the past! Don't live according to the philosophy of someone else, but according to your own heart, to what you Feel!

Follow your intuition, your feelings, and don't nip every experience in the bud by an over-dominance of your "thinking": offer yourself the freedom to live, to freely breathe, to follow your impulses in a cheerful way; FEEL in your Self those awareness-powers, your creative energies, and allow them to flow freely! Don't resist your natural longings: dare to experience yourself. Don't look at things with blinders on; don't restrict your life to small-minded theories, to prejudices.

Break through that hard rind and free yourself: be open to all the beautiful things in yourself.

Once and for all, spit out that which is negative, those self-condemning thoughts.

Also allow unconscious forces, deep-hidden emotions, to come freely to the surface, and observe them, work them out, let go. No longer flee from these forces, these feelings, in yourself: they are a source of energy. If you acknowledge them, if you no longer turn away from this spontaneous power-source in yourself, then you can — in warm acceptance of yourself — purify these energies, transform them into creativity full of a zest for living, into joyful action, into spontaneous participation with nature, with Life.

You no longer have to carry heavy burdens; you no longer have to accept the leaden lid on your Content. Look deep inside yourself and discover that secure Basis, your everlasting Self, which awaits your orders: take your life into your own hands and call up powerful energies from your deepest Self so that every part of your body will be reborn.

Spastic paralysis

Swallowed up in emotions, in pain and powerlessness. You feel bound; you feel stuck, in spite of your enormous longings.

You'd like to reach for others (sometimes with Power), for something far beyond you. You have an enormous urge to make everything subject to your Eye, to go on, to take up ever more space with psychological greediness. You feel weak, but inwardly you resist this powerlessness: you don't acknowledge your gentle emotional world. In pent-up aggression you wish to pierce your prison wall with your fist. Frustration, ambition to organize things with "manly" toughness, to get a powerful overview and control over your business or over people. You are pregnant with yourself, but don't allow yourself to be born. You direct all your attention outward. You don't live from out of your joyful core; you forget to enjoy. Your emotional content overburdens the structure: the foundations shake because you "hold on" to everything. It becomes too heavy for you. Powerlessness - Power.

Let go! Work out your emotions; turn deeply inward and discover your gentleness! Now allow yourself to enjoy, and free yourself of those tensions. No longer look and control things outside of you, but feel the language of your heart. Take away the veil from your gentle emotional core; show yourself the way you are; confront yourself with your gentle, female side. Find rest, feel relaxed in that safe basis of your Living Self. Remain here-and-now, don't direct yourself toward the future nor toward that which is distant; allow everyone to go his path; don't meddle; save yourself through inner liberation.

Be good and gentle to others; radiate instead of wanting to grab or show. Don't force anything. Your life is soft and malleable: work on it in self-assuredness. Stand still for self-analysis, in peace, and let everything and everyone go. Trust will be rewarded.

PARANOIA

You see things that are not there; you feel like you are being pursued; you are constantly on guard; you are distrustful; you are filled to the brim with anxieties — all because you don't trust your deepest Self. You're not really completely honest with yourself; sometimes you look for ways out in order to escape certain situations; you misuse certain forces or characteristics in order to be ahead of others.

You are being confronted with the dark side of yourself, with your anxiety and your deception, with your deepest emotions, with your aggression and your powerlessness, with your desires and your spiteful anger toward others: as a reaction to your own small powerlessness, to your feeling of inferiority or fear of failure. You are constantly fleeing from deep, unconscious powers in yourself: you are afraid of your feelings! You don't at all trust yourself!

Perhaps you've been confronted with manipulation, with heartlessness, with condemnation of your gentle beautiful feelings, and with reproaches for your healthy, powerful energies. You've begun to experience yourself as being threatening; you've begun to experience the world as being more and more unsafe because you already didn't really feel safe in yourself.

Exaggerated negative expectations and anxieties flood your brain: you bottle up your emotions instead of surrendering calmly to them. You don't dare to surrender, however, because you fear you might be grabbed.

You vomit because of an aspect of yourself that disgusts you; you push important energies, emotions, underwater — as a result of which anxieties pop up, like a boomerang. But then it seems as if this threat comes from the outside, while in fact it's you who are the bird of prey which is on the lurk; not a claw will touch *you!*

The healthy mind is being overpowered by your feelings, which overflow after a suppression. You offer enormous resistance to a complete breakthrough of your spontaneous energies; you put yourself into the electric chair instead of freeing yourself. You flee from the absolute truth regarding your person; as a consequence, you no longer see the truth in the outer world; your imagination runs wild in an exaggerated way. You don't love yourself, so therefore you suspect that others can't love you, either. Deadly fears torment you. You want to get a grip on, and power over, others — over situations, over yourself — before you might become the victim. . . . You have insufficient solid ground under your feet, too little earth-atmosphere in your being; you flee into unreal images, which violate the truth.

Your negative convictions regarding yourself, regarding life, call up negative circumstances in life, which then give you a confirmation: "See, I was right." But in fact, it's you yourself who has called this situation into being by your negative, anxious expectation pattern.

Grounding! Become aware of your own strong, safe Basis, your deepest Self, upon which you can always count and which does not die. Create a beautiful life yourself, by a positive expectation pattern, and get yourself out of that prison cell of delusion. Nothing in your life "just" happens; everything that happens to you, you have first called it up yourself.

Feel the warmth of your heart, your gentler energies, and allow the "female" intuitive element into your life as an important aspect of it; integrate all emotions and powers from your deepest "I" and no longer take flight from them. Look very closely inside yourself and know that you are good, that nothing inside you is terrifying. Acknowledge your Sun-center, your mastery; take up your scepter in a self-aware way; realize your worth. Be honest with yourself and with others: dare to open yourself up in love toward yourself, toward others. Knowing your divine core, feeling trust in your deepest "I," and loving your totality, without any longer taking an attitude of refusal toward an aspect of your Nature: that will drive away anxiety and will allow you to look with an honest, open perspective, toward the outer world, toward life.

Make yourself warmly welcome in yourself; don't be afraid of unconscious terrain; what "seems" dark is undyingly light and beautiful! No longer flee; free yourself; confront yourself with the depth of your being, with your emotions; let them come through, and work them out.

Welcome in yourself the caring, the motherly, the gentle, the nourishing, the producing — and allow it to find its balance with the "male" aspect in your existence. A balanced life without suppression: a self-assured "I" as the central axis, without anxiety.

PARATHYROID GLANDS

Overactivity
hyperparathyroidism

You absolutely would like to break through with force, and that *has* to be, and that *will* be: in that regard you are hard, angular, and sharp with yourself, with grim stubbornness: an inner aggressive urge. You WANT to realize and manifest yourself in *one* certain direction, You think it's absolutely necessary; you compel yourself to do it. But — you can't. Much goes against you. You don't give up; you would row upstream! Force — opposing force. Is it in order to prove yourself to the outer world? Or have you chained yourself to the norms and laws your parents dictated to you: "Only if you achieve *that* in life are you a good and successful human being." You feel so powerless not to be able to realize your ambitions: your deepest Self has called up setbacks and disappointing situations in your life (Read Part I), in order to make you stop and think about your *true* nature, your disposition, your *real* longings and talents; to make you stop and think about yourself. Because the ambitions you are striving for are a slavish product of "what others expect from you," or "how others perceive you," or "what you have to do in order to be a respectable human being." Change your direction and live from out of yourself! Inwardly you have known for a long time that the path you are following is not the *real* path, but a giving-in to others: you exclude yourself. Something doesn't want to come along, and you push, you push — it's no use: a waste of energy, and blindness. Stubbornly you keep it up with blinders on, not looking left or right; if this goal isn't reached, or if you don't satisfy this requirement for yourself (for instance getting a certificate), then you no longer see the sense of your life. You ignore your real longings; you think you have to be strict with yourself and that you

don't have the right to enjoy, doing things and experiencing things you love. Self-suppression. You think you MUST do things, MUST be there for others, and you are in the last place. And if you build a career, then this will actually be to satisfy the wishes, the expectations, of others. Because, after all, aren't you only a "nothing"?

Follow that stream of your own Nature: don't allow all your creative energies — which sprout out of your deepest feelings and abilities — to burn away. That which you want so badly, that for which you fight, is perhaps not at all good for you! Stop, and change your direction. Look at your own basis and stand in your own shoes; live from out of yourself. Believe in the beauty of your nature and allow it to come out! The only thing you HAVE to do is be faithful to your own nature. Build your strong structure on your own basis, not on the existence of others. They don't know it better than you do, though you often think so: stand up for yourself and enjoy your own being. Stop breaking yourself down, stop constraining yourself to satisfy others.

Insufficient activity
hypoparathyroidism

You feel ringed like a bird and stuck; you don't see which direction to take. You feel desperate, powerless: you want to satisfy others; you pay an enormous amount of attention to your partner, parents or friends, but you force yourself in these relationships. You try to force things. Powerlessly you try to reconcile, but you don't succeed at it. You hold on too much to your fellow men instead of developing yourself! You concentrate too much on others — and you feel sad, sometimes aggressively desperate, because you ignore your own being in this way. You much too little have your own life in hand; you allow yourself to roll on wheels, as it were. Where to? You feel like a hanged person, full of emotions.

Place the center in yourself. Only from out of this core, from concentration in yourself, can you experience joy. Two people can love each other, in freedom, only if in the relationship both partners have an independent awareness of their own worth and each partner is faithful in the first place to his own nature. Dare to be yourself! You are allowed to be different, to have different ideas as a child than your mentors do. Manifest this. Parents of these children will respect their children all the more as separate individuals with specific characteristics! Parents aren't authorities. Are you so sad because others don't love you, because you don't live up to their expectations? Love yourself, follow your nature: then these people who "agree" best with your nature will automatically appear on your path. A true relationship isn't in blood relation, but in the spirit, in the heart.

PARKINSON'S DISEASE

Directing energy in the wrong way: wanting to control everything and everyone, getting things under your control instead of actively building up your existence in a powerful way.

Wanting to be the best, but not really being able to *do:* powerlessness.

Not being able to truly react; the inability to come to true self-realization. Were you brought up in a too-severe, restrictive milieu, where one especially looked for "achievements," or where you felt as if you were suffering the chopping block, under the pressure of a strongly demanding authority above your head? Or have you been forced, belittled by others? Have you felt powerless and hurt? If so, this was the consequence of your own underlying convictions.

You always know better; you probably criticize others; you want to be cock-of-the-

walk, but emotionally you feel broken, not able to satisfy will and desire. Power — Powerlessness.

You are like a butterfly, one half of which remains a caterpillar: anxiety prevents you from growing *yourself*, from transforming. Wanting and not being able to.

You have no faith in your deepest Self: you want to place everything under the supreme control, the supervision of your Eye; you would get a hold of everything and everyone and push them in this or that direction instead of going on *yourself* in a well-determined direction!

You can't, and won't, loosen your grip; in a cold sweat you cling to others; an urge for power, but so powerless. Because of these fears and your desperate urge to dominate others, you actually create in your life negative situations which only give you more feelings of pain and powerlessness.

Let go of others and turn full of trust toward your deepest Self. Discover your Heart: place all longings and desires under the authority of love, so that you can live in contentment with yourself. Not wanting or doing any more than calmly contemplating yourself and solving the conflict of power-powerlessness.

Arrive at real action from within, not because you have to prove yourself or because you have to find your security outside yourself! You can calmly relax, feel sheltered in your inner Self, in that immortal core. Don't be afraid, don't place yourself higher than you feel, stay close to yourself, make yourself sweet and small: in the child in yourself you will discover the real grandeur of a human being, of yourself. Gentleness, spontaneity, freedom for you and others, the playful enjoyment of every detail in nature; concentrate yourself in your heart, allow feelings to flow freely, let go of cramped thoughts, turn your eyes only to the beautiful Now, and don't reach for tomorrow.

Don't long for more than joy and for being yourself. Solve that inner conflict; come out of your confusion: you are good and safe the way you are, independent of others. Give, and you will be given that which is good for you. Don't seize or grab, but trust. Don't try to anxiously "control" situations, even though this is "with the best of intentions." Trust; let go of everything and everyone.

PERITONITIS

On the one hand you are sharp and destructive toward yourself; on the other hand you are angry, aggressive, with everything and everyone: you don't have a clear view. You feel exhausted, sometimes indifferent: "Let them do to me what they want; I'm not worth anything anyway." You are sooner absent than present in yourself. You'd like to flee, away. . . . You belittle yourself, and you feel condemned by others.

You'd like to change and achieve, to seize and desire so much all at once — in order to satisfy the norms you have created and to which you think you have to answer in order to be considered a complete human being. All this because you feel so insignificant and such a failure. A burden presses in your lap; you focus too much on the less important things, while higher awareness energies can't come through as a result. You attach too much importance to outer values, to what others might say, to your body, which has to answer to social norms, etc. Your natural being can't exist freely. You have put on armor that is too tight! You feel powerless — in the grip of others. You no longer can keep a hold on these emotions, you can't let go of them — your resistance breaks down.

Arrive at rest and relaxation: you are peaceful and good in yourself. Accept your unique Being and dare to show yourself the

way you are; feel safe in yourself, your strong Basis, and then push the curtains aside in order to also experience, as a liberation, that great space outside of you. Bite into your life, bring yourself to realization, and don't be disturbed by the criticism of others. Look very close at reality and no longer drift away into false daydreams. Stop your self-destructive thoughts and your feelings of powerlessness, which lead to having a critical tongue to others. Place fully inside you the power over yourself, and stop living according to the rules of others. Your life is a wealth if you create it yourself, a disaster if you doubt all your possibilities. No longer allow yourself to go along with the flow of water, not knowing where it will lead: nothing can happen to you just by accident! Get a hold of the steering wheel.

PHANTOM PAIN

A body part that in (memory) thoughts is still present, for instance after amputation, can call up pain because it is actually being "created" and isn't really gone.

In fact it's about an emotional pain which reflects itself in the physical (or thought physical) body: inwardly you feel powerless, unable to get a hold on your life, on reality. You don't SEE clearly what's going on with your inner being; so you will see things outside yourself that are not there or that are different than you think. You have the feeling that you can't really live from out of yourself; you'd like to reach much further than you are doing; you'd like to walk, to go onward. . . . Know, then, that these feelings are asking for inner advancement, *for you to enlarge your space — psychologically, and also with respect to your content* — and that they are not asking, first of all, for you to physically walk. Here, it's about an inner call that asks for liberation from your inner, impotent situation and dependency on others; it asks for a sober, clear perspective on yourself and a deep confrontation with your deepest "I." You felt anxious, dark, powerless, and hurt by others.

Now arrive at inner Sureness and get a hold of your life. Allow your awareness to be open and reach as far as possible. Explore all spaces with your inner abilities and broadly expand your life. Know yourself to be powerful in yourself, and make an end to the pain and lies. Discover the truth in yourself.

emotions, and allow everything to flow, so that life-energies are no longer blocked and you will be more confronted with the joy of life: then feel the warmth in your veins. It's the appreciation and love toward yourself which will allow you to sense the triumph of life. In your life you have to be "the first one"; now place the kingship in yourself, on earth. Don't be anxious: nothing negative can happen to you; devils exist only insofar as you create them; you are able to build up your future the way you want to. Don't allow yourself to "be lived," but get a hold on your existence with both hands.

PHOSPHORUS
Deficiency, insufficient assimilation of

Insufficient presence of your deepest soul content in your body here-and-now.

You pull your personality back or down, as it were: you admire others, but you yourself feel too feeble, too flexible, lacking a strong backbone. You feel ringed at the nose, as it were, forever ready like a horse to its master. After all, you feel powerless to really take the rudder in hand *yourself;* you aren't aware enough of your consciousness powers; you too easily go through your knees; too little "I"-awareness. You'd allow yourself to merge with something bigger, something misty or abstract — ultimately you'd become a zombie and no longer feel yourself on this earth. . . .

So become aware of your Self, of your body, and don't float away in the air! Get both feet on the earth and feel the power of your muscles, how you are master over your body and your life. Find the golden balance between rational, conscious thinking-patterns on the one hand and your intuitive sensitivity on the other hand, no longer suppressing either of them. Powerfully carry your energies, your

PLAGUE

You see life as a dark event.

Powerlessness, anxiety about being dragged along with an enormous current against which you can't stand up. Belief in the insignificance of the human being, in the "contamination," in death (See also Infections). The heart, the love-energy, is insufficiently developed; cold anxieties, self-negation, sacrifice, a feeling of being a victim. Belief in the inability of the human being to take his life in hand in a self-aware way. Belief in the possibility of being seized by the hand of fate, or by a punishment from god.

You allow yourself to be swallowed up, without having any hold, in an anonymous mass-happening, because no "personal-heart-energy" is being developed out of faith in your own divinity, because your feelings are so anxious and petrified, because you are convinced that the Plague can strike you, because you don't believe in the natural immunity of every human being. You don't believe in the power that lies within you: you place all power outside yourself; in this way you are being seized, because you don't get a grip on yourself.

You don't need anything else but Faith in your natural immunity and warm Love toward yourself and humanity. Trust in your own pure, sound, honest energies. Nourish the longing to Live and let go of needless emotional burdens; relax your stiffened muscles; leave behind old anxieties and resolutely dare to go on toward a new life, full of light and joy.

POLIO
(See also Paralysis)

Suppression of your feelings: you put yourself on a chain.

Deep-rooted feeling of powerlessness and anxiety. A feeling of imprisonment, fear of being crushed under an authority above your head. "I can't, I don't dare." Insufficient self-appreciation, you disapprove of yourself. On the one hand you look for a hold outside yourself; you anxiously reach for the arm of your mother; on the other hand you'd rather run away fast. "You are not going to get me!"

You look for shelter against outer threats, or against that which you perceive to be threatening, because you are so sensitive and vulnerable; you flee.

Wanting and not being able to; with anger toward life, unable to find support in yourself, you don't know very well which direction to take. You let yourself be influenced by books, philosophies, views of life, or authority, but emotionally you don't see a way out.

You consider the world hostile; you are born with a knife in your hand; possibly with unconscious memories from some remote past, you aggressively and guardedly step into the world. This resistance against life on earth has as its deepest cause: not trusting the deep roots of yourself; anxious powerlessness.

You don't dare to stand on your own feet, and you are angry with the people who take hold of you. You feel so insignificant that you anxiously hurry to prove yourself — sometimes in competitions, sometimes in wanting to deserve affection: "I have to be first, because otherwise someone else might pass me by, and that is life-threatening!" In extreme anxiety, you feel an imperative urge to be first.

Emotions dominate your life, but you experience yourself as emotionally paralyzed; your self-awareness has no grip on your unconscious energies. Nevertheless that is the message of your illness; transformation of consciousness, allowing all feelings and beautiful energies to flow freely, without fear!

Don't be afraid of your deepest powers, nor of life: give your feelings freedom, don't paralyze yourself, relax, discover your possibilities. The powers, the deep emotions which offer themselves, will transform into energies which will make you grow and evolve. Come out of your hiding place; discover the emotion, the happiness, the warmth, the secureness in your Self.

Dare to dig very deeply for your roots, and rouse yourself! Wake up from your stupor, allow your complete emotional world to blossom! Discover that spaciousness in yourself, which offers you all freedom to move; discover your rich emotional tones and make contact with your heart in an intense way. Feel that warm security in your deepest Self, that eternal living core. If you long for Life, then regenerating energies will cure you. Stand on your own feet, autonomously; become aware of those primal powers in you and be proud of yourself! Bring yourself to realization in a self-aware way! Take the hand of your fellow man in friendship; no longer feel threatened; descend on earth, participate in life, and build it according to your longings.

Don't allow yourself to "be lived," nor stay at the surface, but dare to discover your depths; allow yourself to be truly born. Be good and gentle; nourish yourself in love; now allow all the hard resistance to fall away. If you trustfully open yourself to life, then life energies will call your body cells to life.

Don't cling to others: your "I" is extremely strong and able to build a productive and powerful existence without help from anyone. No longer block your life by paralyzing yourself via negative convictions regarding yourself. Rouse yourself to life!

your basic structure; acknowledge your Worth, and let go of negative thoughts regarding yourself. Don't stagnate in immobility or downheartedness. Feel the earth under your feet, and come into motion. Free your head of the overburdening of thoughts! Live, and enjoy with your feelings, your body, your senses. . . . Let go of everything and everyone and trust that that which is good for you will appear on your path — on the condition that you open yourself to new things, to the positive. No longer bottle things up, and allow emotions to flow freely, without anxiety. Nothing inside you forms a threat.

POTASSIUM
Deficiency, insufficient assimilation of

Resistance to your feelings; emotions are being held back, and your head is like a mill that turns and turns, frustrated and aggressive, because you refuse to go On! You refuse to acknowledge the Worth in you; you break yourself down! An unbearable burden, but you don't give up; the resistance is great: you refuse to see and do what's best for you; a stubborn, willful holding-on as if your life depends on it.

A form of self-destruction: you don't let go because you experience yourself as powerless and inadequate, as unable to build up your life in a self-assured way; you are not standing solidly on your own feet, you anchor yourself in the past or you cling to others. Aggression! Because you think you can't go onward — impatience.

You are so afraid that if you would allow your feelings to flow freely everything would overpower and crush you; that's why you tighten the belt too much regarding your emotional experiences.

Assure a healthy balance in yourself between spirit and body, between feelings and thoughts. Feel the strength and safety of

PREGNANCY, CHILD-BEARING
If necessary, see also Vomiting during pregnancy, Postnatal depression, Cracked nipples and breast feeding difficulties, Diabetes of pregnancy

Pseudopregnancy

You don't really take your place; you don't stand solidly in your shoes; you are lacking firmness.

You'd rather hide behind a false attitude. You don't know very well who *you* are, don't really live in your own body here-and-now: you take on an attitude. Possibly you identify with many different people, play many roles, don't live from out of your deepest core. Everyone can "penetrate" your personal terrain: you absorb influences, habits, behaviors of other people. Who are you then? You imagine many things, pure fantasy; you experience again and again another imaginary reality, and every time your body adapts to it.

You "fill" yourself with everything and everyone except your own "I."

And still there's Resistance inwardly! Resistance to your own feeble, chameleon-like feeling of absence. Sometimes you can no longer endure it that others have such an influence on you, sometimes push you back so much that you have no say whatever. But you don't ski forward: you go around in a vicious circle.

You are pregnant with YOURSELF, but you don't allow yourself to be born.

Your energies turn inward. Who are you? Where are you?

Take your place in a self-aware way. "YOU ARE"; this is your life; no one can push you away from here. Close yourself off, determine your borders regarding others, and come into yourself, solid as a rock. Feel strongly established in your own Basis, your living Self, and LIVE according to your longings. Identify yourself first and foremost with your own "I" and then open yourself in a radiating way toward others. Don't take on an "attitude"; be yourself. Go outward, come out of yourself: allow yourself to be born! Look closely inside yourself, be realistic, stand with both feet on the ground.

Miscarriage, threatening

A full-grown fetus will be born at the moment when both mother and baby are psychologically ready for it. Certain entities which wish to experience living as a fetus in the mother's womb for only a few months will automatically be attracted to a mother who, in fact, is not completely ready to bear a child; or to a mother who, in order to come to spiritual growth in herself, unconsciously calls up a spontaneous abortion as a psychological experience. When the mother lives consciously, this will not happen; resolve these unconscious shortcomings!

Don't constrict yourself too much; don't brace yourself! Do you experience your feelings with uncertainty when it comes to yourself or your motherhood? Do you wish to give "life"? Live fully, then, yourself! Are you inwardly not convinced that the

timing is ideal to bear a child now? Do you wish a baby to compensate for — or to fill — your "empty" personal life? Don't suppress your own strong energies! Express your feelings and emotions so that suppression does not lead to an explosion on a physical level. Don't be too cold or too hard with yourself. Do you have the anxious feeling that you always have to stand up for or defend yourself? This is only a consequence of not trusting your own strong foundation. Do you fearfully close yourself up? Do you cling to others?

Achieve good self-support; relax. Open yourself up, unlimitedly, in all directions. Give freedom and joy to yourself and your relations. Achieve a generous exchange of feelings. Be tender and warm to yourself. Dare to bite into life, into its enjoyments. True love toward yourself drives away all anxieties and their consequences.

Inwardly liberate yourself from all pressure and self-limitation; solve in yourself the suppressed longing to "be free." *You don't have to immediately solve all inner problems; let go of them all and quietly be convinced: it's all right like this — everything will go the way that is best for Life. Your faith will direct the physical process.*

Miscarriage, premature baby
(See also Miscarriage, threatening)

The psychological situation of the mother as well as of the child requires a termination of the pregnancy: for the moment, it is better this way. For the little one it is often only a game, just having a glimpse of this life, and then going back again; he chooses to wait with his incarnation. Sometimes, however, it has to do with holding on too strongly to the world that is not three-dimensional — resistance to earthly life.

Mother also has something unresolved to deal with. You experience your own situation as a psychological prison; you are forever stirring the same pot, nourishing the same thoughts; you feel an irresistible urge to free yourself, to break out! An urge for liberation, flying from here to there: you search outside yourself too much; you become aggressive and tense — you should place the Center of your life in yourself, but you direct your life toward others too much, toward the outer world. There is no real evolution or progress in your life; you begin to break out in revolt. "Now it is enough!" You can no longer handle it. You push away. . . .

So it is necessary to preventively take your life, in all freedom, into your own hands and to steer it in the direction you wish; don't anchor yourself with structures that are pushed upon you by others. Achieve peaceful self-contemplation. Or is it the pregnancy itself that overcomes you; would you prefer to wait?

Toxemia of pregnancy, or pre-eclampsia

You can't yet handle yourself very well, and now someone else has to be added to it! You are not really master over yourself. You blame your feelings of imprisonment, of being constricted to pregnancy, but you yourself were already in the "prison" of yourself before you became pregnant. Now, there's even more of an urge to Free yourself! In an aggressive way you want to tear yourself out of this feeling of being stuck.

You haven't really felt safe in yourself before your pregnancy; now anxieties are even increasing. On the one hand you don't know very well what's happening there inside your body; you don't have a grip on it. Unconscious emotions pop up; you feel threatened. It's as if you are suffocating and gasping for breath. Anxiety about Your death, about death of the fetus; anxiety about not being a good mother or anxiety about not being able to handle it anymore.

You are at odds with your feelings; you're not really firmly standing on your own feet. You feel tossed from here to there,

as it were, ill-treated by others; you can't defend yourself; they do what they want with you; you're too absent in yourself. You feel unsure, nervous, unbalanced, overwhelmed. Your self-aware "I" doesn't seem to be really present; you feel submerged in emotions.

You are angry because of your powerlessness, angry with those who are allegedly restricting you and doing you an injustice, but it is yourself that ties you down so anxiously — because you don't trust in yourself, because you don't really believe in your worth and your possibilities of self-creating your life, independent of others. You hide behind a partner, a mother — you suffocate yourself in this way. You start to revolt against this, but you don't bring about actual changes. Sometimes you still feel like a child; a second child being added to this through your pregnancy might form a threat because you then have to share with someone else the attention that goes to you. On the other hand your longings are so intense, you take this responsibility so seriously, that you constantly worry anxiously about it ending all right. You poison yourself with the accumulation of all these emotions.

You feel so unprotected and vulnerable. You gasp for more space for yourself.

Inner liberation, self-realization: the keys to relaxation, to detoxicate.

You feel oppressed by your emotions, by your anxieties and uncertainties: solve this and the danger will disappear. Turn toward the Light, the joy and life in your heart: there is no reason at all for panicky anxiety. You are master over your body, over your existence, if you take up the scepter. No longer allow yourself to "be lived"; trust in your Self; nothing negative happens if you haven't first wanted it. Turn inward, close to yourself, and decide what you want; do you wish a smooth, healthy pregnancy and delivery, then you may easily surrender to those longings, instead of anxiously tensing up. Reality follows your convictions and longings: now dare to take your life in hand, YOURSELF, and long, create the most beau-

tiful! Discover the peace and safety in your Living Self. You are naturally protected if you don't fight against it, if you no longer doubt: about your inner powers and the possibility of creating your existence yourself and guiding it into the right course. Relax; enjoy life; don't fret; give yourself faith; take up the space you need; don't cling to your partner, but do at any moment what you feel you have to do so that you will be at peace and be happy.

Child-bearing: exaggerated pain, complications, breech birth

A belief in suffering and death. Fear of dying; fear that the baby might die. Since childhood you have been made to believe that mothers will suffer at the birth of their child, that they bear the child but that in the end they will have to let it die again. Here lies the deepest pain, which unconsciously penetrates very strongly. You feel at the mercy of something that is beyond you; you grimly try to remain standing. In fact, you don't allow your Self to be born: the baby was there to fill your own emptiness; now you will be confronted again with your own emptiness. You hold on to things too strongly, aggressively, anxiously. A fearful urge for possession. Accentuation of the negative side of life: death, chilliness, loneliness, pain. You have not yet offered yourself the Freedom of life, the true joy of life. You don't trust your nature. You even think that you have to protect yourself against devilish, powerful forces, which come as it were out of yourself; you fight against your labor pains, but you don't realize that it is death you are fighting, and that the only joyful birth is the one by which life, in joy, without pain and death, is placed at the center for you and for the little one. An accumulation of suppressed emotions and a feeling of powerlessness to control the process result in an anxious grip on the baby and also on the

people around you. You anxiously clench life in your hands; tension; you cannot let go of the baby.

You will attract a baby who has its specific reasons for ending up with you — with this anxious nervousness and mistrust, which it also experiences inside itself. It, too, is on its guard and clings fast.

When you allow yourself to be born out of the cocoon, when you realize the fullness of yourself, when you trust your nature and allow your feelings to flow freely, when you turn toward life instead of toward negativity and death, when you trust your intuition and acknowledge your mastery over your own life — then the baby will thankfully experience an influence from your transformation. Don't hold in energies, but let go; relaxation; that peaceful, safe feeling in yourself. Allow yourself to be born, not to die but to live in joy! The baby will follow your example. Don't cramp up; give birth to life in gentleness (See also Part I).

Afterbirth; not, or only partly delivered

Keeping everything shut in a cramped way, putting the brakes on it, holding it back.

An unconscious longing to hold in the baby, to hold on to the prior situation, because you don't dare to allow yourself to be born. You don't give yourself the chance to be born in the fullness of yourself, in the joy of life. Possibly, you have allowed yourself and your evolution to be "frozen" during the pregnancy — with precisely this situation as an excuse. You don't dare to really be yourself; you don't dare to really live; you are afraid of deep emotions and life-powers in yourself. You insufficiently believe in yourself. You stay closed, refusing to go on in life; possibly, you are afraid of confronting problems, and you anxiously stop yourself from going on. What now? Fearlessly dare to let go: create your life in a self-aware way, in joy, because happiness rests in your own hands. Don't get stuck in the past: go on with a perspective on renewed life! Fill yourself with the fullness of your Self.

Hemorrhage after giving birth

In an anxious way, you try to embrace everything emotionally, but that is difficult. A sadness, being left with a feeling of emptiness; the little one has been born. You wish, perhaps unconsciously, to remain in the condition of pregnancy, at least emotionally. Now, you are again totally confronted with yourself. It seems hard for you to come close to the baby, but you cannot experience yourself in Unity: you have a strong need for love; this love cannot be filled by either your husband or the child. You deserve at last to approach *yourself* in love. Your sadness was already there before pregnancy; possibly, it seemed that the coming baby would solve all your problems. Your loneliness, your lack of warmth, can only be resolved within yourself: don't expect from others. That which is good for you will come to you by itself when first you achieve inner harmony and come very close to yourself. The new situation brings along a nervous bond for you and the baby; you don't feel very safe; the apparent distance which is now between you and the baby seems like a break. No: this is about a clear demand from your deepest Self: no longer stand at a distance from yourself, from your body. You experience your balance to be rather shaky, unstable, because you are afraid to go on in life, because you are insufficiently aware of your powers, because you expect more from your partner than he can give at this moment.

*You can only grow toward happiness — toward a true love relationship with someone else — if first of all you truly love yourself, if you no longer have a condemning or negative attitude toward your inner or bodily being. It is now necessary that you take re-sponsibility for your life and for the little one. Don't expect anything, but **give**; bend in warmth toward the little one that you, yourself, still are, and toward the little one in the cradle. Dare to go onward in all power, let go of the past. Mortal fears can torment you, but know that life is joy when you give yourself the right to truly live. Don't build your thoughts on negative experiences from the past, but let yourself be reborn now. Feel free; no longer burden yourself with dark thoughts. Your life rests only in your hands; banish death and sorrow from your life, as being lies. Begin again. Feel safe in your own warm nest and offer the child a life of its own.*

PROSTHESES, IN GENERAL
(See also Teeth and Breasts)

No matter if it's regarding hip, knee, leg, or arm prostheses, man should make thankful use of it. It's not "just by accident" that a certain person lives NOW and that he — if he feels it's necessary and good for him — makes use of a prosthesis. The less inner resistance there is against it, and the greater the love with which one does this for oneself, and the stronger the faith that everything (possibly an operation) will proceed very well, the easier this person makes it for himself and the smoother everything will evolve. Of course, the important thing here is: "Why did I lose this body part?" or "Why was I born with, for instance, just one leg? What does this say about my conviction pattern, about the lessons I want to learn about myself in this life, and how will I adjust my life's course in a healing direction? What does the leg (the knee, the arms, the hips, etc.) symbolize?"

Look this up in the relevant categories, without self-accusation. You can start every day with a clean slate, or make yourself follow a new path!

Evolve in love, work on yourself, and gratefully make use of a prosthesis when you think it best. Also, know that outer norms are of no importance for life. When, for instance, you feel good and are able to move well in life with one arm, or with one leg, then this is okay! Also, if for instance you have received a hip prosthesis and someone tells you it will definitely have to be replaced after 15 years, then know that a future is not "determined," and that you can completely alter this course of things by living with the most positive convictions. When living in faith and love for yourself, working inwardly on the symbolism of the concerned body part, everything will go very well. Also know that the scientific technology of which you gratefully make use — as well as the speed/quality of inventions — forever grows and improves. There will be many new things created under the sun: not only through science, but also via the human brain. Don't exclude any possibility beforehand; live according to the conviction that everything will go well the way it can go, now, and that in the future more beautiful, miraculous things may happen in the field of scientific inventions and new technologies as well as in the field of human energy and transformation.

Live according to the expectation that it doesn't have to be "difficult," that evolution will be wonderful, that you don't have to suffer. In the meantime, understanding the language of the body part concerned, and evolving . . . in this way everything will proceed optimally!

PYROMANIA

Desperately looking for yourself: "Who am I?" A part of your personality takes possession of your total being because you have suppressed this part for too long.

Unconscious energies slowly pile up without being consciously experienced or worked out or being transformed into creativity: a shadow mountain slowly piles up before the sun, your conscious "I," until it overpowers you and you have no more say over it. Suppression of deep feelings, of healthy aggressive powers, ultimately leads to compulsiveness. *Possibly* you were brought up in a milieu where you were not at all appreciated for your feelings, your inner worth, but where one especially paid attention to outward appearances or to your ability to achieve. Where you were taught not to trust your feelings, your natural powers. Haven't you encountered any real love yet? Were your gentle feelings of love, as well as your potential energies, suppressed? Finally, you feel like you are just made out of wood! An inner urge to escape out of this wooden framework; your volcanic powers turn outward; you throw off your white cloth, in which you felt imprisoned. Your frustration now flames up into fury; now you experience yourself as a monster that has been locked up for too long, while actually we're only dealing with an enormous revolt against the suppression of your feelings and powers.

You are afraid of your natural aggressive powers, afraid of your "I," of your energetic Self, afraid of the depths in yourself — and you suppress it all. This leads to dividedness.

On the other hand you feel powerless, a victim of others, unable to be yourself, angry because of your powerlessness, angry also with your feelings, with your gentleness, with the "female" aspect in yourself. You'd carve your heart out, because you don't really dare to love yourself the way you are; you think you are no good.

You don't feel a solid basis under your feet, don't experience a firm structure in yourself. Possibly as a child you have satisfied the expectations of others more than having really lived from out of yourself. You don't know who you really are; you are afraid of what's under your surface; anxiously you hide the deepest part of yourself; you break out in a cold sweat. You feel limp and weak, unable to keep control over your "dark" side; you try to suppress it as long as you can, till this aspect takes control.

Aggressive thoughts and the intense longing to still discover your feelings, to be able to be intensely moved by something, to find yourself in this excitement, to fill yourself with agreeable, pleasant emotions; you light the fire. As strongly as your fire is being suppressed, that is how high the flames burn in the stable.

A safety valve for the powerless fury of not being able to be yourself; anger about being a victim, but a longing to still be able to experience yourself in an exciting way. A way to free yourself from too-great a pressure of tension: fire.

Light the fuse in your reality: break away from your frustration; if you are angry, then dare to speak. Free yourself from your limitations by allowing all your feelings and energies to flow freely.

Become yourself, you are not bad; in you there's no single power that works in a threatening way as long as you don't suppress them! Allow energies to be free; allow them to grow. Feel safe in your own solid basis and don't bottle things up; don't hold on to your powers until you explode; transform them into creativity. Allow yourself to break through in daily life, without having complexes. Lovingly acknowledge your beautiful content; don't be angry with yourself, nor with those who hurt you. Manifest yourself in self-confidence and don't satisfy external expectations, but integrate that part of yourself which you suppress — also your gentleness. Arrive at contentment in yourself. The excitement to be yourself; the intense joy of life, without your needing a help to achieve this; the discovery of your real power, of the mastery of your Conscious "I" over feelings and unconscious powers, no longer condemning or suppressing them. Pyromania disappears with inner peace and the freedom of being yourself in totality, with the loving acceptance of every aspect in yourself.

R

RABIES

Reckoning with your own powerlessness, with the power-game inside yourself: you are angry with the little child inside you, who feels powerless and hurt.

Possibly, you have actually been hurt psychologically by a person on whom you depended. You have depended again and again on a certain authority — as a child, on your father or mother; later, on your friends, your partner. You are extremely angry about the vulnerable position you are in, about your attachment. You don't build your life on your inner values, but rather on your image, on a facade of stalwartness. You are disgusted by your own weaknesses and sensitivity. Anger at those upon whom you feel dependent; you'd like to smother them because you, yourself, feel so smothered in circumstances of powerlessness and dependency. Because you feel so full of anxiety — by yourself, alone — you are submerged in the authority above you, in the relationship, or in your outer image. But this frustrates you; you become furious with this authority, with this relationship, with powerlessness itself.

Old authority, old indoctrination, the laws that governed your earlier life — you would like to pull them out, like a rotten tooth! Your head is a red-hot chaos. Sometimes it has to do with a psychological reckoning with a person who previously has hurt you, when you were small and helpless: incest, sadism, etc. As a reaction to this, you become very hard and aggressive, yes, even sadistic toward yourself, toward others. A black hand strangles your sensitive heart. Now you want to get them. You could broil somebody on the spit, but in fact you feel as if you are the one who's being spit-roasted. Someone has browbeaten you, and now you could beat someone on the head. You could be extremely aggressive sexually, but it is a reaction to your "emptiness."

Allow your emotions to circulate, don't block them. Express your anger, sadness and feelings of powerlessness. Your despairing rage won't last; other feelings will follow if you simply dare to look at all those emotions.

Let go, then, of what you have to let go: know yourself to be safe at home inside yourself. Become conscious of your human worth. Know yourself to be safe in yourself, in your body, in your nature; don't live in your "thoughts." Relieve your head. Push through, in active self-manifestation, from out of your deepest Self. Come first to reconciliation in yourself and mark off the borders of your emotional terrain, for only then can you get into contact with others.

Arrive at insight, at understanding, and know that your powerlessness was the original cause of all the sad facts in the past: you have attracted them to you. Liberate yourself from previous thought-patterns and life-patterns — radically.

REFLEX SYMPATHETIC DYSTROPHY

mostly after a (possibly mild) trauma, often of the wrist or ankle: persisting pain, swelling, sweating, stiffness, vascular symptoms, skin changes, progressive osteoporosis and atrophy

You hurt yourself! You are sad about yourself; you are angry — and therefore you would destroy yourself. This self-destruction, this self-poisoning can only be stopped by you, YOURSELF. It can very well be that other people "hurt" you, but this then is only a result of your self-destructive feelings and thoughts. There's something in you such as, "I don't want anymore." You'd like to cut off your hands because you are angry and sad. "I can't do what I want anyway; I can't have or achieve what I want." The most important lesson is that of gratitude: the joy of Life, of Being the way you are. You want to "hinder." Leave life Free!

Your Soul-core sends you good life energies, but you REFUSE to accept them. You close yourself off to them; you don't want anymore: in fact, you refuse Love of yourself!

Why be so hard on yourself? Why not open your arms wide and welcome yourself in warm Love? Why close yourself off? In this way, possibly, you also push away other people who would like to be very close to you. You are a good human being; you need to know that every day you can start your life with a clean slate, without blaming yourself about the past, without feelings of guilt, without thinking you have to punish yourself. In the NOW you can give yourself all opportunities to open yourself up to Life and Love, so that you can let go of the desires and the "wanting to have" (possibly wanting that *others* will acknowledge you and give

you love), so that you can think of yourself as a Good human being.

Don't cut yourself off from all the beautiful paths! No longer punish yourself. You don't need to be destroyed! You need to stop destroying yourself — psychologically, emotionally; as a result, your body won't be destroyed either. Don't expect anything from others; don't be angry with others, because he/she doesn't want to give what you don't want to give to yourself. Turn around! Don't fight against life's Energy inside you, which likes so much to send your body healing forces: only your destructive feelings block this system, hinder this healing from taking place by itself. No longer fight *against* yourself!

Would you like to withdraw angrily, like a turtle under its shield, angry with Life, angry with yourself, angry with everything and everyone? You, alone, can give yourself Life; you need to make Peace in your Heart. No longer withdraw, but fully enter into the light of existence. Take up your space in a happy way, and heartily offer yourself an existence full of love. Give yourself the opportunity for life, and "allow" the life forces to heal. Don't close yourself off from tenderness, from that which is dearest to you, from that which is most beautiful in life. . . . Don't turn yourself against Life in anger, resentment, or dissatisfaction, but pull yourself out of destructive habit-patterns. You, alone, can "allow" your body to restore itself to prime health — or hinder this process with feelings of hatred, aggression: "I will punish you," etc. Let go of everything you have desired or longed for outside yourself — and begin now to generously *offer* yourself everything, with a Heart. If you call a stop to the destructive urge in yourself, then the results will be visible very quickly: IN your body, in your surroundings. Don't resist taking the necessary turn in your life, and opt now for Building up instead of Breaking down, for love instead of hate, for a "Yes" instead of your "No."

466

RESPIRATORY TRACT

Ailments, in general

Do you put yourself and your fellow man into a cell? Do you smother yourself with negative, anxious, or angry thoughts? Anxiety about a power that is stronger than you — about a threatening superior force. Fear of being grabbed, while in fact you keep yourself prisoner. Unconsciously, you are convinced that you are unable to live autonomously, that you can't trust your Eternal, strong Self; you then make yourself dependent on others and "claw" onto them, so that in this way you suffocate yourself. You deny your complete psychic space and you also wear blinders to that which is outside you. Does your life stand or fall with one philosophy or do you suffocate yourself in prejudices? Perhaps you neglect your Living Self-Core and place Authority outside or above you. Because deep inside you dwells the conviction "I cannot" or "I'm not allowed to be free," do you cling to people who limit you? You become angry because you feel yourself being suffocated by emotions of fear, power-and-powerlessness.

Freedom and autonomy! Sail under your own steam — Explore space without self-limitation. Find the balance between your thinking-pole and your emotional-pole. Grow toward harmony in your relationships. Daring to open yourself, without prejudices, to all emotions, knowledge, information or experiences that present themselves inwardly and also outwardly.

Feeling yourself safe and in peace within the broader framework of your total, living Self, realize that your Consciousness is open and unbounded. Anger and anxiety are but expressions of feelings of powerlessness; seize that power IN, and over, yourself.

(See also Lungs.)

Asthma

Anxiety; inner tension. "I am almost NOT. I can't be here, I can't live." Indefinite life anxiety that something threatening might stab you in the heart, that some monster might crush you. The feeling that something or someone overpowers you. Fear of one's own driving force, of one's own Sunny "I." Out of fear of yourself and of your inner powers, you might turn off the main road, flee. Like an ostrich, you can hide, in structures, in laws, under the Authority of a person or a system. Thus, you feel protected and don't need to go *to your own essence,* because you are afraid of that. In this way, you suffocate yourself, don't allow sunlight in your life.

Children often look for something to hold on to — for rescue — in a father or mother figure, in an Authority that substitutes for their own "I." This has a suffocating effect, and it is most assuredly so when the parents themselves are fearful, which might enhance the child's feeling of insecurity. It sometimes happens that parents exercise an exaggerated mothering, or suffocating, Authority, because they don't succeed in truly living from out of their own safe Basis and in converting their energies into self-development. Still, the cause of the disease is always to be sought for in the psyche of the child itself, or in the psyche of the person himself. The child is too fearful to take up its own space, and its mentors don't always encourage it to do so because they also have difficulty daring fully, without fear, to manifest themselves as autonomous beings.

You feel "pulled" onto the earth and then pushed into life, but you don't comprehend "Why? Where do I come from? What is life?" Mortal fears and doubts; babies unconsciously arrive in this milieu, where they are confronted with the fearful doubts of their environment, which offers a reflection of their own anxieties.

You feel unable to live, and you recoil, fleeing from yourself. You live in a mixture of truth — reality on one side, and on the other side dream, illusion, nightmare, unreal fantasies. Because of anxiety, your imagination goes wild. You try to keep your emotions in balance, but it all slips away from you. You feel nervous, bound to a chain, and as a result your natural spontaneity is inhibited. You would sooner experience yourself as a victim on the defense than acknowledge the Mastery in yourself. Instead of seizing the horse by the reins, you unconsciously long, as it were, for a winged horse to come and rescue you from the fire. You are always watchful, in a defensive posture, on guard; you want to destroy the unknown danger that is about to take you by surprise, but you don't see clearly where it is.

To here, and no further! Out of fear of losing yourself in the cold nothingness, you are anxiously marking off borders toward your deepest Self, toward your inner powers and emotions, toward others. Exaggerated, anxious self-control; accommodating yourself to others too much at the expense of your own nature; always doing what another commands, like a slave in a straitjacket, and with rebellion, powerless anger, as a consequence. Powerlessness: because you don't find yourself, because you don't trust yourself, because you don't dare to fully take up your life space.

Stand still now, by yourself; don't run away any more! Life is safe when you, yourself, take it in hand, when you discover how you attract situations as a consequence of inner convictions: your creative Consciousness is master of your life. Trust this imperishable Basis in yourself; you are not doomed to be a lifelong asthma sufferer, nor to be dependent on medicine. Now give yourself all the space and let your energies come through freely. When you decide "I am master of my existence," you will create your future in the direction of the joy of life. Asthma indicates the denial of the immortal essence, of this creative source inside yourself. You are not dependent on others; you smother yourself with "thinking and fretting" because you deny your own divinity. Anxiety indicates that you are not on the right track and need to bring about changes. So, come, in love, toward yourself, free yourself from your shackles, bestow trust upon your living Self. Anxiety and disbelief are the hindrances to your happiness. Come to pure Self-acknowledgment as an "I"; let go, and love yourself infinitely. Trust, Believe in your Basic Power! The eternal being you are will never die; give yourself all opportunities for an open, liberated, earthly existence. Become Master over your life!

(See further, Part I)

Parents of children who suffer from asthma can, through self-examination, find out to what degree they also have to resolve the above causes in themselves.

Bronchiolitis, infant

Although the psycho-emotional cause lies in the baby itself, with this disease we sometimes see a reflection of the mother's psychological situation; then the causes below count for both:

Resistance, desire to break through! "I feel like a tiger behind glass.

"Let me go! I'm suffocating here."

Experiences the world or the environment as oppressive, hostile.

Feels oneself locked up and dark, desperately angry, in a structure that is too limiting.

Both baby and the person who brings him up have to dare to take up their psychic space: let all your feelings flow quietly, make them known, and don't suppress them.

Baby has entered the world with the unconscious conviction that the world is hostile toward him, or that he will be limited in his search for freedom; at this moment the parents have a similar problem. If they give themselves more room, then they will make space for the child.

Take a good look at how both of you are suffocating yourselves, and change your convictions now; calmly bring about changes in your life, liberate yourself.

It is your anger, not that of the world.

A solid grounding and realization of mother's safe self-assuredness will bring rest. No smothering affection, but an open atmosphere in a home of warmth and — above all — trust in Life.

Bronchitis

It is getting out of hand; you have already experienced too much tension and sorrow. Pain, sadness, powerlessness; you feel stuck. Inner revolt — anger because of it. You are full of energy, which is pushing under the skin to make its way: your deepest "I" asks for action, advancement, and joy of life! But you don't navigate a clear course, and you don't see a goal or direction. You even refuse to completely stand on your own feet, and then you are angry with your surroundings! Even if you somehow do want to, you don't feel able to live from out of your Self. You doubt your powers and possibilities. Nevertheless, you are full of potential talents: you become angry because of your powerlessness when it comes to self-realization.

With regard to children:

Suppressed anger, sadness, and tensions between the parents or in a wider family relationship make feelings of anxiety and insecurity stronger. Thus, the aggressive powerlessness of the parent can influence the bronchitis of the infant in a negative way (although the deepest cause lies in the child itself).

Too young to choose its own way, it follows, from sheer necessity, the footsteps of others, even though this can go completely against its own "nature." The feeling that one *must* go in this or that direction hurts and leads to frustration and feelings of limitation. The child sometimes has the impression that its existence is pointless, and it feels unac-

knowledged as a separate personality. It can feel suffocated, and now has to learn to find — to express — "ITSELF" . . in joy and contentment regarding its "I."

When you finally become kind to yourself, you will also receive joy from harmonious communication with others. Don't vent your anger at others: believe in yourself and break through!

You are very pregnant with your Self: let all your talents and possibilities be born. Don't be angry with others; don't desire, but BECOME yourself! Let go . . . .

Concentrate inside yourself and feel your strong basis, independent of others and full of willpower. It is not, first of all, the material situation that limits you, but your inner imprisonment! The outer circumstances are just a consequence of your inner expectations from life. Change your expectations. Don't close yourself off from new, higher insights, and live according to them. Bring peace to yourself, and your surroundings will evolve into harmony. First and foremost, come to thankfulness for life, and don't desire anything in anger! Take up your SPACE, in happiness, "you" as "you," without nailing yourself down in suffocating thoughts. You **are** *free when you unburden yourself from oppressive thoughts and emotions!*

Cough, in general

A stop, a revolt, a refusal to go on this way. An alarm signal to the outer world: "Now, it has been enough. I surrender. Do nothing more to me or the bucket will overflow." You might collapse at the knee.

You intently demand attention from your surroundings: "Do you see me? Do you love me? Because I consider myself to be only so so."

Nervous feelings of "being stuck" in a certain thought-circle or life-situation.

"I have now experienced enough; I stop it." Feelings of martyrdom, a mixture of sadness and aggression.

You hold back, you don't express yourself completely. You also hold back your aggressive feelings. Perhaps you have been pliable for too long. Now you are revolting against it. Irritated, suppressed anger: toward yourself because you don't express yourself as you would like, or toward others, because you "are" not yourself!
Instead of being straightforward, you perhaps have been too hesitant, and this yes/no attitude of yours disturbs you. And now it is enough.

*Don't block your energy flow, let everything flow freely. Be yourself, dare to stand up for yourself; always determine, yourself, how far others may go with regard to you. Don't **let** yourself "be lived," but determine, yourself, the direction of the stream of joyful energies. Observe everything quietly, from above, without emotion; get a perspective and go decisively onward. If you don't feel loved, this is primarily because you don't appreciate yourself enough; you push yourself to the side. Don't listen to know-it-alls; follow your own intuition. Don't let your shoulders droop, let your motor turn powerfully. In this way, the battery charges itself. Don't doubt, for then your motor will stop. Liberate yourself, voice it, don't allow yourself to be dominated and don't grasp for people or things yourself.*

Shortness of breath

Emotions — oppressive experiences from the past — are being held on to. You don't have a liberating, clear vision of yourself and your life; you prevent yourself from breathing "freely." Painful or *black and nervous thoughts* prevent you from truly going on in one chosen direction. You stand still now, weak in the knee, feeling too-little supported. You are cut off too much from your feelings, your intuition, your nature, your body. Often, lack of self-confidence; you allow your life to be too dependent on the expectations of others. You squeeze yourself into a straitjacket in order to please your relations or to respond outwardly to specific norms.

Dare to dig, dare to look at your deepest feelings. In what way do you feel yourself oppressed? Let yourself go, let yourself grow in all directions — Warm yourself; by nature you have a firm basis, which is your always-growing, strong Self, an open, free "I." Integrate every part of yourself, don't close off your outer ego from its basis. Guide your feelings and thoughts with authority: confrontation and elimination. Purification, liberation. Being "you"!

What you feel counts. Not what others think of you or expect of you!

Live in a calm, forceful way, from within, without rushing yourself, without fretting. Don't exert yourself or move in a way that doesn't really agree with YOUR NATURE. Be faithful to your SELF!

Read more about this in the book *Large, Beautiful, and Healthy.*

Suffocation attacks

Fearfully fleeing pain from the past that is pursuing you. The burden is getting too heavy — you would like to disappear. Inner aggression. You don't see clearly at all any more, and that hounds you. You inadequately realize your personal worth, don't really think you deserve to live. You get excited about futilities, about facts with which you actually have nothing to do. You might fanatically and blindly fight for an ideal. In order to still give credit to your unappreciated "I," you assume an outer role, as a hero, as Santa Claus or Joan of Arc. Being stuck in your problematic situation, denying your own authority, you will, with a torch held high and in an often aggressive way and self-projection, condemn social or personal difficulties. You who strive for good, but whose own chair is empty. Fear. You feel strangled, and would like to break out in one way or another. You still feel too small, are still stuck in the past, and you look up too much to your parents, to leaders or authorities outside yourself. You can't really evolve further because you neglect your own Authority, and you constantly go right on without seeing yourself. Sometimes, you flee past the borders of life, suffocated and dead. Sometimes you look for excitement to fill up your own emptiness.

Be filled with true joy, real happiness; build upon your self-appreciation. Stand still and SEE yourself and the others well. Wrench yourself away from the web of fleeing, anxieties, and self-delusion! Acknowledge your mastery, and then you'll experience your own creative forces and will no longer flee from Life: seize it and take it in your own hands. Don't let yourself be smothered by happenings from the past, nor by idealized, unrealistic thoughts that are but an escape, nor by authorities outside yourself. Was the truth sometimes hard? Don't run away from it. Confront yourself with it: accept it, and then work it out. Don't flee from your emotions, your burdens: resolve instead of suppress!

Tracheitis
inflammation of the windpipe

Inner collision; you feel bound and would like to break out. You are completely stuck; it takes the breath away from you. Heavy, pressing feelings: on the one hand, you'd like to powerfully grasp something or somebody and cling to them; on the other hand, by doing so you suffocate yourself. Deepest cause: *Where* are you? Where is your self-aware "I"? Do you, as a result of a feeling of weakness, bind yourself?

Let go and look at yourself in a "Lighter," more loving way.
Direct the beam of light toward the inside instead of toward your relations, and come to inner self-liberation. Quietly observe your emotions, work them out, and let go. You are

stuck only as long as you allow yourself to be held, or as long as you, yourself, keep on grabbing. Rise above all this with the power of your consciousness. Independence, alone, leads to freely chosen, wholesome relationships.

THE LUNGS

Psychological correspondence

The ability to unlimitedly experience your "I am," to break through all time-and-space barriers, to experience higher energies, to experience your nature in all freedom. This is how our lungs would speak:

"Words are only words; the content counts. With united powers we create a new earth with eternal life, not death, as the guideline. The heart will break through its imprisonment.

Take your vessel and navigate under your own powers where your Living Self Wills."

Ailments, in general

Going against life itself, contrary to the flow: toward death. You don't take responsibility for your life. You flee and deny your living Self. You doubt yourself, afraid of not being emotionally able to handle everything. Then again, you overconfidently wave the scepter of fleeting values, and grasp for power over others instead of placing the power inside yourself. It is all useless.... Self-destructive. The creativity, the powers of your spirit, remain completely unused, paralyzed. You doubt your unlimited possibilities, your strong basis, or you live superficially like a clown with deep anxiety of "falling." Sadness, powerless anger. Do you give up your space to another person, or to an idol outside yourself? Do you live anxiously, cut off from the divinity inside yourself?

With a strong will to live, courage and power, you will break through all barriers of limitation. Enjoy life itself. Direct yourself deeper into yourself. Joy and wealth live within you. Realize the endless range of your Self and follow your inner path.

Peace, freedom.

Place yourself in the center of your existence! Ban suffocating emotions and thoughts from your life. "Fill" your lungs, not with sorrow, but Breathe for yourself and LIVE! Don't "Fill" yourself with endless fretting and brooding. Enjoy life in Thankfulness!

Lung cancer
(See also Cancer, in general)

You feel cold, chilled, sad, without love — you believe in Evil. You are angry about wickedness; you think too much in black and white and are often narrow-minded in your judgment of others. But for the most part, you won't speak up, hiding your opinion. You would like to have the power to destroy the devil, so to speak. Do you feel yourself to be a bit devilish? Do you judge others about things which you find yourself frustrated with? You unconsciously project your feelings: with stone-hard self-willed force you'd like to bang aggressively on the table and condemn, in a discriminating way, certain people or groups as "bad." But you bottle it up, this hard criticism.

We are dealing here with inner powerlessness: your personal frustrations, denial of the warmth of your own heart, the deep anxiety that you might be totally wrong after all, that after all no god exists in heaven. . . .

The old structures and values upon which you have built your life are possibly being attacked or deemed worthless by certain people: therefore, they compose a threat to your existence! Out of the fear of no longer feeling the ground beneath your feet, you develop hatred and ill-will toward them. Finally, you let yourself go in bitterness. It all makes no sense any longer. Do your children, your partner, not live up to your pre-established ideals? Then the cause of your disappointment lies in the fact that you projected your personal expectations on them.

In your life, you are in the center, not your children; they choose their own life's path! You allow your healthy living space to be taken up by others or by your negative brain-concoction, and you forget what Life is. Do you long for death? The choice is yours.

Express your feelings, your sadness; voice what's bothering you and no longer bottle it up. Discover the harmony, the rest within your Self: Come to accept yourself; make peace with yourself and others. Fighting wickedness with wickedness only makes the situation worse inside and outside yourself. Integrate all feelings, also your body, as something good inside yourself. Have you been condemned by others because of the fact that you still consider yourself to be bad?

Are you stuck with "longings" that you find "bad"? Everything is human, everything is evolution: arrive at mildness and understanding. No person or system can tell you what is good for you. No rule can limit you. Only the law of Love counts. You see "wickedness" around you and you suffocate yourself in it; you keep yourself fixated on the negative projections of your personal longings. Don't focus on other people; find yourself at last and liberate yourself from these self-limitations and prejudgments. Don't hold on to others. Come to yourself in peace. The divine is inside your Self. Space! Freedom! Joy!

COPD
chronic obstructive pulmonary disease
Chronic obstruction of airflow in the lungs because of EMPHYSEMA or CHRONIC BRONCHITIS

A Plutonic pressure from your depths; you are being obliged (by that which is deepest inside you) to rise up from out of the deepest foundations of yourself. Perhaps it seems threatening sometimes, but the objective is that you will transform yourself, that you definitively wake up from your hibernation, from your underground existence, in order now to begin to live above ground, completely... yes, without "holding back," without self-inhibition or keeping on living in concealment... that you would "be" yourself.

You show, perhaps, the white sails of your boat above water; you really would like there to be peace, but you yourself are for the moment still in the hold of the ship, "under water," in the midst of emotions — deep underwater energies flood you. Possibly you don't show anyone how deep it really is stuck. You don't really see clearly, and you feel overwhelmed with sadness... definitely, if you keep living there, under water.

Why don't you allow yourself to be "born"? Why not sail ON the waters of life in unity with your upper sails, showing yourself, manifesting yourself in healthy pride regarding your "I"? Don't you dare to? Do you fear that if you reveal yourself completely, with your total being, your emotions, it will make your boat capsize?

Many unpleasant odors come up from your depths; the smell of the past, the stored-up evil in yourself; resentment, anger, sadness, and powerlessness... fermenting, looking for an outlet. In fact, you escape self-realization and remain stuck in the muck of the past. You just keep hiding in the subterranean part of yourself. It's time to start looking for the daylight of your being and to rise above water with your feelings and thoughts in an honest way, so to come finally to a clear vision, a solution, in dialogue with life, with others. No longer keep your feelings hidden, come above water with them.

Now, show yourself in all clarity and let go of the Past! After all, as long as you turn to the past you will feel sadness, because it has passed and no longer belongs to "life."

Free yourself from burdensome thoughts and heavy emotions and turn toward Life. Let go of everything and everyone... free yourself completely from oppressive thoughts, of heavy emotions; live in peace with yourself. Become yourself, in the happiness of YOUR "I." Energies that purify now look for their way... allow them to flow through! Free yourself; offer yourself that inner freedom. No longer dwell on dark emotions and thoughts! Don't suffocate yourself any longer.

Go onward! Apply ALL those energies — "like an express train" toward your future, in evolution, with speedy force, with super-fast energies that now "happily" concentrate themselves inside you: at least they know now "where" they are going!

Toward self-realization, separate from whomever or whatever. Separate from a past. You liberate yourself, free yourself. You whiz onward, and these *energies that turn and turn* do so much good for you (and your body). You now feel how life is on your side, how life forces fill every fiber of your body with happiness. In this penetration, in this Uranian liberation, you search, very powerfully, your way through life. Now that mass of energies is being used in a constructive, advancing way — now they no longer flood you like a kind of threatening emotional power; now they smell strong and fresh, because you no longer turn yourself toward the underground, pushing yourself in anger, powerfully and devilishly downward.

You pull yourself *above the water surface* and purify yourself from all heavy, dark emotions and thoughts that just had a suffocating effect on you. You pull yourself up and offer yourself a swift sailing in the space of life. That joy and that immeasurable feeling of freedom INSIDE yourself for being able to be who you are, having freed yourself from all darkness; a constant, consistent going-onward in a new direction, unhindered by anything or anyone — yourself included. Nothing in you can hold you back any longer, and you feel happy and free! You no longer hold yourself back in any way; every power-pressure on yourself, every sinister perspective on life has disappeared. You have taken the second chance with both hands. Complete Love toward yourself, complete softening, complete happiness for your existence, without placing conditions on life, on these or those people from your surroundings.

You now see CLEARLY into yourself, into life, into your emotions (read Part I); you understand why something has happened, why everything is the way it is in life; you also know that you have your life in your hands and that nothing happens by "accident." In this complete understanding of yourself, in understanding others, you can let go — and firmly go onward: the air flows freely and powerfully through your lungs, unobstructed, now that you have freed yourself!

Lung embolism

Inner collision. On the one hand you feel powerless, feeble and without will power; you anxiously keep hidden in a corner because of fear that if you come out of your hiding place you might find death — that coming out will have final consequences.

On the other hand, you are stuck with pent-up aggression, a clenched fist in your pocket; you hold back all your energies, but inwardly there develops a longing for more power, including power over others, because inwardly you feel so powerless.

Inner revolt: "Stay away from me, or I will. . . ." And then again, you'd like to draw others toward you (or tempt them or blackmail them).

The game of power and powerlessness, of anger and anxiety, develops deadly negative energies. Your gentle inner being, your sadness, all your feelings — they can't outwardly manifest themselves. You pose, as if you are tougher than you really are.

Find rest, and trust your spacious, large "I"-power. Show yourself the way you really feel; no one will "seize" you. On the contrary, in gentleness and love you will come closer to yourself and others. Experience the calmness in your nature, the peace in yourself. . . .

Emphysema

You carry a heavy load on your shoulders, and you don't see a way out anymore. You constantly go around in the same vicious circle. You feel threatened by fears, deep emotions. . . . You might suffocate. Sadness, anger, rancor are all held in too long. An accumulation of overwhelming energies. This requires self-realization, working things out, and a conversion into creativity!

Afraid to lose power over yourself completely, you unconsciously refuse to take a close look at these emotions. And, for the most part, you even hide them from the outer world.

Let the air out of the balloon before it explodes. Let your energies go, and also your anger: open up your feelings to yourself. Look at them. Don't, because of fear, put on an act. Manifest outwardly the way you feel inwardly. Anger, as a consequence of powerlessness, is nothing to be ashamed of! Observe your feelings and "loosen" them up. You only become stronger by doing that. Action, creativity, and relaxation.

Lung fibrosis

Like a bird, hung on a string, you rob yourself of freedom. You stay put, refusing to bring about changes in yourself. You lower your head and don't want to go on. Self-destruction. Poisonous, dark thoughts. You believe in the ugliness of yourself, of life. You conceal yourself; you don't really show yourself. You feel guilty, ashamed of yourself, powerless. In your thought-emotional world, you needlessly carry a load that is too heavy, but you refuse to throw it off your back. You hold on to the past. You thrust the dagger inward: "I'm simply bad, ugly or a failure. The products I bring forth, the emotions I feel, are of but a low caliber." You are angry with yourself. Your head, your thought-world, are squeezed into an iron harness; you are so hard and negative to yourself. You feel pursued by destiny or by a curse, as it were, but you don't realize that it is all about your own poison. You don't really listen to your own nature, to this inner wisdom; you'd rather listen to what others have to say about you. You can heartlessly distance yourself from yourself. You are afraid of this deep, emotional world inside yourself; you condemn your emotions and yourself. You allow yourself to be influenced too strongly by indoctrination from your childhood, which reinforced the detrimental convictions you already had about yourself.

Don't fight against your nature: listen to yourself. Don't be afraid to walk new paths: follow your feelings, your intuition. Go along with the supple inner flow of your nature and don't be afraid of emotions.

Bring yourself out, don't hide your emotional world so much. Confront yourself with the powerlessness within yourself and break through all this via transformation: tear out this old tree and replant it in new ground. Burn the past; no longer smother yourself with negativity. Start again, free! Make peace in your heart; come to rest within yourself. Get on your horse; self-aware action! When your deepest feelings tell you that freedom and joy lie to the right, don't go to the left with your thoughts. Don't fight against your happiness. Be open to the most beautiful powers in yourself; stop self-destruction. Make everything lighter for yourself.

Pigeon breeder's pneumonitis

An emotional life that is too tense. You are so afraid that you want to shield yourself, as it were, against not only your own nature — which you mistrust — but against whatsoever imaginary danger. Possibly, you cling to others, to a religion, or to a superstition.

In fact, you constantly shield yourself against your own Self, against your natural feelings; you are afraid of the powers inside yourself. You spasmodically hold on, because you consider yourself to be rather brittle, vulnerable, unstable, and unsafe. It is as if you could fall at any moment and break — as if the ground could disappear from beneath your feet. You forget to truly live, to enjoy, to use your energies in free creativity.

Build upon Self-authority. Laugh copiously, with your lungs wide open, and see the relativity of things. Joyful and carefree, step into life exuberantly and enthusiastically, without anxieties. See how foolish and needless your anxieties are. Trust in the Sun, in the natural beauty of your Self. You are safe in yourself. Let the vibrations of your laughter and joy purify your lungs. Live from out of yourself!

Pleuritis, pleurisy
inflammation of the thoracic membrane

Nervous, contained aggression; you would like to realize yourself, manifest yourself, but you don't dare to or cannot. In unsureness you hide your true longings and ambitions; you are not sure whether you can trust your feelings or that which you would like to do. You accumulate emotions and frustrations; you feel unprotected and unable to guarantee your own safety. Because of this you might push yourself to the background and do a lot for others, yes, showing yourself outwardly to be stronger than you really feel. Anxiously holding yourself back — oppression. You'd like to grasp for something beautiful, an ideal, instead of allowing everything to evolve quietly from out of your solid basis, here and now.

Know yourself to be protected by that powerful energy-source in yourself. Don't stay sitting there, but stand up straight and go on in self-confidence. Dare to express to the outer world your worth, your possibilities, your longings, and don't hide anything from yourself. No longer be angry with yourself about this powerlessness; now allow yourself to grow in love, no longer holding yourself back, no longer suffocating yourself. Allow it to come outward — speak and act!

Pneumonia

You feel overwhelmed, in a deep sea of emotions, and can no longer tell where you'll end up. No longer with a real goal or vision. Originally, you were so full of longings, but now you recoil, hurt, like a martyr. Life does not answer to your real deep longings, not to what you "want" to do, nor to your wishes regarding love or relationships. You feel limited in your life, you are so tired of "not really living."

At birth, you found yourself in a life that doesn't really suit your true nature: an unconscious choice. Thus, you are obliged to liberate yourself from the track of parental authority in order to begin freely choosing your own life. You feel helpless, however, sometimes apathetic, sometimes angry again — because you keep suppressing your own "I." Your head feels like it's been cut out of wood, and you are frightened to death of true life: an independent choice made from within your Self! Relaxation, pleasure, happily experiencing your nature — these no longer exist. Energy-blockage: you refuse to really communicate any more, neither with your deepest Self nor with others. Anxiety. Like an ostrich, you plod along. . . .

You no longer really see or hear. You feel you have been pierced by a sword, unable to live any more. Possibly, you are hiding in a job that doesn't really suit you. Your energy flows away . . . you feel no life, no more power. Still, you would like to live, but *differently.* You would like to free yourself. Inwardly, you have high aspirations (aspire — breathe), ambitions, projects you want to "conquer," an inner call to Action. But you can't bring it to realization; you experience yourself as if on a foundation that is too weak. You cling to helpless infancy.

You look to hold on to something outside yourself instead of putting your Self in the center. That with which you "fill" your life appears so unauthentic and senseless that you would like to spit it out!

Being too severe, too hard on yourself — sometimes caused by feelings of guilt: "If I don't kill myself with work the whole day long, or do this or that, then I'm a bad person." You do anything but follow your own longings; you are not faithful to your nature. The body bears the consequences of this situation.

Babies, children with pneumonia: the above causes are sometimes experienced by the parent(s) as well. Then resolve these inside yourself; and in this way you will also help your child.

Choose another way! Simply get out from under it! Open up your horizons, choose your life direction for yourself, now. Don't let yourself be shaped by tracks or holdovers from the past, or by a partner, etc. Build a new life on a stronger basis than before — upon your deep, powerful Self. Pull your roots out of the old earth and sprout up elsewhere. "Behold the Man, the Human Being": let him be, completely, and comprehend his worthiness. Don't turn away from your own divine source. Let that inner fire warm your body. Become aware of every cell in your body. Use your senses intensely: don't turn away again. Direct your convictions differently: in this way you attract happiness, joy, and new paths to yourself. Disbelief blocks your life. Thus, finally, acknowledge your Self.

Benign tumors in the lungs
(See also Tumor)

Sharp, aggressive thoughts, inner anger, Frustration. As a consequence of black, poisonous thoughts — of critical feelings toward others, and as a reaction to your own feeling of powerlessness — you want to rage like a fool who has lost his senses; you'd like to begin chopping with an axe and destroy. But you keep it all inside yourself, often even wearing a friendly mask. You expect things from others, instead of opening up yourself; you want to attract people instead of giving yourself. You don't love yourself enough, and you search after compensation for this in relationships.

Acknowledge your "inner" leadership. Don't desperately look for self-affirmation, don't expect that certain reactions of relations will be the way you'd like them to be! Let everyone be free, and also let your suppressed energies be free. First of all, remain steadfast, self-aware, on your own "I"-basis. Your powerlessness is the real evildoer — get rid of it. Find yourself being borne up by love within yourself and radiate it toward others instead of wanting to grasp or "to expect." What you give, you will receive. Love yourself because of yourself. Don't blame others for your lack of self-love. Relationships will never bring you happiness if you don't first appreciate yourself.

RHEUMATISM, IN GENERAL

You exaggerate: you lift loads that are too heavy; you think you *have* to do too much. You prove yourself with deeds that are tough, showing a spectacular capability for endurance — by carrying lots of emotions, like a martyr. But, finally, it all weighs too heavily upon you, and you collapse; you ache.

Inwardly, you feel small, but you might be dreaming of big things: in this way, you arrive in a sphere of unreality; you no longer see the world around you the way it really is. Your life and the people around you don't answer to your longings — although often enough you say what you *want*, with a criti-

cal, pointing finger. Because of this, you'd rather not say anything, and you remain dissatisfied, sad and disappointed — poisoning yourself with powerless aggression and heart pain that go inward.

The deepest cause of your problem does not lie with others or with your unsatisfactory life circumstances, but within yourself: you don't give yourself the warmth and love you so need. You attract negative life circumstances because you are convinced you don't deserve love and happiness, because you are convinced that man is a victim of circumstance, and that he can't determine his own life himself.

In order not to feel your insignificance, you perhaps camouflage yourself in a splendid outer display, or in exaggeratedly hard work, or in risking your neck by the performance of dangerous routines — trying to show yourself as stronger than you really are, in fairy tale-like dreams, holding on heroically (next to a so-called inhuman partner), like a martyr, etc. Possibly, you place yourself within severe norms and structures. You want very much, you go beyond your powers, until everything overwhelms you. It is as if you think you can earn love in this way, and still you don't receive any more love than you did before.

Sadness weighs heavily on you. You don't really live Consciously from your sun-center; your anger is but the inability to truly, through your powerful "I," come to self-realization. It is you who doesn't offer yourself what you need: loving acceptance of yourself, as you are. As you don't accept yourself, so do you also want to change your environment. But know that your surroundings will only change when first you take another direction.

Don't float in the air, don't build any dream castles, don't let your energy flow away, come close to yourself, here and now; be satisfied with your little space on earth. Stand sturdily, with your feet on the ground, discover your Worth. Resolutely take your life in your hands now and create your life yourself. Don't **let** it all happen to you. When you turn toward yourself, in love, then you will attract other situations. No longer poison your blood with sadness, false expectations, and reproach. But live from out of your sun-center, your heart. Be present here, strongly concentrated in your body. You don't have to prove yourself, don't have to be tough; you no longer have to behave like a victim — perhaps to gain attention and admiration from others. You are good the way you are!

Now, dare to live spontaneously, from out of your emotional core; satisfy your longings, no longer be hard, not to yourself or to others. Accept the unique nature of every human being and build your new world from within, from out of your heart; beautiful expectations will call up beautiful life experiences, but don't try to "change." Call up that which is most beautiful for you and close relations, and that which is beautiful will come to you; but in a way that is best for everyone. Let go of worries and tensions!

Enjoy life. Don't lay punishment, limitations, or strict rules upon yourself. Let go of gruff, critical, disgruntled thoughts, because it is you who have called up your circumstances. Changes here will come about when you live, more concentrated, in yourself! Creating your life joyfully from out of the here-and-now, let go of everything and everyone, take pleasure in the simplicity that is in yourself.

When you are satisfied with your "I," and with your particular Nature, then this joy-energy will chase away all pains, then you no longer will direct yourself toward others, toward distance, toward that which is not here, now. Instead, welcome yourself in the here and now: free yourself from the prison you have created. Do so by taking yourself, step by step, out of this martyr-pattern, by taking your own life in your hands, little by little — by offering yourself love, pleasure, and relaxation! Don't expect anything from others,

don't drive yourself so hard any longer. Don't bottle up your feelings, live your life to the fullest, in your own way!

RIBS
(See also Skeleton, fractures)

Broken ribs

It all became too much for you; you "break" out of a situation you can't handle. Emotional pressure. You take up only a small part of your space, of your total being. You cling too much to superficial or external values. Because you ignore your inner Authority, your deepest Self, you'll try to cling to a beautiful social image, a busy career, materialism, a shining outward persona, a demanding sport, "beauty contests," etc.

Your torso bursts from stress, from superficialities; your deepest Self asks you to give more attention to deeper values and to your accumulated emotions. SPACE for your *true*, pure self.

Possibly, you want above all to pursue outer Authority, and this can lead to a collision, to an inner resistance to others, an intense emotional desire to break with existing power structures. Because you are not conscious enough of your inner Power, you place all power outside yourself; as a result, not only do you feel threatened by other authority, but you also can actively oppose competitors or another authority — your teacher, your partner, etc.

You can become entangled in a battle which is too burdensome for you. You can take an exaggerated amount of work on your shoulders, so that it becomes very difficult to bring it off or to manage.

Anxiety, tension, stress, anger, opposition, an unconscious longing for liberation from this situation. You tie yourself down, you fixate on a certain something. You are not flexible and supple! An accident does not just happen, a fracture is a symptom called up by your deepest Self to make you Conscious of the above-mentioned facts.

It was time for you to be wakened up! Only a shock can bring you to yourself. It is not superficial outer authority that counts, but deeper inner authority. True power over yourself: how you create your own life.

Every human being creates his own circumstances. Become conscious of this.

What your heart feels counts; the outer form is a manifestation of your inner soul situation. Don't attach too much importance to insignificant aspects of life. Take up your true space, now.

Don't suffocate yourself with inner struggles, with defiant thoughts, but free yourself from a life-view that is too narrow. Free yourself from a life-philosophy that is too limited. Allow your ribs to open flexibly, in love toward your deepest Self, and toward others. Don't tensely tighten a rope around your chest, as it were, by holding on to untrue values. Come to inner peace. Let go. Suppleness, space. . . .

Bruised ribs

You feel oppressed, suffocated, at your limit, hurt, pushed into a corner. Suppressed aggression, powerless anger, sadness — which is all becoming too much for you.

You feel incapable, unable to bring yourself to realization; you feel fearful and confined; you retain your emotions too much, holding on to them, being locked up in yourself.

You flee from yourself, hide yourself, allow yourself to be pushed aside; but inwardly you cry out in pain and powerlessness. You wrap yourself up, as it were, in order to protect yourself against your environment; you feel as if you are without oxygen, wrung out and weak.

You don't feel supported by your own strong structure; on the contrary, you might let yourself be pushed over. You don't get a grip on yourself.

Emotions and suppressed powerful energies are dominating you.

Become master of your own life and take over its rudder. Feel the power of your deepest Self, know you are supported and protected within your Self. Cast abroad your energies, your creativity, your possibilities, your talents; free yourself from all needless burdens and bring yourself to self-realization. A concentration, a coming together of powers within yourself. Mark off your own terrain; don't allow others to penetrate your private terrain; determine yourself with whom you wish to have contact. Organize your life yourself; don't allow yourself to be hurt. Take up all of your wide space; feel that inner warmth, your potential energies. You are not weak, so go on! Let all the sadness drain away, and build up your life in joy. "Stand back, please, 'I' am here": not coercively, but with love and in self-respect. In this way, others will respect you.

ROCKY MOUNTAIN SPOTTED FEVER
tick bite fever
carried by ticks infected with Rickettsia rickettsii

As if sitting on the back of a big goose, you take a flying dive down to earth, very fast; you don't know where or how it will end . . . anxiety. You no longer can act as if nothing's the matter; you no longer can "hide," act as if you don't know: time to examine deeply yourself and certain things, in all honesty. You no longer can escape from them.

You possibly live according to the conviction that there's constantly dirt and unpleasant things inside you and around you, as if you constantly need to wash yourself clean; a vague unconscious fear of "something." Because you have lived too much outside yourself, because you are too little INSIDE yourself, because you believe too little in your goodness: possibly you have avoided certain things in yourself, have hidden certain things you thought didn't become you. Know, then, that you are a Human Being with gifts and shortcomings, like everyone else, and that you always, and every day, have the opportunity to start again, as long as you don't present yourself outwardly as being "better" than you are, as long as you are honest: that, after all, is TRUE beauty; that's honesty and openness.

This ailment, therefore, calls you to come into your body as fast as you can; identify completely with it: becoming ONE with yourself; no longer living in inner division or two-faced, nor latching on to someone else because you don't trust yourself or your content, nor do you think of it as being really good. Become more CONSCIOUSLY present in your body. Become present in YOURSELF. You are one, forthright. Comfortably establish yourself in yourself. Did you assume the thoughts or life pattern of someone else, and were "you" not YOU?

Did you tie yourself to someone else like "a Siamese twin," and do you now have to detach yourself, *really* having to stand on your OWN feet — separate from someone else — and become YOURSELF, Autonomous? You now look for safe shelter; you withdraw; you encapsulate yourself under a safe roof, but at the same time you lock yourself up by doing so.

Pull open that zipper of your tent and radiate outward. Step out of your seclusion, and radiate life with all force! Manifest yourself! Allow energies to radiate outward from within, and give yourself the chance to get "through" *to the outside. See how beautifully the sun shines, how good life is. Feel safe. Have done with putting on an act or a show in public (giving yourself an image that you are not); now you go to your true unique home . . . close to your TRUE "I." Total relaxation is the result, but at the same time this means a confrontation with yourself: here you will finally find peace. No longer run away from it! You feel: "An old period is now being closed. Now it's up to 'the REAL Me' and Life." You are Absolutely determined. And you rely completely on yourself and choose to make a totally new start!*

You BURST with stored, honest, authentic energies in your being; therefore, break that tightly stretched girdle around your being and allow steam to escape, allow ALL those energies in your being to flow freely, largely, spontaneous and forceful, honest, and without detours. Phew! A mass of energies that accumulated for too long is being let out; things that have been kept in for too long are being released . . . and you feel like you are becoming "purer" now that this can all flow away freely out of you. A cleansing, a relief, a liberation, a being able to breathe freely again: now that you very honestly, without inner feelings of dividedness, show WHO you truly are, separate from everything and everyone — you as you, direct, without detours, without being two-faced, without secrets. You know that everything is allowed to be there, that old instinctive patterns can transform themselves into new consciousness forces. Out of this marriage, this UNITY in and with yourself, forces are being applied immediately in service of truth: toward healing.

Without detours, direct, without wanting to stick your head in the sand, without avoiding or hiding layers in yourself: you honestly reveal who you really ARE — reveal this to yourself, first of all, and also to others. You rise up like an eagle, as reborn, happy and thankful for who you are, full of UNDERSTANDING and love toward the complex situation in your psyche. It now becomes simpler — as long as you push yourself out honestly, without detours, without maintaining the conviction that you are not allowed *really* to be yourself. Evil destroys itself, and good is being stimulated and keeps on growing. The growth, the purification of a wonderful autonomous self-thinking and self-creating Human Being! Your brain now functions in a creative and inventive way: from out of your Being, from out of your (now) heart-warming vision of yourself and of Life. *The show is over now . . . you are "truthfully" YOURSELF.*

S

SADISM

The deepest cause of this is a feeling of deep Powerlessness: you feel small and weak. The little one feels itself grow when it can read someone else a lesson! You have two faces; you experience a duality in yourself. You don't really want to be seen the way you feel inside: like a poor, sensitive, vulnerable victim. You are afraid that you're not really worth more than this poor wretch. That's why it's necessary that you wear a Mask or build up a second personality around this sensitive core: the mask of the tough brute. You'll identify yourself in such a way with this Powerful Mask, so that you sometimes "become" completely like it!

Possibly you have been confronted very early in life (as a result of the convictions with which you were born) with the power-structures of your mentors, the educational institution, other children who teased you, etc. Acting sadistically gives you the feeling that you belong to the world of power-systems, where mentors have a grip on their children instead of respecting them according to their own natures. But now you are one of those powerful Authorities; now you are the representative; now you are the Big Chief instead of the poor wretch you used to be.

The less you saw the sense of things, the more you had to listen and obey others who could do with you what they wanted, the tighter the straitjacket became, and the less you could stand on your own feet — the more frustrated you became and the stronger grew your inner revolt.

Also your feelings were never really satisfied; again and again you have bottled up your emotional longings and kept silent about them, ashamed as you were about your "weakness."

Your positive fire-force, your creative energies, your sexual longings, were being smothered in the all-overpowering feeling of Powerlessness.

You grow up with suppressed feelings, rubbing your hands together out of nervousness; you don't know what to do with yourself; you think you are bad, inferior, and incapable.

But because you feel so dependent on others, on love, you'll hide this weak little heart. You come outward with force and fire like a superman who thinks himself the Powerful one, like a ruler over others. You feel so strong when you can show your powers. Unconsciously taking vengeance — also on painful experiences from the past. The victim with which you are dealing is in fact "YOU." You are hurting yourself; you are the one who's suffering; you are destroying yourself, as others have destroyed you.

Sadism isn't only "punishing," but also "self-punishment." Because you don't really love the little child, the true, gentle soul in Yourself, you might like to murder it. You take pleasure in projecting the little one inside you outside yourself (in the form of another person) and then maltreating yourself.

Often, you experience extreme pleasure by doing this: a pleasure that is a result of your emotional frustration.

Turn everything around and you will have the "cure": experience that fundamental power in yourself in all the deeds and tasks

The Key to Self-Liberation, Christiane Beerlandt © Beerlandt Publications

you perform in your daily life. In self-awareness and pride take your life in hand; no longer bottle up healthy natural forces inside you; in particular, place inside you all Power over yourself, not in others; no one can tell you what to do.

Now accept the little sensitive child in yourself and no longer reject it; don't put on a mask; you are not powerless!

Don't work off your frustrations by getting stuck in unconscious processes: become aware of the fact that you used to be mocked or psychologically mistreated by others because you were born with the conviction that you are a Zero. The cause was lying inside you; you have attracted people who reacted to this, which of course doesn't make their attitude right, just as your behavior now isn't right, but all of it is human.

Solve your problems by stepping out of the vicious circle: finally value yourself according to your Worth; make yourself welcome in a warm and loving way.

Become aware of your inner grandeur. It is not the outer world or the outward Authority that counts, but your inner Authority, the powerful Source in you which enables you to change your life, to create it yourself.

Don't allow yourself to "be lived" by passions that are the sign of a lack of Consciousness.

Transform yourself; lustful feelings, obsessive thoughts and urges will disappear as a result of Self-respect and true love toward yourself.

See also: Exaggerated Sexual Desires.

SALIVA, EXCESSIVE FLOW

Strong inner agitation; eagerly awaiting the "fulfillment" of your longings (your self-manifestation, getting your share . . .) Overproduction of energy because of emotions.

You are functioning especially for the outer world. An urge to exist for the outer world; sometimes wanting to manifest yourself in an exaggerated way to the outer world, on the pulpit, or by going around with a feathered hat.

Anxiety, fear of not being able to satisfy, of failing somewhere, of being condemned, etc., for instance at an exam, at the dentist, on a podium. Tense preparation.

Often, you're already busy with your thoughts beforehand, perhaps in stress; an energy development that is very strong: ready to attack, to act, to speak; possibly you perspire; you brace yourself.

Your fruitfulness, your potential qualities, your emotional content, are "bound" and confined. You tensely check yourself; you want to do everything right but sometimes you doubt yourself; in relation to the "task" you have to do, you produce an extra amount of "energy," "nervousness," and "saliva."

It's as if you say to the outer world: "Please acknowledge me. Do you think I'm all right like this? Will you not punish me?"

You live with bottled-up feelings; you don't live your life to the fullest. You too little express yourself in a spontaneous, natural way. You control yourself; you are too passive, too tense, too pent up.

If you exist more WITHIN, and FROM OUT OF, yourself and no longer worry about what the outer world has to say to you; if you follow your Nature more instead of planning with your thoughts, eating up your feelings, then you won't develop any needless energy. Be yourself, don't worry about things, live according to your feelings, not for the eye of the camera.

Live now and not tomorrow. Develop your "male" aspects; self-assuredly stand with both feet on the ground. Be faithful to your Self! It's not the form, but the content that counts.

Dare to give in to your longings to enjoy the beautiful life; say what you have to say, don't repress yourself. Allow healthy ag-

gressive forces to come through freely, don't hold things in. Don't immobilize yourself in tight armor, in a controlled straitjacket. You are good the way you are. Come to rest inside yourself, but manifest yourself outwardly the way you feel inwardly, without anxiety.

SALIVA STONE

You don't feel able to satisfy your enormous longings.

You remain "folded closed"; you don't really reveal yourself; you don't dare.

Holding on to things or people because of fear; you worry about what you might be "short" of. You want to "fill" yourself in a greedy way with everything and everyone; you rush around in a nervous way because you don't feel safe and sound in yourself. You are overwhelmed by a multitude of emotional impressions: you hold on to those things outside of you, especially to those which are light, beautiful, and giving hope. You long for, and desire, a lot, but you can't take it in; you don't succeed in breaking through, in fully participating in life. You are stuck, in spite of your enormous needs. You don't succeed in getting out of your burrow-of-frustration. You are afraid you don't have enough, afraid of being pushed into a corner materially as well as emotionally. Your "holding on" hinders a beautiful evolution.

Become solidly Grounded. Your urge for fulfillment serves in this way as a compensation for your own feelings of emptiness and insecurity. Liberate yourself; establish yourself firmly with both feet on the ground; don't rush around any longer, find rest in yourself. There's plenty for everyone. You, yourself are the most important supplier for yourself: of attention, warmth, permission to calmly enjoy — discovering the warmth and beauty in yourself. Don't look for it outside your-self; that which is good for you will come to you by itself. Let go of that passion and those desires: they are only signals which make it clear to you what you especially deny in yourself. Look for it inside yourself; no longer go on in order to "fill" yourself, to grab on to things outside you; feel your own fullness! No longer bottle up your creative energies: express yourself, go on, unfold your talents! Bring about changes in outer circumstances if necessary.

SALMONELLA INFECTION

Salmonella infection has negative consequences only if psychologically there was already a breeding ground for it.

You feel emotionally overburdened with inner tensions! You experience yourself as being too feeble and weak; you think you have to protect yourself against something or someone outside yourself. Possibly, there's an anger present in you because of powerlessness against authority, against that person you think is "above" you. You don't acknowledge your inner Authority; you feel bound to others, to a situation. You want to be free, but you can't; you feel like you are in the grip of others. Emotional pain, an emotionally burdened head, aggressive powerlessness to a more or lesser degree. You're not really yourself; perhaps you manifest yourself as tough and proud outwardly, but in fact here it's a self-protective attitude: you think you have to defend yourself against others because you experience yourself as being unsafe and not really sheltered in yourself.

You don't really speak for yourself; your mouth seems chained, powerless, unable to express your anger, to say what's sticking in your "stomach" or what's burdening your "liver." Nevertheless, this situation sometimes makes you sick.

For some time, already, you have felt unpleasant and knotted up; your feelings don't find their way out enough; you feel bad in the light of the sun (the authority) outside of you but you're not able to make contact with your Inner Sun.

You experience yourself as an emptiness, filled with small "irritations." Via this infection the psychological and physical detoxifying can begin if you become Aware of the cause of it: the beginning of transformation.

Speak: say what bothers you; free yourself from ties which are too oppressive. Become your own master; no longer feel like you are bound. Express your feelings!

If you experience the force of your deepest Self, if you make yourself welcome in love, then you will come into open friendship with others — then you'll no longer feel threatened. Immunity is natural to you: anxieties and self-depreciation will destroy this.

Now digest and work out your emotions and acknowledge your worth as an autonomous human being.

Come to inner liberation of that to which you have held on for too long: no longer poison yourself.

The intruder will disappear quickly if you proudly take up your space! Transformation!

See further the category Infections.

SARCOIDOSIS
formation of "granulomas" (i.e. accumulations of inflammatory cells) in various organs

---

Your "I" can't exist in a self-aware and autonomous way: you hold on to people and things outside yourself. You allow yourself to be dragged along by the flow; you don't get a grip on anything. Anxiety, without a solid sure Basis. You allow others to treat you as they like; you allow yourself to be strongly influenced by people or systems. You don't really make decisions about your life yourself! Your attitude is rather bland, and most of the time credulous; you might go along with someone else too quickly because you don't, after all, believe in your own Power.

You'll feel attacked or hurt by others because you allow yourself to "be lived" by others.

Primitive emotions can overpower you. You are not at all aware of your divine worth as a Human Being; you'd sooner adore an Authority outside yourself. You smother yourself by suppressing beautiful human consciousness-energies and creative forces. You'd sooner allow yourself to be directed or even riled up by others. You don't use your own brain enough. You refuse to really stand on your own feet, to live an independent, personal life; you allow others "to penetrate" your personal terrain.

You are not a poor martyr; turn yourself deeply inward and feel that firm Basis of your inner Self. If, in a self-aware way with love toward yourself, you take your life in hand, anxieties will disappear. Border off your terrain and feel your own power center. Step out in complete self-confidence; no longer allow yourself to be controlled by others.

Critically determine your point of view, yourself; make a choice; create your life yourself according to your longings. Creativity of an active spirit; stand solidly in your shoes; take your life firmly in hand and, from out of your consciousness, determine what you are going to make out of it. There's nothing that will drag you along if you decide to lead your life yourself. No single Authority has any power over you except for your inner divine Self. There is no wiser leader other than your deepest Self; trust in this, and resolutely go forward on the path that you Consciously point out.

SCHIZOPHRENIA

The schizophrenic splits himself up because he thinks he has to defend himself, because he positions himself on the alert, in a camouflage system toward himself, but also toward others. In fact he plays a game of attracting-rejecting; he provokes and draws like a magnet, but at the same time he isolates himself in loneliness. Here it's about an inner Power-game: alternatingly, more or less power is given to this or that part of the personality. In this way, he thinks he is at the rudder of a complicated system, with which he also can keep his surroundings in his power: no one can grab him because "he" is never really there; "he" can't be held responsible because, after all, it was that other small part of his personality! An escape, a camouflage.

A constant "flight," also, away from that part in himself that he might experience as "bad, malignant": deep unconscious emotional currents, sexuality, suppressed emotions, frustrations — he designates a part of himself as Bad.

He runs away from it, especially because he might glorify and idealize certain other characteristics: he wants to live up to the requirements of being a holy one or a Napoleon, he would desperately strive to be splendid, out of the ordinary, good and high-minded — but he experiences in reality that the "bad" part in him constantly has to be fought back or at least watched closely. A part of him engages other "smaller parts" (different personalities) to be on the lookout in order to protect him against threats or "incorrectness." In this way he exercises a constant supervising function on the "bad" part of himself. This bad part however can also send out its pawns, and soon he will find himself with a complete army to deal with. But HE is the strong one, and in this way has Power over himself!

Looking at things from above, as it were, he neglects the little things, the weakness, but also the normal, natural longings in himself; he escapes into an unreal position of superiority — until this construction collapses and the war is lost by the Handsome Knight: all the suppressed parts of himself burst out like a volcano. In the chaos he loses all control over himself.

In daily life, when everything seems to be "normal" with him, he can never be good enough in his own eyes: he'd like to do great deeds, yes even do stunts in order to get appreciation and admiration from others because he doesn't get love from himself, nor appreciation. "Do you see me? Do you see how good I am? How beautifully I play the piano?"

He challenges himself; he plays a game here in order to let his good side come through as strongly as possible.

In the meantime everything that lies beneath or behind this is "forbidden terrain": anxieties, feelings of guilt, and especially experiences from the past, play a role here. After all he carries inside himself negative convictions regarding certain characteristics in life, which especially make him condemn himself. Anxiety, taboo, suppression. A dark, secret domain inside him: that's what he is afraid of. He is convinced that a human being has "good" and "bad" inside him; that he constantly has to be mistrustful of a part of himself. He mostly experiences dark and sexual forces, but also spontaneous, natural forces, as being "bad." These parts in him all play a "Role": he braces himself against them, flanked by the knights of the good. In other words, he doesn't accept himself in totality, in love: he was born with these anxious convictions. Of course he will attract, therefore, circumstances which will give him a reflection of his inner division.

So, he can let himself be born to parents who are, themselves, contending with the problem: "I as a human being am sinful and bad; I have to beware of my nature; touching human 'flesh' (affection, sensuality) is sinful, etc." Frustrated parents who, for instance, have known a religious atmosphere in their youth, where hypocrisy, the tight uniform, strong rules, and commandments were prevailing. They didn't love their nature, they couldn't offer true love to their children, stiffened and unauthentic as they were in themselves: our schizophrenic, having similar convictions regarding the human being, will be born in such an atmosphere in order to finally be able to make an end to this problem! But the "cause" always lies in the human being himself; milieu or education can only strengthen or weaken this.

His problem however is often also the problem of the parent(s): all together they might strive for a solution, a healing. Their frustration and negative convictions and his: a throwing off of masks is necessary.

He's afraid of himself. He thinks he can do harm and also be punished (or murdered) for it by others: therefore he hides. Suppressed parts of himself can surface like outbursts of desperate fear or fury, and also in the form of "voices," such as "demonic commands"; words and deeds can appear to him as "not being his"; possibly, one experiences him as a "possessed being." He can make illusionary predictions or bring to the fore all kind of things which are "real" in his mind but, in fact, they are compulsive texts or deeds which are brought out by a "sub-personality." He will hear "someone" talking to him, telling him to do this or that; he will allow "someone" to use his hand to automatically write things down — but this "someone" is the outlet for the suppressed part of him, which now surfaces in a commanding or compulsory way. Messages from the Holy Mary or a UFO-ship, complete visions and films, it can all happen.

He's looking for Love outside himself, but considering his negative self-condemnation he'd sooner be born to parents who can't satisfy this profound need; he will thus be confronted with his powerlessness.

He will be the best, the model child, in front of his parents or mentors: he suppresses his deeper disposition, his nature, in order to satisfy others. In this way, he still feels powerful. He's so afraid that other parts of himself might break through: in this way the process of division comes to be.

He makes demands on himself in order to be "good," so that one will "like" him. This game can last a lifetime without being noticed by the outer world. In many, the game "breaks" when overburdened — for instance when they enter a relationship with a partner or someone who loves them, so that all parts of the Self want to be involved.

He needs to discover that love-force in himself, and also in the ones who love him. One can give him the following message: he is good, nothing in him is "bad"; that he is allowed to completely be himself; that his previous convictions — "that one has to watch out for bad parts in oneself" — are false. That self-affirmation, and the game of attracting and rejecting, in himself as well as toward the outside, is not necessary. That he doesn't need to flee from himself nor from his nature. All parts are allowed to melt together into one Unity: he no longer has to hide himself! He may take total responsibility for himself, without anxiety.

It's the repression of a part of himself that leads to extreme reactions.

No specific power should be attributed to sexuality or to the unconscious unknown.

He needs to accept his vulnerable depth, approach it gently; he should know that deep inside him there's a Core that is good and trustworthy. That all forces are allowed to express themselves freely. That the Ideal for every human being is: "to be Oneself as completely as possible." In a self-aware way, he may stand at the rudder of a reliable and integrated ship, trusting the machine-room, without the captain having to bother with it. Everything goes along smoothly as long as one doesn't consider oneself bad or insufficient or powerless.

The Conscious "I" has power over itself, lovingly carries responsibilities, and accepts its sensitivities, its longings, its specific natural disposition. In unification the anxieties disappear.

You are good the way you are; you no longer have to flee.

Schizophrenia is the result of negative convictions regarding yourself: alter these misleading convictions and become healthy. Trust your nature and its forces!

Thankfulness for your total Being, without giving power to desires means the beginning of the solution.

SCIATICA

The prince prefers to stay a frog: you deviate from your straight path, from your essential being. Perhaps unconsciously, you have created all kind of constructions or structures, which now determine or restrict your existence, as an evasion of having to live completely from out of your true nature. Finally you get entangled in these self-created diversion-maneuvers: "Where are you now?" You think that your true "I" is not worthy enough to be the way you are, or to spontaneously live the way your nature wants it to be. You hurt yourself, out of Anxiety.

An *enormous* energy is locked up within a forced structure: can it not but ask for liberation? You pull yourself down by your hair: you deny the deeper values inside you, your spontaneous creative energies, your feelings, your very personal urge for action, your longings. . . . It's all being pushed to the side; YOU BUILD YOUR LIFE ON A "SIDE TRACK." Unessential values, such as image and Money, can become number one. Until your deepest Self, your sun-center, comes to the surface and demands first place: it "radiates" you awake, with

pain, however, in order for you to listen. Are outer image, urge for achievement — satisfying the expectations of a society or acquaintances, materialism — of primary importance in your life? Are you imprisoning your nature by not trusting in your inner Authority? Do you tie yourself down and listen to the Authority of the outer world, to norms and laws which have to determine your life? Do you not dare to determine your personal path in an honest, direct, and resolute way, from out of your inner Center? You just keep on functioning in a world which doesn't really go with your natural disposition. Do you want to prove yourself? Then you don't have any awareness of your personal worth, you doubt it; you look for everything outside yourself. Anxiety causes you to direct your consciousness to things that might offer you some security, because you don't find that security in yourself! There, the prince remains a frog, because he denies his golden worth! You sense, however, that there is a duality inside you: living really from within or hiding yourself in a masquerade? It looks a lot like "hypocrisy," but still here it's rather "anxiously making sure you are safe."

A nicely divided structure, in perfect balance, constructed in all honesty around a powerful center: your life can only be flowing and in a healthy balance if you dare to trust in your Basis, your eternal living Self. A flexible structure which doesn't restrict but leaves room for a free flow of energy: experience your talents, your possibilities, your natural wishes . . . For once be completely honest with yourself, with others; take of the protecting mask and dare to show yourself the way you are. Don't play a Role; don't hurt yourself; don't cling to something to hold on to outside yourself, but look for that divine source deep inside you. Exchange tinsel for inner wisdom and give free existence to higher intuitive energies beside the pure rational; offer your consciousness powers a place of honor, and stop praying to a golden calf. Experience your total Nature and no longer hide behind a screen. Life is light and joyful. Why do you make it so hard? No longer flee from the essential truth deep inside you; in all honesty come away from that side-track; play all your strings and choose the HIGHWAY.

SCLERODERMA
**chronic disease with degeneration
of the skin, joints, internal organs
(such as the esophagus), and blood vessels**

You live, as it were, with a metal helmet on your head as a defense because you don't trust the world nor yourself. You don't feel safe in your deepest Self; as an exaggerated reaction to a supposed feeling of threat, you become very tight. You feel yourself to be but a wretch, a handicapped person, a clumsy human being; probably, you also consider your body to be ugly or a burden.

You don't really love yourself, don't love your body: you look at your body from a distance; you feel barely able to carry this "body."

A feeling of inability, of emptiness, with thoughts of the end of life instead of enjoying life to the fullest now. Sometimes you'd rather not be here, because you don't really live from out of your heart, from out of your joyful core. You deny your worth, you'd sooner hide. Do you think yourself so inferior, so unworthy? Are you afraid of your natural feelings? Do you feel threatened by those spontaneous forces in your deepest Self? Why don't you dare to enjoy the sensorial things, your physical experiences, deep feelings? Are you so afraid of your deepest Self? You don't give yourself a chance for a spacious existence. You don't dare to get into open communication with others. You don't dare to really show yourself openly and honestly because you think you are just nothing. You withdraw yourself. Your energies burn away on the spot, precisely where

you're standing: you pile up those beautiful creative energies, those feelings, without utilizing them!

You allow yourself to "be lived"; you allow yourself to be cared for by others: because you are convinced that you can't take care of yourself. You destroy yourself: are you so angry with yourself, with life?

Manifest yourself in all openness; become aware of your Worth and joyfully take up responsibility for your life. Life is not pain or sadness if you stop considering yourself as something threatening! Your deepest Self is good and safe, offers you a solid Basis; trust in it. Allow your feelings to flow freely; no longer block yourself. No more self-condemnation: in all warmth, welcome yourself and look very close inside yourself. Discover your rich unique content and no longer underestimate yourself.

No longer hide; show your true face and allow yourself to enjoy the here-and-now. The people surrounding you only respond to your feelings; they are not the cause of your problems: you call up circumstances which are a confirmation of the degrading opinion you have of yourself. No longer allow yourself to "be lived," don't feel inferior; break through this self-delusion. Allow your body to calmly relax; nothing can threaten you. Firmly take the rudder of your ship in hands and know that positive expectations directed to the future will bring you joyful experiences. Feel welcome among people, but first and foremost cherish yourself in love. No longer stand still! Productivity with heart and soul; an honest participation in life. In this way, flowing energies can transform your body into a healthy condition.

SCRAPES, GRAZES

Perhaps you feel wronged: "That's not fair." But you make compromises with others, with the outer world, and by doing this you betray yourself.

You feel powerless in this situation, drawn along by others without your being able to really be yourself! You can take on a forced friendly attitude, while inwardly there rages a revolt, an anger. You can nod, "yes," because you don't feel able to say, "no," although you would like to.

Inwardly, you feel too weak and too small: you too strongly live according to others. First, you wait for the reaction of others, until others either reprimand you or reward you. In that way, you allow yourself to be dragged along, because you don't acknowledge your strong inner Authority! For you, it's important what one thinks of you.

Your feelings are bound — their nature is determined by others. You don't fully live the way you feel inside. You don't really get a grip on the situation. Your powerful Mars energies just run out of you because you don't really call on them: healthy, natural, aggressive forces are being denied; feelings are being bottled up. You allow yourself to "be lived" too much. You feel you are the "victim."

Here "I" am! Solidify your feelings under the safe roof of your Self.

Know yourself to be inwardly protected; be yourself, without putting on an act or holding back.

Others will only scrape you if you position yourself as powerless. No matter if you feel the scrape of a spike or of the fingernail of your friend, the cause doesn't lie in the outer world, but in you.

You think you are vulnerable and weak: change this opinion and experience yourself, express yourself, the way you feel, one hundred per cent, without compromises! As long as you experience yourself as a victim, you will attract circumstances which will brand you as a victim. Become yourself; no longer deny your inner forces, and in all honesty bring yourself to realization.

SCURVY

Inner emptiness; you ignore the fullness of yourself. A feeling of powerlessness, anxiously reaching for a hold, for Authority outside yourself, for a fetish, a god, a human being — because you don't acknowledge your "I"-worth. You feel unsafe inside yourself; you are cut off from your deepest Self, from your divine intuition. Perhaps you hide your sensitivity — your anxieties and unsureness — behind a tough, overly dominant male behavior! But you feel unstable; you can't go one way or the other; you feel stuck. Sometimes you might force something with all your might; you'd like to destroy yourself and others in an aggressive, primitive way. You are silent; you bottle up your tensions and your anxieties. You don't see the sense of things anymore; you drown in emotions; you consider life only as a threat. You go about in a self-destructive way; you might jump overboard from the ship. As a human being, you feel so small and powerless.

Come closer to yourself; don't fixate on one point outside yourself. Feel safe in your deepest Self; accept the gentle, intuitive, "female" feelings in you.

Discover the many possibilities in your being and don't doubt the ability of the human being to create his life himself. Speak, express yourself, no longer bottle things up; allow the steam to escape! Get a good hold on yourself and feel the Force of your Consciousness. Be resolute, proud, self-aware, protected in yourself; stand firmly on both feet; say what you have to say; acknowledge that which is warm and kind inside you; soften the hardness. Know that your basis is very large and solid; don't bottle up aggression; transform primitive emotions and instincts into Insight and Awareness. Become master over yourself and over your instincts. You are not "at the mercy of": you call up your own experiences yourself, so create beautiful circumstances. Replace anxiety with trust: knowing that no Destiny or god outside you decides about your life. In a self-aware way take the rudder in your hands!

SELENIUM
Deficiency, insufficient assimilation of

The cause of this lies in Fear, mortal fear. You see everything too black; you already take precautions against danger, you are armed, at the ready, to defend yourself against evil! Confused thoughts, dark imaginings, sometimes paranoid, nervous panic. You imprison yourself; you keep yourself within a tight structure; you don't allow yourself a flexible and free existence; you are afraid of having the rug pulled out from under you. Emotions are overwhelming you; you can't keep it in hand.

You are afraid of your own dark feelings, of the obscure unconscious inside yourself; you can't trust it. You live as if on a time bomb: at any moment a disaster can happen (you think). . . .

Confrontation with your feelings; don't look for shelter, but revise the situation you are in and gain an overview. Dare to look at your deepest feelings; accept them and deal with them; let go. A more playful, lighter, joyful life! Life is not a nightmare, unless you turn it into that. Nothing can overthrow your powerful structure in the process of incarnation! Trust in your Living Self. In optimism, create your life yourself.

Become master over your feelings. In a self-aware way, follow your life's path, without hesitation; nothing threatens you if you don't call it up. A sense of reality: stand with both feet on the ground; feel safe and protected in your deepest Self. Don't flee from life: dive into it, without fear!

SELF-MUTILATION

Self-hatred, an urge for self-destruction. By nature, you already feel hurt and pained; you have attracted people who hurt you because you already positioned yourself as a suffering victim. You don't allow yourself to live, to be happy. You are convinced that you have to suffer and undergo pain, and that you have no right to joy. You sink into sadness; you no longer see any sense in things; you'd prefer to sacrifice yourself on an altar to some god because you think you don't deserve any better. You want to punish yourself; you think you are bad and ugly. The psychological pain and self-hatred is unbearable; the external self-mutilation is only a reflection of this. You are mad at yourself; psychological self-destruction, self-liquidation. You are so afraid that you will be swallowed up by a stream of anxieties and that you will no longer be able to handle it. That's why you take the handle in your own hands; you are ahead of the mortal fear.

Healthy aggressive forces, creative energies, and spontaneous expressions of feelings are not allowed to come through; you suppress that which is most beautiful inside you. You don't allow yourself to live.

Take out the sting, which is very deep in your skin. In love, turn to the little child inside you and allow those gentle feelings to blossom. Offer yourself the warmth that you have missed so far. Every human being is unique and worthy.

Don't be afraid of those feelings inside you; stop being angry with yourself; direct your feelings into pure channels. Take good care of yourself; listen to your heart and be the Savior for yourself. You are king, but you refuse your crown.

Get both feet solidly on the ground; be master over yourself. If you hurt but one part of Nature, in this case yourself, you hurt the Entire Nature. Have respect for the divinity inside you! You are allowed to live; you have the full right to be happy. Don't doom yourself to being the ugly duckling. Or will the duckling ultimately discover who he is: a royal Swan?

SENILITY, DOTAGE

You are too much in the "spirit." The deepest Self, your inner source core, directs your life in an automatic way. You *allow* yourself to "be lived"; you no longer hold the rudder. There used to be a spontaneous exchange between your Conscious "I," here-and-now, and your deepest, inner Self. Now you let yourself go, and "unconscious" parts of you take over the rudder. You are no longer really here. You now experience everything on another level. You prefer to experience

yourself in a sphere of childhood because then you can shake off all responsibility, because then you'll receive all the attention and care, which gives you a peaceful and safe feeling. After all, it's your anxieties and insufficient trust in yourself that make you flee into this unreal world.

You didn't have any say anymore; you felt powerless; possibly you felt rejected by others, but in fact it was you who didn't really like yourself. In this new dimension you can have a grip on others; you do receive attention. In fact you are looking for the love and the warmth you have denied yourself, which you have missed in life: you rise into a spiritual realm in search of gentle, harmonious feelings. But you don't really *live* anymore: you are much more unreal than a "child," but the spheres you are looking for are best reflected in childlike behavior.

You can, if you want to, now turn back — "descend," with your feet on the ground, feeling safe and protected in a calm and peaceful environment. You are allowed to belong. . . .

Reconciliation, merging of heaven and earth, enjoying the here-and-now, consciously being yourself.

SEX, HORMONES, SEXUALITY

The continuous primal Creation event

Now let humanity wake up out of its age-long sleep of "unconscious programming" and create a life, a body, which will have more true joy. Becoming conscious also means, among other things, "no longer being slave of so-called unconscious drives."

The solution does not, however, lie in the *suppression* of longings or desires. The

transformation of unconscious instincts into Conscious experiences full of love, and into true joyful creativity, happens via the clear Insight of the human being, in Himself, via true Love toward himself. The closer he comes to himself and the less estranged from himself the human being feels — no longer feeling powerless regarding himself — the more calm, the more at peace, he will feel, and in turn the more powerful and self-aware and loving he will be toward others, without violence or the misuse of power.

Sexual glands and hormones;
Becoming Conscious

As long as we don't have clear insight into our possibilities, as long as we don't live "consciously," we let ourselves go along in primeval systems, in unconscious processes, upon which we count out of habit without consciously bringing about changes.

In this way, we think we are subject to certain "impulses" or sexual passions that happen to be there and determine our being. As long as we stay convinced that the unconsciousness, or subconsciousness, is stronger, or that it determines our life now, we doom ourselves to slavery, to being victims of ourselves.

In ignorance, this lie was kept alive by, among others, many psychoanalysts.

The truth, however, lies far beyond such pessimism!

Humanity, indeed, has until now been a victim, because it had these kinds of fatalistic convictions.

Our brain can be compared to a computer; it's also being directed by the "I," a master.

It is indeed so that certain older parts of the brain carry in them the more primitive, life-preserving reflexes and instincts, very ancient information on which the human being (and the animal) unconsciously calls in case of life-threatening situations; sexual stimuli for the perpetuation of the species, the feeling of hunger, etc. Certain new brain parts show a more evolved brain pattern: a human being can think, make plans, analyze, come to creative emotional development, etc. In this discovery, Science is not wrong.

What is not acknowledged, however, is that our Living Self — the Consciousness that lies behind matter — constantly directs our brain. The true master, the director of our body, of our glands, of our brain, lies within us: the Conscious "I."

The more we become aware of this, the more we will stimulate our brain toward further growth; on the other hand, it's thanks to the presence of our body and of our brain that we can come to the further growth of consciousness. A strong awareness of our eternal Core of Consciousness which lies behind the body, as well as the awareness of the possibility of offering this Core of Consciousness, this soul, this eternal Living Self, formidable growth in a physical body, and the striving toward "unification" of body and soul-core, ultimately can lead to the coming about of a new body, of an immortal, earthly creature. Our nerve system, the brain, the enzymes — but also especially the glands and the hormones, not the least of which are the sexual glands and sexual hormones — play a very important part in this growth.

Our Conscious and Unconscious convictions direct our glands, our "old parts of the brain," and our hormone secretion.

The "I" is the director of the total happening, of the complete hormonal system. Do we, out of habit, depend on old, unconscious programming? Or shall we now consciously start to direct our body? Isn't it about time that we resolutely reprogram ourselves and the world, away from sexual compulsions and violence?

A concrete example here is the following (see further the category Testosterone): as a man, are you convinced of being a poor human creature who has no grip or power on his personal life? Do you actually feel like you are a nothing, and are you looking for confirmation that somewhere you do possess worthiness? But except in Image or sexual desire you don't find yourself? These feelings of inferiority and emptiness, of doubting yourself — doubting your content — lead to an overproduction of the male hormone Testosterone.

Testosterone, in classic science, is being considered to be the carrier of sexual impulses and male characteristics: by overproduction of Testosterone the sexual impulse will become stronger, and in this way you will keep going around in your vicious circle of emptiness and worthlessness, until you become aware of your divine inner worth. Become conscious of your own fullness; make an end to compulsions.

Transformation: programming – deprogramming, unconscious – conscious

Our body constantly reacts to psychological changes. Unconscious or conscious psychological reactions bring about changes in the "chemical composition" of the blood, which, in turn, influences all body parts. Certain parts of the brain are being activated; the hypophysis receives all these signals and will secrete hormones (like the FSH by the woman or the ICSH by the man.) These hormones will, in turn, send out other stimuli, and, for instance, will activate the sexual hormones in the testicles, the ovaries, or the adrenal glands.

Hormones and nerves are important messengers. Hormones carry "spiritual messages" to all parts of the body. If the hypophysis receives a "message," then this will be transmitted to the body.

Our psychological condition influences the body. *If we wish to transform our body into a powerful carrier of eternal, lasting health then it's of the utmost importance that we take up our Mastery and Consciously give new, healthy convictions to our brain and hypophysis.* For instance, if we are convinced that, in a process of decline, we will live till about the age of 85 and then will have to die, then the brain will send signals to the glands (hypophysis, thymus, pancreas, etc.) and they in turn will send the message of "decay" to the total body.

Our genes and cells have been given *codes* psychologically and, also psychologically,

the codes can be *altered:* via the Conscious "I" and its union with the body, we are able to bring about change. Also, the sexual glands and hormones are carriers of powerful, psychological energies which, in self-aware creativity of the human being, will prove their usefulness in the transformation into a new body.

In the genes, in certain parts of the brain, are engraved very ancient convictions, reflexes, compulsive actions: they push "life" into certain patterns. As conscious people we now have to realize that we are not victims of certain convictions (and therefore programming) which mankind had in the past! We can direct our computer and, if needed, deprogram it! Why is it necessary that all women in the world "have" to menstruate? Why should one person "have" to have power over another through sexual temptation or abuse?

Why should we have to be faithful to tradition and die?

Creation Powers

Let's step out of this enslavement, in love toward Mankind.

We are not victims of the accidental functioning, or not functioning, of glands or parts of the brain! Our glands and brain need to be under the supreme command of our Self-aware "I." The more consciously insightful we become, the more we get a grip on the so-called old instincts that in olden days actually were needed for survival of the species, but now are no longer. Anxiety and aggression were the arms against death; sex assured continued existence of the species, etc..

Now we can "choose" to transform instincts into higher awareness, into open creativity. We can now choose to experience sexual pleasure, but on the other hand we will start to feel the full functioning of the sexual glands in a new body, and the first step we will make toward this is: "liberating ourselves from being enslaved by someone else, and thus becoming completely autonomous"; and secondly using or developing these enormous sexual energies for emotional creations, for new experiences in the area of consciousness, creativity, and love.

It's not about "sublimating" sexual desires, but it's about a transformation, or usage, of these powerful impulses (hormonal, et al) in our body in order to reach new experiences in the area of "living," feeling, creativity, communication with people on a different and happier level. Pleasure then makes room for joy, for true "happiness": a larger, more free feeling will be the result of living on this new level of consciousness. Not obscure, but very personal! Not heavenly, but consciously on a New Earth.

No experience of sexuality without pure Love.

The transformation of a herd animal into an individual; from zombie into divine "I" experience. Saying goodbye to emptiness; going toward powerful self-assuredness; from loveless gratification toward loving intense joy.

Let us direct our brain, our hypophysis, in the direction of a conscious development of large, very open, energies. Let us realize that our brain and the hypophysis are in fact waiting for the moment that we will give them a much more beautiful role than we have given them so far!

A New Body
Hormones as carriers of inner messages, as powerful impulses of consciousness

Our body: an atomic power-center

The consciousness of the human being will bring about new vibrations, which will make it possible to bundle forces into a concentrated form (our body experience). Con-

sciousness cultivated on the pillars of Insight and Love.

The hormonal system, the nervous system, and the functioning of the glands will have a very directed, concordant task to fulfill in the evolved body: an especially powerful body in a new dimension, in which all forces are bundled together; out of which will radiate one consciousness energy and whereby one can immediately perceive the forces and possibilities of the divine Self.

A loving atomic power-center. These seeds lie within us: they will only be able to germinate in people who are open to Abundant Insight and Love.

The possibilities that come out of this are endless. That's why humanity can, and will, only gradually call up and integrate new energies so that a New Earth, a new humanity, can be born without mistakes or forcing things. The misuse of power or destructive action will no longer be possible.

The human being calls up new energies in himself and in the world and creates, in such a conscious and loving way, a New earth, a New human being, who will rise far above judgment and conviction.

This new dimension — in which harmony, thankfulness, and joy go hand in hand — means the end of the "old world," without the world having to be destroyed: transformation of mortality and finiteness into an immortal dimension of human being and planet; becoming aware in the light of the total cosmic happening.

With the power of Consciousness and Love, the human being will come to be in charge of an inner atomic power station: every cell in the human body has the capacity of explosion, of fission, of fusion ... enormous potentials which can exist only under the loving eye of the human being.

Remembrances in the "human memory" of very ancient civilizations that destroyed themselves, of civilizations that in certain areas were technically higher than ours, but, because of discord, destructive emotions wiped themselves off the map — these remembrances lead to the fact that Humanity has taken precautions to avoid such kind of catastrophes in the future. These precautions live deep in your soul, in the "unconsciousness" of mankind itself. Strategies are being called up worldwide, without the earth being destroyed.

Happenings are being called up all over the world, which will force people to look inside themselves and begin to search for the true causes of sorrow and violence, for the solution.

For this, no sad dramas need to be experienced! The sooner a human being finds *the path to his heart,* acknowledging his true, divine autonomy — coming to true Insight and awareness — the sooner he will banish all suffering and sorrow from his life.

Ultimately, the Earth can only be populated by people who try to achieve peace and harmony in themselves and with others.

No single fact justifies the use of weapons, war, or violence.

The atomic power of the human being can only be used by those who don't misuse it, by those who strive after harmony and only feel thankfulness about this force of life in themselves. *Here, it's not about "magnetism" the way animals and human beings have "used" it throughout the past,* and are still using it in healing processes and such. Nor is it about ritual initiations, nor about so-called wonderful magic tricks in order to make jewels or other objects materialize out of nothingness, etc. — these techniques were, and are still, being used by people who posses "power over matter," but it has nothing to do with the "new joyful dimension, in which every human being will be aware of his loving divinity and will grow toward a New Body in freedom and independence." *New energies are waiting to be used: every simple human being, without privilege of order or tribe, of race or color, of leader or pupil, now has to make a choice. The only attached condition being an openness to Insight and Love, and a willingness to work on this.* If the most "powerful" guru blocks himself in a narrow spirituality, then he hinders himself and others from truly entering "into" the paradise of the New Earth. *True spirituality is in the spontaneity of Life itself, in the becoming aware of the Power of your being, with both feet on the ground, in Faith, in Love.*

The earth won't destroy itself; humanity won't either. But a natural selection will happen: *self-selection.* Do you or do you not choose a beautiful, new Earth, a new dimension, in which live goodness and harmony? No one obliges you to this, but the most beautiful and highest energies that we call up in order to build a New Earth in a new dimension will, automatically, no longer attract those entities that have no longing for this evolution for themselves, or will not allow them to be born anymore. There are plenty of other reality systems in which they can find what they want. *It is, however, our fullest responsibility to create a new Earth on which the chaos of violence and death, pain and epidemics, war and sorrow, will disappear.*

Sex, aggressive violence, pain and crime, often lie very close to each other. Potential sexual powers, hormonal and other chemical substances, will be at the service of the building of our "New Body." Both parts of the brain will start working perfectly together and will be ideal channels for **1** concentrated Self, our "I," which will leave earthly mortality behind and which radiates like a warm red sun that will never set. Not necessarily through spiritualization or via the development of a kind of energetic light-body, but by employing the concentrated energies in a self-aware way, which is only possible through "alchemical" fusion, as it were, of sensitivity and mind, of intuition and thinking, of consciousness and unconsciousness, of wisdom and Love. *Every human being is capable of it* if he is simply open to it. Ask — and it will be given to you by your Self to yourself!

Read more about this in the book "New Days" by Ch. Beerlandt.

FEMALE GENITALS

THE UTERUS

Psychological correspondence

The uterus is the microsymbol of the divine, shoreless Cosmos, in which creation constantly takes place and grows. Experiencing the unlimited space of your consciousness. . . .

An unlimited feeling of joy. You are being born, reborn in yourself: in this birthplace, the womb, as a receiving channel for very broad light energies that live on several levels of consciousness.

The feeling of: "I feel at home in myself. Safe." You can mount this saddle and develop creativity. Beautiful awareness energies, pure, clear; higher radiation powers are being received here from your deepest Self.

The faithful, loving, being-there, for yourself in the first place: with happy light energies the child in you — which you forever are — is being cherished in the "mother." The gentle, flexible, unlimited, sensitivity.

A basis where whirling energies, Action, Creation, Creativity, Self-development, are being born. A pure source which carries love for life inside. A meeting point of the "male" and "female" principle.

Here grows the Fruit of psychological productivity. It's a radiating Source of strong light energies, which through their enormous potentialities bring about a movement that allows the Activity, the Coming to be, the Manifestation, to happen. See there the Yang in Yin, or plus in minus, no matter how you call it.

The "female," receptive principle on the one hand, and the "male," active principle on the other hand: both present in every woman! The female sex organs and sex glands, in their totality, symbolize, on the one hand, the enormous urge for creativity, and on the other hand the large receiving station for higher energies.

Interaction between both creates constant growth and production.

The receptiveness of the uterus is there first of all in order to be filled with the personal creativity and active growth of the Woman herself! In order to bring together the so-called male and female element, or the passive and active principle, one will form a Unity, a fullness, in oneself. One doesn't have to attract a sexual partner from the other gender in order to obtain a balance between plus and minus. It all lies in every woman, just as it all lies in every man.

Ailments, in general

Shutting yourself off from those illuminating awareness-energies: you see everything black.

Do you hold on to the past? Do you clutch on to something? In this way you can't be reborn in yourself; in this way no creative fruits can come into existence!

Why do you reject the child you, yourself, are? Why so cold with yourself?

Offer love to yourself and don't first of all expect it from others.

Fill yourself with the powers of creation, with feelings of self-appreciation.

Superficial sexual experience will not allow you to experience the Fullness. This Fullness, this happiness of satisfaction, you will *really* experience it only if you first give your "I," in an independent way, the unlimited freedom to experience joy in your Being, in your creativity. Only this Fullness of your Self, in which female and male elements are in harmony, will lead you to true love with a partner. Often, this means dying in yourself and rising up new again, and this time on your own solid Basis and on a higher consciousness-level.

Open, unlimited consciousness, on a strong "I" basis.

Open yourself up to that mass of energies which are ready to be directed. Break open your borders in joy: your uterus will be liberated from an imprisoned, black feeling.

Cancer of the uterus
(See also Uterus and Cancer, in general)

Having no more contact with Life itself.

Disenchantment.

Sadness, sentiment, emotions — look at me, I can't go on anymore.

Ever and again, you have looked for support outside yourself; now you have lost this hold (a partner, a task, etc.) Or your prayer for love has not been answered.

For too long you have carried needless burdens. You have given much of yourself; much you have cherished, much you have mothered — but only in order to feel love.

If you don't, first of all, *really* love yourself, your partner will also disappoint you. Possibly, you feel deserted.

A pessimistic vision of the future: life won't offer you anything anymore. . . .

Neptunian blindness to seeing the truth the way it really is.

No longer believing in your personal creativity.

You have lost all contact with your Higher consciousness-energies! You experience yourself as only weak and incapable. You deny the enormous regenerating energies in yourself.

Drag yourself away from this dark, false life's perspective! Finally, be reborn in yourself, and offer yourself the Love you so long for. Feel the strong true Light in your inner Power-source.

Allow your feelings to stream out; look at your emotions, allow them to flow — trust this process of letting go. Dare to let go of everything in order to make a place for renewing energies. Become aware of your worth and your possibilities of creating your life yourself according to your longings: independent of others.

You only need Power and appreciation from yourself, not from others. You will experience their love only when you first completely acknowledge yourself, your personal nature, your unique being.

Nothing just "happens" to you: this illness asks you to acknowledge the child inside you. It feels like it's being neglected in a room full of smoke: open your windows, look very far, and allow your child to explore this unlimited space.

Your uterus is no closed up cell, but is a powerful generator, for self-healing.

Cervical cancer
cancer of the neck of the womb

Flooded, overpowered, by not really being "present" in the Fullness you are; this asks for a complete entering into yourself, into your body, for a transformation. Become master over yourself and guide that mass of energies in your being. Don't just sit by and watch. Old structures and habits need to be thrown over. Joy about your Being is asked for! *Don't ALLOW yourself just to "be lived"* like a zombie, like a robot, according to the standards of others or of things that are not of real value. LIVE yourself, stand up straight as a HUMAN BEING and consciously become the Leader over your energies!

You have not "participated" enough in yourself, placed yourself out of doors, as it were, outside your true body.

A mass of energies, creative forces, and emotions inside you now asks for transformation, for you to take up Mastery over your life, your body, your energies. So, no longer just look at yourself from the outside, but enter into yourself and identify yourself with the Inner Power Source that is inside you. Become master over your existence and no longer keep looking on, standing at the outside of yourself.

Small puddles of water run out from under the front door, as a result of a water leak in the house. You come home and get a scare: the Plutonic water pipes have burst, as it were. Symbolic of: you are convinced that Something or Someone — a danger of emotions and feelings and desires — can overpower you, become master over you, that you won't be able to handle this mass of energies and emotions, that you will be *overpowered*. This is not true . . . as long as you live the way life asks you to live. STAY CLOSE TO YOURSELF and ALLOW THE CREATIVE FORCES TO CONTINUOUSLY FLOW THROUGH YOU IN A FRUITFUL WAY; use them for creative self-development! For productivity! DON'T ALLOW YOURSELF TO BE OVERPOWERED BY ANYTHING OR ANYONE; *you are master over your existence, over your body, over your energies.* The safe "basis" lies inside yourself.

You don't allow the past to submerge you either: you are "with" yourself! You have a need to come very close to yourself, and your body begs for it. You have too long hesitated to enter "inside," to take part in yourself, in your full body of flesh and blood. Now, no more hesitation; when you are "with" yourself, you will never have the feeling that something in yourself, or someone else, can overpower you. After all, you now make yourself master over your life, over your feelings. YOU take a hold of the Scepter and know that you are the loving Shepherd over your existence, who leads his mass of sheep-energies in the right direction.

The Path you have to follow doesn't have to be "hard" the way you are possibly convinced it is (for instance: strict diet, sex against your will, emotional boredom, family problems, work, etc.), but it is so soft, as soft as sheep's wool and as fresh green grass, as long as you are convinced of this. For, your reality you create yourself. So, no thorn ever again has to prick your skin; never again do you have to stray from the highway of life: you determine your "borders"; you live from out of your broad being, not from out of "possessing" and "seizing" and "self-negation as a Human Being," because this goes together with anxiety and sadness and feelings of being a victim.

Don't fill yourself with something or someone, but fulfill yourself; allow creative energies to flow freely; use them in a sensible way! You now direct your life energies with force and determination. You know that everything will happen at the right moment. You let go of things and people around you!!! (Whoever seizes can be "seized"). You know how to say, to formulate, everything at the right moment, without having been preoccupied with it beforehand. Your path now becomes gentle and noble. Your path you make yourself, and you make something beautiful of your future: this conviction you now root deep inside yourself, and it will be that way. No single other conviction is stronger than this, even when doubt surfaces sometimes. This can never trample the fundamental conviction: "My life becomes very good, beautiful and gentle!"

Knowledge of deep, old issues now becomes very useful: you have known for a long time, from the beginning of your existence, from your "birth," that at one point you will (have to) choose to never again suffer, die. So, this step now takes place.[1] A thorough transformation pushes itself through. Arm in arm with the people you love, you go onward, and you never give up! You are optimistic. Beautiful it is. . . . Feet[2] are happy and thankful(!) that they are allowed to go, that they may bring you to the places where you have to be on this earth. Your heart sings of joy and nothing can be ruined anymore.

You still feel halfway in the eggshell, like a chick thrown upside down into the world. As if you have no say over yourself, over life inside you. You feel overwhelmed, overpowered. Know, then, that this will last only as long as you look upon life as: "I am powerless, and life is an incidental happening."

---

[1] Read more about this in *New Days*.
[2] Read more about the symbolism of the feet in the chapter concerned.

On top of it, your head weighs too heavy — indoctrinations, age-old thoughts, possibly from a long-past life . . . it seems it all lives in your high-pressured head. You'd like to undo your Living Self from those old thoughts — from that old world in which you still dwell with convictions — but you think you are powerless against that which has forced itself inside your head, against everything that presses on your head. You want to get out! You want to free yourself! You want to undo yourself — be it unconsciously, which is why this signal is there now: to make you conscious of it — from an old structure of being trapped, from that which has been planted on and in your head! With all your might, you'd like to erase all you have ever seen, heard or done, etc. You no longer want to hear anything about it. Possibly with fury and sadness, in helplessness, you want to erase in order to start again with a new slate.

Know, then, that everything you have attracted in the past was from a feeling of (power-)powerlessness . . . and that now you need to stand up as a Mighty Loving "I." You have nothing to expect from others, but have everything in your hands; from now on you can attract circumstances that will only give you joy, that give you everything your heart longs for. But, then you do have to BELIEVE in the Power of the Human Being you are and really have to RISE UP as a reborn "I," no longer regarding yourself as just one of the "mass of little people" or a powerless victim. Begin anew.

In this case, healing often goes together with "literally" announcing a new Beginning in your life. . . . Be joyful about yourself! Be thankful about your wonderful Being. Don't get angry about what is not, what has passed, but understand in mildness and gentleness . . . don't feel vengeful and bitter, pained, because of the pain someone has caused you. After all you have attracted this yourself. Now understand yourself, understand why . . . and LET GO!!! Enter into yourself in the greatest love and no longer

ask yourself the question "why." You know it; it is for you to finally realize that YOU deserve to be loved, deserve to lead a wonderful life. Realize that NEVER again do you have to attract, or burden your head with, unpleasant things.

Make an end to the powerlessness of the past (and possibly the "power" with which you unconsciously or consciously have "drawn" others to you) and in a powerful way become *master over yourself*: NOW. Take the worthy Scepter in hand and magically attract that which is most beautiful for you, FOR this is the way things energetically work! And especially open up your HEART, and love will pour out of you, true love will flow toward you. However, as long as you remain living in anger and bitterness, in the system of power-and-powerlessness, this will cause confrontations that bring up feelings like impotence, fury, bitterness. This is no longer necessary. YOU have understood and definitively got rid of every negative conviction. You now go onward without looking back, in the fullest self-respect. This is the only way!

A *new Beginning* goes together with transformation, with the birth of your true "I"; as a human being who realizes that he stands as a worthy Master, at the Head of his energy content, and has his life and health completely in his hands.

Ectopy of the uterus neck
red spot around the uterus mouth,
made up of mucosal cells of the inner uterus wall

Your life is like a winter sleep; your body is not really inspired by your Conscious "I." With a passive and resigned attitude you wait, indifferent, not really motivated in life. Inner energies don't get a chance to break through, since you are not interested in building your life yourself; energies are spreading out. They spiritualize, impersonalize, decentralize themselves because you don't take up your central space. You don't really live; you allow yourself to "*be* lived."

Mechanical sometimes, like a puppet, you let yourself be ordered around; you don't set any bounds on others. Do you consider yourself a worthless, wilted wallflower, who has no say in her life? Would you sooner believe in "fate" than in the possibility of creating your life yourself?

*Determine what you Want and what you Don't want; action, dynamism, liveliness, movement! Feel strongly concentrated in yourself and no longer allow yourself to **be** lived. Dare to wade through emotions, and use inner powers to build up your life. Constantly regenerate your body through a loving presence in yourself. The body immediately reacts to the conscious or unconscious impulses and instructions of your Self: in a Self-aware way, take your life in hands and discover the richness of it.*

Uterus inflammation
metritis
(See also Uterus)

Suppressed anger. You feel hurt. Pain, being overpowered by others. Pent-up feelings; hidden aggression, even if you don't really know why. You don't unconditionally accept the joy of life: you ponder things too much, you make heavy weather of certain emotional matters.

You experience an inner division: you turn away from the gentle aspect in yourself, perhaps you even have a dislike of yourself or your body.

You project yourself often onto your partner: you are angry with him but, in fact, the cause lies in you. Self-condemnation of your weakness, of the anxiety of being who you'd like to be. Dissatisfaction about your exterior or your life's circumstances. Feelings of inability to create and to realize yourself.

Sometimes, you become hard and blame others, but actually it's powerlessness regarding yourself. Do you bang your fist

hysterically on the table? It's about powerlessness.

Build up your life! No longer frustrate yourself. Be your own boss. Flexibly let yourself go; don't slow yourself down! Don't close yourself off from your feelings of being nice, of affection, tenderness. From out of a strong energy basis, stand up for yourself and discharge yourself in creativity instead of piling up aggression.

Give to everyone what they deserve, but first of all give yourself what you need: self-protection and self-appreciation, by acknowledging your powerful "I." No longer vent your powerlessness on your partner: stop considering yourself "bad."

If you are being raped, then this is because you refuse to direct your own forces, and because you mistrust your deepest Self. Find again this trust in yourself! Assume your Leadership!

Myoma of the uterus

You are not really here; something else is taking your place. You have withdrawn, away — anxiety.

Perhaps you have fled and are no longer living from out of yourself in a motivated way.

Fled from a life that doesn't really interest you, fled from life circumstances which don't offer you real satisfaction.

Are you living without a soul, superficially? You have no contact with your basis, with your deepest "I." Nor do you really choose your path in life: you are barely there.

Because you actually feel empty, you anxiously grab for something that "fills" you up: a job, a "teaching," an "ideal," which REPLACES your core!

You draw toward you; you attract occupations and activities to fill your emptiness. You become "occupied" with negative thoughts or happenings.

In your center you grasp "hold" of something or other (the myoma) instead of acknowledging your own creative force, your sun, as a center pillar. You are possessed by something or someone, by anything but yourself.

Your consciousness doesn't guide your life; you too much allow yourself to "be lived." Are you a parrot, who imitates everything her mother or friends do? Do you live superficially or in an unauthentic way, according to narrow-minded, social, external norms?

CONCENTRATE your spiritual energy in your body!

Feel how you can take your life in hand with your power of consciousness and your longings! Don't let yourself be lived by assuming a slavish follower's — or superficial — life's attitude. Place yourself in the Center.

Build true wisdom inside you. Come to more profundity in your outlook on life.

Listening, seeing, and being silent; pondering and calmly ruminating, contemplating.

Bring your feelings into perspective, also the anxious grip you hold on things.

Allow your Self to be born!

Don't allow your body to be possessed by a replacement of yourself. Radiate, give — in joy and action — to the outside world. Trust, and let go of everything.

Allow pure, authentic, creative powers to be born out of the depths of yourself!

Prolapse of the uterus

The following causes are often being kept in, not expressed.

Without using your mind any longer you unconsciously want to surrender to an exaggerated, reckless, conquering, stormy behavior. Everything is allowed! No more norms, no more laws! An enormous frustration, a longing for Space, freedom — for being able to fly like an angel. Your longings go wild in an uncontrollable way.

You would like to reach far and high and grab, but it all slips away from you. . . .

A giant source of energy radiates its forces outward; like a dragon, you feel the need to storm forward and blow up bridges!

An inexhaustible urge for freedom, which takes on outrageous proportions because of a past suppression that was much too strong; supremacy of your own creativity

You are allowed to jump out of the plane, but carry a parachute! Protect yourself with healthy contemplation. No longer bottle things up. Let off steam; erect your building, stone-after-stone. A healthy balance between feelings and mind!

Use all energies in healthy creativity; don't slow yourself down! Realize what forces you have inside you, and use them in the right way, not in a self-destructive way, nor destructive toward others.

Fighting for an ideal is good, but first and foremost place it into your own life; and, steadily, in an uninterrupted tempo, row toward it.

Transform negative forces into positive Action.

Tipped uterus
(See also Uterus, in general)

You are filled to the brim with feelings, but you're not getting a grip on them, a perspective on them. You feel suppressed, imprisoned, and unable to build up your life from within yourself. Frustration: "I can't." Feeling subordinate to Authority. You'd like to go onward, but something holds you back — after all, you feel inhibited by your own emotions, your anxieties. You feel your aggression and would like to spit it out! But you keep in your feelings for fear of being roasted yourself. Sadness turns into anger. Real action doesn't happen.

Give yourself freedom: dare to come out with your feelings, your talents, your creativity.

Pay no mind to what others say; acknowledge your worth yourself.

Carry yourself lovingly: acknowledge your "female" characteristics, your feelings, your gentle receptivity, and allow this to be guided by a powerful will. Stop suppressing your emotions! Let them flow freely, deal with them, and enjoy!

OVARIES

Psychological correspondence

A safe feeling, trust in your dual unity: the power of the merging of the male and female aspect in the Woman, which leads toward Creation. On the one hand, inner divine wisdom, fundamentally intuitive, the gentle heart that is open, flexibility in evolving, daring to let yourself be taken up into the large space (See also Uterus) of your own being; the potential source of creation. On the other hand, Powers to create; you are leading creative processes, solidly taking everything in hand in self-aware resoluteness; experiencing the oneness in yourself and, with accuracy, being able to determine your life's path; self-manifestation in fruitful unfoldment of your potential talents.

Victory over all anxiety and panic, over death, through the growth of autonomous self-awareness, which creates its life itself and takes it in hand a hundred percent: rest, joy and peace because of one's own Space; trust in the relationship with your deepest inner Self and in the relationship with others.

Ailments, in general

These are mostly caused by enveloping oneself too strongly in a second "skin," into a mask, in a false role, in restricting armor. Anxiety is the origin of this. Anxiety about your own deeper feelings, about a "dark unconsciousness" — instead of becoming Master over yourself. You think you have to protect yourself against yourself, also against others, against "evil" or illness. . . .

You experience yourself as being so tied down; you don't at all dare to follow your free nature and your urge to create. Suppression of creative energies; being swallowed up in emotions; getting no conscious grip on your life. Are you afraid to be cursed or grabbed by the neck by others? Are you so much restricting your living space? Do you fanatically renounce certain things or do you actually anxiously cling to certain supports? Instead of coming to full creativity and liberation, you encapsulate yourself with all your potential talents. You don't believe in your own Authority; you are afraid of authorities outside you.

Now, manifest yourself from within, from out of your TRUE "I."

Underproduction or no production of egg cells (and still a healthy production of energy on a physical level caused by sexual hormones)

Cause: a blessed immersion into Life itself; intense creativity and cheerfulness; fully living your emotions without frustration; constant creative awareness powers; no longer being stuck in the sheer sexual or physical; joy which is very intensely experienced with the heart, the Conscious spirit; joy which goes far beyond pleasure: happiness beyond all time.

The functionings of the glands and hormones immediately result in these liberating energies, in these spiral forces, and no longer have to be at the service of the production of egg cells. True fertility on earth.

The cause of (over)production of egg cells

A frustrated feeling; as a woman you experience yourself as subordinate to the "male aspect" instead of integrating this aspect in yourself.

Keeping your creativity and your experience of relationship strictly limited to physical sex without bringing to realization the deeper unity in yourself! In other words, as a worthy personality you remain absent — your Conscious "I" is not allowed to exist; you submerge yourself in a partner you "need."

Exaggerated flexibility, loose sand that flows away under a foot. . . .

Allowing yourself to be driven, or taken for a ride instead of taking the rudder of life in your hands! Nervous tension: you feel "imprisoned" in the system, and you would unconsciously like to break out, but you feel too small and powerless; you don't do anything. . . .

Flesh without consciousness. Body without a head; emotions without a heart. Being emotionally at the mercy of your "unconscious" contents. . . .

Therefore, now take in your hands, yourself, the right to decide; consciously become master over yourself and transform unconscious power fields and instincts into creativity and conscious Love.

Replace the sadness and the attachment from the past with true joy, wisdom and autonomy. Sun and self-confidence!

Make use of your energies in a conscious way, and take up all your space!

Estrogen hormone:

"Under the POWER of,"
or
"bringing the divine AUTHORITY in yourself to realization in a CONSCIOUS way."

What is your choice?

Psychological correspondence, function

On an unconscious level:

Powerful, crushing forces which need to be used in a constructive way.

It symbolizes the dominating Authority, the large, coercive space that takes possession of you and says, "Here, this is where you are supposed to be. I am the powerful!" These have been unconscious compulsive impulses of the woman in the past: propelled onward by these enormously powerful energies, she lets herself go, blindly sitting on an arrow which has been shot at a goal, reckless — does she feel vague anxieties because she doesn't know where these forces will lead her?

Something seems to constantly and rhythmically be pushing on your head, like an automatic printing press; you can't do anything about it; you are at the mercy of a compulsive up-down-up action; resistance is of no use; it crushes you with merciless force. You allow yourself to be led by this iron-like, dominating headmistress's behavior in yourself (unconscious forces); you experience it as something you can't escape, something devilish, or something divine. . . .

Energies which, because they are not being used on a conscious, creative level, have a strong effect on the physical, on the character, of the woman, on the uterus, on the sexual life. A compulsive, programmed function directed by the old coded system in the unconscious part of our brain computer.

In the woman who is full of love and who comes to awareness:

Impelling forces transform themselves. Under the authority of the Conscious "I" estrogen will contribute to a psychologically open, blessed, joyful space; she is a blue force, as it were, which leads to liberation of enormously beautiful emotional experiences.

A force which kills or restricts, yes, gives anxieties as long as you don't clearly direct it from within your "I." A force which participates in the process of the monthly cycle which so far has fitted the framework in which babies have been born in order to have to die 80 years later! An energy which works psychologically impellingly, if you don't become Master over yourself!

Now, allow this process to radically turn itself around for the good of the total world of women.

Here, it's about the most beautiful Forces that lead toward higher consciousness experiences, toward wonderful creativity, toward pure love, if the woman no longer allows herself to be led by a "dark unconscious part of herself," which she would have to obey!

The woman who places the divinity in herself and only brings forth fruits which, in their turn, don't "have" to die.

If she wants a physical or sexual relationship, if she wishes to ovulate or wishes to bear a baby in the way that is known thus far, then this is now good if it happens without compulsion: free Choice, yes or no.

Big changes can follow, however, in the awareness-process of the woman regarding "bearing children," sexuality, creativity.

Space, relief, softening, an ability to explore the depths; the ability to reach a broader, intuitive spectrum (taking off the blinders on your eyes), an energy (also in the male!) which stimulates looking further, enlightening, gentle, emotional flow, a catalyst in the unfolding of loving, caring feelings. This all has to do with estrogen: if we no longer allow ourselves to be led by an authority outside ourselves, by the Authority of our inner Unconsciousness! We are not victims of unconscious forces if we transform them into Consciousness: out of this transformation comes happiness as a replacement for anxiety and sadness.

Psychological cause of underproduction of estrogen

You don't really dare to manifest yourself, to go on in life; and you withdraw. Not wanting to be or to do. Afraid, cowardly, anxious — you flee from that which is earthly, from Life here-and-now; you barely breathe in air; you hide in a psychological diver's suit, in an illness via which you don't really have to be here (for instance dementia), imprisoned and anxious. Nervousness; more spirit than body.

Psychological cause of estrogen overproduction

You are too flexible, too subject to unconscious impulses; you can give in blindly to sex, to sadism, to superficial pleasurable experiences. You have no backbone, no conscious Will; you let yourself be led like an automaton or like a zombie — by others, or by your own compulsions. Reaction to your feebleness: you become hard! You might also go through life apathetically, indifferent, like a limp rag, but you don't really live! Perhaps this is precisely the reason why you would look for exaggerated excitement: because you feel so empty and absent in a Neptunian way. You storm through life but you don't know "to where." Where is your conscious "I"? In desperate nervousness, in search of yourself, you might work this off in an iron-hard way with the whip of criticism, an aggressive flow of words, (possibly sadistic) sexual pleasure. The sexuality is possibly mostly in your head, but the true joy of the physical experience or of general creativity — that you can't reach. An exaggerated manifestation in the flesh, in the material world; an absence of self-confidence that is based on true "I"-consciousness!

Estrogen is constantly being produced in order to offer you the Authority which lies inside yourself: reach for those Forces within you, and become aware that they bring power and softening into your life, if only you would step away from the conviction that you are a powerless being at the mercy of unavoidable impelling powers in yourself. They ask for conscious use and transformation: become master over your own energies and be open to higher consciousness experiences via creativity, via sensorial joyful experiences in life, no longer restricting yourself.

Progesterone hormone

Psychological correspondence

The experience of unity of soul-body in a peaceful, harmonious way; every cell of the body is strongly animated by your consciousness. The dynamic of the bodily energies themselves: a comfortable feeling to the tips of your fingers, to the ends of your hair, as it were, when, with a powerful will, you very self-assuredly are strongly concentrated in your body. Rock-steady convictions, belief in life. Unfaltering inner forces. Merging of spirit and matter: this stimulus is also important in the "process of incarnation" — not only of yourself, but also of a being who wishes to be born. Inviting impulses to "come in," into the material world, in which you feel so peaceful and safe. Production of this hormone becomes less necessary when this feeling of being welcome in your body, in life, has taken shape in a solid way.

If, on the contrary, you take distance from life in a cold way, if you are far away from warmth, blood, and heart; if you are up high and are cold, at a distance from that which is earthly, from your body — then you unconsciously call for more progesterone.

Be full of faith, proud, calm, without anxiety; be aware of your worth and develop pure energies; take distance from death.

Stein-Leventhal syndrome
polycystic ovarian disease (PCOD)

You live hidden underneath false layers; you don't really live from out of your emotional world. You are like a puppet that once in a while plays in the theater. Although you seem cut off from your actual core, deep inside you hold on to emotions from the past, without anything being really worked out or something new being born. Feelings are so deeply hidden that you don't even know you still have some of them; you can appear indifferent or apathetic, without your own will to live, because you just "accumulate" (emotions and thoughts) instead of achieving innovative creativity. You don't really live; you have your mind on false perspectives; you eat and sleep and do your duty. But where are you really hidden? Where is your true "I"? You live too much for the approval of others; you are dependent on it. But you stand almost outside of life; you are present here as a shadow, not as a woman of flesh and blood.

You carry painful memories, against which you now especially want to protect yourself. You don't give yourself a chance to be born. You hide behind a superficial attitude. You live according to the judgment of the outer world, or of one "godfather" or another. You don't have power over yourself; you live deeply hidden in yourself, sterile and quietly submerged.

Transformation! Look at the sadness and the emotions you have hidden, even if it hurts you: work them out and give yourself the chance to come very close to yourself and to grow out of the passive and suffering phase. Turn back inside yourself and puncture all those accumulated pain blisters; puncture your sadness and no longer allow it to have any power over your existence. Now be good to yourself and know that if you no longer place the authority and power over your life outside yourself, then you will be protected in yourself, because here lies precisely the cause of sad circumstances and the sadness which you previously have attracted. Therefore, don't hide any longer, but become aware of your power and dare to bring out your femininity, your feelings, your spontaneous energies. Production, action, openness: from within your true core. No longer live at the surface of your existence, but discover the joy in your deepest Self.

Come to life! Liberate yourself: even if you have suffered a lot in the past and have accumulated negativity, this isn't a reason to not live now! Begin anew.

Ovarian tumor
(See also Tumors, in general)

Dissatisfaction with your situation now, but you don't bring about any change.

There's nothing the matter, allegedly, but underneath your tight, smooth face, behind your silent, ascetic mask, anger rages! Suppressed aggression, not being able to achieve real decisiveness, action, or self-manifestation: creative energies are being suppressed. You'd blame others for this! The little child inside you is so sensitive and feels hurt — you push away this gentle aspect of yourself: you are furious, and you cackle without laying any eggs! "We'll see!" — that's what you think, but you don't actually do anything.

Mostly, you manifest yourself as being tougher than you are; you hide your true sensitive nature.

You should go on, evolve onward, and achieve full development of your creative possibilities, but you stay where you are, in a "controlled" way.

Is it perhaps to please others, to satisfy the longings of a person you think you might otherwise lose? Or do you wish to be "accepted" by the outer world and are therefore holding back? Are you hiding your feelings because of this? Is this why you are restricting your life? Do you feel so weak and don't dare to really live? This all ultimately means you are very dissatisfied with yourself: find out the reason and bring about changes in your convictions regarding yourself and possibly regarding outer situations.

Dare to be yourself; no one else but you has to be satisfied with your self, with your deeds. Have a big cleaning inside yourself and remove all piled-up aggression and sadness: integrate the little gentle lamb in yourself and let aggression out in active power, in creativity, in resolute enterprise! Trustfully, let yourself go and live in the way that goes with your true nature, without restraint. Allow love to guide your thoughts and a structure will follow by itself. Therefore, don't place a restricting structure upon yourself — seen from the outside or meeting the norms laid down by others. No longer block your advancement. Resolutely make new decisions which will give you a feeling of liberation. Bring about these changes in your life, in your thoughts, changes which are necessary in order to feel content and happy inside yourself.

MENSTRUATION

The monthly cycle of the woman comes from a very old conviction system in Humanity, from the times when gods were paid with blood sacrifices, when women had to pay their toll with pain and sorrow. The unconscious, programmed system doesn't need to exist in this way forever: "brain," "glands" reprogram themselves consciously or unconsciously. The cycle doesn't need to continue existing in this way in the future. Evolution will go hand-in-hand with the general growth of Consciousness.

In the traditional framework, we can name the following as causes of menstruation problems — although menstruation doesn't have to be a "problem" at all. Grow! Create! Go onward!

Nuisance of excessive menstruation

Menstruation indicates to you — and at the same time is a call — that you must open yourself up much more to your creative, powerful, glowing warm energy, which wants to come through; you hold it back somewhat. A demand from your deepest Self to fully exploit the creative possibilities in your brain, in your (creative) sexual glands: to come to a powerful "I"-awareness; not experiencing yourself as a servant or victim. As a woman, fully experiencing on the one hand the "male" assertiveness, the natural aggressive forces — that which is self-manifesting — and, on the other hand, allowing the free, happy, emotional current to flow through yourself.

In you lies the possibility to produce electric energy, to become the creator of a joyful, happy world: create it! Don't feel sad, but treat yourself as a Worthy human being.

We are not here first of all to bear children, but to create a reality of peace and happiness without the spilling of blood. This energy of joy lies within you, unused. Allow *yourself* to be born!

In order to avoid the painful flowing of blood inside and outside you, you need to orient yourself toward the beautiful and not toward the negative. One doesn't build a new, beautiful world — you don't build a joyful existence — by turning to suffering, pain, sorrow, etc.. Therefore, create your own happiness; no longer allow red tears to flow, but know that it has to do with red forces which wish to reveal themselves: a demand "to create" *yourself* even further and to get rid of all needless burdens. Create a sunny existence! If you have held on to sadness for too long then it will come out now.... Are you living too passively, surrendering to others instead of to your powerful "I?" Do you feel weak, powerless? Do you not you stand up for yourself enough? Do you allow yourself to be bossed around? Possibly anger, aggressive outlet, deep anxiety.

Therefore, develop a powerful, joyful, creative flow inside yourself.

Experience that primal power in your being, and bring out your energetic qualities; don't hold things in, don't bottle things up. Lovingly, radiate your energies outward! Don't shroud yourself with sad, melancholy isolation: stand up out of this negative self-programming of the female race, and build up history in a more enjoyable way.

Become relaxed, restful in yourself; now let go of all negativity, of all sadness: your life is a joy if you, yourself, ask for it. Experience Mastery over your Life in yourself.

Menstruation problems, in general

Anxieties, an aggressive resistance against one's own weakness and powerlessness, against the female or physical sexuality; emotionally bottling things up; burdening oneself in an exaggerated way by thinking or fretting; shame, guilt, feelings of being a victim. Giving more power to death and sadness than to life and joy.

Self-liberation! Dare to be yourself, active and self-aware. Don't be hard on yourself, but allow emotions to flow freely. Surrender to your inner gentle, receptive energies: balance between the female and male aspect in you.

Don't try to grasp everything with your rational mind. Trustfully open yourself up to your deepest Self, the intuitive, so that anxieties will disappear.

Make use of your energies to create! Creativity!

Egg cell, ovulation and monthly cycle;

"CAN BUT DOESN'T NEED HAPPEN"

Unconscious programming, habit: the Menstrual cycle, passively allowing or . . .

The monthly cycle is an age-old phenomenon stored in the "unconscious" human memory. In the beginning of the existence of the human race, the human being — closely bound to nature and gods, in full worship, and loaded with anxiety and feelings of guilt — threw himself at the feet of Something or Someone much grander than he.... He made blood sacrifices.

The human being was full of reverence for the divine Phallus, but he was afraid of that which was hidden and obscure — the sensitivity, the female aspect in himself, cut off as he was from his own inner depths. . . .

(Here, we speak about the first phases of a new human race, not about previous civilizations, the numerous previous races which populated our planet.)

Still today, in certain primitive tribes, the menstruating woman isolates herself from the rest of the tribe during the period in which she "sacrifices her blood" to the gods — considered to be not pure, doing penance, the symbol of non-integration of both the female and the divine in the Human Being.

Certain "old" parts of the brain have coded mechanisms, habits, traditions. The total body of the woman obeys unconscious commands from the brain for as long as she allows it. This programming, this unconscious conviction that "a woman *has to* have a monthly cycle, an ovulation and a monthly bleeding," can however be reprogrammed, consciously or unconsciously.

The conviction that a woman has to suffer, that she has to have a monthly "fertile" period — why does this *have to* be? As a result of this slavish following of age-old patterns, people have "babies" like cubs in starved, underdeveloped population-groups; millions of unwanted children are begotten, often without the presence of love. Slavery, habits, unconsciousness, sexual compulsions.

It's time the woman becomes Conscious! She will begin to direct her processes *herself*, and in the light of love and creativity! Classical science has seen, in the menstrual cycle of the woman, a cooperation of several physical elements as follows:

The hypophysis gland reacts to impulses from, among others, the hypothalamus (via the releasing hormones) and because of this produces the Follicle-stimulating hormone and the Luteinising hormone, both of which have a specific influence on the ovaries, via the blood, with regard to the forming of the hormones estrogen and progesterone and the release of the egg cell, among other things.

What has to be realized, however, is the Consciousness-power that lies behind this whole process: "unconscious" programming in an ever-repeating rhythm of about 28 days, until menopause begins: this is also a coded conviction.

In other chapters, you will see how hormones are powerful carriers of consciousness impulses; every woman can decide, freely and consciously, what she will do with it.

Instead of going on in a rusted, sclerotic pattern, she will discover the possibility in herself of coming to an enormous creativity and consciousness development. Red flow will make room for delightful blue energies! But likewise it can be that transformation of consciousness goes hand in hand with a persisting cycle of construction - withdrawal/bleeding. This is different for everyone!

Or — a conscious choice

The production of egg cells under the stimulation of glands and hormones was until now an unconscious, blind collision of the nose with the pole. . . .

In the conscious woman, however, the action of estrogen and other hormones — the energy that is produced in order to form egg cells — will have a very specific function: a powerful, turning, enormous energy which symbolizes divine creativity, which represents the "birth of the human being in himself," which represents the true earthly incarnation of a divine being.

There doesn't *have to* be "ovulation" (but it's okay, there's nothing wrong with it!): in the first place, it's about the new creative energies which are being brought about by the consciousness, and thus are being transferred to the glands, hormones, nerves, etc. . . . Electrical impulses are being released in the light of the Conscious spirit of the woman, and now ignite enormous energies in order to come to positive creativity: the woman arrives at transforming instincts and consciousness energies into actual creation. These creative actions can manifest themselves on many levels in her individual life as well as in relationships with others: on the playful level, on the level of love, on the artistic level, etc.

Via this unfolding of productivity, she will more and more find herself. . . .

This becoming conscious is necessary if the woman no longer wants to be a slave of the "past," of unconscious programming — if she no longer wants her "being" to be restricted to superficiality.

Only then, when she manages to unite the "male" and "female" aspect in herself, when she allows unconsciousness to be taken up into consciousness, when she finds the Unity (see also Ovaries) in herself, only then will she be able to have a loving relationship with a partner, man or woman. If she places the active, creative mastery in herself and does not first of all project it on a man or counterpole, then the gentle, receptive, sweet Moon will no longer feel sad, melancholy, lonely — no, this moon, this "female aspect" will find itself sustained in its radiating, golden, warm Sun! This self-aware sun-power will no longer tolerate the sad moon assuming the upper hand and crying out monthly her slave-like sadness or feeling of "only partly being". . . .

Joy!!! Then bleeding only means cleansing, leaving behind. . . .

When the unconscious intuitive feels taken up in the warm power, in the conscious Heart!

The woman is stuck with the egg — let her allow herself to be born! Decide yourself, in wisdom; don't abandon this "power of decision."

In unity, in love toward herself first of all, the woman will herself decide consciously in what sense, and whether, she will or will not "rest" or be "fertile." Anyhow: come into the Fullness and Joy of yourself, with or without bleeding. "BE" in this Faith, as a masterful, creative Human Being: that is the main thing!

Hormonal production offers positive, joyful creativity: it's up to the woman to orient this herself. This hormonal production is, however, first of all directed by the Consciousness of the woman; if she lives in Balance (body/soul, male/female, sun/moon, intuitively/ rationally) and longs to evolve into further creative awareness, then she will stimulate her glands in a positive way. . . .

It's all not as difficult as it seems: it's good that you, as a woman, become aware of this "unconscious" situation and cherish the

intense longing to solve this situation and free yourself from a too-restrictive pattern in order to discover your wide range of possibilities. The physical answer will follow your question, your longings, your convictions. . . .

Woman, create your life yourself — in joy, and don't leave any constructive possibilities unused!

Consequences

The female organs will undergo changes as a result of this natural, conscious intervention; certain parts will be reshaped by new vital cells. The endocrine glands in their turn will undergo changes.

Changes in a positive way concerning stability of the thinking faculty and the character.

This is not a futuristic vision, but a perception of changes that already take place in certain women as a result of becoming conscious.

Menstruation; trust in your Nature and Growth . . .

It takes time; it's about a process of life-renewal on the one hand, and allowing that which is superfluous to die off, to flow away, on the other hand.

As long as it's necessary for the well-being of the woman, bleeding cycles will occur regularly or irregularly. This depends on the nature of every individual woman; every human being is unique. Therefore, don't consider yourself "abnormal" when it's different with you. After all you are not a herd animal. It speaks for itself that, in cases of abnormally strong/long-lasting bleeding or terrible pain, you can ask to be "diagnosed" by a physician and so arrive at an understanding of the cause and a healing.

Certain women have no "bleedings" for years, and then all of a sudden they do. Trust your nature in the "spontaneous" purification process when necessary.

Don't absolutely "WANT" menstruation to disappear, because this then means "desiring." Evolve; live according to Life, according to your heart, and you will see and feel whether it's good or not if a bleeding happens to come. Trust your developmental process, go onward on your path of life! Live lovingly and consciously, not like a slave victim, but definitely from out of your worthiness, uniting the "man" and the "woman" in you in a balanced way.

Premenstrual syndrome
**several days before one's period:
pain, emotional confusion, tension, etc.**

The cause of this signal? You furrow your brow, as it were. You don't really get it, don't quite understand: because you think you have to grasp everything with your "thoughts" right away. You have to learn to let go and trust that at the right moment you will understand — intuitively, emotionally, and also rationally — that which is at this moment not yet completely clear to you. Not understanding, you look. Something is very unclear and you want to "comprehend" it. DON'T WORRY SO MUCH! Don't sit fretting, thinking, and in the meantime remain "Unmoving!" Energies that flow through your liver now drive you onward, asking for energy to be allowed to flow through! *Don't stand still in thought; don't try to comprehend; but LET GO and RELAX your brain.* What you don't understand now may be as crystal clear as limpid water tomorrow. You fixate ever and again upon the same point, and you don't let go; you dwell upon it, you worry unnecessarily. *Look at the BRIGHTER SIDE, at that which is happy, don't get stuck; release yourself from this fixation and go onward on your path of Joy! Go through life more light-heartedly and trust that no problems need to cross your*

path![3] You see things as too dark, too sinister — and in these sinister anticipations you of course attract things that will give you confirmation of this. In this way you make something heavy of your life. Life by itself doesn't offer you any burdens. *Let go and go onward!*

You hold on to too many things; you attach yourself to dark expectations; you need to look at life in a much lighter way. Don't in this way hold back the energy flow in yourself; allow that energy to flow freely through you. SURRENDER TO LIGHT-HEARTED JOY FOR YOUR BEING! As a result, no toxic matter will pile up inside you; you won't block energies, won't experience dark feelings. Free yourself from this closed circuit — this "dark" outlook on life regarding certain points, possibly points on which you have fixated for too long. Don't blame those points as the cause of your sinister feelings. They are, after all, the result of not SURRENDERING UNCONDITIONALLY and TRUSTINGLY to that which is beautiful, light, happy in YOURSELF! Therefore, no longer look for problems; don't *expect* them.

Start with looking at life in a HAPPY, LIGHT way and expecting it to be so — and the circumstances you experience, whenever you experience them, will be pleasant!

* * *

You droop; you feel somewhat despondent, caved in; you don't see the sense of things. Especially not when confronted by a mirror in front of you: "Who am I after all? What shall I do with myself?" A kind of discontent or disappointment with who you are. When you have lost courage in life in one way or another (for instance with children, or with material things, etc.), then this is the result of a more deeply rooted fact: that you are not really happy "with yourself." Don't fix-

---

[3] In this respect, read the symbolism of the Grapefruit in *The Horn of Plenty.*

ate on the outer form: eternal youth and beauty (in the true sense of the word) grow from within. The outer appearance is of so little importance and is only a result of inner changes. Trust life: the physical shape you develop is good for you, with or without wrinkles, spots, etc.. Everything will grow to more life, no matter how, if you believe in the victory of life over death, of health over illness and deterioration. NOW, CONTEMPLATE![4] Goodness and beauty go hand-in-hand; don't fixate on appearance and norms, on the idealization of sham images in society. *Stop the basic discontentment in and about yourself.* Now, come to total JOY about yourself! This can only happen when you tune in to the DEEP FOUNDATION, to the deeper WEALTH of your being — and don't get stuck to the unpleasant, dull, superficial side of existence. Change your convictions! Not "Just who am I?" but a jumping-up joyfully about WHO YOU ARE, and for the fact THAT you are.

Are you dissatisfied with yourself? Do you think you fail in some way, or think yourself ugly, bad? Then begin to develop in your heart gratitude for the fact that you are ALLOWED to be, that you are ALLOWED to exist as YOU! Out of this *vibration of thankfulness* regarding yourself, regarding the fact that you are allowed to live on earth in your highly unique body as "I," you will attract pleasant situations!

Do you not see any sense in things sometimes? Would you like to leave it all behind, abandon it and forget . . . run away from it? Do you perhaps want to be like a rooster, proud about its exterior? But do you feel an inward discontentment BECAUSE YOU ALWAYS DENIED THE WORTH OF YOUR CONTENT? Because you haven't acknowledged and experienced enough the DEEPER VALUES of life, of yourself, and because as a result of this you also disapprove of your exterior? Time to start searching for that DEEPER SOURCE OF

JOY which originates in your heart, that source of thankfulness, of happiness, for being YOU, separate from outer images, achievements or whatever. You don't shine on the outside, but you go searching for the true MEANING of your existence, for the MEANING which lies INSIDE you: that Fullness of experiencing yourself, of being able to live your life to the full, of feeling yourself — is wonderfully beautiful! Therefore, don't TURN YOUR BACK to your true, wonderful Being; acknowledge yourself from within. Don't live according to norms and expectations from the outer world, from society, and from that voice inside you that unconsciously has been indoctrinated and has connected itself with all this! Listen to goodness, to the golden heart — from here you will develop your true authentic beauty! There is no distinction to be made between truth, goodness, and beauty. Every other form of beauty is false, and has to do with sham. Therefore: come out of your previous shell, and now show yourself from within, no longer looking in the mirror or bringing yourself "into question," no longer being discontent because you have placed this or that DEMAND on yourself, which you can't fulfill.

You now have to let go of this form of desire, once and for all. Come to your true, inner center in honesty, in harmony, and try to always stay close to this feeling of truth. Get rid of your complaining layers and replace them with happy ones, through the joyful, radiating force of your heart. This happiness will work infectiously on your surroundings. Everyone, not in the least yourself, will profit from this happiness: about YOUR BEING THE WAY YOU ARE, and no other way! Content, the exterior closely connected to the deep Inside; no longer shut off from your Inner gold. You plainly radiate it, as a good human being. Every confusion disappears in this *fundamental self-acknowledgment: inwardly and outwardly woven together in unity; no dividedness in this, no sadness or discontent . . . because you are so happy about Who you are and How you are as a result of this "unity force,"*

---

[4] Read more about this in *New Days*, chapter 8.4

directed joyfully from within! You now know that you are allowed to let the male and female in you exist, in balance, that not one outer norm counts, that only the honest externalization from an INNER NATURE into form will create happiness. You now live very PROFOUNDLY from within ... you don't have to be "Snow White." On the contrary: the Prince and Snow White are parts of one and the same person, who artificially was split up, whereby a he-man and a frail woman were created and: Oh, goodness, if you didn't answer to one of those two images! Now, it's up to you to deal with this syndrome of *dividedness,* which for so long has been afflicting mankind: be yourself, with male and female forces ... and kiss yourself to Life!

From this loving embrace with yourself you will also be able to experience wonderful contacts with other "complete human beings," in true goodness and beauty, not in false appearances and dissatisfaction. Be yourself in a powerful and happy way! Allow the volcano to boil and burst in exuberant life enthusiasm for the deep foundation full of life forces, which it experiences in itself! Don't feel superficial, weak, discontented, thinking you don't live up to the demands or expectations you place on yourself: JUST BE YOURSELF, but DEEPER, from WITHIN. The male/female/human goddess stands up, unified, and dances with Joy!

MENOPAUSE, CHANGE OF LIFE

The true beginning: the birth in oneself. The inner Self calls the woman to be the "white bride." Physical changes now offer her the possibility of realizing in herself the ideal reconciliation between earth and heaven, between matter and spirit, or soul and body: thus to allow higher consciousness energies to come through in the name of Love.

A spiritual wisdom which reaches from the dark depths of Pluto to the highest spheres of joy. There is nothing, no level of consciousness, that is not accessible to the '

human being who orients himself in love toward beauty, purity, the joy of Life.

Higher, beautiful, light awareness energies can be experienced in a body that isn't burdened any longer by painful, sometimes compulsive, programming from the past.

This new state of being can present itself at whatever age. A chance, more than ever, to go the path of immortality; to definitely say goodbye to death. The transformation toward a new material body.

Problems with this menopause?

The cause lies especially in your associating menstruation and being "beautiful and young." Your beauty as a human being has only started to grow now! It is you who condemns yourself or who doesn't think yourself good enough; you wrongly think that you now are heading toward death, or at least have to become weak and sickly.

You take off your crown as a worthy being: Why? Your life will now actually be enriched because of a better, stronger balance between the male and female elements in you, on the condition that you continue to build up your life, Self-aware and powerful, with authority. That you don't stamp yourself as being old and burned-out; that you develop your creative energies outwardly, in a useful way; that you don't cling to a one-sided, limp, and weak femininity, and refuse to let your strong "I" exist; that you don't feel like a poor victim without a basis.

Decalcification of the bones (osteoporosis) or other ailments are being caused by your psyche, by your convictions of degeneration (see the category Osteoporosis.) You can direct yourself toward death or toward eternal health: the choice is up to you!

Hot flashes and other discomforts during menopause

So far you have insufficiently, or not at all, placed Authority IN yourself. You have made the sense of security and "survival" dependent on things or people, systems, gods, and idols — outside yourself. You have allowed yourself to float along on instincts, more or less, instead of taking your Life in hand in a self-aware way, unafraid, and Trusting in that basis of Fullness in yourself.

Time for Transformation! Everything lies in your hands: how do you deal with these red energies inside yourself? Don't flee! But bring about changes, fundamentally! Now LOOK closely at how life really works.

It's as if you are afraid of what must come; as if you need to "secure" yourself against an approaching catastrophe. You perspire because of it; you hurry, instinctively, in order to quickly find a safe shelter.

You hurry onward, like an Ostrich who so far has not been able to, or has not wanted to, gain clear insight into life, because it allowed itself to be RUSHED ONWARD by a kind of "instinct," instead of taking its life in its own hands, in a very concrete and SEEING way. It is necessary that you now transform your instinctive powers into Consciousness-energies. *That* is the objective, *that* is your task now. An emphatic CALL from life inside you to transform yourself to a new, higher Level: and this will be beautiful!

In order for you to come to a Greater Awareness of *how* life really functions, so that ultimately you realize that you have EVERYTHING to say about your life and are much more capable than you think. The old instinctive, anxious, self-securing pattern (which is present in you to a certain extent) now has to be left behind completely! There, where you previously were blind or didn't want to see — there, where you placed Life, your life, in the hands of one or another Power (abstract or concrete) outside yourself . . . you will now have to come close to your real Power Center, to the Authority inside yourself. Become aware of your Possibilities. Letting go of power and of a hold on others, things, and people, and fully learn how to deal with your energies in a totally creative, conscious way, in total TRUST,

unafraid, full of love, from the knowledge that Your Life lies in Your hands, that you only need to realize and to see *how* life really works. You no longer look anxiously for a Power outside yourself, nor will you feel weak or unable or "inadequate," while "filling" yourself with others. A call from life to bring to realization the AUTHORITY in YOURSELF, to begin to feel comfortable IN yourself, on your secure basis, to start taking your life into your own hands, to break with every primal instinct. Arriving at *true* creation! Energies ask for a kind of "transformation." Your major glands, your complete being, will become like a golden, radiating source if you now go onward in full force, from your Heart, from an awareness of completeness, from your inner Authority.

You know that you have time; you don't need to force anything, except that discomforts ask you to do something with yourself now, in a Conscious way, to no longer hide yourself from the true, divine powers that want to manifest themselves. Therefore, no longer deny that fullness. Open yourself up to the Ability that lies inside you, the Ability to transform to a New Level. This often asks that you shed the Old Skin, that you become aware of the male-female powers in your being — the divine, primal powers inside you — that you begin to manifest yourself as a FULL HUMAN BEING. You are not at all a powerless female who needs to build her life on instinctive, protective, securing, reproductive, surviving or escape patterns. After all, as long as you do so you can begin perspiring as a result of deep-rooted anxieties "that now everything is over for you." This is a lie which "death" inside you wants you to believe, but LIFE inside you tells you something completely different, tells you that something completely new is beginning to happen, if you now listen to the powers of truth inside yourself.

You are not a "female" — you are a HUMAN BEING, in its totality, the female and male aspect united in one. You are not at all dependent on the power outside yourself, nor do you need to maintain a certain power in order to secure yourself against any disaster or accident that might happen to you. You no longer need to look for SHELTER with someone else, with a human being, authority or system outside yourself. You need to come to the realization that the end-less shelter — safe, eternal and delightful — lies within your own divine source, in your inner Central Power Base! SAFETY LIES INSIDE YOU: therefore no longer anxiously flee from things, but develop yourself, unfold your totality and begin to discover who you really are. Then all fear, every insecurity, will disappear: the Secure Basis lies inside yourself! Now, arrive at the INSIGHT that you have your life in your hands. You take leave of not wanting to look at that greatness in yourself, at that great human depth in your being. You no longer maintain that instinc-tive pattern of the "female animal" in your-self. You apply the primal powers in a won-derful creative process: a great event in which you become who you really are! Don't get into a panic; don't be afraid. Expe-rience the signs as signals that inform you that you may raise yourself now to a totally new stage. You are undergoing a metamor-phosis and the end result will radiate golden happiness . . . if you want it to be so. You acknowledge the divine Authority in your-self. You trust with your heart your Ability to lead your life toward eternal happiness, and as a result, brain, glands, hormones, etc. are being brought in for a transformation process, after which you can only come out enriched.

Trust in this and live according to the conviction that YOU alone are master over yourself. Let go of everything and everyone outside yourself, but now bring yourself to realization . . . as living only under YOUR OWN AUTHORITY. Only then will the glands, hormones, cells, etc. understand that they are in the service of Life, in the service of a life that can be eternally beautiful. You BELIEVE in your FULLNESS. Body ele-ments no longer place themselves in the service of "survival," of instincts, but in the service of "life," of a creative, creating proc-ess. Become who you are! Listen to your Heart, to your Inner Authority. No longer place yourself under any other Authority than the inner authority that is WITHIN YOU; do what you feel you have to do: live according to this truth . . . and things will go well for you!!

*   *   *

Initially, you feel driven by an energy that seems to push you ahead: hurry, you can still be in time "inside" the ark, before the rain starts to come down . . . driven by a kind of instinct, by anxiety. This anxiety is there only as a "signal" to indicate to you that somewhere you are wrong. Your soul-center sends you anxiety in order to tell you that you need to RAISE yourself, that you now need to look more clearly at your TRUE "I," at your possibilities, which thus far you have underestimated. You are not an animal that anxiously must run from forces above or out-side itself, that needs to cling on to things or people outside itself! Here, the Life Energy speaks, your inner life-center, which wants you to go on, which wants you to go onward on your life's path . . . but at the same time asks you to start seeing CLEARLY and . . . not to run away from true awareness.

Even if you don't really know why, trust that those energies manifesting themselves inside you are allowed to be there, that it is good they are there. You need only to HANDLE them, to USE them, not by "holding yourself back," by "slowing your-self down" instead of truly going forward — an evolution that means Elevation and Total Acknowledgment of your being! This means: now come to the Insight of how life really works. Know that every human being is able to take his own life in hand and direct it; to consciously create his life himself. Not by practicing positive thinking; no, anything but placing yourself somewhere and begin-ning "to think"! But through a metamorphosis from animal being to Divine being, through dynamic, richly Conscious Participation in yourself, in the life forces within you. In this way you will no longer have the feeling that you are overwhelmed: you become master over your powers. You no longer have the feeling that you have to FLEE from any approaching disaster. On the contrary, now for once you are going to look in a very conscious way at Life, at the possibilities present inside you and inside all people. You are going to deal with life forces in an aware way.

Firstly, you need to let go of everything that you hold on to in thought and deed; secondly you need to completely get rid of every form of "negativity," of expectations of illness or death ... so to finally replace this with the conviction that everything inside you will take place in a very harmonious and lively way if you live according to this beautiful conviction,[5] if you start to bring yourself to realization as a worthy Human Being and no longer stay stuck in a male-female pattern, if you no longer just remain stuck in the superficial side of your Being!

Life circumstances are the result of your expectations regarding life, of the unconscious or conscious driving force that you place behind your energies. Therefore, choose the best way, the one way that leads toward true, happy living.

You shouldn't "flee" from life, nor from yourself; you may look at your own Body as if at a sun-drenched "ark," in which all energies seek their way and will find it — on the condition that you open yourself up to it. You now need to bring yourself one step up, further on your path of evolution. Don't hold on to things and people outside yourself; no longer look for shelter in things or systems outside yourself. You are safe within yourself: you are not allowed to run away from yourself! On the contrary, this signal indicates that you may participate more and fully in your total "I."

Don't behave like a scared ostrich, but open yourself up to the truth, open yourself up to truthful energies that want to manifest themselves with full force. Don't keep yourself frail, limp, unable or weakly feminine — on the contrary, allow all channels to open themselves wide in order to allow your very strong primal forces to flow freely in a male/female powerful way! You should not be "well behaved"; you should not remain waiting for things to happen; you definitely should not "draw in" and expect your fulfillment from "the male element" outside yourself. You need to build your life on the Inner Authority, not like the incapable "animal," but like the divine human being who thankfully and lovingly takes life in his own hands! Anxiety disappears by transforming instincts into consciousness and love. Therefore, don't draw in, but give, don't fill yourself up ... but fulfill yourself. Become aware of your creative possibilities to make an eternal, wonderful happening of your life.

You need to live according to the truth, to give, to allow energies to flow with full force; not taking in anything, drawing in anything, waiting for someone else to acknowledge you or reward you! *Give,* do, create, act from out of your Heart ... and you will attract, as if by itself, beautiful circumstances on your path. Allow that honest flow of truthful forces to stream out of you, glowingly! Don't remain "just half a human," in the background of yourself! A period of renewal is coming, not of deterioration or decay! Choose in Joy regarding yourself, applying all your energies in the name of life. Don't remain thinking, fearing or lamenting, but GO ONWARD ... so that the energies, led by a conscious, living human being — you — can have a constructive effect! This cannot happen if you flee from your deeper self, if you don't start to build fundamentally on your own basis, if you run away from yourself instead of developing trust and doing something with it ... with those beautiful life energies.

Don't hold on to the superficiality of yourself, to the exterior, to the material things or the things behind which you used to

---

[5] Read more about this in *New Days*.

hide . . . but expose yourself the way you are, in ESSENCE, and take away all masks. Become who you really are! Show yourself in full form; show yourself to the earth in happy roundness, as a HUMAN BEING (not like the restricted "female," be it somewhat "sophisticatedly" represented in a society of "human animals"), and enjoy every fruit that wants to manifest itself from out of you. Allow true creation to be born! Take part in the creative process that only can be led by Humans who have become Conscious. Take part in the world celebration where there doesn't have to be hatred, complaints, mourning, sadness about things that happened in the past.

Only an intense participation in Life, in yourself, in the NOW! Anxiety and instinct go hand-in-hand; becoming conscious and love go hand-in-hand with the Awareness of Fullness of the human being . . . and with fearlessness.[6]

*   *   *

On the one hand, you keep the sword at the ready, like a knight in self-defense; on the other hand, you stand stock-still, like a great "Y" with two antennas, the tree trunk solidly planted in the ground. Instinctively, *fearfully,* keeping yourself rigid and still: as if the slightest movement might mean danger! Such a *tight, petrified, still, posture indicates anything but a true, living, flexible, aware "Human Being."* In life, you "stand to attention"! Tense, on guard, tight. You don't — or don't sufficiently — trust your own deepest power source, because so far you have not tuned in to it enough, or not at all. You have lived too much at the surface of yourself, too much "toward the outside," too little acknowledging the Inner Authority.

Why do you attract this kind of a signal?

So that you will throw away your burden in order to definitively break with every *forced* attitude (placed on you *by yourself,*

possibly all through your life). As if you could exist only as a soldier in uniform or as a mannequin in tight, close costume, as a marionette or pawn within an authoritative system, etc.! . . .

You make a backwards move as it were. The female aspect, tight and tense, outlined and structured according to old habits (or perhaps to current fashion patterns). You suppress the warm, round female element, the soft flexibility that feels free and loose, supplely expanding and relaxed. You seem to want to accentuate and expose yourself as being "flawless" or "perfect" according to certain norms! Like an "Eve" tight in a suit, suffocating, in irritating artificial nylon stockings, the legs properly crossed in the posture one is "supposed" to be in. Artificially giving yourself a superficial facade, speaking in a way you are "supposed to be" or "should appear." A kind of dividedness; one part is unauthentic, false, for outward appearances, away from your TRUE INNER original NATURE!

Break through this false "armor," which you are not, which just sticks to you like a "mask." Show your true face in real, natural, human form. *No longer take on a "form" that you are not; no longer "behave" yourself . . . but BE, completely, your NATURE the way you essentially are.* Go and search for truth and live according to this truthful energy which dwells in all that is alive. Don't try to achieve or show off, nor to act chic or to pretend you are a movie star; don't surround yourself with attributes that only show how you want to exist as an "image" or with a tight outer appearance. No longer draw in. Don't pull things (or people) toward you. No longer try to impress anyone. Be honest — your first original Nature!

Active and dynamic, pure and original the way you are as "YOU," not in a "ROLE" or a "partial aspect" of yourself. *Throw off every falsehood, every binding that suffocates you, so that energies can flow freely, dynamic and honest.*

---

[6] If you want to know more about *how* you can determine your own life, then read the first part of this book.

OTHER AILMENTS OF FEMALE GENITALS

Endometriosis
presence of uterus mucosa in the "wrong" places (e.g. ovaria, intestines, etc.)

For too long you have let yourself droop; you swallow everything without question; you accept things from others; you let others treat you the way they want — because you doubt yourself: "I can't do it anyway." Your backbone melts away like chocolate — because you don't acknowledge the sweetness in yourself. You experience your own basis as being limp, you feel as if you have no strength and have no real solid structure in your life.

Often, this happens after a long period of pain, of sadness, or disillusionment or (self-) humiliation; you have sunk very low, and now you offer resistance to raising yourself up. Still, there's a question of inner, repressed aggression, and because of it you might vomit, might be disgusted! First of all because of your self-negation, of course, although you might blame others for it.

For a long time you have wanted to break through, but you constantly hold yourself back because of uncertainty: you pile up feelings, emotions; you swell up because of restrained energies and creativity. You allow yourself to "be lived" by others, and then all of a sudden you might spit it all out on them!

And so you run in place, in inner conflict, without making any progress. Remaining inside yourself or realizing yourself outwardly?

Confirm your own individuality: you are you! Clearly mark out your personal boundaries in self-respect and don't allow anybody to enter uninvited! All pain and sadness, all disillusionment in your life, have been called up by your uncertain attitude regarding your self-esteem. Arrive at powerful self-

manifestation, and now allow all energies to freely flow out of you; no longer hold on to your emotions; let go of them, and break through in a creative way!

Adhesions of the Fallopian tubes
(possibly causing tubal occlusion)

You are not occupied with the core of yourself, of life! You "follow" instead of creating your own life. You allow yourself to be lulled to sleep by the Words or Authority of others in such a way that you don't really take responsibility for your life. Facade: But where is your Content? Outwardly achieving; answering too anonymously to materialistic or religious laws. . . . Perhaps you work hard, but there's no question of Female, Individual Creative forces under the guidance of your Self-aware "I." You are too gray, too hazy, too impersonal. Possibly, you live in a very superficial way and consider life simply a game; true joy escapes you. You bend under the influence of your surroundings. You don't resolutely choose a highly personal life. You feel too incapable of solving your own fundamental problems. You look for a hold in a partner; if need be you'd allow yourself, against your will, to be used sexually, as long as you can grab on to someone, because you have no grip on yourself, no insight into yourself.

You look up to others. You let others treat you the way they want: "and you won't do this and that . . ." You obey orders.

You are not honest with yourself, nor with others.

Don't live "just like that" or always adapting to the outer world. Contentment and joy about yourself! Make an end to that Neptunian haziness and take up your central space.

Get a perspective; build a beautiful, clear, pure structure in your life; become master over your existence. Don't waste your time: use those energies as true creative sources. Let go of others; live from out of your own Authority. Really live from out of yourself, from out of your feelings. Allow higher awareness powers to come through and don't underestimate your worth!

Vaginal discharge

You are sad; you long for love, but what do you expect from others if you don't love yourself? You don't live honestly from out of yourself! Sometimes you surrender to a man submissively, sometimes like a hypocrite, sometimes like a mechanical puppet. You "play" with Life in this way. You have no real contact with your deepest emotional core; you don't experience yourself as being taken up in Love, not by yourself, nor by your partner.

You are too "absent"; you don't reveal yourself outwardly the way you feel inside; you sometimes use your body like a machine. Possibly, you let yourself be used sexually; you don't really get engaged with your heart!

Perhaps you "use" your partner; maybe you manipulate to get something, or "as a compensation": that's why you put your dead body at his disposal.

Here, it's often a lack of self-respect in the woman; she doesn't like herself, and she spinelessly gives herself to someone without being aware of the fact that she hurts her Self. It seems to her that her partner mistreats her: she's now fed up with it — inner anger now ferments!

Her own creative and self-realizing energies aren't allowed to exist: she plays with fire; her own life isn't being valued sufficiently; her body and talents are being looked down upon, or wasted.

Your "I" seems to be absent — you feel inferior; you withdraw from the here-and-now; you just let things happen — you keep your deepest Self hidden. Certain women feel that because they are "women," they are less worthy than "men": fatalistic and passive, they will go along with the whims of their partner. Inner sorrow boils up in powerlessness.

Lovingly, becoming present in yourself, your body. Allow Life to be really born! Feel your beating heart, your warm, earthly nature, and love yourself. In this way, allow the white-cold phantom to be replaced by a full-blooded, straightforward, unified you! Be your own guardian angel and border off your terrain; protect yourself. Step out of this dead, unauthentic life and dare to feel yourself deeply! Don't hide yourself, but speak and create; stand up for your rights and don't accept anything that goes against authenticity, love, or truth. Value life fully; feel the power over yourself which no one can take away from you if you will only acknowledge it. The attitude of a partner is only the result of your self-negation. Now allow your energies to blossom freely!

Vaginal dryness

A refusal, a withdrawal. Here, it can be a "no" to sexuality, but because of a feeling of guilt one yields to penetration. It is possible that, as a woman, you want to prove to yourself that you are still "young and attractive" and therefore you do your best to bring up your own sexual longings, while in your heart you'd prefer to experience your creativity in another way. Or are you afraid to lose your husband? Do you want to prove what a good wife you are? You'd prefer to slip away, but anxieties prevent this. Here, it can also be a refusal toward "life" itself; you suppress all your creative energies; you expect so much from life, but you don't get to bring it to realization. Possibly, you are not honest with yourself, with your partner, with others. You think you "have" to succumb in order to be accepted, but in your play-acting you feel cut off from your true Self. You build your life insufficiently on your own Authority; you don't enough live spontaneously according to your own feelings. The "thinking," the dreaming and imagining, the brooding, the development of all kinds of head energies, predominate over a joyful, physical participation in life.

A demand of creative development, of awareness-expansion: of listening to your own nature and not to that of others. If you live in harmony with yourself, honest with your feelings, only then can you make your fellow men happy, like yourself. Sexuality is only one of the many ways of expression, but it's not essential; a man who thinks he absolutely "has" to have it is not yet ready with himself. Be faithful to yourself; allow yourself to really live in joy with that which is earthly — the sensorial beauty. Say "yes" to your natural longings, say "no" to the unnatural, to self-restriction, to self-obligation!

Allow all life energies to blossom freely and in a powerful way bring yourself to realization.

Vaginal infection
by Gardnerella

Actually, you are sick of pleasing others and forever being at their service, making sure they have everything they need. And you yourself? You feel left out in the cold. Because in your heart you still feel like a baby, dependent on others; unable to make use of powerful energies for your self-realization.

Warm-red energies are being blocked; you live only according to others, not according to your nature. You cling to others because you don't feel safe on your own feet; because of this you would "sell" your body in exchange for safety and affection. For you close yourself off from your nature, from your feelings; it seems as if your body sometimes is separate from your feelings. You are not one with your body because you close yourself off from this in an anxious way, possibly because of painful memories from the past. You want attention and love from others, because you don't really believe in yourself: you feel like a small donkey that is waiting to be jumped on. Then it carries the burdens. You cage your nature; you are not honest with yourself, with your partner. Outwardly, you do your utmost to please

others, but unconsciously aggressive, revolting forces accumulate. You have played your role long enough for the public, for others; your nature now asks that you finally listen to yourself. An irritated, impatient process. It seems as if you are in the grip of others; a dead-end process against which you unconsciously revolt. You feel cold, without warm love. Do you possibly accuse your partner of having sex with you without respecting you as a complete human being? Then, first of all, you should blame yourself for this: don't you love yourself? Don't you dare to give yourself what you deserve? Are you at a distance from your body? Do you think yourself ugly? In a jungle of emotions and sadness, you feel safer being a parrot in a cage; you look for shelter in this imprisonment, but you participate in life in a too-passive way, unauthentic and sterile. Are you disgusted about certain things and don't dare to say no?

Stand up for yourself! Make an end to your old ways of living, and make your own rules now. Stop playing tricks to please others, and listen very honestly to your feelings. Be faithful to yourself and don't allow your behavior to be directed by anxieties. Love for yourself ultimately triumphs over everything and will attract or transform the partner, who really suits you.

Give yourself all opportunity to blossom. Allow powerful Mars energies to flow through, and build up your existence in a personal, autonomous way, without constantly wondering if it will be good for others. How long will you leave yourself standing in the cold? Every human being is unique and worthy in his own way, inwardly and outwardly: in love, come to yourself, and warm yourself without self-condemnation. Be honest with yourself and with your body.

Build your life strictly on inner wisdom and dare to say "no," when your feelings tell you so. Support yourself!

Vaginal or labial cysts

Duality in the emotional world: you don't accept or acknowledge yourself the way you really are. You are anxious; you feel dependent on others; you look for confirmation outside yourself, and you might start to play a Role, or you might not spontaneously present yourself the way you are, because of fear of not being accepted by others. Also, sexuality can become a "game" of self-affirmation (see Nymphomania. Don Juanism).

You are so afraid to let go of the other person that you'd rather play an act in order to hold on to that person.

Also the sadness and the anger as a result of experiences from the past are hard for you to let go of — you look too much to the past; your head burns with sad and angry memories.

Or do you play the role of Zorro or Superman? Do others have to believe in you, because you don't believe in yourself? Are you therefore building a job or function of responsibility in order to be adored as a hero, because you don't love yourself enough? You exert yourself to find affirmation in such a way that you swell up with cramped emotional accumulations.

You are good the way you are! Dare to breathe freely! Open your hands to others but don't grab on, don't force things. Independence and self-confidence; feeling happy and free about and around yourself: you don't "need" anybody! First love and accept yourself: only then a happy relationship with someone else will be able to develop itself. Shake off the past from your shoulders and know that the pain which was inflicted upon you in the past already was a result of your inner convictions regarding yourself, in which you were stuck, namely: "I am Just worthless." Open yourself in all honesty and let go off all dark thoughts and feelings . . .

Feel your strong Powers and create! Experience the oneness in yourself: your earthly life built on your fundamentally strong Basis. Take your life in hands yourself.

Vulvar problems

You feel scared, small, and vulnerable; emotionally you close yourself off because of this. Because you are not aware enough of your personal Forces and don't allow them to come through enough — because you deny the leadership in yourself — you may attract someone in your surroundings who gives you the feeling that you are being strangled, as it were: you have no more room to breathe; you would like to withdraw completely; perhaps you play an exterior Role and hide your vulnerable "I." The cause lies in you: a shortage of self-assurance. Because of this, you can no longer open yourself up emotionally toward others; this would only be a "rational" opening-up. Perhaps you don't at all dare to stand up for yourself, and you let others treat you the way they want. You are too much in the spirit, too much in your head; you are on guard against earthly Life, against the love-exchange with others.

You are too little in your own body; you are anxiously on guard. Painful memories from the past have a hold on you. You don't dare surrender to your Self, to your nature, in Love. You are afraid of just being yourself.

Possibly you experience sexuality and feel how your Heart doesn't agree.

Find the balance in yourself: a conscious soul in the body, a complete presence of the heart, warmth in your body. Don't withdraw: dare to sit solidly on your basis and stick up for yourself if necessary! Take good care of yourself and welcome Life, Love! Allow all your forces to come through; no longer hold back; cherish your nature and completely open up your emotional world to yourself. Dare to communicate freely with others; don't be afraid to manifest yourself. Make an end to the convictions that you are weak or that the outer world poses a threat. Outer circumstances only follow inner convictions!

Pain of the outer female sexual organs (vulva, clitoris)

You feel pushed aside — approached in a way that is not loving.

Often, this is a result of not daring to stand up for yourself or not being straightforward, or a hypocritical submission to the sexual game, while your heart is not there. Perhaps you were treated rudely: because you have been suppressing your own "I"-forces for so long. Anxiety and uncertainty. Therefore, stand up for yourself and become aware of your worth and your possibilities as a human being. Only when you respect yourself will others respect you. If you waste yourself, others will take advantage of you. Therefore develop your creativity in a self-aware, steady way, and dare to build up your forces! Be pure and honest in yourself; acknowledge gentleness and love.

Mucous membrane polyps of the female genitalia

Because of fear and inner uncertainty you hold on to many things: you don't dare to trust your own nature. Spontaneous energies and longings are placed in a tight framework. You follow laws and rules within a severe structure.

You feel unsafe and threatened: because of this you might look for strong pillars outside yourself and perhaps will come to adore certain people or systems who will dominate you or bind you. You cling to things or to other people.

The influence from outside is too strong because you are too little inside yourself and you believe too little in your own possibilities. True inner feelings are barely allowed to exist: they always have to step aside for outer or social motives, for material interests — mostly in order to satisfy the expectations of the outer world. You refuse to follow inner laws. In this way, you knot yourself up; you don't really look out of your own eyes, but out of the eyes of others; in this way you suppress yourself, lead a false life, in fact, and will develop a false growth, literally (a polyp) and figuratively.

There's a division in your existence; you see double images: from out of the eyes of others, from out of your inner Self.

Therefore, come toward unity in feeling and action! Allow your energies to come through in self-confidence: feel strong on your own basis, with your feet on the ground! Experience your fundamental powers, your original nature, and no longer block the activity of these sources in you. Allow yourself to become free and spontaneous, without heeding the outer world. Be very honest with yourself; let go of your fears. Life is safe if you seize it with both hands and build it yourself. True evolution, using all your energies instead of false growth and dependency on others.

Fungal infection of the female genitalia
candidiasis
(Read also Fungal infection, in general)

You feel incapable, "seized," and left behind — as a woman you feel hurt, mostly in a love relationship, possibly sexually.

It's really about the bottling-up of your own natural energies, instead of daring to fully experience yourself in self-aware action! You don't really dare to come into contact with your deepest core, don't believe in it enough. Your powerful Mars energies, your self-manifestation, are being suppressed by you! You might show a friendly face to others; you might give in to things that disgust you; you don't really stand up for yourself — but inwardly things are starting to bubble and gnaw away. You feel like you are being seized by the neck; sadness piles up inside you. You force yourself again and again instead of truly living from within your own center. Emotions and suppressed creative energies overflow — you can't handle it anymore; it becomes too much for you. Perhaps you blame it on the behavior of your partner, but it is you who needs to resolutely determine your life and your personal boundaries!

But do you feel too small, too inferior, like a rag? And do you therefore spinelessly allow yourself to be treated so? You carry needless emotional burdens!

Self-respect! Become aware of your worth as a human being and call upon the self-protecting forces deep inside you. Don't lock yourself up; allow creativity — and especially feelings — to flow through: they will confront you with your core. Come outward with your true "I," with your true longings and thoughts; don't play-act. Dare to voice yourself completely, and don't do anything you don't want to do.

Others will respect you only if first you acknowledge your value. Now, come to full development of yourself, and don't direct your life first of all toward your partner: if you take care of your happiness, then your surroundings will undergo the necessary changes for the good of all.

Itching of female genitals

Aggressively nervous thinking about. . . .

You are angry, you experience yourself as a victim, and you'd like to break out with all your bottled-up aggression! But you "think" too much instead of "doing."

Here, it's mostly about suppressed feelings directed at your partner.

Energies are ready to break through, but you keep yourself encapsulated; your forces remain suppressed, and you lead them toward one point — about which you would then make yourself angry instead of coming to true self-realization!

Irritation, probably toward your partner, because you have perhaps allowed yourself to be treated unjustly, or without love: self-protecting energies now orient themselves in an aggressive way. But the true cause lies in the fact that you don't take your life autonomously in hand enough, don't really live Consciously enough, or are not enough present in yourself. You feel bound, seized, your sadness looks for a way out and turns into aggression. Why don't you love yourself? Your patience has come to an end: your inner Authority now asks for a breakthrough. Now, actively take your life in hand!

So far you have managed to fill up your emptiness with "others": therefore don't be angry if this self-negation has called up a dissatisfying relationship.

Energetic powers of creation, creativity: you have repressed it all! This asks for liberation! But you just fret instead of acting, creating. . . .

Allow all energies to flow freely, and no longer stop yourself from developing spiritual and awareness powers also: let yourself go, and produce flexibly. Action! Experience all the forces in your Self, and arrive at complete self-manifestation. Don't get stuck in silent reproach, in negative thoughts. Throw yourself open! In creativity! Speak with your partner in open, true communication and lovingly care for yourself.

In the first place come home to your own feelings, in gentleness, and don't expect anything from someone else. Only when you are completely, Consciously, present in yourself and no longer "need" others, will you be free, and in this freedom you will be able to love yourself and others.

As long as you refuse to come to complete self-fulfillment, beyond the material or the physical, then it's better not to come to sexual intercourse at all. First come to deep emotional experiences, to large creativity from within yourself, because here lies the true cause of aggressive projection toward the outside: arrive at active, Conscious self-realization!

MALE GENITALS

PENIS

Psychological correspondence and function

In a negative sense
The penis represents surrender by the man to the domination of destructive aggression and sexual compulsion. The man who, as a victim of self-negation, degrades himself to become an instrument of unconscious motives, of bestialities. The denial of self-worth; the rejection of his true, divine forces. Sexuality will then be an outlet for his own frustration and emptiness: the penis then represents the channel through which negative emotions such as "losing oneself," self-destruction, or the violent urge for power over others, etc., find their way out. The instrument through which sadness, pain, passion, aggression are discharged in the form of urine or sperm, a gray powerlessness. Sometimes, one is desperately looking for self-affirmation, a search for oneself without end and without solution.

Step out of this vicious circle and first of all come to self-contemplation: the discovery of your true forces, worth, and possibilities is very necessary. Only after all that, can sexual energies be experienced in a totally other way, in completely satisfying feelings of joy, be it via physical love experiences or via energetic experiences which represent inexpressible happiness and creative development.

Sexual experience without first having come to acknowledge and love one's own core leads only to "filling up" one's own emptiness: a bottomless vat that never will be able to carry true happiness within. One "needs" someone else in order to still feel one's worth somehow. An instinctive urge for satisfaction because one ignores the call for something much more beautiful.

One thinks — also in many sects — that "free love" means the true liberation of mankind: here the human being is misleading himself. Nevertheless, this is an understandable reaction to many religious systems which are afraid of anything that has to do with feelings, femininity, sexuality, etc.

In a society where fanatical leaders are being called up, one can go beyond this duality only by rising to another level: the experience of Oneness of the Human being, in the first place of himself! And, as a result, in a true love relationship with the other.

In a positive sense
In the New World, the penis symbolizes the powerful experience of oneness, experienced by the man in himself, without taboos, without frustrations.

Once one has come to "fulfillment" of oneself, sex is no longer an "absolute necessity," but a "possibility."

When, in oneself, integration of the rational and the intuitive has been reached, of the total emotional world — when the total space of "the Human being" is being realized and taken up on a spiritual-physical level — then the man is also able to have contact with a partner in a loving way.

The penis therefore is a symbol of the man's powerful, pure awareness of safety in himself; directed toward the earth, and thanks to this strong, self-assured grounding, it is able to be fertile. Fertility, productivity on many terrains, making use of an atomic energy, driven by consciousness, and able to direct physical, but especially awareness-, powers toward creativity, toward loving care and responsibility for others. This is the symbol of the penis. A man, who — instead of being at the mercy of his powerlessness and frustration — brings forth beautiful fruits because he now rows with his own oars, making conscious use of his potential divine forces, instead of allowing himself to float along on the sea of unconsciousness, of sleeping, threatening anxieties and passions.

For the health of this organ, it's necessary that the man take up his total space.

There doesn't "have to" be sexual unification with a partner in the physical form in order to be completely happy. One *can* have sex, but doesn't need to.

Pain or illness of the penis indicates that one closes oneself off from Life, from broad light, from oxygen, from the wealth of energies and feelings in oneself — if one restricts oneself to physical patterns or to the purely material, or to sex without a deeper feeling of love, or to sex without "feelings" being involved in it, or to structural rules, or to the damming up of one's own potential possibilities.

In other words: the penis that is detached, so to speak, from The Human Being.

Forcing yourself into a restricted space which isn't good for you, instead of liberating yourself completely, leads to constriction (see also the category Foreskin). Dare to blossom freely, trusting in your strong, inner Basis; then the poisonous substances and the ashes of spent fuel will leave along the safety valve that the penis also is.

Stand powerfully, full of trust, on your own feet, and navigate full steam ahead! Proud independence, being proud of your Nature, and in oneness with your physical body, with your Feelings! A beautiful, blessed state of awareness reached via the use of energy, called up by your Consciousness and then physically produced by your sexual glands and hormones: this doesn't have to be experienced in the sexual deed nor in sexuality or masturbation, nor in certain eastern yoga techniques.

Of course, this is all possible, but making use of the "blue" very open, caring, loving, creative energies has, in its full experience, nothing to do with sexuality as such. It does have to do with the feeling, the experience, which lies at the basis of THE PRIMAL CREATION EVENT: an inherent divine feeling of creativity with an immense potential Power!

In the woman this is reflected in the "uterus" and the ovaries; but here in the man as well as in the woman it's about symbolic reflections, and such a powerful creative ability is present in every human being, independent of the presence or absence of certain organs. It is true, however, that by removal of one part or organ, the psychological function immediately can be taken over by an other element of the body.

Glands, hormones, and sexual organs are channels by which we can come to an enormous development of energies and the release of them. These are channels which our Inner Self — the eternal, individual power-source behind our physical body — uses in order to allow new energies to come through.

The more we are aware of the unity with our divine Self, and the more we consciously direct our body toward a new dimension — where aggression and powerlessness no longer exist, where harmony is found within ourselves — the production of hormones by glands will become ever stronger and more efficient, and a man's production will become stronger on many creative levels.

Constant, higher, luminous energies that make one free and happy, and also can exist independent of sexual experience.

Foreskin problems, hardening, inflammation

Unconscious feelings of powerlessness, sadness, frustration, suppressed aggression: you would like to break through, to widen your borders, but you feel stuck — you keep on thinking, and you are more floating in the air than you are on the earth: feelings are being strangled. Your spiritual energy is too strongly present in comparison to your earthly "nature or physical awareness." Partly not-being, a passiveness: you should be getting through something, but you remain immobile — your strong, energetic "Mars" powers turn inward instead of developing themselves outwardly.

In unsureness (you are like a little boy revolting against a bossy mother) you close yourself off; there's a resistance but you don't yet see what way to go, and until then you keep hiding. . . .

This, however, leads to self-electrocution: as you don't operate your own "resilience" and flexible energies, you don't reach liberation. You close yourself off in self-restriction, in unconscious anxiety about getting hurt, not believing in your own "masculine" or powerful, active possibilities, having no clear view of your own Content: you are at a distance from yourself, from your own nature, from your feelings. You don't only close yourself off from yourself but also from others — there's an unconscious fear of being "grabbed" by others, and then of losing the authority over yourself.

Sometimes, there is a remembrance of painful, sad experiences from "a" life, having to do with relationships; because of this you now (inwardly) would like, with all your aggressive force, to smash earthly, bodily contact, the exchange of bodily feelings. As a reaction to your sad experiences, you have pulled your root out of the earth, as it were, and trampled Venus into a thousand pieces.

This unconscious anxiety and pain poses a "Halt!" regarding others. Then you should know that you have already attracted the experiences from the past on the basis of your underlying expectations, thoughts, and convictions (such as: "I am caught in the clutches of the 'female grip,' I am powerless," etc.).

In this attitude of self-defense you ultimately deny your own body, your own flesh and blood: you are tense, and you are not good to yourself.

The deepest cause lies in the conviction that was at the basis of your sad experiences; insufficient belief in your Self-worth, and not believing in your active, powerful qualities — because you don't "know" yourself — lead toward the basic conviction: "I have to protect myself because my content as well as that from other people could possibly be threateningly bad! I cannot completely trust my feelings — I have to watch out for others, because I'm so vulnerable, and they could hurt me. . . ." And precisely this anxiety has called up painful situations in the past.

Why bind yourself so anxiously, when Uranian energies ask for liberation?

Why make yourself so "hard?" Why "narrow" yourself so? Fixating on this with your thoughts will lead to "inflammation" on top of it all.

Don't tighten yourself up so much: enlarge yourself!

If you ground your roots deeply in the earth, then you can go forward with forces rich in energy, and you will be able to calmly relax inside yourself.

No longer flee from confrontation with your deepest feelings (don't stay closed at the surface) and with nature, flesh, the earthly, the feelings around you. No longer live only in your head; bend over the brown sand — be good to the small earthly things; dare to enter into deep communication with your nature. The unconscious anxieties and defensive mechanisms having nothing to do anymore with the reality of the here-and-now: now become master over your compulsive behavior-patterns which overpowered you until now. Open up the curtain, and no longer strangle your emotional world with an iron thread, within a hard structure which doesn't allow flexible existence. Now become a Leader over yourself, so that the fear of true emotional, intimate contact with others will disappear.

First of all, find reconciliation in yourself; no longer hurt yourself; get a good hold on yourself; dare to fully feel all your emotions; no longer run away from the most sensitive part of yourself. No longer stay coldly distant from your own nature, from your own body, from your own penis — stop rejecting it! Follow your nature and don't feel threatened by it.

Hardening asks for "softness and flexibility"; the lock is allowed to be opened. This can only happen if you become aware of the valuable content of your treasure chest full of gold. Believe in your Self!

Narrowing of the foreskin is not "bad" or "unhealthy," and always has its reasons: often it has to do with a "healthy" adjustment. Namely, the female aspect in the man now asks for development in the psyche. Don't force anything.

An operation isn't "obligatory"; feel free inwardly.

*Love is what really matters; you **can** have sexual experiences, but you don't **have to**.*

TESTICLES

Psychological correspondence

The testes are comparable with the ovaries of the woman. Every man has the "female" and the "male" qualities in himself; so does the woman.

In order to keep a healthy balance between both aspects and still keep the outer characteristics one hundred percent male (or female), hormones and other substances in the body fulfill a very specific task.

On the one hand, the testicles represent this "female" aspect, psychologically and physically: a contained, warm, potential energy; receptively being open to awareness-impulses (hormones and other messengers which react to our conscious and unconscious psychological signals), the cradle for the birth of the sperm, the "gold." On the other hand, sperm cells and hormones are produced here in an active "male" manner under the direction of the feelings of our heart as well as of our convictions, which all lie at the basis of this. After all, it's these convictions — the unconscious emotional life and the conscious longings of the heart, the positions we take in ourselves — which stimulate the Hypophysis, the adrenal glands, and the testicles in their production. Sperm, hormones and other substances are being produced in the testes under the command of conscious and unconscious factors: optimal production, a healthy condition of the testicles, will be achieved when, in the man, Unity is experienced between the male and female aspects, between the active, decisive manifestation and intuitive, sensitive, gentle qualities. In the testicles one will find the reflection of the Fullness of the human being who allows himself to be directed firstly by the warm energy of the Heart, there were yin and yang merge, where there is no more dividing line between the divine and the human: this Unity in every man leads to golden productivity, to beautiful creations, to new consciousness energies.

If a man denies in himself this divinity, the Basis of his existence, the eternal living Self — out of which the body has grown after all — and acknowledges only his body or his animalistic sexual urge, then he leaves unexploited the enormous potential of creative energies on many levels.

If he only acknowledges the male element and denies the female, then he burns his potentiality into ashes; or if he suppresses his action and his conscious urge for creativity and keeps wandering around in emotions — without resolutely going onward — then he denies the male element in himself and he will die off. A balanced production of "golden energies," thanks to the loving acknowledgment of his worth as a human being: in this way a man knows himself to be protected in himself, without anxieties. . . .

Direct symbolism

A safe, protected feeling inside yourself; daring to bring your deepest forces out and to manifest yourself in productivity. Giving a warm feeling to yourself and others. On a self-confident basis, daring to go on, to work on, letting your engine run at full speed, swimming onward in Life; a many-sided, creative development, without anxieties. Handing on this rich creativity and sharing it with others. Not frustrating yourself by suppressing feelings and creativity. The courage to go onward, to create from out of your deepest Self: overcoming doubts and allowing emotions, energies, to flow freely, without reservation. Victory over: "no I don't dare. . . ." Once you go on, you will experience nothing but liberation and relaxation. An experience of unity in yourself: potential emotional content (the "female aspect") and decisive creation (the "male aspect"). A fullness which reaches far beyond animalistic sex or making children.

Ailments, in general

The anxiety and vulnerability of a man who denies his inner Power, of a man who considers himself "weak" or considers his power only "physical" or "macho," superficial.

Illness or pain indicate self-underestimation here; he feels anxious and vulnerable because he cuts himself off from his deepest "I," from his intuitive, inner source. Perhaps he positions himself in subordination to others, or to an authority outside himself, without his being aware of his full worth. Or does he only prove himself in sexual achievements, in a job or a function with a Feather in his hat. Inwardly, does he feel small? He knows the game of power and powerlessness, but the true, large creativity on the basis of his enormous potential energies is unknown to him. A painful shrinking of his existence to the superficial, to the materialistic or animalistic compulsiveness, to the strictly rational, excluding the beautiful, deeper emotional life.

A feeling of not being safe: "They are going to grab me, hurt me, break me emotionally." Anxious mistrust as a result of closing himself off from his own deeper Source. He cuts himself off. Feelings are being put behind locked doors.

Small, cold, unpleasant, vulnerable, powerless in a dark world: those are the consequences of being at a distance from one's own divine Nature. The man experiences himself as empty, as a vat of feelings which need to be mistrusted; he feels at the mercy of others, weak because his Conscious "I" is absent.

He'd like to manifest himself outwardly to the outer world! But his mouth anxiously gasps for breath, because inwardly he feels small. He can't really stand up for himself and say why he feels so hurt. So he will hide in a role, in a certain attitude or in a boxing glove (the fucking), frustrated. Perhaps he turns away from contact with others.

Solution: see the category "Testicles, psychological correspondence and symbolism."

Sperm cells

Psychological causes of overproduction

Primitive instincts and desires control your life. You are not aware of values and possibilities in yourself: you are fixated on others; you would "draw in" relationships, attract others, want to feel as if they are in your power.

A feeling of emptiness, powerlessness, or of "being at the mercy of your own emotions, which you are not able to handle," so to speak. This leads to aggressive behavior, which can get out of hand.

Psychological cause of underproduction or no production

Anxiety, unsureness, feeling threatened.

Often you are afraid of your own emotions, of your Natural longings. You think you are "bad" or at least susceptible to being seized by deeper feelings inside you, which you distrust.

Or you feel oppressed, suffocated, in a certain situation, in a pattern of life that thus far you have maintained (contrary to what is sometimes being said, tight jeans are only a reflection of this, but not the true cause); you want to break out! You would like to get free from a terrifying, lonely feeling — they will get you, you feel bound. You experience life as a dark tunnel. Where did you come from? Where is the end?

These deep-rooted emotions have a paralyzing effect on productivity and creativity.

This symbolizes the anxiety in the man about the "female" aspect in himself, about the "Unconscious," about the emotional world. The male and female aspect can't get into harmony with each other; he would run away from the intuitive, emotionally rich aspect, sometimes also literally from a relationship with a "woman."

Balanced production and positive psychological correspondence of spermatozoa

When the intuitive, emotional aspect and the rational, logical, sober aspect reconcile with each other — when the "man" and the "woman" in every human being merge into one — then this will lead to a new consciousness; then this peace will give birth to a higher level of productivity in the head, in the heart. Then one doesn't "need" one's partner, but is able to really love the other person. With the Force of the "I"-consciousness, the man throws from his shoulders, in full freedom, the dark threat of the unconscious or the emotional: there's nothing that can threaten him! Black and white kiss each other; yin and yang are taken up in each other. Or: the conscious and unconscious intertwine on the basis of a very strong Trust in the forces of the autonomous, Self-aware, creative "I."

This unity in himself will lead the man toward creativity on a high level: there is creation in the head, in the heart — this brings about beautiful fruits. The living, the exploiting, of these forces rich in energy, will offer the man beautiful experiences in the area of general awareness-creativity as well as in relationship experiences: an experience which goes far beyond the physical, which can be experienced without or with the bodily contact of both partners. The fruits that come forth out of such relationships are then creations, or children, of happiness, of harmony, meant for life, not for death.

The sperm cells as such can be implanted as physical seed in reality, but it won't be necessary anymore: children can be born out of the corresponding power fields (in the man as well as in the woman) as products of true love-energies, no longer as products of sexual intercourse on the physical level.

There can be an ejaculation of sperm, but it isn't a necessity. The creative energies, the consciousness forces that come free — an activation by the "I" of the hormone and gland system — don't ask for a sperm ejaculation; it's allowed, but it's of no importance. The child can be the fruit of a loving human creation, not of the necessary merging of the sperm cell and the egg cell in the physical form. But the future is not "fixed" or "predetermined." May everyone listen carefully to the signals Life itself emits, and act upon them; then everything will go brilliantly.

Testosterone hormone
male sexual hormone

Overproduction of testosterone: psychological cause

You don't take up your worthy place as a Human being: you feel like a zero in an empty barrel. You don't come to true productivity; you leave your beautiful, creative energies unexploited; you live like a "zombie" or like a slave of society, stubborn, obsessed by superficial sex or by other "fillers of emptiness" in which you can't find true happiness or real satisfaction, because you keep yourself cut off from your deepest Self, from your deeper emotional values, from your Powerful inner "I." You don't really live consciously! You allow yourself to "be lived": unconsciously.

Your body, the glandular system, works as a feedback system in reaction to psychological impulses. If you are stuck with feelings of living in an unconscious, or senseless way, then this situation is being transferred — via registration in the brain — to the hypophysis, which can automatically react to this through producing, for instance, the ICSH hormone, which will stimulate the testicles to produce the testosterone hormone because this hormone is exactly the bearer of very broad, powerful awareness-energies. One can translate these energies into Self-manifestation as a reaction to the feeling of being a "zero." The man, however, often translates this overproduction of testosterone into exaggerated or frustrated deeds; instead of this, he'd better use these energies freely for the building up of his self-awareness with a greater consciousness of his own divine worth. In this way, he can finally come to greater fulfillment of his value and to productivity in life! Becoming conscious, insight: the only solution here.

Underproduction of testosterone: psychological cause

You are not enough present in your body, too much in the spirit. Powerless anxieties. You are not really present on earth, often out of fear of the decline or destruction of life, of all earthliness. . . . Your hands are cold and absent, instead of your experiencing life with your flesh and blood. You don't get a grip on your earthly Self.

Perhaps you fear (unconsciously) that if you surrender completely to earthliness it will hurt you all the more to have to leave it behind afterwards: fear of pain.

Possibly, you hallucinate; you are too much with your head in the clouds, your feet hardly feeling the earth. Perhaps you see devils or negative punishing gods, who don't at all exist but perhaps you were taught that way — and the anxiety makes you withdraw into an unreal world. You have turned away from reality or from earthliness.

Do you flee from "the human being in his natural body?" Do you flee from contact with others? Do you flee from love: love for yourself and others? Helpless.

Balanced production and psychological correspondence of testosterone

A great, powerful, roomy feeling! You posses the ability to break through all limiting boundaries and to Live in a self-aware, resolute, and autonomous way! Daring to bring yourself into contact with your deeper feelings, with your instincts, beginning to experience them consciously, and transforming them into bright consciousness forces! Experiencing the earth in an intense, sensorial way (smelling, tasting. . . .) and experiencing optimal cooperation between your body/feelings and your consciousness/mind.

Allowing your outer ego to exist in harmony with your inner Self: not taking on an "attitude," no macho behavior, not trying to "fill up" emptiness with things or persons outside yourself or with "outer" activities, but living from out of your deepest "I." Inner sureness and awareness of your worth! Allow your feelings to open up freely; don't block yourself with reactions of fright or flight.

Dare to begin relations with others from out of this powerful "I"-basis; don't lock yourself up in an ivory tower, nor in unauthentic, superficial behavior.

A balanced production of testosterone indicates the flow of unconscious forces toward a conscious experience, in a gradual process. It indicates a constant transformation of hidden emotions and subterranean instincts into great, expansive energies of awareness! At least if you wish it so. . . .

Epididymitis
inflammation of sperm duct near testicle

You cherish the gold outside you instead of being aware of your own worth. You restrict your life to a half-black, cold, sober, material, deathly, surly, severe, or stingy affair, where there is no room for true warmth or joy. In your existence, a stern Saturn plays the lead; you will fix your attention on duties, Authority, on structure. Merciless toward yourself and possibly also toward others: you seem to be closed off from your heart, from your core of consciousness. You hurt yourself; true life-motivation is absent. Even if you are angry, you will destroy yourself inwardly, instead of bringing it all out. You call up false gods in life (money, religion, authorities) instead of discovering your own wealth; you keep a piggy bank instead of exploiting your potential talents. You dwell upon certain negative things so that you hinder yourself from evolving.

Warm joy: you are allowed to belong! Don't stab yourself to ruin, bring out your aggression, speak. Deal with your emotions, your experiences, your pains, and see how you, yourself, with your negative attitude regarding life, have attracted negative circumstances. Look at life now in all its richness of color; come to joyful creativity! Revise certain things; don't dwell on the negative, because in this way you just reinforce it. Don't crunch your teeth until they break, but chew everything thoroughly: digest that which you now are needlessly holding on to. Produce, go on! Acknowledge the sun in yourself, your worth.

Orchitis
inflammation of a testicle

You are cut off from your personal "power center," from your fundamentally strong Self.

Tensely, you keep yourself standing; you might force yourself (perhaps like a hypocrite) to come outward in a certain way, without daring to reveal your true nature. You hide your feelings, and you act like nothing's the matter. You might present yourself as stronger than you feel inwardly. You feel wounded; someone has hurt you but you "stay friendly" toward those who have pained you. Inwardly, however, you fixate your thoughts with vengeance or in powerless fury on that which has hurt you so. (You'll pay him back for it!) Your thoughts are heavy and suffocating: with held-back aggression you direct them toward "others," instead of realizing that it's first of all you who doesn't live in openness and honesty. After all, the true cause of your pain lies in yourself "closing yourself off, hiding yourself behind a protecting mask," by not daring to experience yourself, your nature, to the fullest! Are you afraid of the reaction of others, of the devil or of one or another religious law?

Your feelings, your spontaneity, are encased in a hypocritical or artificial structure which ties up all nature.

Unconsciously, you'd like to shoot at those who dare to permit themselves to live naturally and spontaneously, at those who might mock you because of your narrow-mindedness or your restricted life. Are you constantly angry? You prefer not to let it be noticeable. . . . But your real creativity in life is being suppressed by yourself: don't blame others! Your powerlessness and anxieties are the principal problem!

"Nature" in all its forms is "divine": don't put up any obstacles against it.

Don't cling to false, superficial, narrow structures or visions. Allow your feelings to flow through, go on steadily, and don't stand still, obsessed by vengeful, or bad, thoughts! See the relativity, laugh about it, and discover the child inside you: spontaneity, productivity — discover your multitude of possibilities for self-realization! Dare to throw yourself into Life without hesitation and don't stay woodenly locked up inside your-

self! Instead of being angry it's better to bring yourself, in all openness, to realization, with all your powers.

Testicular tumor

You don't dare, or you refuse, to look at your personal power and possibilities! Bottled-up energies, kept-in forces, repressed action — suppression!

Your spontaneous feelings ask for a full and free existence, but they are put within a metal mantle, in a structure which is too severe. Your valuable energies flow away like liquid gold in a sewer. You don't allow yourself to be faithful to your true disposition; you are now estranged from your own nature; perhaps you feel totally separate from your body.... All your precious energies are burning up: you don't come to real development of your talents. On the contrary, you allow others to direct your life; you feel hurt, but actually it is you who are wrecking yourself by suppressing healthy, natural aggressiveness, action, emotions.... Your creativity is allowed to exist only in a very limited way: "narrow spirituality" or "narrow thinking."

You live and exist only via a structure, a job, or a system, but you are cut off from your strong Basis, from your foundation on Earth! Perhaps you have a big mouth but don't really come to true action! Possibly, you live spiritually, or in the head, to such an extent that you have swept emotions and earthly experiences to the side!

Don't deny the essence of your being; experience your human existence in its entirety: live your feelings and allow all those emotions to flow freely — come to respect yourself and live from out of the warmth of your heart, not from rules and regulations forced upon you (by others or by yourself).... YOUR ESSENCE!

Don't suppress your very personal, powerful, fiery energies; don't be afraid of your nature; build primitive forces into Conscious creativity!

If you choose Life, then stop self-destruction. No longer refuse to look at yourself and all your Forces!

Testis, undescended

You'd prefer to hide yourself behind a shield, anxious, on guard. You experience the "descent" into life as a limitation. Your emotions and awareness powers are only allowed to exist within certain boundaries, and that frightens you; you bring yourself into question because of it. "Can I trust myself?" Fear of pain; life frightens you somehow: in a war zone you might build a bunker. You feel suffocated, without room to breathe. If you were born in a milieu where one is a slave of Image and outer appearance, of structures and laws (for instance the baby *has* to drink something every four hours, etc.), where, because of their own oppression, parents unconsciously radiate powerless aggression toward you as a baby, then this will just enhance your feeling of being strangled. But you actually call up this situation unconsciously in order to deal with your anxieties.

You feel oppressed in life and vulnerable. You mistrust yourself; actually you are not open to love; you'll be angry and will protest against the person who, according to your feelings, smothers you; a pushing away, a refusal. You even suspect the mafia to be behind the village fair, hypocrisy behind formality; anxiously, you look in all directions. You are also afraid to do wrong; possibly this is reflected in an upbringing in which you are not allowed to cry too much or show your emotions, in which, as a child, you have to keep yourself properly to the rules; possibly your mentors suffocate themselves in this way. In an anxious way you hold in your emotions. Don't you think yourself to be good unless you answer to the expectations of others? Are you ashamed of yourself? Don't you dare to freely take up your room to breathe?

It's necessary that mother and child listen to their nature and don't force themselves within tight, structural laws. Every child has its own disposition and requires a unique way of being handled. Here, the emphasis will be on safety, Trust, on the one hand, and natural freedom on the other. Every human being has to determine his own boundaries, to take his time, not to withdraw in himself, but to dare push through to the outside when the time is specifically ripe for him. This shouldn't be forced. If the parents also build their lives on inner wisdom and seek their safety in their deepest Self, not being afraid of truly being themselves, and living according to their own unique nature, then the baby will receive good influences, then it won't be so afraid anymore to descend into earthly life. (Although it has to be emphasized that the "cause" lies in the psyche of the child and that no "blame" has to be put on the parents. Read more about this in Part I, the category Children.)

PROSTATE GLAND

Psychological correspondence and Ailments, in general

Acknowledgement of Divine Mastery. No self-degradation.

Knowing for sure what direction you want to take without inner contradictions! A feeling of thankfulness and peace about yourself, about your Being. Awareness of self-worth. A beautiful flow of energies (feelings, action, etc.) and a free discharge of too much, or of waste matter, after a balanced digestion of experiences, of emotions.

Daring to be yourself in all openness; being immediately able to clear up problems or hidden things in the light of your Consciousness! Not living in chaos or confusion; not allowing yourself to be pushed to the side by others or by your anxieties. Self-leadership! TO BE — without desires. Being HUMAN — not an animal.

This gland is a *Guardian* at the threshold; it takes care that a man exploits to the fullest, or transforms, his gathered experiences and the forces produced by him; it makes sure that he, in full awareness of his personal values, does not waste any energies, does not develop an excess of self-destructive feelings, nor throw away into oblivion his divine nature and emotional richness. The prostate: a self-controlling function in relation to the inner, spontaneous Authority that every being carries within himself. Only this inner Authority will know whether feelings are being suppressed or not, whether in a disdainful way, one bypasses the human, joyful longings for enjoyment, for truly Living and creating on many levels! If one listens to another authority instead of to one's own inner Knowledge — for instance to the authority of know-it-all leading figures in communities or systems who would put a human being on chains by forbidding him to do this or that — in that case the prostate gland will react. Do you look more toward suffering and sadness, punishment, self-castigation, obligation, structural restriction, to what society or others oblige you to do or forbid you? Do you refuse to listen to your natural, inner Authority? Then a free flow will become impossible.

Do you degrade yourself? Don't you know that life means JOY? Do you deny your personal longings and your feelings? Do you suppress your emotions or creative energies? The prostate watches, and no longer allows things to go through, if you keep breaking yourself down in this way! Do you limit your life to "thoughts" of sex, to materialism?

So be aware of your Worth; put on your royal crown and — only under the mastery of yourself — allow all feelings and creative forces to flow freely now, without frustration or self-restriction! Don't hold on to things or persons; don't block things; discharge your feelings; don't "constrict" your life; listen to your inner voice — be faithful to your nature, to your individual disposition, which no one can experience in your place. Don't live like an automaton or a robot, nor like a Spirit.

The prostate sees that a balance is kept between bodily experience and awareness-energies; one doesn't *need* to be sexually active for this! Physical awareness, the experience of "matter," always happens in relation to your Consciousness: Being, creating, enjoying — an intense presence of your "I" in your body.

Neglect neither one: achieve unity in yourself, and certainly don't withdraw into a spiritual ivory tower. Live with both feet on the Earth! Only when you are completely present in yourself and dare to acknowledge the worth of your nature in an autonomous way, will the prostate then sound the triumphal bell, and poisonous matter will rather quickly, without any problem, be able to leave the body via the urine.

Don't hurt yourself: experience yourself as a worthy human being of flesh and blood! Come to clear insight into yourself! Stand up for your personal rights; dare to unfold your energies, and don't allow yourself to burn away — don't allow yourself to "be lived," but blow the big horn yourself! Replace chaos with peace, and "forbidden" with "permitted" . . . TO LIVE!

Superficiality with profundity!

Desires with Enlargement of your Consciousness, and with emotional experiences that are "full of Love"!

Cancer of the prostate
(See also Prostate, in general)

You restrict yourself; you flee! Like a fish that just blows bubbles. . . . You lower yourself.

You put on blinders; perhaps you escape into material comfort or in one or another fake existence. Perhaps you seem stalwart and strong to the outside, as if your delicate emotional life doesn't exist, but in fact there's sadness in you; you resign yourself to it.

Instead of fully rowing into the stream of life in a resolute way, you undermine yourself — you close your eyes to what you don't like to see, but you don't really react from within your inner soul-center!

In fact, you feel incapable, unable to live to the fullest; you experience yourself as inadequate, not able to — perhaps you complain about "sexual inability," but then this is only a camouflage for your true inability: your inability to experience your *true* forces. Or do you possibly restrict your life to thoughts about sex? You are anxious about being yourself! You don't allow your deeper emotional world to come through: you are afraid of it. You are convinced, in fact, that you don't have a solid basis: you deceive yourself into thinking that you are weak and unable to truly manifest yourself as a worthy Man.

You restrict your life extremely: you neglect your feelings; you suppress actual creativity; you slump into boring routines; you don't dare to push back these borders because you don't trust your deepest Self.

You refuse all contact with your fundamentally strong inner Self; a refusal to see your own divinity. On the contrary, you'd sooner see yourself as bad, or perhaps even as having devilish characteristics. Powerlessness, anxiety, pain, sadness.

You close yourself off and refuse all growth. Stopping is as good as killing yourself.

Where is your powerful, self-aware "I"? You degrade yourself unreasonably! You are filled to the brim with emotions and creative potential, but you prefer to stay blind to it. You break down your Worth as a human being; your self-negation leads to inner tensions and bottled-up emotions.

The zipper of your beautiful emotional world has been closed mercilessly; you have hung your powerful "I" on the peg.

Do you feel guilty? Do you think you are not worthy of Living? Why do you take away your right to thankfully enjoy life?

Acknowledge the totality of your being-HUMAN! Enjoy with your senses, explore yourself and the world around you. Come to open creativity and take up all your space. Dare to dive into your emotional world: surrender to it. It will be your rescue and your healing. Via this emotional flow, you end up close to your deepest Self, the eternal living Self, which constantly directs your body.

Break with negative and anxious convictions regarding yourself and Life; they are lies. Don't restrict yourself to the surface, to structures, to the mechanical or the sexual; discover your wealth of feeling and share it with others. No longer lock yourself up. Allow all your emotions to flow through without hindrance, don't bottle up or hoard, but in self-confidence discover your possibilities. Action and expression: but not at the "surface." Deepen your existence.

Hypertrophy
of the prostate
enlargement

You keep fruits and productivity outside yourself; you don't integrate it. It seems as if a punishing god or Tribunal will judge and decide your life; this Eye you might place outside yourself in the form of severe laws, in an Authority above your head, but first of all it is present INSIDE yourself. This means that you keep a close watch — possibly also recalling indoctrination from your youth — that "female" characteristics (See Left Body Half), your natural feelings, intuitive creativity, physical enjoyment, stay strictly separated from you; in other words a split appears.

In this way you have an ailing communication with yourself, with others, even if it seems to be different.

This can lead toward frustrated thoughts concerning sexuality, because of which you will condemn yourself even more and will tighten the reins of your nature. The other extreme is also possible: you restrict your "potency" to sexuality or thoughts about sexuality and material things. In so doing, heart and feelings are being suppressed.

You are too distant from your own nature, from your beautiful emotional life; a disturbance in the contact with others is only a result of this. You smother the child in yourself; you live very strongly in your head with worries and thoughts, but it seems as if your head is cut off from the rest of your body, just as your thoughts seem to be cut off from your deepest content; a rude interference in yourself. Are you possibly afraid of your deep feelings — of those inner forces — because you condemn it all as being bad and frivolous? This is because you deny the deep values of yourself, because you refuse to open yourself up to intuition and consciousness powers which go beyond the rational mind, beyond business or one-sided "spirituality." You deny the unity between body/feelings and Consciousness. You deny your creative ability to self-create your life. With limited thoughts, you see life as a Calvary, which needs to be suffered, without your being able to do anything about it. You don't really live from out of your true nature. You are a wicked Stepmother to yourself!

You force your life into structures and norms; you check yourself, as it were, with the chronometer. The way a hot-air balloon finally lands on the earth, so does the prostate call you back to your Nature, to your earthly being, swollen from thinking and poor in Life: listen to your feelings, to your body, to your true creative forces. No longer be so distant from your earthly being; allow fire-red forces to escape into true life.

Listen to what the child in you longs for and allow it to enjoy, to eat sweets, to be cheerful. Follow that spontaneity in yourself; don't be hard and restricting, or critical and reprimanding, toward yourself.

In anxiety and tension you have fled from yourself, possibly into the narrow spiritual domain, possibly into the materialistic or purely primitive domain. Both indicate only an escape from your original safe nature.

You cut yourself off from that divine basis in yourself so that you no longer trust life, and in fear need to look outside of yourself for a "god" (for instance, the god of materialism, of sex, of. . .), who then again will burden you with certain obligations and rules. Step out of this armor! You fall down under the cross you want to carry yourself: Why?

When you place the Authority in yourself; when you listen to your nature in all openness; when you dare to fall back on that fundamentally strong Core inside you; when you are honest with yourself and with your feelings and no longer flee from them; when you take off the sterile garment and dare to stand naked in your Nature — then the prostate will relax again, because she, as guardian at the threshold, watches that the Male and Female element in you live together in harmonious unity. A solid, big building, your Male "I" amidst a paradise of natural plant growth, (your sensitive, fertile, female characteristics). Be fertile: all those potential forces inside you, your rich emotions, your talents, your expressive possibilities, your creativity, the sensorial richness of earthly life, all fragrances and colors, enjoyment — give openness to your Fertile, powerful Self. Open all the windows instead of locking yourself up in your Tower.

In order to have a healthy prostate it is necessary that you break through a Wall, so that you come close to yourself, so that your emotional life becomes complete Movement instead of immobility.

Inflammation
of the prostate
prostatitis

You are looking for happiness, you pursue it; you can't find it because you look at everything from below and because you are looking for it outside of yourself. You don't really live in warmth, in joy about your earthly being: you don't allow your true Mars powers, your consciousness energies, to flow freely, because you fixate yourself on things like money, prestige, possessions, or, possibly, superficial sex.

You don't really live from out of yourself; you feel imprisoned, isolated, because in an artificial way you separate the female and male aspect in yourself. Helpless, sad, you can't get a grip on anything because you cut yourself off from your deeper feelings. You are afraid of your emotional forces. You are not really present in your body with a warm heart.

With cold feet, separate from the warm earth, with worrisome negative thoughts, you allow your life to flow toward death: you deny your deeper worth; you are not really productive. You close yourself off from others; you get excited about futilities; you linger over unimportant things, you pass by the real life; you live in confusion, and because you cut yourself off from your Basis, you will bring yourself into question: "Who am I really?" Have you become like a parrot who says what others say, or an anonymous citizen with many faces but who refuses to acknowledge the unique greatness of himself? You look for a hold outside yourself, and you anger yourself about things that are really unimportant in life. You experience frustration; productive forces ask for an actual breakthrough of yourself, on many levels, no longer treating your feelings in a stepmotherly fashion.

This can only happen if you live in joy and thankfulness regarding yourself. No longer restrict your life in this way, controlling it tightly, but dare to accept your femininity, your feelings, and to express them. Don't immobilize yourself but open the sluice and allow emotions to come through freely; let go of sadness from the past and turn toward the Present. Sensuality, earthliness, the sensorial, enjoyment of food and drink, of music and flowers, of your body, and of communication with others in a loving, affectionate way. Render yourself the honor you deserve, and stop looking upon yourself as a "low" being; acknowledge your worth and your productive possibilities. Now bring yourself to realization and transform bottled-up aggressive forces into action and fruitful self-development. No longer doubt your worth; dare to be open toward your deepest feelings; look for happiness in yourself, not outside yourself. Thankfulness for life itself. In mastery, you lead the natural forces; you participate in a joyful way in the earthly existence in the flesh. You don't lock yourself up in your head. Give yourself the chance to spread fertile seeds on many fields: discover your depth, your talents, your wishes, your longings, your pleasure — on the worthy level of Love and self-respect.

INFERTILITY, STERILITY

The ingrained conviction-system of Humanity says that women have to bear children, and that this is possible thanks to the fertile sexual relationship between man and woman. Because of these convictions, women think they can't get pregnant without this sexual relationship.

Such convictions work in an indoctrinating and restricting way, but they are no "absolute truths"! Neither is it necessary that a woman MUST have children in order to be considered a worthy human being even though small-minded society often expresses condemnation. This is nonsense, restriction, which humanity now has to abolish. Sterility asks for your SELF-ACKNOWLEDGMENT, for LIVING YOURSELF.

If one absolutely wants a child out of urgent emotional needs, or because one wants to "have" it, then this is in fact not so good for the child! If a child is necessary to fill up our own "needs" or even our own "emptiness," then it's better not to bring a child into the world.

True fertility means: "the acknowledgment of one's own creative forces, active productivity on several levels." If one isn't able to fructify or become pregnant, then this is a clear signal from the Living Self, in which one always can trust.

Know that when you don't get "pregnant," your deepest Self is not allowing it because at the moment it is not good for you. Several reasons, be they unconscious, are causing this. Perhaps you have unconsciously chosen completely different, large goals, whereby you will be fertile in a very broad scope: don't cling to obsessive thoughts about "pregnancy." Follow your nature: follow your primitive, spontaneous natural forces without placing yourself under the "spell of a so-called curse," which you call up yourself, without tightening yourself up emotionally through fretting and brooding. Trust in this: if you are not fertile in this area, then this clearly has its reasons without your being "inferior" or "bad" or "incapable." That has nothing to do with it. First and foremost, it's a sign for you that you have to be completely open to yourself: feel the fullness of yourself; offer love to yourself; allow your spontaneous, natural forces to exist freely; don't restrict your life to "working," to "caring for others," to "satisfying the needs of your partner, the people around you," but *live* from out of yourself and enjoy! If one "needs" someone like a "baby" in order to be really happy, then something is wrong. You need yourself: no longer fixate on the ancient, inveterate conviction that one must have a child before one can be completely happy. Every child is an individual by itself, and is no possession, but is an autonomous being — no matter if it concerns your own children or the children of a "complete stranger."

Almost always, this is forgotten. A child is no possession. The children of the world are also your children, just as if you would have borne them yourself. It's exactly that strong dependency — the emotional tie which is too strong between mother and child — that hinders a child from growing up in its own autonomous Force, aware of the ability to constantly nourish itself from its inner Self, without having to feel "lonely" or deserted.

Love doesn't ask for an "emotional" tie, for a "blood-tie," but asks for an exchange of unconditional loving feelings between two beings, without harrowing dependency!

Acknowledge the joyful child in your own inner being; receive with open arms the children of the world, who are nobody's possession. Live and enjoy. If it's good that you "physically" bear a child, then you will become pregnant in a spontaneous way without your having to do something special for it, such as taking hormones or having special checkups performed on you. Neither the age to become pregnant nor the age to die are determined: it tends toward infinity. Let go of it all; in joy, concentrate on the Now; trust in the inner reasons that prevent you from being pregnant. No longer feel yourself in the grip of a fixation; let go of these thoughts, and build the solid foundations of your own house. You are "without child" not because you are doomed, but because your Living, divine Self has other beautiful intentions: another fertility now has to be recognized. Spread your arms wide, opening yourself to all possible experiences; know that, when it will be good for you to be pregnant, you will be. Make an end to ossified, rusty convictions; don't put limits on your life, nor on the duration of your life, nor on your "fertility" or creativity. Completely relax, enjoy life; don't exert yourself for anything; follow your longings; never force yourself. Your nature shows you the way; it knows very well what it does. . . .

PUBIC BONE

Psychological correspondence in women as well as in men

Protection — safety — shelter — covering. . . . Pain or ailments of the pubic bone

indicate insufficient faith in your own self-protecting energies; you are afraid that someone might hurt you on the intimate or sexual level. Have you allowed someone to penetrate into your most intimate emotional life? Do you feel, as a woman, to be the slave of a man (or vice versa)? Do you feel used? Left alone? Do you have a hollowed-out feeling? Then fill Yourself with the security of those self-protecting forces. If you trust your own invulnerability, then you won't be hurt as long as you don't wish so. In a self-aware way mark off your terrain and don't suppress your creative energies.

SEXUAL HORMONES, IN GENERAL

What is "too much," what is "too little"? It's not up to the human being to start placing himself above Life and beginning to determine how and what the human being is supposed to be. . . . A black-white separation between "man" and "woman" is absurd, and it also stamps people in an unhealthy way. Every human being does well experiencing his own original nature, without attaching norms to it. Why does a man have to be muscular? Why is a woman not allowed to have a beard? Let's not limit and suppress ourselves and put ourselves in boxes.

"TOO MUCH" or "TOO LITTLE" therefore means: one experiences, inwardly as well as physically, an unpleasant unbalance because of health reasons.

The term "man" means the human being who is born in a body with outer male sexual characteristics, and "woman" means that human being who is born with what we thus far call a "female body."

"Man" with too much male hormone

Causes:
The "unconscious" life, the spontaneous child inside you: you are not interested in it, close yourself off from it. Hard self-manifestation. You think conceitedly that you can do without others. You take who you want: you draw them toward you. You are especially interested in your own well-being and in the superficial, physical life. You work and live in business and administrative material frameworks, being heedless of emotional worlds. Cut off from your source, from your Living Self. Stubborn. Are you so afraid of your deepest Self, or are you blind to it?

Dare to relax, to acknowledge the child inside you. Dare to be open to your deepest feelings and all that is hidden under the surface. Feel flexible in your own skin; don't be too hard, not with yourself, nor with others. Surrender to your gentleness, your heart, your intuition, to your total self.

Become Aware of your divine forces of creation, of your wide spectrum of creative possibilities.

"Man" with too little male hormone

Causes:
You can't make any contact with your Self, as it were, with your earthly Being. You feel just like a sugar doll, powerless, unable to fulfill the task or obligations which you require of yourself. You would force yourself then, would reach further than you can — with cold, long fingers you would "grab" for something, for someone, in order to rescue yourself or defend yourself. Sometimes this feeling of powerlessness makes you aggressive! It can degenerate into lust for power, into sadistic power-games, etc., because in your heart you feel as if the world mistreats and misuses you as a child. In fact it is you who doesn't feel able to deal with a strong, mature world; you think you can't handle it all; you feel so insignificant — helpless, at the mercy of others.

Don't take it out on others; become aware of your "I"-worth!

Let yourself stand up and leave the power-game alone. Self-manifestation from within your deep awareness of self-respect. Working out traumas and thoughts of inferiority.

Place all power inside yourself: don't allow others to have a grip on your life.

"Man" with too much female hormone

Causes:
You feel small; you'd like to hide behind a camouflage-screen; "A man is not allowed to be afraid, a woman is. . . ." An escape from the male aspect, from the hard father; you don't see the sense of things anymore; you feel powerless and defenseless. You'd rather identify yourself with the small, shy woman, who's fleeing from the threatening, dark shadow of the male aspect, which might crush you. You'd like to call up a physical way of rejecting the hard, male aspect in order to keep it at a distance (odors, development of breasts, etc.)

You feel ashamed, unable, an old man — you don't know what to do with your gentle feelings, with your female aspect, but still you'd like to be taken hold of by others, loved by others; on the other hand you are afraid of being "grabbed"; inner confusion and self-doubt.

Acknowledge to the fullest your own gentle, sensitive nature as a man: for that you don't have to be born as a woman!

As a man you are allowed to be gentle; don't flee from it, but also acknowledge the powerful, active, manifesting part of you.

"Man" with too little female hormone

Causes:
Self-betrayal: you deny your divine, deepest Self; you are at a distance from your deepest emotional life. Your attitude is sometimes called arrogant or conceited, also because you appear so hard, so functional or mechanical, so critical, cold. You are so hard and demanding on yourself that you can come into an extremely tense situation; you no longer breathe freely, perhaps you suffer from hyperventilation. Your outer ego is clear, but where is your deeper personality? Why this prohibition sign? Do you look down on the female aspect? Are you afraid of your feelings? You don't know it yourself anymore, because you gradually sink deeper into the ground, into the structure in which you are imprisoned. Perhaps you look for shelter in the woman outside of you; you "need" a partner because in fact you feel one-sided and weak.

But the woman you embrace will be just as one-sided, and you'll be "needed" in her life: this can't be called love. Possibly, you experience yourself as a tough gorilla; perhaps you feel like you are bad and obliged to behave only as a macho or bully. Because you don't know whether you have a deeper, gentle side and whether you are allowed to surrender to it?

"Woman" with too much female hormone

Causes:
You would like to come into action, but bottled-up emotions keep you from it.

You stay where you are, too immobile, but with inner tensions; knotted up in the stomach. You keep on thinking and brooding. Inner conflict: your thinking keeps you from intuitively and resolutely following that path that is best for you. You doubt yourself too much; you don't see your content clearly: "Who am I?" Your Self-aware "I" is too absent.

Action! Organize your life; make a structure, in balance, and don't neglect the intuitive nor the rational while doing so. Self-assured decisiveness. Onward!

"Woman" with too little female hormone

Causes:
You stay closed up, with inner aggression. On the other hand you lack a binding factor, a center in which your existence should be concentrated. Degeneration, as it were; a letting-go of necessary, powerful energies.

A woman who no longer takes care of herself, perhaps because she has put her life again and again at the service of others: now you are stuck, sad, disenchanted or dissatisfied, half dead — because you would like to reach for others and cherish them, but to Open yourself up is difficult for you.

You are stuck fast, still, empty, and dry: your "I"-force ebbs away. You live at a distance from your own gentle feelings. Don't you think it's worthwhile to live for yourself?

Become aware of all your feelings: be OPEN to your rich content, to your Worth; don't make yourself hard. Dare to cry — don't bottle it all up until it becomes a big cake of suppressed anger and irritation.

Be happy to be able to offer your helpfulness to others but also be sensitive to your own needs. Develop again your flexibility; become supple. Be present in your feelings, and Consciously get a hold of yourself. Discover fruitful productivity and come to life: experience those creative energies in your womb and radiate them out from your concentrated "I"-center. Carry your scepter like a queen.

"Woman" with too much male hormone

Causes:

With blinders before your eyes: you hide yourself from your gentle, sensitive side, which you possibly condemn as "weak." In certain cases, this can be a reaction to the fact that you have been taught that "The man is strong, and the woman is his subordinate." Or is it an anxious reaction to being at the mercy of a man, a father, a partner, who can do with you as He wants?

You experience yourself as powerless; you see no more sense in it; you hardly feel yourself anymore — you feel like you have to let go of your grip, but you might fight against it! From fear and powerlessness, from anger, you would like to grab on to everything like a crab. A hardening, an inner self-restriction: your femininity, your receptiveness — you act like it doesn't exist, you flee from it.

Perhaps you now cling to outer toughness, to proving yourself; you blow up your ego; in outer pride you fly high above the ground like a circus acrobat to show how good you are — in the meantime you pierce your own, small, sensitive heart.

You ARE beautiful when you are gentle, sensitive, and feminine: no longer run away from your deepest inner life. Come toward yourself in gentleness. This powerful female aspect in you is open to beautiful emotional experiences: don't look down on them.

"Woman" with too little male hormone

Causes:

You hollow yourself out; you too much make way for others to make room for them.

You are just at the service of — in sacrifice. Finally, you feel powerless and without a hold, because your earthly structure, your backbone is too light. Too flexible, too unearthly, too much "spirit" and hazy softness. You allow only light and feelings: your head, full of light, is much more present than your body. You are searching, groping, but too feeble; you can fall down at any moment.

Come to active participation in the joy of life! Show your teeth, beat the tom-tom! You dwell too much in non-three-dimensional worlds, in the so called "unconscious" spheres: allow this to become balanced with your Conscious presence, here-and-now. Every human being, every atom, has this double structure inside: unconscious/conscious, receptiveness/action, spiritual-awareness/matter; allow the second aspect to exist!

SEXUALLY TRANSMITTED DISEASES
(See also Part I: Infection and contagion)

Genital chlamydial infections

Anxiety, sometimes in a panicky way; nervousness, desperation. Anxiously running away from deep emotions, from aggressive and sexual forces in yourself. You are afraid of being overpowered by these forces; you are also afraid of being crushed by forces outside you, by a partner, by sexual aggression. Distrustful and tense, you await; in a loveless way you feel pushed over by someone else. Help! Afraid of something dark and threatening in yourself, and as result also afraid of powers and forces outside you. Afraid of compulsions, of perverse or sexual compulsions in yourself, which seem to have power over you. Afraid of the powers in you. You ignore the most beautiful feelings in yourself; you mistrust yourself; you actually push yourself to the side, lovelessly. You *allow* yourself to "be lived"; you deny your own mastery.

Trust your nature; unafraid, dare to be yourself, so that bottled-up emotions and forces don't pile up until everything comes apart at the seams. Enjoy life, without anxieties or destructive aggression: respect the sanctity in yourself.

Offer yourself and others true appreciation. No longer look at life as a black threat; enjoy the sensorial beauty, in all freedom. Don't let yourself be oppressed; you are master over your existence at all times. Handle those feelings and those creative forces in yourself in a productive way. There's nothing in you that is bad, if you stop looking at yourself and the world as something negative.

Evil exists only where there's a shortage of love and insight: in love, make yourself welcome. Only if you love yourself, will you be able to experience honest, worthy relationships. Stand in the center of your existence.

Gonorrhea

You want to prove yourself, almost reckless.

You constantly ponder your worth — you doubt yourself; you look for confirmation in your relationships, in the outer world. Feelings of inferiority and often severe condemnation toward yourself: "I am nothing, I can't do anything." Because of your feelings of powerlessness you look for affirmation outside yourself: in an exaggerated or excessive way you want to get power over others or over certain situations. You want a lot — you try to embrace a lot of things with your arms, thinking you are going to conquer the world. Perhaps you no longer see reality the way it is; you have too much on your plate; perhaps you puff yourself up too much; you want to achieve and put up a bold front, but

actually you can't come close enough to your personal, deep, power source. You don't *really* speak for yourself; you can be angry, not realizing that this is caused by your feelings of powerlessness and self-rejection (a "zero," looking for fulfillment).

Now, dare to simply see and accept yourself the way you are, without wanting to wear a big crown; live from out of your deepest Self; your unique being is irreplaceable, this counts for all human beings. Don't look for confirmation outside yourself: in love, turn toward yourself, toward your body. Place in yourself all power and authority over you and don't reach for power outside yourself. Pleasure, satisfaction, will follow if in self-contemplation you will discover your worth: no longer condemn yourself — your specific characteristics are all allowed to be there; don't suppress any part of yourself; freely dare to thoroughly FEEL your own being and to develop onward. Take away that forcing, that lump in your throat; allow your emotions to flow freely, don't be afraid of yourself, and speak; dare to express yourself the way you truly feel inside, including your uncertainties. Now, abandon the "camouflage" behavior.

Genital herpes

Afraid of disappearing in the claws of "sex" or of a "partner, who can swallow you up," but this is just a result of running away from yourself.

Anxiously escaping your own nature, your physical (and sexual) feelings: because you don't dare or can't surrender to yourself, to your own feelings. Your convictions, your controlling thoughts, prevent it!

Afraid, unsure, not with your feet solidly on the ground; you don't trust your own nature: you would like to tie it down! That's what you think.

Unconsciously, you are so afraid that if you would surrender to your emotional longings the world would collapse and you would be the first to be destroyed. Indoctrination that "your body is dirty" leads to a certain reservation, to self-blockage. This not only hinders you from fully experiencing yourself, but also from entering a close emotional relationship with a partner.

It is you who fixates on "sex or no sex" — for your partner it is perhaps the deeper "love" or the beautiful emotional exchange that is of importance, but you perhaps blow up in yourself the thought of sex because of your anxieties, your complexes, your feelings of guilt.

You experience your physical body as a burden; you feel "seized" by the animalistic aspect.

Your deepest Self calls up this illness because inwardly you aren't completely ready for a true "love relationship." First, come back close to yourself.

That which is being suppressed can pop up like a little devil: integrate all your feelings; acknowledge your body. You shouldn't have sex if you don't wish to! Consider in how far you withdraw onto an emotional island as a result of indoctrination. Or is it because you feel obliged to somehow want to experience sex while your deepest Self says "no," because you first should come closer to yourself? What doesn't do you any good are the barriers you put up in the communication with Yourself and others. In this way you hinder in yourself the free circulation of all rich feelings.

Without holding back, fully surrender to yourself; your nature is beautiful in all its aspects. You don't have to be afraid of any punishing gods or of a curse that will overpower you if you cherish your body and your feelings. Action, self-manifestation, in the name of joy and love! Free yourself!

Only if you come to full surrender to yourself, if you trust in your own basis, if you love yourself, no longer condemning any aspect of yourself — only then are you ready to experience love with a partner; without fear, without harboring any feelings of guilt. The

"God sees you, so don't . . ." —this pointing finger *— lies in yourself, is a part of yourself. Come to totally accept your complete nature; love yourself and dare in a self-assured way to express yourself outwardly!*

Pubic lice

You don't accept yourself completely the way you are inwardly and outwardly. You are ashamed and you would like to hide. You are afraid of confrontations with your body, as a human being, with your deeper feelings.

You feel uneasy in yourself; you unconsciously fear being confronted with something evil or devilish, something ugly in yourself. Perhaps you consider your body to be ugly. You feel anxious and threatened; not only by your deeper Self, but also by the aggression of others — because you repress your own proud forces!

You allow others to direct your life; you let yourself droop; you don't dare to stand up for yourself. In sadness, you put yourself at the mercy of others. You don't really dare to make contact with your deep, strong "I," and because of that you can't really communicate with others; you run yourself down; you think yourself to be just "miserable" — you feel Vulnerable and grabbed by the claws of other people, but in fact you also are grabbing for a hold . . .

Cut the umbilical cord between yourself and others. Dare to be very closely present in yourself, and don't reject your good core. Make yourself welcome, with open arms, and love yourself the way you are. Don't identify yourself with foolish, condemning norms the way they have been proclaimed by certain persons or institutions, which don't allow people to exist freely in their unique being.

*No longer hide from yourself, inwardly or outwardly. Replace sadness with pride and openness. Look under the surface (and not constantly in the mirror): make contact with your soul and feel how **your** complete per-*

*sonality **penetrates** into every fiber of your body.*

*Arrive at complete acceptance of yourself and be proud of your **true** nature: from an ostrich to a free bird. Autonomously!*

Syphilis

You throw away your talents, your deeper feelings: you look for self-affirmation in sexuality. The game of sex is an escape without any emotional depth. You puff yourself up in the manifestation of the flesh: it remains a superficial, empty decoration in your life. The true art of living, the contents, your true feelings — those you don't dare to experience in a relationship. You are not honest with yourself; you don't dare to truly unite with a partner out of Love. You want to gain power or prestige or you want to prove to yourself who you really are — you want to be "best." Therefore, be correct with yourself, with others. Take away the mask and take off the showy artist's hat; paint your life with a deeper perspective.

Dare to warm-heartedly and solidly unite with yourself and don't waste yourself away. Value life according to its worth and don't lose yourself in an endless series of unsatisfying games. Do you think yourself so worthless? Come to true Self-Awareness.

Trichomoniasis

Fundamental anxieties; you are on guard against an indefinable, threatening danger. Fear of yourself, of deep emotions; feelings of guilt; fear of punishment. You are afraid of doing something very wrong. You don't trust others either. "What's hidden behind someone's smile?" You are at the ready with a pistol behind your back; if someone will hurt you, you will be the first to defend yourself. Also in sexual relationships you can feel "taken," especially if you don't experience sex with real love. Because you use the other person, you are afraid of being used.

Because you are not completely honest with yourself, you are afraid of a mean face behind the friendly mask of your partner. Possibly you have problems with sexual "deviations." Do you feel guilty about this? Are you afraid that someone will accuse you? You feel nervous, not at all at ease; sometimes you would like to vacuum the past away, as if it had never been there. Deep emotional anxieties, a feeling of not being safe, as if at any moment the bridge under your feet might collapse, because you don't really build your life on the Authority of your Self, on Love.

You are not at all a sheep for the slaughterhouse: free yourself from the bondage in which you imprison yourself. In all honesty come close to yourself, respect yourself. Trust in your Living Self chases away all anxiety. Don't allow yourself to be manipulated, don't manipulate yourself. Dare to put the past behind you and don't blame yourself for the things you have done. Now come to insight, allow yourself to grow toward sureness, and autonomy. Break with every power system.

(See further: Sexuality.)

PROBLEMS CONCERNING SEXUALITY

Impotency

Is no illness, is not unhealthy.

Your Self calls you to develop your Inner worth, your inner Authority! Insufficient awareness of your inner power. You'd like to manifest yourself outwardly more and more in an upward trend, so to speak, but inwardly you feel unsure.

You think you *have* to satisfy certain conditions in order to be acknowledged as a "Leader" or as a "Great man." You are afraid of failing in this.

You "think" too much; perhaps you become obsessed. You think too much about others, about their needs, or about what they might say.

You are filled to the top with emotions, but you don't dare to let yourself go. You don't really dare to show your feelings. Your thought-world governs everything. Instead of first thinking of yourself and enjoying, not attaching yourself to "a burden, a task," which in fact isn't a burden at all, you fixate anxiously on that which supposedly *has to* be.

Nothing is obligatory; even sexual contact is only one of the many possibilities of expressing your love. No single expectation-pattern is important! You need to live from out of your deepest Self. Potency is always present. Don't force. Let it go from your thoughts; within a true love relationship impotency is of no importance.

Sexual impotency is being called up by the Living Self in order to make you pay more attention to psychological values so you become acquainted with love, intensely and honestly, full of joy and harmony. Now, do without sexual intercourse. Now, allow the inner Authority to grow; discover your inner possibilities and the creativity of your Consciousness on many terrains and then you will understand why you are allowed to be sexually impotent: thus to get to know your total space; thus to discover your worth; thus not to limit your existence to the material and the sexual; thus to meet true love for yourself and others.

A human being is no animal; animals or people who wish to act like animals seldom have the problem of impotence. It's exactly because you unconsciously call up beautiful and deeply human values, because you are sensitive, that you experience impotency. Don't doubt the reasons; develop your inner abilities! Don't *think* too much, but dare to be yourself, to live, without looking at the expectations of others. Creativity on many domains!

Frigidity
no sexual desire

The sexual glands and hormones can function either as powerful, creative energy sources or as stimulators in sexual intercourse between two people or in individual experiences.

Frigidity is no illness, no abnormality!

If, at a certain moment, the sexual desires disappear, it's in many cases because of a powerful Consciousness-development in which all energies, from out of a worthy self-awareness, are engaged in a creative process. Sexuality is okay but is not necessary.

One doesn't have to feel frustrated if the "excitation" is absent.

Sex is only one of many expressions of love; it isn't a necessity. If your body says: "I don't at all feel like doing it," then you should never force yourself in order to please someone else, because then you deny yourself. Nothing "just" happens. If it can't be for you, then your deepest Self definitely has its reason: listen to it.

Do you not experience true love? Do you feel used? Do you feel hurt, sad, and therefore you turn away from sex? Or: don't you love yourself, your body, and therefore do you push others away from you?

Do you not at all experience pleasure because you are not really sexually interested in this relationship or because you don't have a need for pleasure in this way? Sexual contact should be a free choice; if you don't find pleasure in it, then don't do it. Your partner unconsciously attracts a partner like you because of very definite reasons. He (or she) will no longer be able to escape into sex; he will be forced to look for himself and no longer find compensation in sex for his own feeling of emptiness.

(See the category Sexual lusts.)

Within an honest, loving relationship one can easily do without sex, if one or the other has absolutely no need for it. Here, it's not about suppression of feelings, but about utilizing energies on a different level. Reproach will only come from the mouth of that partner who absolutely wants sex because he hasn't found himself yet, because he perhaps feels rejected, because he experiences himself as inferior and finds self-affirmation in sex. In this way, the partner is being "used" or "misused" to satisfy one's own needs.

Unconsciously or consciously one longs for an "ideal" affectionate emotional exchange, where it's neither a question of a power-game nor "having to": that's why one can (unconsciously) resist any kind of sexual intercourse, that's why one can be "frigid," when one senses "here it's about satisfying one's needs." Then you are normal; then the other one is a slave of his passions. A man, as well as a woman, who thinks he or she has to use the blackmail method: "then I'll go to someone else" — or someone who acts *as if* he/she enjoys it, isn't honest with himself/herself and uses the other person in a (power) game. Illness can be the result.

Frigidity is not a sign of being "unhealthy" if you are in loving contact with yourself, if you don't reject your body, if you are not emotionally at odds with yourself, if you don't regard your body as dirty, if you don't turn away from it, if you have a good relationship with yourself!

Don't be at a distance from your body; firmly plant yourself in the earth; free yourself from "obligations" and "anxieties." The day that you "might" again like to have sex doesn't depend on someone else, but on your evolution and your choice.

Sex is not a necessity or an obligation, but it is allowed: when experienced "in Love" and honesty. Never give yourself without your heart, without experiencing joy.

Trust that if sex is good for you, you will at that moment attract a situation which will let you know. First, come to complete self-

realization: then, something else will come first, instead of sex. And possibly in the future you'll once again long for intercourse. Don't plan, but follow your heart, your honest, inner feelings.

Allow your energies to blossom freely; create your life full of self-confidence; now open yourself up to new things. Sexuality the way it has been experienced through the ages "can" take on another form in the light of the cosmic happening; so don't worry, and live in joy, in love!

Vaginismus

Anxieties, deep emotions, lack of self-respect, resistance to those who might hurt you. You think you "must" have sex in order to be accepted as "normal." You close yourself off; you really don't want anybody to "take" you sexually.

You feel imprisoned in the web of the relationship, perhaps even full of guilt feelings because you, yourself, have spun the web like a femme fatale.

An inner conflict of wanting-not wanting. Do you use sex as a form of self-affirmation or "holding on to" someone, and not as an expression of love or of wanting to enjoy yourself? You are not enough yourself! You allow yourself to "be lived" too much: you'd give your body, at a distance, without really being present with your Consciousness.

Your deepest Self says *no* to sexual intercourse: therefore don't do it, even if it is just to please your partner. Are you angry with him? It's you who allows him! Become yourself; be completely faithful to your nature, to your longings, and your feelings.

Sex is not at all necessary; there are other possibilities to develop creativity or to manifest love. If you only "do" it in order to gratify or keep your partner or to punish yourself, then you don't give a chance for physical growth of yourself nor your partner.

Allow that dark stream of emotions to flow freely away, and don't bottle up anything.

Come to respect yourself and become conscious of your worth. Only lift that beam that you can easily carry; never force yourself; do only that which you, as a total human being, like to do.

Gain clear insight into the relationship; sex is not necessary, but is allowed. Is there question of real love? Come to higher consciousness and don't hold back: say what you have to say; no longer hold back your feelings and thoughts; express your emotions, your anger.

Be proud of yourself; no longer give yourself sexually when you feel that emotions are in the way. A true loving partner can live without sex.

The more Consciously a man lives, and the stronger his inner awareness of worth, the stronger he will be able to experience, in totality, Love and beauty. He will find his energies and his joy in wonderful creativity and in the warm feelings of love for the woman he loves. Sex is then allowed, but it's no necessity for him, either. You now have the ability as a woman to allow yourself and your partner to evolve to a deeper and higher level, by being faithful to yourself, by not doing anything against your will, by growing fully in consciousness of the Worth of your Self! Feel those consciousness powers in yourself; create, be joyful, mark out your personal boundaries; don't look for confirmation outside yourself, but allow your life to blossom on a much larger level, from out of your sun-center!

Let go of your partner; love knows no "bonds." Love does know "faith": you are there for one another, with or without sexual experiences.

Inability to achieve orgasm

Orgasm by itself doesn't have to be connected with sexuality; the highest, most joyful point, a sphere of light and happiness can be reached without it having anything to do with sexuality as such. The body can form a way toward this, but it's not necessary. The

partner can go along on this path, but that is not necessary either.

There is nothing the matter when one can't experience an "orgasm" within a sexual relationship, and it isn't necessary either. A gradual growth toward ever-greater awareness can ultimately lead toward the warm feeling of fullness in yourself, a broad cosmic experience of life, a concentration of pure joy of Being.

That one needs a "partner" or "sex" in order to reach the climax of joy is not true. The all-penetrating consciousness, the complete surrender to yourself: the path toward this is different and unique for every human being.

That "sexual rules" would be tied to this is very limiting. Whoever can't experience an orgasm within the sexual game, actually doesn't have to worry.

Determine your point of view; feel safe inside yourself; choose sex or no sex. Never feel obliged to have sex if you don't intensely long for it, orgasm is not a must. The most beautiful, highest pinnacle of joy can be felt in your own unique way; sex is no must for this.

You have ages to gradually grow toward ever-greater consciousness experiences. Let go of everything, no longer think of it, don't exert yourself for it; be happy and creative in a thousand domains! Allow all your energies to flow freely, and follow your path intuitively.

Exaggerated sexual urge, sexually aggressive

Powerlessness, anxiety.

You are afraid that others might hurt you, afraid of being tormented — you are so mistrustful and suspicious with others, but first and foremost with your own deepest content! The look in your eyes is nervous and paranoid: you'd flee from yourself! You don't at all dare to trust in yourself, "because you are certainly very bad." Your feelings are dangerous and form a threat! Therefore it is not surprising that aggressive behavior occurs particularly in men, because they especially have learned to keep hidden, and mistrust, their emotional world, their intuitive channels, their deepest emotional ground! They might even become furious with this terrifying emotional world, which they don't want to know anything about; and therefore this suppression of their own most dear feelings leads to violence, mostly directed toward a personification of this suppressed part of themselves: the "female" or the "child."

Even in the sexual act, he stays at a distance from his deepest Self as well as from the woman: he is involved from far away, at a safe distance — afraid of confrontation with deeper feelings, with his own deepest "I."

The solution here is acknowledgement of the emotional world, of the inner heart and outer behavior. Carefully daring to explore your deeper feelings, so that you can conquer the mistrust regarding yourself.

No longer fear yourself or others: come to peace and relaxation, come very close to yourself; nothing in you is bad or should be avoided!

Only by denying or suppressing a part of your feelings will this end up in frustrated behavior. Sense your deepest emotions and don't suppress; become aware of your worth and no longer feel threatened by others. It is you who threatens yourself by not allowing your higher creative energies to come through, by not believing in the power of your Conscious "I." Accept the child, the woman, the vulnerability, the sensitivity, in yourself: make yourself welcome, in Love. Place all power over your existence in yourself.

Allow creative forces and feelings to exist freely, separate from desires.

Read the categories about Sex and Hormones.

Exaggerated sexual sensitivity, sexual compulsion
Being quickly sexually stimulated by influences from the outside
(See also the category Sex, Hormones, Sexuality)

You completely merge into others, in the world outside yourself — you, yourself, just feel like an inferior being. You'd prefer to suck in others, so to speak, and lose yourself completely in anonymity or non-being.

As a child, you have placed yourself strongly under the authority of your father or mother; you were under the "power" of. . . . Now you are still under the power of. . . .

You suppress your own authority, your deepest feelings; you push yourself away — there's resistance to experiencing yourself in totality with all your forces and all your emotions. You merge yourself like a helpless fetus into "others." Still, you are unconsciously looking for yourself, not for the partner; here, it's not about love, but about being dragged along like an unconscious personality, who for the sake of self-gratification would look for the other person in a primitive urge for pleasure and intoxication.

You allow yourself to be pushed along like a sailboat by the wind — you allow nature, your unconscious instincts, to take their course — you feel so incomplete, so inadequate or just half. . . . In this unsureness you grab on and would "suck in" in order to feel more complete, in order to somehow be able to feel your worth.

You feel yourself to be in the grip of unconscious emotions; you are not master over yourself; your personal structure is flexible, bendable in an exaggerated way: after all, you don't believe in your own power and force, in your higher consciousness-energies.

You feel tied, powerless, but as a compensation for this you might act with crushingly aggressive or sexual behavior: image and self-affirmation. In fact, under this hides the anxiety of being yourself crushed by others, by an authority; the anxiety of being swallowed up, and at the same time a deep longing to melt away completely — in short, a paradox.

Autonomy! Powerful self-awareness and faith in your own worthiness and possibilities; a conscious experiencing of your deepest Self, independent of others: this pure self-awareness leads toward your no more experiencing sexual stimulation, unless you yourself consciously call this up or allow it.

Via the unfolding of one's own Consciousness-energies and productivity on many levels, the frustrations and the longing for gratification by elements or people outside you, will disappear.

The stronger you experience your Fullness, the less you ask to be "filled up." If you come to complete awareness of your self-worth, then you will choose freely, without compulsion.

Exhibitionism

You feel like a wooden puppet; you look for excitement to wake yourself up to life. Affirmation of the outer Ego is still better than the inner feeling of being a Zero. You feel like your own prisoner. You cling to others because you are too absent in yourself, because you don't really live consciously, but rather you exist in a feeling of "stupefaction." You don't get a grip on yourself; you are sensitive and devoted, but you are the slave of an unconscious motive.

Why? Because you are afraid, because you don't allow yourself to openly and freely experience love or feelings of love. You don't dare to have a true, intimate, close confrontation — not with others nor with yourself. You don't really run away from yourself, but you are searching for yourself. You don't stand solidly on your own feet; you look outside yourself for confirmation of your existence.

Your "I" lives too unconsciously; you can't really bring yourself to realization in life; you look for excitement, satisfaction,

outside yourself because you experience yourself inwardly as Empty.

Exhibitionism offers you a possibility of breaking out of your prison walls, of feeling Powerful, as a compensation for your inner feeling of powerlessness.

But the power exhibition runs out of hand; it's stronger than you, yourself, because you refuse to acknowledge your worth, because you keep pushing yourself away, because you don't give yourself the opportunity for a powerful, conscious existence in full daylight.

Frustrations seek an outlet. You allow yourself to be dominated by unconscious desires and urges instead of taking up your mastery in a Self-aware way. Apparently, you don't have a grip on your nature.

You doubt your possibilities; you feel inferior; perhaps in this way you take revenge on that which you experienced in the past as painful: a motherly, dominant authority possibly has "grabbed" you too strongly. Other causes from your childhood are undoubtedly recognizable. But the happenings from your youth are, in fact, already a Result of convictions regarding yourself — with which you entered life as a baby. You were born with a feeling of inability, with a feeling of lovelessness, with powerful energies, but with the feeling of helplessness regarding the utilization of these powers in self-manifestation.

Feed that wooden puppet with inner fire, not with outer compulsion. Come to life in yourself: you are not made out of wood; you are worthy. Come out of the darkness; acknowledge yourself in Love. Action, self-realization, doing, giving to others in love, no longer hiding your feelings. No longer frustrate yourself; free yourself by becoming Aware. Become master over yourself, over your nature. Realize yourself in daily life and dare to express yourself, to show yourself, the way you feel. Experience your feelings, your longings, not sneakily but with your total being. Respect yourself and others.

(Read also the category Compulsive acts.)

Become aware of the fact that the shock, or the powerlessness, of the one who sees you is a reflection of the degree to which you feel "taken": no longer doom yourself to being a prisoner, no longer doom the other person to being a prisoner.

Openly express your feelings in your relationships: don't hide yourself.

Voyeurism

You feel small, clumsy, and afraid, like a child, unable to truly live yourself, to manifest yourself like an adult human being; you think you don't fulfill requirements. Unsureness. Dissatisfaction with yourself. You experience yourself like Don Quixote; you don't really know who you are. You cling to false values, to norms that are unimportant, but for you they are important.

You don't get a solid grip on anything; you feel unstable on your own Basis.

You look at life through restricting glasses; you fixate yourself on that which is sensational in order to compensate for your own feelings of emptiness and Absence. You don't really live as if you are Conscious of your worth — on the contrary, you instead feel like a "little dog."

Hesitantly, you remain behind the curtains of Life; you don't dare to realize yourself, not in contacts with others either. You don't get a grip on your feelings; it's hard, or impossible, for you to express them or to share them with others.

On the sexual plane you are afraid to fail; you fantasize yourself into the role of a hero, or you like to identify yourself with the person you are spying on; you let yourself merge in this, or be taken up into it, because you experience yourself as being a Zero. Frustration.

Self-realization! Get both feet on the ground: be yourself! Look at life in a broader way and don't hesitate to free your energies. No longer oppress yourself; allow your feelings to exist freely and experience

them to the fullest, don't hide. In the process of becoming Conscious you will realize that you fixate yourself on filling up your so-called frustration void. Now turn yourself inward and discover the large range of possibilities in you.

Self-respect. Self-appreciation; daring to show the way you feel inside. A triumphant victory over yourself: being directed toward beautiful energies inside yourself, toward the true joy in your heart, no longer toward compensating fillers of emptiness. Take up your space without hesitation and LIVE in all openness! Don't allow yourself to BE lived: no longer identify yourself with others. You are good the way you are!

Don Juanism

You don't know who you are; you are searching for yourself. You don't dare to show your true core, because of fear; you hide behind Don Juan behavior. You are afraid of your deepest core, also afraid of death: you flee! Help! You raise a flag which attracts attention, but it's in fact a flag which asks: "Say, then, who am I?" The flag flutters in vague, misty clouds where you dwell. . . .

You experience instability inside you: the result of not finding a firm structure, solidity, a strong center in yourself.

You move on wheels, as it were, from here to there, following others with rolling eyes; you have to follow, because you experience yourself as empty.

Perhaps you have filled yourself with philosophies, with theories, with a technique, with a system, but you float in this as in thin air; it doesn't really come from yourself; these are just things to hold on to; it doesn't really satisfy you.

Psychologically, you feel impotent, naked, shabby, and old; you flee from yourself to others. True Authority in yourself is being denied!

You don't feel real love for yourself; you don't have a clear view of love in general.

You allow others to direct your life, powerless as you are to make contact with yourself. As Juan you prove to yourself that you "still" exist in Life as a human being. You look for acknowledgement and confirmation in others, because you underestimate yourself.

You assume power over others for as long as you do not assume power over yourself, while at the same time you reject love for yourself.

Place the center in yourself: experience the core of your deepest Self. Don't live under the influence of others but from out of a concentrated "I." Acknowledge your worth as a human being and open yourself up in love toward yourself. Don't look to compensate your own emptiness with relationships, but turn inward and open yourself to your fullness! In self-confidence build your own existence; no longer filling yourself again and again with the words and bodies of others. You think you are fleeing from death, but in fact you are turning away from life. Immortality lies in you, yourself: the independent authority, the Power to self-create your own life in a worthy way.

No show, but self-respect. Self-confidence, belief in your possibilities, independent of others. If you lovingly appreciate yourself, you will meet stability and joy. You don't need acknowledgement from others: acknowledge yourself, and you won't need appreciation from others anymore. Don't look for it outside yourself, but within yourself.

Establish yourself firmly in your own roots!

Nymphomania

Inwardly, you feel handicapped, incomplete, psychologically impotent; you look for self-affirmation. You show off your body, you take power over others: in this way you no longer feel powerless. You fill your emptiness with the attention of others; you feel

yourself being filled up in a powerful way by others, because you experience yourself as powerless and without inner Force. You "feel" yourself only through others; you don't feel able to stand independently and resolutely on your own feet. You don't allow yourself to really exist!

You want to feel, through others, that you are "desirable," that you are "worthy"; you use others for this, others use you. In this way you prevent yourself from building a worthy existence.

You limit your life to a game of attraction and rejection, of lust and desire, of having, possessing and — inner loneliness.

True joy you find in the fullness of your existence. Now allow your forces, your feelings, to live from out of your heart, not in the first place directed toward others. Self-respect! Discover love and affection, warm giving. Dare to experience yourself as a worthy being, independent of others, filled to the brim with possibilities, no longer being fixated on futilities, superficialities. Find satisfaction in yourself through resolute self-manifestation: don't hesitate to develop your creative possibilities. Be honest with yourself and don't grab for others; experience the power-center inside you; make yourself welcome, so that you no longer ask others for confirmation. Your life is like a bottomless vat, dark and eternally empty; replace this chill, this cold attraction, this suction force, by warm productivity, by tenderness and attention to yourself. No longer deny that which is most beautiful in you.

Onanism, self-gratification, exaggerated

Inwardly you feel small, dependent, powerless; you don't feel able to build your existence in a straight line. Emotions and energies are being bottled up: you underestimate your worth; you don't dare to manifest yourself fully as a Conscious human being.

Somehow you prefer to stay in the shelter of the past, when you were still a baby, because you don't see very clearly how otherwise to realize your creative energies. You go around in a vicious circle; you don't succeed in bringing your emotional contents nor your talents to realization in the outside world. You don't really feel safe yet in the outside world; you look for an escape-valve, an outlet for your bottled-up emotions and seek compensation for your feelings of inability. Too little independence, not really self-aware, a kind of imbalance in the sense that you don't allow yourself to fully enjoy life; that you block yourself; that you don't really dare to be yourself; that you hold back; that you perhaps question too much what others think of your "exterior" instead of just enjoying all aspects of life, from out of your heart. . . .

Work at your emotional ties; free your feelings; express yourself; develop your creativity; experience those forces deep inside you and bring them out. Manifest yourself, full of self-confidence! Self-gratification is not unhealthy, bad, or sinful, but it does indicate a "retention" of creative energies, of feelings. Growing up to adulthood, the growth toward Self-awareness, means awareness of your autonomous worth; it also means integration of your feelings in the light of the Sun, your central "I."

Don't allow either one to lead an independent existence, but merge them together. A powerful "I," propelled onward by inner energies, emotions, longings. . . .

Don't lock yourself up inside yourself; dare to manifest yourself; don't bury your talents in the ground.

Read also the category Sexual Lust, exaggerated, and the category Testosterone (sexual organs).

Dare to take up your full space and allow the bud to open up; dare to enjoy yourself as a totality. Don't restrict yourself: now allow your energies to flow out freely without holding back. Sexual self-gratification indi-

cates an insufficient use of your creative energies and emotional forces, not living to the fullest, toward the true joy of life, toward happiness. Become aware of the strong Structure inside yourself; experience the oneness inside you as an autonomous being; in proud self-realization transform all dormant and pushing energies into action. Don't suppress your creativity. Feel safe in yourself and leave the cradle. . . .

Incest, rape
(See also Pedophilia)

The victim

First read Part I, the category Emotions.

The victims of incest (and rape) are stuck with a deep emotional trauma that seems to destroy their complete life, and that is very hard to resolve apparently. This is because the victim is convinced, and stays convinced, that the trauma is *a consequence* of an act of incest (or rape). As long as one holds on to this conviction, the trauma just can't be resolved. The child *is born with* this trauma, and the experience of incest is only the occasion through which the trauma surfaces in order to be able to resolve it once and for all. As long as one doesn't realize this, one can't get rid of the inner problem.

That's why it's of no use to endlessly involve oneself in therapies such as regression, hypnosis, or rebirthing. This counts for all emotional traumas. Unmasking of the inner state of being of all people involved, which was the true cause of the happening, will lead to a solution.

INSIGHT into "why" one attracts such a painful situation, unconsciously . . .

You were born in these specific family circumstances in order to once and for all deal now with your unconscious inner conviction: "I am just a victim. I am not in charge of myself. I am not complete, and I need to fill myself with others."

You live in and through others; you don't experience yourself as an autonomous "I." You experience yourself as a victim, at the mercy of other people's whims. Unconscious power-attraction toward others because you don't lovingly assume power over your life.

Where *are* you? You are not yet really present in yourself. You live with your consciousness not concentrated in your body. You are pliable, flexible, and too easily influenced; you allow yourself to "*be* lived." You think you have no right to determine your own life. A lack of self-confidence; too little awareness of your own worth, of your own rights. Your spiritual energies "centrifuge" as it were, don't bundle together into a self-aware force. Powerlessness, not being aware of your inner Power. You are not really yourself; you live too much according to others; you have no contact with your own warm feelings, your heart; sometimes you experience yourself to be like a piece of wood.

Anxieties; you bottle up your emotions; you don't really feel your heart beating, because you don't acknowledge yourself in love; you bring yourself into question; you don't yet know your true natural disposition. That's how you were born with the anxious conviction that you always have to be fleeing from others, that as a victim you are easy prey for others; you were born with very little awareness of your personal worth, filled to the top with anxiety and doubts.

Incest victims are born as beings who are Anxiously fleeing from themselves. Now they are being rudely awakened: a forced confrontation with their "I." One can't flee anymore. The naked truth regarding oneself: "I feel cold, small, sad, vulnerable, without love, and I can only exist thanks to, and via, others." Especially in the sexual relationship can one then totally "lose" oneself. One is afraid to become oneself as an autonomous "I."

For the most part UNCONSCIOUSLY, strong, drawing magnetic-telepathic impulses are being sent out, no matter how small the being is: "I cannot, and don't want to, exist 'by myself,' I take you, I want to lose myself, take me." An unconscious refusal of transformation with all the painful consequences thereof: unconscious or conscious seductive energies are being sent out.

One feels cold because one flees from oneself, because one doesn't give oneself love, because one's heart remains cold; one longs for that warmth. One unconsciously refuses to become oneself; one thinks one can only find warmth and security in someone or something bigger and stronger, although one also feels fear of this.

Sexual organs and glands are symbolic of Creative powers (See the category Sex Organs.)

If, however, one suppresses oneself as an autonomous, independent being — denies the authentic creative values in oneself — if one refuses transformation (allowing oneself to truly be born), if one refuses to acknowledge the power in oneself, then one will remain stuck in the phase of sex and power. Instead of becoming oneself, one powerfully and anxiously draws (mostly unconsciously) others "in" with a powerful suction force, so to speak. Whoever reacts to this — the rapist — is stuck with the same kind of problem. He also "loses" himself in the sex and power game because he doesn't believe in his autonomous self-worth, because he denies himself warmth and love, because he wishes to force it from others by using power, and because he also experiences himself as a victim of his own past.

Both long for warmth and love, both feel undervalued, both ask of the other to fill their own emptiness. The rapist avenges his own powerlessness.

Come to clear insight of the underlying causes of the happening. Finally step out of your role of victim, and transform! It is not rape that is your deepest problem (it's already a result) but your (possibly unconscious) refusal to transform toward Mastery over yourself. You are not pitiable, but you are "worthy," although you perhaps become angry when one tells you that you are no unfortunate victim of circumstances. You have suffered because of it, but your personality suffers a lot more under your refusal to become your Self as an Autonomous individual. Therefore, discover your inner powers, and allow your "I" to be born. Once and for all make an end to your role of being the victim, as well as your role of a Sad and Powerless person. Realize how necessary it is that you, without the support and attention of others, first acknowledge and appreciate yourself in Love.

Build up your solid Structure and live according to inner Authority. Transform powerlessness-and-power into pure inner force; manifest yourself in a creative way and feel the warm sun-flame burn in your heart in order to pass it on to others.

Give, *don't draw. Is your body "manipulated" or has it honestly grown out of your inner life source? Time to honestly look at yourself: read about this in the book "Large, Beautiful, and Healthy." Offer love, don't anxiously flee. Be yourself, don't lose yourself in others. Don't get stuck in the negativity of the past; instead, concentrate on that which is positive inside you. Take full possession over Your life. Let go. True love is now your salvation; lift yourself up toward this feeling of freedom.*

Parents of incest victims

One will not condemn them, but will urge them to arrive at Insight and understanding of the Situation. After all, they have been born with a psychological similar problem to that of their child(ren.) In order to solve this problem, they all have looked for each other in this life, be it unconsciously.

They all struggle with a feeling of inferiority, of weakness, of inability.

Because father is born with a low self-image, he will be born in a milieu where parents have approached him in a possibly ty-rannical, aggressively dominant way — a milieu in which he has experienced coldness, harshness and humiliation. He can feel anxious and inferior with people his own age.

He constantly desires objects outside himself because he inwardly feels so empty and worthless (See also Part I, Desires). He denies the strong, Self-aware Man (even though he can act outwardly as an inflated Image or tyrant) as well as the small, hurt child inside himself. He experiences himself as powerless and places all power outside himself, because of which he constantly loses himself in desires. He's been born with a feeling of zero worth, and he further destroys himself. His behavior is only a result of inner negative convictions regarding himself.

Because he is angry with the powerless, vulnerable, small helpless child inside himself, he closes himself off from it in an aggressive way, and projects this inner problem on the victim.

Mother is born with a victimized feeling — just like her child — and, as a result of this, she'll be born in a milieu where one doesn't respect her true worthiness. The confrontation with the truth is too painful for her, because of which she often closes her eyes. Because of the negative convictions regarding herself, she will attract a father, a husband, situations, which are a reflection of this.

That these facts occur is, in and of itself, only a result of the deep-seated feeling in all parties involved, of not being worth anything. Therefore, the problem needs to be solved via a thorough revision of identity in all. A puncturing of the lies, according to which they would be only victims (mother, child), according to which they are zeros who can't do anything but "fill" their lives by desiring objects, instead of beginning to discover the fullness and true beauty in themselves (the father). Making an end to silence and secret behavior; complete openness, without forcing the person involved, is necessary to come to an evolution and a lasting result.

But especially: don't expect anything from others, not even an "admission of guilt." Let go — look at the deeper causes inside yourself, resolve things and go onward on YOUR path.

Pedophilic rape
(See also Incest)

The big man has much pain and might vent these emotions on a child. He feels hurt in his "male ego"; possibly, he was overpowered, hurt, or dominated, misused in the past, but these facts were called up by him, be it unconsciously, because of his inner feelings of powerlessness, of feeling unsafe, of anxiety, helplessness, emptiness, guilt.

An inner conflict: on the one hand, the big man is the small, powerless child, himself; on the other hand, he treats this "small being" in himself mercilessly hard. He condemns himself as being bad, rotten, and helplessly pathetic. With a sadistic attempt for power, he might overpower that small soul in himself, but he projects it outwardly on a child.

He "desires" that which he has rejected in himself: the full body of himself, the sensitive softness, the female element, the child element — he doesn't really accept this in himself, because it's weak and vulnerable. The excitement rises the more he fills up his own "emptiness." But inwardly he still feels as vulnerable as that part of himself that he doesn't really accept. He doesn't allow himself to have a full life: he's filled to the brim with feelings, deep emotions, longings, creative energies, but he doesn't really believe in himself!

He feels stuck, pestered, and mistreated: in desire, in the lust for power, he wishes to lose himself further — until "nothingness"; he unconsciously wishes to be swallowed up completely by the suction force of sexual attraction. . . .

The endocrine glands, the sexual hormones, react very strongly to the feeling of inability and the "Absence of the living 'I'-center," but instead of transforming extra energy into self-realization, one allows oneself to be drawn along through the sexual game, in order to fill up this emptiness. Inwardly so small, outwardly so big.

He doesn't love himself. Sex replaces love, but it's like a bottomless vat.

He doesn't at all feel warm and sheltered. He's afraid of his feelings; he holds back his deepest feelings, until he looks for an outlet.

It's good to realize why there are feelings of lust toward a child: don't condemn it, but come to understand the real cause. Thoughts are not "acts." Pedophilia doesn't at all have to lead to actual sex: turn inward and come to self-study. Now accept the totality of your feelings; acknowledge the female, the child, element in yourself and welcome it warmly. Strongly feel the Power over yourself; you are not powerless. Be gentle and good to that which is small in you, and come to true Self-love. The stronger the awareness of Self-worth and the clearer your Self-awareness, the weaker the lusts.

SHOCK

Nothing "just" happens. What's the cause for someone attracting a "state of shock?" For too long already you have lived in a state of "stupor"; you haven't understood the forces of Plutonian transformation. You don't really live from out of your Self! You have suppressed your feelings, your forces, your energies, your aggression. Anxiety, also about death. You have lived in a way that was too unauthentic, possibly adapting too much to others.

You felt too oppressed, somewhere in life too "tied down," but you didn't bring about any change in this: refusal to change, to transform.

Do you allow your life to be too dependent on others? Do you allow yourself to be "dragged along" by life? You are stuck with deep emotional experiences, but you don't allow your "I" to exist fully in the here-and-now. Perhaps you fly right past life while working, but inwardly you are filled to the brim with sorrow, powerlessness, and tension. You are being awakened by something that emotionally shakes you up.

Time for transformation! Take the burdens from the past off your shoulders: now allow all feelings to flow Freely, allow everything to come loose! Speak; don't hold back: express your emotions, your aggression, your anger, your sadness, and your Powerlessness. Come to life by finally allowing your feelings and your forces to flow freely: look, hear, and feel with all your senses in an intense way. No longer live in a stupor; feel the warmth of other people; don't coldly close yourself off from yourself, from warmth and tenderness. Solve all your anxieties, including those in connection with death. Don't allow yourself to "be lived"; get a good hold on yourself; don't allow yourself to be dragged along by the stream of life: build your existence in an active way. Individual awareness, strongly concentrated in your body. Discover your deepest Self and live according to your Will, according to your longings. Now place yourself in a loving way in the center of your life. Now allow yourself to be truly born like a butterfly coming out of a cocoon, having left the caterpillar stage behind.

SHOULDER

Psychological correspondence

Symbolic of the security of the child inside you, carried by a powerful, Conscious "I." Symbolic of taking up your large living space, with self-aware pride. Symbolic of the safe and peaceful feeling inside yourself.

Life for you is a radiating giving, a joyful self-manifestation, a loving openness toward yourself and others.

You carry your Content, your feelings, very supplely and strongly; you don't bend under the weight of emotional burdens. Rational and emotional worlds are in balance.

Symbolic also of the freedom of being able to radiate your energies in all possible directions: continuing on your main course with ease and agility.

If you believe in your goodness, in your deepest Self, then you will be able to carry a lot, also for others: you can put things in perspective and gain a clear view of everything in order to arrive at solutions. You acknowledge your worth; you have the ability to digest emotions quickly, without creating obstacles.

You respect your limits and those of others.

You don't dominate; you don't totally withdraw into yourself: a healthy balance in communication with others.

Ailments, in general

Anxiety. You don't really feel safe inside yourself. You might withdraw into yourself like a hermit or like a fugitive, sad and afraid. Or you might frenetically try to keep yourself standing under heavy burdens, perhaps sticking out your chest toward the outer world in order to camouflage your powerlessness, in order to keep a certain grip of power over a situation or on others.

You can sadly droop your head and your shoulders; you don't really believe in your inner power. Emotions are flooding you. You have already absorbed too much; you can't carry it all anymore. Burdens are becoming too heavy. Do you close yourself off to others or, on the contrary, do you absorb too much?

Do you feel anything but protected in yourself, and are you constantly looking for ways to protect yourself? You don't have any faith in your Basis; you feel you are on unstable ground. Anxiety, unsureness, and sadness weigh you down. Tensions.

You don't have a clear perspective, not of yourself, nor of your life's circumstances: this asks for a solution. Emotions are being bottled up, not channeled.

You doubt your worth, underestimate your possibilities.

Shoulder pain
(See also Ailments, in general)

Life weighs heavily on you: why do you burden yourself so? Why all these heavy worries? Does the anxiety press on your shoulders? You are bossy with yourself (perhaps also with others): you oblige yourself to do this or that, you "have to" do it; again and again you put up conditions for yourself in order for you to be able to accept yourself. You carry needless burdens: you block feelings and intuitive forces. You don't allow your nature to exist freely, flexibly, and relaxed!

You take burdens on your shoulders that are not at all necessary. Do you demand that you achieve or that you satisfy others? Do you want to manifest yourself as bigger and stronger than you inwardly feel? Do you demand too much of yourself? Misusing power regarding yourself? Don't you believe in your inner force, and do you therefore force yourself? Do you make yourself dependent on others? A feeling of powerlessness. Do you overload yourself with futilities, with details? Do relation-problems weigh you down? Do you think, brood, so much?

Anxiety about the future: don't you trust life very much? You hurt yourself!

Find the balance in yourself, and with a clear overview make yourself Master over your problems. Let go of all that is superfluous. Achieve no longer: accept yourself unconditionally. Your life is Joy if you create it yourself in a Self-aware way, if you no longer hold on to a Fate or an imaginary

danger: you can direct your life, without misery. Discover this power of creation in yourself; intuitively follow your path; don't bottle up your feelings. You are good the way you are: feel safe and solid in the Basis of your deepest Self. Throw those needless burdens off your shoulders. Live spontaneously, free and happy, like a child.

PSH
periarthritis scapulohumeralis, inflammation of tissues surrounding the shoulder joint (tendons, bursae)

Because you don't have faith in your Basis (symbolically, the lower back), you take too heavy a burden on your shoulders. You actually don't build enough on your Self, don't really evolve from out of yourself; you don't achieve emotional growth; you hold on to a lot of personal energies, emotions, without resolving them. On the contrary, you try to embrace everything with one swoop of your wings; you reach far beyond yourself; it seems as if you flee from yourself by doing this. You take everything too broadly, too largely, including certain responsibilities (which lie outside of your domain); you run ahead of yourself by reaching and grabbing as much as you can outside of yourself.

Because inwardly you just feel rotten and anxiously tense, you try to resolve this by following and carrying the entire world with your "controlling thoughts." While you are suffocating in your emotions, you might outwardly, silently, thrust out your chest. Because you don't acknowledge the Authority in yourself, you will try to retain power, or to keep everything and everyone under your wings, though it might be in the name of love or sacrifice. You don't do yourself a service by doing this; in a heated, tense way you accumulate emotions; you try to reach ever farther and for more and more, far ahead of you; your thoughts are meanwhile going around like crazy. Your personal creative energies, here-and-now, are being suppressed.

Exaggerated worries about others or being tensely directed toward everything and everyone, except toward yourself, indicates only that you are fleeing from yourself, from your emotions. You don't live enough in a self-aware manner; you live too much in your "head"; you walk right past your emotional content.

With your head you create enormous masses of energy, but not for the good of your own development. You storm ahead with your thoughts, while you can't yet plant your right foot firmly in the ground.

(See Right body half.)

Energies and emotions are "stuck": free yourself from them; this can't be done by reaching further outside yourself, but by waking yourself up. Even a donkey trusts its nature and doesn't carry any more burdens than it can. Listen to your feelings! Relax; quietly turn inward; let go of those burdens; accept your emotions and allow energies to flow freely under the Authority of your Self-aware "I." Be more gentle with yourself; see how you have neglected yourself. Take up your own shoulder-space, but no more: become Conscious of your worth; know that anxieties are not necessary if only you trust in your Self (See Anxieties) Don't block your powers and your feelings in a burning head, nor by overburdening yourself in the service of others. Allow yourself to evolve from out of your natural disposition.

You don't have to safeguard yourself, nor to prove yourself to the outer world.

SINUSITIS

You feel "seized by the throat," especially emotionally, but you remain silent, like a Sphinx.

Who or what to believe inside or outside yourself? You see stars; you don't have a clear perspective! You keep yourself too tightly bound; you live controlled within an iron structure. A powerless sadness. Pent-up aggressive forces. A feeling of being "stuck" in something and not being able to go onward. For instance in a relationship: you don't dare to live completely from out of your nature. Deep-seated anxieties about your own inner Self prevent you from truly evolving in life.

The powerlessness makes you "reach and grab" strongly for things or people outside yourself. You allow your life to be too dependent on a partner, on your children, or on an Outer function — self-affirmation in a social position, in a role with a proud Image, etc.

You have immobilized yourself in a Role, an attitude, a way of life in which *you* don't come into your own. Again and again you have poured water into the wine, made compromises, or sacrificed your life for an "outer" or ambitious plan, but your inner emotional world is being suppressed.

Sometimes you are overcome by a powerless sadness, an anger, bottled-up aggression, mostly directed at your partner or at one of your fellow-men, but don't fool yourself: here in fact it's about the revolt, the inner resistance to "being stuck" yourself. Your aggression, your angry outbursts, are directed toward others, but it's about the powerlessness of realizing yourself, of experiencing your feelings as a total human being, powerless to step out of the iron armor in which you have imprisoned yourself.

Sinusitis breaks through when these tensions become too great; bottled-up healthy aggressive forces, natural feelings, and longings ask for attention.

A call from the inner Self so that you would fully acknowledge your nature, that with your "thinking" you'll no longer castrate your nature, that instead of thinking yourself black, fixating on the negative, full of anxieties, you now will make and end to this dark situation.

You are afraid of that which is deepest inside you; you don't trust your own disposition — that's why you cling to something or someone outside you, by which you block yourself.

Anxiety about not being able to keep everything under control, anxiety about being "dragged along," fear of pain, anxiety about someone or something "grabbing" you. These sometimes very vague anxieties come from your depths and tell you simply that you are not really on the right path! You block your healthy energies; you are looking for safety outside yourself or in a strongly structured life, in an existence restricted by rationality, in a Function, in a relationship, or in material things, but your Self doesn't really get a chance to manifest itself from out of your spontaneous nature. You tensely hold on to that which you "have" today, because you don't DARE to live according to your spontaneous longings.

Perhaps you might "give in" too much, or even completely, to your partner, out of fear of losing your safety: in this way you deny your nature. Sadness, powerlessness, and resistance to this, without you necessarily speaking up (it's mostly a silent sadness) are the results of your self-restriction.

You feel "tied down," actually want to break out of this, but you don't see how to or where to, and you remain silent. Powerful energies are suppressed in this way! This inner tension, bottled-up aggression, leads to "inflammation."

You are like an ostrich, but with your head anxiously turned away from yourself. Afraid of the depths within yourself: therefore you anchor yourself in a safe system, without daring to go out of it anymore! You rust in habits. You no longer grow; you hurt yourself because you hinder yourself from transforming, from using your forces in a positive, spontaneous way, from developing emotionally.

You look at life too one-sidedly, purely rationally; you don't trust your intuition, although the greatest wisdom can be received via intuitive channels: you resist the divine, eternal part of yourself. You smother your-self in a "world of thought" without depending on the Basis of yourself; of course you then look for support outside yourself. You have no faith and therefore you get excited about a hundred things, until your head might burst! That's why you walk around, inwardly tense, with a feeling of being unsafe.

*Doubts can lead toward your not daring to really live from out of yourself, toward your living more from out of your Image or your false pride than with heart and soul. In this way powerless fury because of mockery, pain, and oppression during childhood can now be projected on a partner. Know that your sad experiences as a child already were the result of **your inner Powerlessness**, anxiety and a feeling of inferiority, through which you unconsciously have called up these kinds of situations. Do you still punish yourself by suppressing your nature? Do you still think that you are not allowed to stand up for yourself? Or are you afraid of your partner's reaction, and therefore you hold back? In this way, you hinder your evolution and make yourself sick. **Negative self-destructive aggression, which leads to inflammation, only exists if you don't respond to those fundamental energies in yourself which present themselves to be experienced. It's of no use, because of this self-negation, to blame others for your bitterness and anger!** Think about why you don't really love yourself, and why you don't dare to experience yourself.*

Your self-suppression calls up tensions in your surroundings. In the first place, love yourself and dare to express yourself! Speak about that which bothers you, and don't walk around "thinking" about it; work things out and let go.

Don't condemn yourself for your feelings, for your nature. Dare to be yourself, faithful to your nature; stop compromising. Also in a partnership true love asks every partner to be "himself/herself," the way he or she is: don't restrict yourself.

And stand up for yourself.

Discover that inner wisdom; allow rationality and intuition to go hand-in-hand;

come to true awareness. *No longer place your nature in a straitjacket that is too tight; relax!*

When you are "stuck" or feel sadness, then this is because of yourself. Trust in your deepest Self, feel that safe Basis in you, let go of worries, don't fixate yourself on problems outside of you. **No longer be hard on yourself!**

Allow gentleness and love in your life, toward yourself in the first place. Become aware of your inner worth.

No one forces you to look at "dark" sides: discover joy in your Self; become more sensitive to that which is beautiful! Enjoy fully with your senses; don't tense yourself up: breathe, smell, taste, and look! No longer lock yourself up in a cell.

Experience the space of your emotional world and trust in these feelings. Come closer to your heart and be more flexible than you have been. **Peace in yourself, rest and safety, trust in everything taking the course it has to.** *Don't worry anymore, and no longer hold on to material or outer values. Everything you need is inside you. Anxieties are not necessary. Bring yourself to realization from out of your longings; dare to be yourself, in joy, and make an end to mortal fear by trusting in your everlasting Core, because that is your only anchor in life. On this, you can build. Now, come out, no longer hide your deepest Self, your feelings! Express yourself, speak: what comes out will not do any damage inside.*

SKELETON

Psychological correspondence

You are the solid rock in the sea of life, in the Light of your Living Self.

In wisdom you give shape to your existence. The skeleton represents the balanced structure in yourself, in your life.

The giving of shape to your individuality: the concentration of the "I"-consciousness in the form, in your existence on earth. The stone-laying, the Basis, the foundation of Love for life. The strength, the perseverance, the sureness, of an unshakable "I," which takes care that you walk that path which connects directly with your true nature. The protecting, safe structure of your deepest Self.

Feeling good ,warm and sheltered; being the way YOU WANT to be from out of your heart, without "bending" yourself too much toward the expectations of the outer world. The way a baby safely rests in its cradle, so you also trust in your deepest Core, your Living Self: the pure faith in this inner soul Core. A structure that is open to the "treasures" of the Self, to the new, joyful Content.

Stand up for yourself, solidly, with your feet on the ground. The ability to go along, to stand still, or to resist.

A clear structure gives room for emotions, without them overpowering you: you don't fight against, but you build your life in a positive way yourself.

Being present in yourself here-and-now; you are not cold and critical, but warm and loving, toward yourself and others.

An harmonious merging of the sober-reasoning and the emotional-intuitive, of the "male," the "female," the child in yourself, without your neglecting one of these aspects.

Honoring your divine Core. Fulfilling your function, your life's task, with joy.

The all-penetrating Light of your Living Self protects, guards, warms you, brings together, arranges into order, spontaneously and optimistically — like life itself.

You carry your content in a self-assured way, conscious of your worth, in self-respect, very close to you.

Ailments, in general

Are you too absent in yourself? Do you float in the air? Don't you really want to manifest yourself on earth? Do you withdraw? Do you feel like a victim, helpless, at the mercy of others? Do you allow others to direct your life? Don't you stand up for yourself? Are you so afraid? Do you think yourself ugly or bad, inferior? Do you take away from yourself the opportunities for a decent existence? Have you no faith in your deepest Self? Do you live on guard regarding others, ready to defend yourself? Do you feel attacked? Are you weighed down with enormous emotional burdens?

Or, do you cling in an exaggerated way to others, to material things, to ambitious ostentation in the outer world? Does your life stand or fall with the acknowledgement of Image? Do you revolt? Do you stand up against established structures, instead of building up your path yourself, in an autonomous way?

Powerlessness, frustration. Do you feel not at all supported in yourself? Do you make yourself hard, rejecting, stubborn, unrelentingly obstinate? Do you refuse evolution, in gentleness toward yourself? Do you feel cold and unloved? Why deny any longer your fundamentally strong Basis? Turn yourself inward, toward your Living Self, and experience the power, the love, the trust in yourself.

Osteoporosis
bone decalcification
(See also Skeleton, in general)

You don't think yourself worthy of fully taking up the place that every human being deserves; unconsciously, you feel guilty, sometimes even actually thinking you are a bad person. Critically judgmental toward yourself, toward others! In this condition of self-condemnation you don't *truly* dare to live. You hinder yourself, you tightly bind yourself up; you do what others (or your gods, idols, society, etc.) tell you to: you have no "character," as it were, no "backbone" of your own (anymore). Those who consider man to be a creature which can barely trust itself and would rather do pen-

ance for its so-called sins, and that the human being is "subordinate" to one or another great force or primal spirit by which he will sooner or later be swallowed up. Punishing almighty gods. Unconscious feelings of guilt. You mistreat yourself, violating your own nature. You would like to *truly* live, but then again you hold back, not allowing yourself to. In fact, you are convinced that you had better beat a retreat (an escape). . . . Now you look upon the harvest of your life: you realize you haven't been able to separate the wheat from the chaff; actually, you still only see the chaff of your life — also with regard to others.

Look in a "healthy," critical way. Don't flee; look to that which is beautiful in yourself, strong, as an unique Individual. Become conscious of the fruitfulness of your "I." Evil, the devil: put this out of your head. Everything in your life is evolution. Nothing has been bad. Begin finally to take your own life in hand yourself and dare to trust your own intuition. Divinity is in you! Build up your talents upon your own authority. No one, no god, no Satan, has any authority over you. Take up, now, your responsibility! With the power of your personal spirit, your body can be regenerated and rehabilitated. No longer doubt these powerful creative energies, which can be directed only by your Conscious will. Concentration of consciousness powers in your body. It is necessary here to have a balance between your intuitive emotional potential and your rational self-aware powers. Now dare to trust your feelings and place yourself high on the throne of human worthiness. Stop condemning yourself. Cherish your body in a nest of warmth and love.

BONE FRACTURES
In general

You experience a feeling of suffocation, restriction, and you want to break out of it! You feel like you are in the grip of others, in the power-claw of authority — but in fact you are in the grip of your own powerlessness, in the grip of your own anxiety that you might be worth "only" this or that. You stand up against an authority, a parent or an oppressing situation; you break a bone. Because you now have to realize that it's about your inner emotional world. The circumstances of "breaking a bone" just don't happen by "accident," but are unconsciously called up in order to make something clear to you, in order to be able to change your attitude of life to your advantage. Inwardly, you feel a weakness somehow: outwardly, you try to prove yourself! You inflate your image; you show yourself to be tough or proud — this happens in your dream world. Instead of bringing to realization the authority in yourself, and really believing in yourself, here-and-now, you dream, often unconsciously, of heroic, romantic scenes or a beautiful role that compels the admiration of others. When you insufficiently value the content of life because you undervalue your own content, and your world is being built as a facade, then you place "power" in others, in society, which can judge you, approve of you or condemn you: you deny the power in yourself by doing this. You might feel frustrated because you think you are in the "grip" of a person or situation. This leads to anxiety, to tension, to aggression!

The skeleton indicates giving structure in space and time: resistance and impatience here, breaking through structures (this is symbolized by the bone fracture).

Place all authority over your life in yourself.

Become balanced, in self-confidence: lean on yourself. Achieve a clear view of the here-and-now, and seize the bull by the horns. Concretely build toward a perspective, and resolutely go that path, but don't allow your joy to be dependent on outer or materialistic values, nor on that which — in the eyes of others — is good or bad, limp or strong. Break through the mask and determine your life yourself. Inner liberation, breathing freely, in independence.

No exterior pride, but inner certainty of your own worth.

No longer doubt yourself; don't force anything; don't try to affirm yourself toward the outside. Outer circumstances that oppress you are only the result of the denial of the authority in yourself.

Tensions, anxieties, and aggression are only signs of powerlessness; acknowledge yourself in love; live from out of your heart.

Skull fracture

Frustration, pent-up fury. You want to drill through things somehow, to push over everything in the little world around you that allegedly was in the way. You now try to force a way out. The truth is that for too long you have neglected the call of your nature; for too long you have been going against the grain. In frenzied nervousness, in powerless fury, you feel "stuck" in a desperate situation; you feel tied down, possibly experiencing yourself as a prisoner of an Authority, of someone outside you, because you don't yet dare to stand on your own feet. You can't yet get out of a situation about which you have been sick for a long time. Emotionally, you are looking for a balance, but you are not very successful, because you experience yourself as still so dependent on others, because you don't yet place the Authority in yourself. The dominant, authoritarian attitude of teachers or parents, or of a certain Authority, annoys you in such a way that you position yourself against it in an aggressive, protecting way, with the helmet of a Viking on your head, as it were.

In this way, aggressive forces work self-destructively. It remains an excuse for not having to be yourself. An inner urge for power, a revolt against the power above your head, not wanting to be bullied: "Get out of my way! *I* am here now." You force things: a fracture.

See how it's you, yourself, who's stuck in yourself. Do what you inwardly feel you have to do. Come to true self-realization in respect for yourself instead of holding in emotions and forces any longer and straining yourself. Know yourself to be safe in yourself. Your inner wisdom points out a direction to you: follow that path which follows naturally from your true nature. Be just toward yourself, toward others. Acknowledge the authority in yourself and no longer slow yourself down. Express your feelings, create your life, build your life on your own authority so that you find rest and relaxation in yourself. Thankfulness for life itself.

Jaw fracture: see JAWS

Spinal fracture of the neck: see NECK

Fracture of a vertebra: see VERTEBRAE

Sternum fracture
(See also Bone fractures, in general)

You feel stuck in a certain situation. You'd like to fight your way out of it, but you don't know how. Feeling powerless to solve it all at once, you'd like to break out, as it were. The person who feels imprisoned calls: "I want to get out!"

You call up this signal — the fracture — in order to start realizing clearly that your heart and lungs want to see themselves freed from an oppressive situation. You are filled to the brim with energies; possibly you'd like to force certain situations instead of understanding the signals, interpreting them, and confidently letting go of them.

An unconscious longing to delve inside yourself, into your heart, into the deeper feelings of love for yourself, for life. It seems as if you are cut off from your deeper love's core and unconsciously you long to make intense contact with your inner heart, far beneath the superficial layers. This basic feeling of being powerless to truly and fully BE from out of the deepest core of your being, can lead to calling up life situations in which a sort of impatient anger, revolt, and aggressiveness is experienced.

You "want something to be absolutely SO," and it doesn't work; this fire of desire only indicates that your "I" desperately longs to be acknowledged by you, in love, fundamentally. Allow yourself to fully BE, in all your width: your heart calls for a free living space, it longs to BE happy and relaxed. Your deepest Self cries, "It's been enough of this!" So, free yourself inwardly and bring about changes in your life where necessary for your evolution, your health.

Come to a deeper awareness, to more depth in your being and give yourself all opportunity for an open existence, without oppression — which you have laid on yourself. You can only revolt against yourself, against certain situations that you yourself — be it unconscious — have attracted. Therefore, solve the problems deep INSIDE you; outer circumstances will change, and you will realize which situations need to be changed as a result of your inner liberation. Stop the conflict in yourself, and come to inner peace by letting go and allowing yourself to BE in all freedom, not wanting to force something from life with might. As long as you feel emotions of revolt and anger, it means that you are fighting against yourself, against life. Let go. Just let yourself BE, and turn deeply inward. Come to a deep, loving reconciliation with yourself, and no longer desire anything outside of you.

Come to the pure happiness of Being yourself.

Broken rib: see RIBS

Collar-bone fracture
(See also Bone fractures, in general)

You would like to fight, fly, kick — bottled-up aggression! Anxiety and sadness. You feel powerless; you don't get a grip on yourself; you are angry about it! You ache for a vast living space for yourself; you'd like to fling away with one powerful grip everyone you suspect of wanting to hinder you — not being aware that you are the only one who hinders yourself from building your life in a calm, self-assured way.

Do you think yourself to be bad, unworthy of breaking through completely? Feelings of self-doubt, inferiority, self-hatred, self-negation — and an unconscious longing to break out of this cell. Resistance, aggression. Heartache. Deep in your heart you yearn for love and gentleness.

Blow off steam. Loosen everything; free yourself from those sad emotions.

Let yourself go for once; don't be afraid of your expressions — and observe your feelings: after all they are based on self-condemnation and on the denial of your sensitive, warm side and your strong, inner Self. Perhaps you projected this on others: now enter your strong, trustworthy "I". Dare to give and take flexibly. No longer feel threatened. Begin with being more open and loving: your surroundings will react differently to that. No longer suppress your energies!

Shoulder fracture
(See also Shoulder, in general)

Do you absolutely not want to lose your control, your authority, your power, your function or your status? You can no longer endure it all in this way; you are no longer master over it. You have grabbed for too much and have reached too far beyond yourself, have embraced too much, in care, in responsibility, in anxiety. Burdens become too heavy. Possibly for a long time you have kept up a big and strong front for the outer world, with a sense of responsibility. Possibly, you have made big achievements, but you have gone beyond your borders. You have been too hard on yourself.

Did you want to prove yourself? By "keeping straight" in the eyes of the outer world, you have suppressed your inner emotional world. You have fought against emotions, against the gentle, female feelings inside you. Possibly, you have fought in the same way against other people. You have

absolutely wanted to keep up something or push something through that would have been better to let go of. Aggressive powerlessness is the result. You have hardly any breath left; you feel smothered under your own emotional burdens. You'd like to break out now, to enlarge your space.

Reasons for the burdens: because you don't experience enough safety in your Self, because you don't have enough faith and confidence in your inner worth, you concentrate all your attention on the outer world; you expect acknowledgement and try to keep everything under your control. You run past your feelings in order to be able to embrace it all. Until these emotions block your path and thoughts, which are too hard, destroy your life.

You need to "break" with this way of life.

Use all the forces inside you; seize power only over yourself.

Turn back inward. Get a solid hold of yourself and navigate through your emotions without any detours, the way a solid ship cleaves the waves. Throw those burdens off your shoulders: feel free and spontaneous in your nature. Feel solid on your own safe Basis, so that you no longer look for affirmation and security outside yourself. Self-development from within; don't reach beyond yourself so that aggressive forces pile up, but let them steadily unfold in this self-development. Don't neglect your feelings; follow the demand of your nature and don't force anything. If you put faith in your Self you will no longer carry needless burdens, especially not for the sake of the outer world or in order to keep the "power." Let go, and be faithful to your nature.

Fracture of the upper arm
(See also Bone fractures, and Upper arm, in general)

Anxiety about not being able to embrace it all: tensely, you hold on to people, to old structures, especially when you feel that they are slipping away from you. Enormous energies turn inward, like a time bomb: you reach for a hold outside of yourself, for a job, a social situation, a relation, etc. — in order to "fill" yourself. You are afraid that these false structures might fall away from you. You allow your life to be controlled by factors outside yourself; you are not solidly with your feet on the ground. You experience yourself as small and powerless and perhaps you have allowed others to grab you by the hair for too long — you are afraid they are going to crush you.

The most important thing in life escapes you, something that doesn't let itself be grabbed, nor forced: love, friendship, self-esteem, trust. You try to keep power, or a grip, "over"; you stand up against people who seem to hinder you in this.

Let go!

Mount the throne of self-respect; make yourself master of the situation! Friendship, love, and one's contents are of true importance; put in perspective the worth of the form and outer structures. The life structures that are good for you will automatically follow on your appreciation of the content; a tight structure or an outer pattern that serves to replace an empty content will break sooner or later. It doesn't matter if your outer world collapses as long as you still stand on your own feet. Your life falls or stands, indeed, with your inner worth and the faith in yourself to be able again and again to build a new and better life. Be master of your life and give yourself all the room you need.

Elbow fracture
(See also Elbow, in general)

You are angry with the Authority above your head, but you can't or dare not puncture it. Your nature was already being suppressed for too long; you want to end your role as a victim; you begin to resist the restriction of your nature; you might offer resistance against established values, norms, or authority-structures; your life was being smothered by outer rules or by demands from your surroundings.

You feel contorted; you'd like to slip away. Your "I" revolts strongly against something or someone. You feel the other person as an intruder in your private nature. You'd protect your terrain with force and aggression. Inner tension. Now you can't free yourself fast enough from this, you think, but emotionally you feel too powerless, too heavily burdened to actually push yourself through. After all, you are not aware enough of your worth; you experience yourself like a victim in the power-grip of people and norms.

Your aggression rages, especially inwardly; you withdraw into yourself; tense, filled with aggressive forces. From under your dark glasses you look angrily at the authority that annoys you. You fire arrows underground. But in the meantime you don't see an alternative for yourself; you are still looking for your direction.

Don't put on a mask; don't be silent in anger, stubbornness, and sadness, but come to open communication and say what bothers you. Trust in your intuition; dare to express your feelings. Go straight ahead on your path and don't look at it all in such a dark and aggressive way.

Give yourself room; don't smother yourself, because it is you who in dependency on others, has restricted yourself too much.

Be open to clear insight and allow intense consciousness-powers into your existence, instead of those negative thoughts. Powerful assuredness of yourself; be aware of your worth. Come to open, honest, smooth contact with others, in supple versatility. Be completely inside yourself without hesitation; don't force yourself into armor. Allow the negative to escape in time, before the cesspool overflows.

Transform powerless resistance into active self-realization.

Forearm Fracture
(See also Bone fractures, and Forearm, in general)

You'd like to break through something with your fist! But something holds you back: you are even a little afraid of it, you "flee" from it. You fear the consequences, the re-action of your partner or your colleagues; you don't know if you would be able to han-dle it. You feel yourself slowly sinking into a swamp, anxiety grows. You stagnate your personal development. You immobilize yourself completely; tensions pile up, and from a feeling of powerlessness you would like to deal with someone in an aggressive way! Unconsciously, you get angry about this unfruitful, unhealthy situation.

Make a decision and come into action; trust yourself and no longer block your evolution. Trust your emotions: allow them to flow; don't bottle them up; dare to express them! Relax, take up all your space and make your opinion and your longings known to others: in the exchange of thoughts and feelings eve-rything will evolve more flexibly than by bot-tling things up in a grim, anxious way. In gentle resoluteness bite into it and flow sup-plely along with the river, with your ener-gies, your feelings. Go onward, break your attachment to past values.

Wrist fracture
(See also Bone fractures, and Wrist, in general)

Too little flexibility; lack of self-assurance: rigid and anxious!

You feel oppressed in a structure that is too tight. Your own "I" is being pushed away. Somehow you don't trust yourself completely. Perhaps there's a very rotten, untrustworthy foundation inside you? You are afraid, as it were, of allowing yourself to come through in a supple way! The situation is distressing you; you want to break out! You'd like to push away everything and eve-ryone you think hinders your growth, takes your space.

You rear up, like a horse. . . .

Allow yourself to be supplely taken along by your own fruitfulness; allow yourself to be guided by your inner forces. Life will appear much lighter because of this faith in yourself. Nothing inside or outside you forms a threat for you: these illusionary phantoms have been created by your anxieties.

You are the master over yourself; follow your intuition; act in a self-aware way, with a free will that can't be stifled by anyone.

Instead of defending: stand up for your worth as a unique human being. Be open to new experiences, don't push them away.

Hand fracture
(See also Hands, in general)

You revolt, you don't go along in this way any longer. Thus far you have "drawn in," taken in, everything and everyone, pain, sad-ness, criticism, as well as those others who have absorbed all your attention and efforts, who have used you: you have allowed all this because you considered yourself a helpless victim and also felt a need to be dependent on others. Like someone born with the sun in Cancer — holding on to so much that he might collapse under it — that's how you feel right now. You now close iron gates so that nothing or no one can enter anymore, no emotions, no burdens, no more words of an interfering Authority. Possibly, you have for too long allowed yourself to be used in the name of love, as if you were a hall-stand or a stepping-stone, while you barely felt yourself supported.

Your "I"-power now wants to break through and make an end to the powerless-ness to exist like an autonomous, self-assured individual. With exaggerated force, your ego now breaks through; you no longer know any suppleness; you are now aggressive in a hard way. For too long you have grabbed with your hands for support, although sometimes it seemed to be the opposite.

Decisively take in hand your personal life: become aware of the warm sun-center inside you. Come to clear insight of yourself, follow your intuition; take good care of yourself. If you are strongly concentrated in your Self, then you will also be able to be a strong, radiating beacon for others. Bend supplely toward yourself, toward your nature. Acknowledge your own fullness, the Authority of your Self, so that you never have to experience yourself as empty and in need of filling this emptiness with everything and everyone.

Radiate health and love toward others; GIVE, without having to swallow or take certain things just because you are in an emotionally dependent situation. You are no victim, but are master over yourself.

Don't allow yourself to "be lived," but work and create; build your life under the sole authority of your Self.

Fracture of a finger: see FINGERS

Hip fracture
(See also Hip, in general)

You have become like an erupting volcano: all pent-up energies now break out.

On the one hand, emotions are going beyond you; anxieties, tensions, sadness and burdens that are too heavy have become too much for you. On the other hand, you have been suppressing your forces for too long; like a snorting bull with held-in, stubborn fury, you finally break through the fence in a sharp, aggressive attack. For too long you have felt muzzled; you are angry with those who have, so to speak, stood in the way of your life. The deeper cause lies in you, however: now you say, "You won't get me anymore, nor restrict me!" But it is you, yourself, who hasn't lived enough according to your own nature, who possibly has too much yielded to others, to the outer world, silent, suppressing yourself — possibly because you don't at all think yourself good enough. Have you not dared to live from out of your-

self? Have you not dared to stand up for your opinion? Have you for too long followed a path that doesn't really suit you? Then you have lived under pressure and tension, untrue toward yourself. Now you stand up, protesting, like a dead person who wants to start living.

Build your life on the strong foundations of yourself. Discover those life forces, the sureness in yourself, and speak; express yourself to others. Stand up for yourself; don't hide, but dare to voice what is necessary, so that you can calmly relax again in yourself. Only count on the Authority in yourself, and come to flexible, clear communication with others. No longer pile up tensions and emotions; at all times dare to be yourself, the way you are. Get an overview and, in spite of protests from your surroundings, don't hesitate to choose your personal path.

Thighbone fracture
(See also Bone fractures, and Legs, in general)

You are afraid that your deepest "I" is bad or weak. You beg or ask or pray to others, to gods; you are completely standing still on the path of self-development. You place all power outside yourself. You are stuck in your past, and you think you can't get out of it.

In the meantime, there develops an inner flow of fury, aggression, emotions. You will take the Law into your own hands! You don't realize that it was your own feelings of powerlessness, your unconscious convictions of "I am the victim," which brought you into a living-space that is too restricting. Sooner or later you will break through: a frustrated volcano!

Become aware of the fact that others, or structures, only restrict you if you first asked for it (unconsciously). Once and for all, come to self-confidence and consciousness;

allow that deep power to penetrate you completely; enlarge your spiritual space. Come to insight and mastery in Yourself. That really offers open space. Action, decisiveness, rest, and relaxation: balance. Nowhere is there an authority higher or more worthy than you, and that worth is in your heart, your soul — your worth as a human being. Create your life yourself!

Knee fracture
(See also Bone fractures, and Knee, in general)

Degeneration of an inner conflict; a fight as it were between heaven and earth. Between the "male" and "female" principles. A power struggle inside yourself: going along with the flow, feeling you have to go in that direction — and then blocking this with resistance! Are you keeping yourself standing in a tough way, or do you flexibly flow along? You bring yourself, your worth, into question — inferior, unsure. You therefore begin to frenetically resist every person you suspect has more grip on you than you have yourself. You remain at the ready, like a roaring lion, in order to resist the so-called "power" of others. You might kick in prevention!

Instead of flexibly entering into dialogue with others, you might sooner feel threatened. You don't trust yourself nor your own Power, so how can you trust others? Then, suddenly, you feel that you are being seized! You can no longer get away; you develop a counter force; you feel dragged along; you resist — then collide!

Aggressive resistance.

First achieve harmony with yourself: solve that inner conflict.

Open yourself up without prejudice; receive freely that which others offer you in words and gestures; calmly go over everything; take a good look at it. Don't stubbornly hold on to established false values

from the past; open yourself up to your true evolution.

Blame your stubborn resistance on your unsureness: feel solid in yourself! Calmly approach new things and especially open yourself up completely.

First, find a solid basis in yourself, only then can you calmly "receive," which in turn will get you further; no longer push it away. Come to fruitful, flexible creativity and communication.

Lower leg fracture
(See also Bone fractures, and Legs, in general)

You feel small, unsure; perhaps you experience the work you do as not being good enough for you, especially because inwardly you undervalue yourself. You revolt against authorities or just against people who "threaten" you in some way in the little authority you give yourself.

You might then begin to defend your terrain in an aggressive way! You'd like to pull down others, kick them, in this power struggle.

Furious, you would even destroy that which is beautiful, because in fact you are angry about your own powerlessness and inability: a form of self-destruction.

You will not easily admit that you feel unsure in yourself; on the contrary, outwardly in a stalwart way you would reach for the top at once and take down any other authority. This desperate revolt means that you want to force things; it's like an outward coup, which can cause you a bone fracture.

Do you experience yourself as vulnerable and fragile? You can't solve this by being aggressive with others, nor with yourself.

You grow to your Peak from within, gradually; surrender to your own strong fundamental force and don't want to be the first in competition with others, but realize all the more the value of your own Energy Field. . . .

Take delight in your life; now be content with your place: if your longings go out to something else, then create new situations in your thoughts; don't force anything. That which is good for you will come to you if you open yourself up in self-confidence.

The world is not hostile toward you; no longer feel threatened; show yourself the way you really feel, and don't hide behind an aggressive attitude: people will only react aggressively toward you if you are stuck with suppressed anger.

Feel sure in yourself, in this way you won't have to prove yourself.

It's not others who are in the way of your evolution, but you, yourself, because of your doubts.

Ankle fracture
(See also Bone fractures, and Ankle, in general)

You feel unable to change direction, although you know this is necessary for your evolution.

Anger, impatience, resistance against an authority or situation that oppresses you.

"One" holds you back, you say, but it is you, yourself, who doesn't dare to change direction.

Nervousness. You are busy with many things at the same time; you search in all directions — "It won't be much longer, just wait!" In the meantime you stand still. "Keep away from me!" you'd say in an irritated way. Because the inner conflict gnaws at you: afraid that if you go onward, or would choose another direction, the roof might come down on your head, so you just keep sitting there — this makes you so rebellious!

Follow, in self-confidence, the direction you feel you have to take; no longer obstruct new paths, your evolution, your growth — by fallacies. Go along flexibly with that which your inner Self offers you.

Foot fracture
(See also Bone fractures, and Foot, in general)

You don't really see *how* to go on, but there's an enormous, aggressive urge to push yourself through.

You resist being stuck, a situation which has been too heavy for you for too long. Dark thoughts thunder in your head. You look for a solution. Inner conflict. Potential energies have been suppressed for too long; you don't have a clear view of your worth and your possibilities. You stand up against people who treat you in an authoritarian way, because you are desperately looking for the authority in yourself. You become stubborn and willful. You even refuse to go *truly* onward, because you think your path does not lie there, where your inner self, your intuition, directs you. You fight; you'd go against the stream and collide with others. You follow everything but your heart; you want to force something, to satisfy certain demands made by your rational mind. You are hard on yourself. The burden that you carry — you can simply throw it off!

See clearly how you restrict yourself; now follow in a calm way the path your nature indicates. Be aware of your true power and go on! Calmly build your structure and in a self-aware way go onward.

Surrender to the natural flow. Now acknowledge your heart, your emotional side. Thankfulness.

No longer fight, no longer carry any needless burdens. Follow that path which is good for you.

Fracture of a toe

For too long, you have lived at the surface of life, or you are on a life's course that doesn't *really* fit you. You feel like you are standing still. . . .

Your energies turn again and again in the same vicious circle; you are stuck in the old mire; you are not aware of your powerful possibilities, or they are being paralyzed. You no longer see any other direction than the one into which you have become rusted. . . . You feel like you are in the power-grip of habit or of your stubborn, retentive nature. In fact, you can't go on, because you don't believe in yourself!!! You don't trust life; you are on guard; you refuse to choose. . . .

Your piled-up energies and creative possibilities translate into aggressiveness! You'd like to cut it off at last! But you cut into yourself and others instead of pushing yourself in a new direction.

For such a long time, you have been covered with dust: when are you going to free yourself? Do you think you are worth merely *that?* Revolt. Unconscious refusal to go any further on *this* path on which you are now stuck.

Look for the core; come to true life and explore all its depths! Choose your true direction and no longer go around in a circle. Break out of your prison and freely build your life. Handle with mastery all those energies in you and make use of your talents. There are indications enough in your surroundings that show you your path — don't hesitate. Go onward.

For a fracture of a specific toe: see the category TOES.

SKIN

Psychological correspondence

The outer sense that lies in the extension of our inner Feeling, our inner perception. The skin senses, feels, sees, and lives: it's a reflection of our inner feeling of Authority, "I

AM." The sureness, the pride you have in your individual worth.

You set your borders regarding others, thanks to your self-protecting, inner Authority: you take care of yourself. You allow the warm sun-rays (the sun, your self-aware center) to warm your skin so that you experience a feeling of coziness, of contentment, in yourself.

This harmony in yourself, between soul and body, this openness to your Living Self will lead to a harmonious meeting with your surroundings, with your friends, etc. In other words, *your skin tells you what relationship you are in with yourself.* Contact with others will be a reflection of this. If you don't hurt yourself, and you respect yourself fully, your skin will gleam in a relaxed way; then you won't get injuries, nor by the acts of others.

The skin also symbolizes the Freedom to completely be yourself — to move supplely in the direction that, deep inside, you experience as being the most natural: like a flower that spontaneously blossoms, not tight or tense, so also will your skin ask for this steady, inner growth, without forcing, without placing yourself in tight armor, in stress, cut off from your inner longings.

Symbolic of inner sensitivity: you allow the breath of life to joyfully penetrate your senses, to the tip of your little finger. Feeling who you are; feeling contact with everything, with others.

The skin quickly reflects communication problems. The mirror of contact with yourself (do you love yourself?) and others. Being aware of your inner wisdom, revealed outwardly. Being open to earthly life, to sensorial enjoyment. Or do you live too "spiritually?"

Ailments, in general

Do you allow yourself, in self-doubt, to be hurt by others? Don't undervalue yourself! Do you feel helpless, naked, at the mercy of others, because you neglect your Living Self? Do you build your life too much on your thinking, on tight structures? Don't you dare enjoy what's earthly — your body? Do you anxiously hide yourself away? Are you not at all Aware of your self? Do you only live for others, allowing yourself to be used for a doormat? Don't you walk *on your own?* Do you lean on others instead of on your inner Authority? Do you think yourself ugly, inferior? Do you flee from yourself, and do you think that others will run away from you? Do you hoard your rich energies? Do you not dare to stand up for yourself, until at last you'll burst because of suppressed aggression?

Look in the mirror: accept yourself inwardly and outwardly; you are worthy of your love. Dare to manifest yourself in self-contentment, without acting or hypocrisy: be open and honest with yourself, with others. Enjoy contact, caress nature, and let yourself be warmed; feel yourself taken up inside your Self! Allow all beautiful consciousness powers to radiate outward through your pores and handle these energies in creativity: don't block yourself! Know that you are safe and sheltered inside yourself.

Rashes, in general

Signals, energies from the "unconscious" force themselves to the surface, to the skin, where they explode in order to make something clear to you. They say to you, "Allow your Sun, your Consciousness, to break through! Dare to be yourself!" But you keep in your creative energies, your possibilities, your consciousness powers, your talents — because you don't feel safe inside yourself.

You not only experience outside Authority (your father, your teacher. . . .) as a threat, but you are also afraid to acknowledge your own Authority! You doubt your worth, your ability; you keep your own sun-center under water. You allow your life to be ruled by unconscious forces, by emotions — upon which you can't get a grip, in your opinion. You can't handle yourself; you feel smothered,

unpleasant, anxious. Bottled-up feelings and potential energies pile up inside you until the volcano bursts open into skin eruptions.

Don't allow yourself to be propelled onward by unconscious forces, by emotions, but come to true Awareness. Don't allow yourself to "be lived" by fate or coincidence, but resolutely take the rudder yourself. Liberate yourself! Allow energies to flow freely under the guiding eye of your Conscious mastery. Don't let yourself be ruled, not by so-called unconscious mainsprings or emotions in you, nor by others. Be productive, acknowledge your worth, and don't stick your talents into the ground. What's being repressed will manifest itself all the more intensely — also via the skin: don't block yourself. You'll only become nervous, impatient, and frustrated if you repress yourself. Listen to the inner authority, to your intuition, and don't consider yourself inferior to those who can teach you something today. Test "knowledge" all the time with your inner wisdom.

Acne, juvenile pimples

In discontentment with yourself. You are not sure about your content, about who you really are. You are greedily looking for fulfillment outside yourself, for a solution to your inner emptiness. You revolt against the authority above your head; you react to your feelings of powerlessness and unsureness with a particular attitude toward the outside. You can come across as arrogant or as a smart-aleck who constantly expresses criticism of others; you may go your own way in a very self-willed manner. This is only camouflage. Criticism, anger, possibly unexpressed. You might get power or a grip on others because you turn away from yourself. Perhaps you think yourself ugly, and you completely bring yourself into question, but outwardly you might present yourself as holy or at least as someone who knows it all already. Inwardly, you sometimes tremble like a leaf. Insecure tension. Sometimes resistance to being nice to others, because you will rebel against anyone who might lecture you, since you already doubt yourself enough.

Let go of being constrained and of that grip on others: allow all impressions to calmly come in, and work out your feelings of dissatisfaction without projecting outward. For this, it's necessary that you trust in your deeper Self, in your Basis.

Thoroughly transform yourself: root yourself, and then no outside authority will hinder you. Let go of that resistance to lovingly coming toward yourself and others.

Dare to express your individuality: don't bottle up your natural longings, your urge toward self-realization, and creativity!

Replace criticism with growth. Come to complete acceptance of yourself. Softening, instead of sharp feelings.

Blackheads

You'd like to hide, ashamed, afraid to speak for yourself in social contacts. You feel unsure and small. You'd prefer to withdraw into the womb. Despite all your qualities and talents, you'd rather remain in the tunnel; then again, you'd like to break through in full force, like a spear, propelled by all bottled-up energies! You just turn with the wind; you have nothing to say, your opinion is not asked for; your surroundings react to your unsureness, and therefore take you for a sheep. You are ashamed to come out with your true feelings, with your worth and your talents, even though you feel deep inside that you have a lot of them. Do others hardly see you? Do you feel alone, deserted, unloved?

It's good for you to very consciously take all responsibility for your life; to make contact with your deepest Basis. To be born truly from here. Rise up out of yourself and come toward new life: surrender to your deepest feelings, to your true nature, which is beautiful and can be seen. Don't hide yourself,

but dare to exchange contacts in friendship, dare to communicate with what you feel. You are equal to others: come to self-assurance and action. Don't allow yourself to be influenced; resolutely determine yourself your life's direction! Get rid of that negative opinion of yourself, that black spot, and manifest yourself without fear. Don't expect others to love you if you hide yourself and don't like yourself!

Are you unhappy with your outer appearance? This is just the result of your generally feeling, "I'm not good enough." Now, solidly plant yourself in the earth. You are unique in your way; be proud of your being!

Birthmarks

A reflection of the inner battle: dependence and resistance against this. The path to incarnation on earth lies in the uterus: you go along with the flow of your mother, but on the other hand you feel grabbed by this, imprisoned, and you wish to push through your own autonomy. You feel "branded" by the bite of the stork, by the power and the characteristics of your mother and you do long for this tie, on the one hand, but on the other hand you feel pain somehow, you resist, you wish to come free, you are even angry — "Leave me alone!" Perhaps you get a good scolding or a smack on the head; you want to get away. No one has to tell you anything after all. You want to burst out like a bottle of champagne, but you are being restricted. An aggressive accumulation of energies, a resistance against any restriction. Wanting to get away, not wanting to get away: unconsciously, your feelings go around in a circle.

Blisters, in general
(See also Hand and Foot blisters)

Blocked energies ask for a breakthrough; your head bursts with tense thoughts, inwardly turned energies, as it were. You are afraid of your deepest nature; you anxiously hold on to everything. In this way, you evolve only shufflingly, hesitantly. You constantly extinguish in yourself the forces, the creativity, your fire — you slow yourself down. You are hard on yourself; you force yourself between lines that are too strict; you tie yourself down in a structure full of "obligations," because it has to be so. You feel so vulnerable: you constantly protect yourself against this. You don't go straight for the goal, or you waste your time in secondary occupations. Perhaps you get angry because of the restrictions you put on yourself. But you are so afraid of those forces inside you, of your emotions, of your fears — you don't trust your deepest Self. "Is there a devil in me? Or am I rotten inside?" You anxiously keep yourself closed, so that you blow up because of hidden aggressive forces. Nor do you say goodbye to painful memories from the past; you can't forget something or put it out of your head: you carry all of it along. You push away feelings, and possibly also Love, from you: you screen yourself from this because you don't dare to live intuitively. You might look at everything in a critical way because you are not at all sure that it's not a threat for you! Still, you long so much for peace, but your paranoid thoughts hinder this peacefulness.

Resolute action in self-assuredness, based on those deep, trustworthy pillars of your Living Self. Authority without fear! Freedom in emotional experience; intuitive choice without self-doubt. Don't exclude a part of yourself. Let go of those thoughts, those frustrations, the past. In an energetic way experience joy! No longer fight against yourself; allow yourself to flexibly flow along with your Nature, and come to feelings of peace, gentleness, and love. Don't fear yourself, don't fear others. Know yourself safe and protected deep inside your Self.

Vesicles (small blisters)

Help! Asking attention from others because you feel too small and too weak. You let others direct your life. You feel imprisoned, stuck; you are being hurt, sometimes you feel oppressed by the warning finger of a mentor (as a child). . . . Sadness; you might wistfully dream of beautiful, fairy-like regions — you are somewhere else with your thoughts; you escape from the present. You flee from yourself, sometimes anxiously. They do with you what they want; as a child you have no say, no authority; you resign yourself to this, because you are not enough present in yourself anyway. Are you in the clouds again or do you play the clown? A clown hides his tears; that's how you carry a mask: you don't dare let your true feelings come through, in part because you are too critical regarding yourself, or: What would "people" say? You don't trust your deepest nature; you don't dare let yourself go, except in a superficial way! You stay closed, hidden, like a turtle!

Feel the warm center in yourself. Stand solidly with both feet on the ground. Live here-and-now. Don't fly away; allow your feelings to come through freely from out of the depths of yourself and experience your nature, your body, fully, so that a balance is being reached in your dreaming, thinking little life. No longer hide your feelings; dare to be yourself, don't be afraid of a tear either. Allow yourself to OPEN UP!

Join the wisdom of your Living Self, via intuition and feeling; don't try to comprehend everything within the rational. Dare to march into life in a spontaneous, impulsive way like an adventurer with a knapsack, full of trust in yourself. Don't look for adventure and for your satisfaction in thoughts, but in true action.

Burst, chapped, split skin

There's no smooth flow of energies because you don't really live according to your true nature; you are not faithful to your nature. You don't show your true disposition — because you are afraid, you are on guard with everyone! You too much "play" a game, you give yourself a role. Inner division. The skin is the "contact-organ." Don't you feel protected enough? Your hands (in the case of chapping) shout this out: "I have pain, sadness, I feel hurt and tensed up in the solar plexus, often in the stomach." Inwardly crying, you hide; you feel so tense that your skin might burst. Do you have painful communication problems with others? Do you live in antagonism with your partner? Then this is the consequence of "the rift" (the split in your skin) that you maintain toward yourself. Do you feel so hurt? You feel attached and vulnerable, but you wear a mourning cap in order to camouflage it. It is possible that you take on too much sadness from others, that you sympathize enormously with the pain of a friend. But you hold on to this sadness only because it is closely related to your own sorrow. You lose yourself in the pain of others, because you are stuck with pain yourself and don't depend enough on your Self-aware "I"! Do you flee from true contact with your body, from the physical in general? Do you feel inferior in your contacts? Afraid others might hurt you? Do you think yourself to be "bad"?

Stretch yourself open all the way! Relax, and take up your space. Open up your lungs! Free yourself from emotions and oppressions: tune in to your deepest, joyful Self. No one can hurt you, if you haven't first unconsciously asked for it. Therefore, be aware of your worth, enjoy making contact with your deepest feelings, your deepest wishes, and be open about them. Speak up, and don't allow yourself to be hurt. Acknowledge yourself with respect — only then will others fully respect you. Your surroundings only respond to your convictions regarding yourself! Being conscious of your own joyful Existence offers true resistance to whatever word or sorrow comes to you from the outside. Give warmth and appreciation to your Self: your sadness will disappear, and others will also warm you with a respectful attitude.
Every human being is "good" in his own way. Feelings of being bad or inferior are

subjective and absurd. Acknowledge the worth of your nature, your body, your skin; dare to enjoy your senses. Come to oneness in yourself; close that rift in a loving way. Make yourself heartily welcome.

Calcinosis cutis
calcification of the skin

In an exaggerated way, you want to protect yourself; you make yourself hard. You see things as being too heavy, emotionally too dark. You allow your own luminous "I" to be obscured by other people, by figures who in your eyes have authority — and because of this you have the feeling you have to turn yourself against them. In defense, looking for shelter, protecting yourself. Feelings of anxiety, doubt, pessimism — the conviction that "life is dark and unsafe."

You are safe and protected IN yourself. Acknowledge the Authority in yourself as a fundamentally strong Basis, and come to softening, peace, relaxation. Nothing, or no one forms a threat for you: blow off those old convictions and live in Trust. Give to yourself; give to others. Only true love brings softening and inner rest.

Skin cancer
(See also Cancer, in general)

Emotionally remaining stuck in the past: an emotional burden. You place Authority outside yourself: you allow yourself to be ruled by an enormous crushing energy, which divides you — the Sun radiates outside you, it blinds you: does this concern your father, your partner, your faith? You feel to be in the grip, in the power. Instead of placing the sun (self-aware worthiness) in your inner center, you allow your life to be ruled by others, by criticism, by social norms, by beauty-demands (Do I look good in the eyes of others? Do I satisfy the requirements?).
Because you deny your inner Authority, you make yourself dependent on others. Be-

cause of this you also feel anxious and unsure. You are on guard against accidents and setbacks; you walk on tiptoe — you don't trust your deepest Self at all! You don't look enough under the surface of your existence. You are always busy providing, or arming yourself against, that which might go wrong. You don't at all realize that it is you who creates your life. Instead of evolving onward, you keep going back to the past, or you waste your energies by fixating yourself on anxieties and worries. You are afraid of those deep feelings; you run away from your own Core.

You can't really show yourself the way you are; you have built a shield, as it were, around yourself. If you don't trust yourself, then you will also mistrust others. You don't dare to live *truly!* Division: inner feelings — outer appearance.

Don't run away from your emotions; don't suppress them: observe and work them out. Build only on your own authority; discover your deep trustworthy Core. Come to full awareness of your creative possibilities and take, in an autonomous way, the steering wheel of life in hand. An openness toward yourself will lead to deeper consciousness. This encounter leads to love and peace in yourself. Not others, but you, have been your own enemy. Let go of the needless burdens of the past. It is not the outer form that counts, but the Content, your feelings: dare to be yourself, without hypocrisy, the way you are. Don't try to answer to the expectations of others, but follow your longings and live in joy!

Candida
(See also Fungal infection, in general)

Enormous energies turn and circulate through and around your body: frustrated, held-in thoughts and longings — but you are unsure; you don't dare.

On the one hand, you place yourself under the Authority of others; on the other hand, this annoys you, and you'd like to

break out. The paradox of the aggressive urge for being yourself and self-suffocation. You don't know it anymore: will you give yourself and open yourself up to others, to a partner? Or will you resist and keep closed? You can't stand an Authority outside yourself anymore, and yet when you fall back on yourself, you again feel so afraid and unsure. In love relationships and friendships you are afraid that if you open yourself up emotionally and energetically toward others you might waste away in flames; and in this way your power, your urge for self-realization, ebbs away under a thick layer of Anxiety!

Too much spirit, too much unconscious forces: free yourself from this, and become master over your life. Come to rest and harmony in yourself. Land with both feet solidly on the earth and clearly determine what you want. Listen to your inner authority. In a conscious way, be present in every cell of your body: don't leave your body unmanned, but take the rudder in your hands. Handle your energies with mastery and transform them into creativity, into action! Break out of your oppressive space. Don't allow yourself to be held back by anyone.

Build your beautiful structures yourself.

Carbuncle
furuncles, boils

Desperate fury because of the feeling of being "stuck." You can no longer handle it: you would like to break away, but you cannot (yet). In smoldering anger you fixate your thoughts again and again on the same points: you'd like to force something; you rebel! Dark thoughts. You try in vain to get a "hold" on something, but you don't succeed very well because you don't get a grip on your inner, unstable feelings; you experience yourself as being aggressive but powerless, for resistance doesn't seem to be of much use. Possibly, you turn, full of indignation, toward those to whom you attribute

Authority — your parents, your employer, etc. — or perhaps you think you have been wronged.

You'd like to see something changed; you pull and tear, but you don't get anywhere. This situation only reflects your inner struggle, the discord in yourself. There is a struggle between that which you rationally would like to do and that which you feel you have to do. You suppress the sensitive aspect in you, the natural, the warm and gentle, your softness. You would rather handle everything structurally and rationally, but then you come into conflict with your emotional world, with your nature. This is reflected in your aggression toward the outer world. You wrong yourself! Are you afraid of your spontaneous inner Powers?? Dare to demonstrate your powers in a gradual unfolding!

Accept every aspect of yourself totally, and also the warmth of your body, your earthly being. Allow intuition and intellect to work together, solve the conflict between Nature and Structure. Allow your natural feelings to flow freely, and a structure will follow out of your spontaneous way of living: feel yourself to be like a child. Be gentle to yourself, don't fight against your natural aggression, but transform it into action-power.

Handle your pent-up energies and allow them to blossom under the authority of your love. Be aware of your Worth! Don't fixate on others, nor on their behavior. Just because you are sharp and hard with yourself, don't be sharp with others. Discover the unity in yourself between the female and male aspects. Come to open consciousness, listen to your intuition, and don't demand that others understand you in your uniqueness as a human being. Dare to be yourself, don't be afraid of inner energies. Manifest yourself the way you inwardly feel — in creative deeds. Don't direct yourself angrily at others, but allow that which is deepest in you to come to the surface. Batter your way through the ceiling of self-limitation!

Dandruff
scaling of the scalp

Suppressed emotions — especially aggression, anger — are seeking their way. You defend yourself against an "attacker," against the authority that, according to you, presses too heavily on your head. A revolt against a dominating factor, which you experience as stronger than yourself (for instance, your mentor, or Something. . . your work. . . .). Fury sometimes, indignation about the pain that someone inflicts on you. Perhaps you feel hurt in your image, or you are obliged to go along in a certain direction, which doesn't at all please you. Your emotions begin to dominate you; you feel a constriction in the solar plexus, you are tense. You revolt, defending yourself in a sharp way! Perhaps you experience a "power struggle" while this is not at all the case. You feel wronged, because you have not yet found yourself. For you want to have a grip on yourself, but your emotions hinder it. You experience yourself to be in a "forced" situation, but it is you, yourself, who creates it.

Grow out of this! Gradually come to true self-manifestation, without forcing it. Allow your powerful energies to freely come out. If you believe more strongly in yourself, if you become Aware of your worth and your possibilities, if according to your own insight and intuition you fulfill the tasks that now need to be fulfilled for your well-being — then you will find joy in everything you do; then you will no longer attract a pressing authority outside yourself (or a pressing Something, such as your duty, your work, etc.), because the personal Authority inside you — if you build your life on it — is the guarantee for a free, independent, and happy existence. Therefore, discover these Forces in you, and use them in creativity, so that you no longer aggressively act in frustration toward others. Don't allow wonderful energies and talents to end up in nail-biting or dandruff. Self-liberation and self-realization.

Skin discoloration
café au lait spots,
pigmentation (red or brown)

You deny the Force from within your deepest being, deny intuition, feelings, your body, the propelling impulses that come from your Living Self. You think you have to regulate, to structure everything with your Head: your rational mind strongly controls your life, while the voice of your natural spontaneity is not being heard. Sometimes your body seems to be "separate" from your thinking-self: a division; you "look" at your body from a distance. You can't, however, hold back with your head that inner urge for self-realization, those active Mars forces. But you are afraid of those deeper forces inside you, afraid also of feelings you consider to be "wrong." Are you programmed in such a way, by a religious or educational indoctrination, so that you feel bad when you feel anger? Are you, therefore, afraid to bring out natural aggression? Were you already born with the conviction that you are ugly, that your body is allowed to be there, but not to be enjoyed? Are you ashamed of yourself, of your feelings, of your body, and do you try to hide behind a (brown) mask, behind your words and your rationally justified way of life? You don't live openly and honestly with yourself, nor with others.

You feel guilty, ashamed about yourself: look at this conviction inside you, which hinders you from living truly spontaneously and free, honestly and open; hinders you from being in close contact with yourself, with your body and your soul's complete content. You feel like a stranger, not accepted by others: because you treat yourself like a stranger. Perhaps the conviction that you are bad, or not good enough, makes you bend toward others. Perhaps you go into a relationship in which you are the slave, in which you allow yourself to be "raped," in which you can't meet true love as long as you don't love yourself in soul and body. Possibly you'll attract a partner with the same inner division: two royal children can't come to each other, because the water ("unconscious anxieties about fully experiencing your total emotional world, your nature") creates a distance between them. You conceal your values, your talents, your possibilities, because you are ashamed of your rich content, as if you are not allowed to blossom! Deep, unconscious feelings of guilt lie at the basis of this: become aware of these sad, self-humiliating, destructive convictions, and make an end to them! You don't think enough about your rights as a human being, and too much about your obligations. Perhaps you are a martyr, thinking you have to do penance in order to earn your life. Sometimes powerless anger seethes inside because of this! The eagle begins its flight in full force with the longing to reach the Top of the mountain, but, ah — he starts to "think." He looks back, he doubts, fears rise up, he's afraid of falling — his thoughts make him return to his starting place. He lacked Trust in his deepest Self, in his intuition. Thus also calls your total being, your body — sometimes inwardly aggressive, because of being suppressed for too long — to be allowed to fly onward!

If you would trust in this intuitive Wisdom, in your impulsive longings — if you allow love for yourself to exist, the Unity between feelings and mind — if you are present in your body with your full consciousness, without looking at yourself from a distance, as if at an object — if you allow the inner, divine forces to blossom into creativity and complete action, then you will never fall, because then your life is built on your unshakable rock, your Autonomous Self-awareness, the unconditional love for all aspects of yourself.

"I Am here, unified, undivided, straightforward, consistent, honest and open. I no longer bottle things up; I live my life to the full, no longer punishing myself. Structures and rational mind will be at the service of my deepest Self-realization and will no longer be obstacles. If I come to inner harmony, I'll come to harmony with my surroundings; I take off my suffocating mask.

"I am MYSELF."

Eczema

Self-degradation, self-condemnation, self-punishment. You degrade yourself to being a penitent, a guilty, inferior being. Refusing to acknowledge your own worthiness; especially contemplating your own faults and shortcomings. Denial of your own larger possibilities. Because one is convinced that one is but a poor servant, or at least a human being with many bad characteristics, one subordinates oneself to an outside Authority. This leads to enormous inner conflict! On the one hand, one refuses to use one's brains, as it were: one carries one's brains in the stomach instead of in the head. One puts a lot of one's energy into activities like sports, housekeeping, administration, etc.; one can even put too heavy a structure or discipline upon oneself!

Habitual, daily, rational use of the brain suits this person. But thoughts keep floating on this narrow level. There's a lot of thinking, especially on the surface. On the other hand, there's that revolt against the self, that itching irritation, that restless resistance coming from the "I": a call to allow larger, higher energies to come through. A call for liberation of the personality, which is imprisoned in a net. The only way out is awareness of one's own worth and opening oneself up to one's intuition, talents, the larger creative potential, higher awareness-energies.

"That's not for me." Shutting off parts of the brain in self-punishment! The deepest Self now protests against this self-negation or against this restriction of possibilities.

(No slavery, but kingship! No endless fretting, nor self-degradation, no more head that becomes mad from pent-up energies.)

The brain is only allowed to think on a superficial level because the governor of it denies the rest of its Contents.

Feelings of guilt, thinking one doesn't deserve "love" from oneself or others unless perhaps one "sacrifices" oneself completely. Not only does one think oneself inferior, but often one thinks oneself "ugly." Here, too, one often assumes that outer beauty has to be earned. One can punish oneself in this case by forcing all kinds of diets or sports-discipline on oneself. One flees from oneself. On the other hand, one inwardly cries out for acknowledgement and love.

Burn these negative convictions with the fire of your Conscious self-esteem until nothing is left, and then rise up like a phoenix out of its ashes! Recognize the lovely, innocent child in yourself, and offer it affection and acknowledgement.

Allow more beautiful, lighter tones into your existence; no longer keep yourself to the ground. Every human being is good, beautiful, and unique, the way he IS. Don't change yourself; accept yourself the way you are and go and discover your larger possibilities. No longer restrict yourself; don't linger, fretting, in this inner conflict (yielding or breaking through) and think back to why you have brought yourself down or restricted yourself. Masses of energies ask for a breakthrough: open yourself up to your intuition, to your longings, and don't allow yourself to "be lived." Create the future you want. Don't push yourself away: make yourself welcome one hundred percent, and now give yourself all opportunity. Don't expect anything from others, but give it all to yourself. Only when you completely accept yourself, respect yourself, and love yourself — only then will you attract people who will approach you with the same positive values. Believe in yourself; allow all itching possibilities to be born freely now — no longer put a damper on them!

Infantile eczema, on the head
milk crust

You live rather unconsciously, allowing others to treat you the way they want. An emptiness, a feeling of absence. You'd like to stand up against those who take care of you, but in fact you stand up against yourself. It's as if your head, your body, is not (yet) really yours (or no more); you feel foolish in your human outfit. You push yourself aside, and as a result you also push others aside. Then again you feel rejected and alone. . . . Inner confusion; in your ignorance, you allow yourself to be attended to by others. Perhaps you think yourself very ugly.

Therefore, surrender in love to yourself and take your place on the throne: become ruler over your life, and feel contentment and thankfulness about life itself. Joy about yourself will lead to joyful communication with others.

Evolve from an unconscious way of living toward a Self-aware way of life! Fully take up your space. Mothers, respect the uniqueness of your child and raise it in a free, open atmosphere, without oppressive authority, but by stimulation.

Folliculitis
hair follicle inflammation

You are at the ready with a defensive but aggressive attitude toward anything or anyone who might threaten you: you are so afraid that someone will (still) hurt you.

Unconscious anxieties rise up because you don't at all feel safe inside yourself. You put up red thorns to defend yourself: you feel as if others have pierced you with knives from all sides.

Fear of profound communication: probably someone has hurt you in a sensitive part of your soul; you shield yourself so no one can hurt you anymore in your most intimate being.

Often, it has to do with imaginary anxieties, paranoia, the result of unsureness.

You, yourself, have unconsciously called up all painful experiences and communication problems from the past. Change your con-

victions; know yourself to be strong on your own Basis; feel protected in your Self; allow yourself to grow in self-aware dignity. Nothing is done to you if you haven't first unconsciously asked for it. Throw away negative (illusory) thoughts and create your reality yourself! Consciously take your life in your own hands and come into Action!

Nettle rash
hives, urticaria

You don't manifest your potentialities. You hide; you don't really dare show who you are. Possibly, you hide behind others — afterward, you would blame them for being the cause of your not being able to manifest yourself.

Bottled-up aggression is the result. You would like to shoot arrows! But you just look on the dark side of things, through a pair of black glasses, as it were; you feel powerless — lost, anxious. You allow yourself to turn on a wheel, a maelstrom, instead of confirming your individuality. Others penetrate your personal terrain; you *allow* them to drill into your being; you keep silent, but inwardly a red-hot flow of anger swirls. You feel pitiable, in the grip of others, while you'd like to be free as a bird. You are cut off from your Source, from your nature; you allow yourself to be scorched by the fire of others, because you deny your personal Power.

Be proud of your Basis, your Living Self, and come to energetic creativity, action! Don't give up; instead of becoming inwardly wound up, it is better to sow your talents. Act, instead of fretting! You are not at all pitiable or powerless. Get a hold on your life with both hands and resolutely direct it in the way you want. Don't allow yourself to be influenced by others, but come into honest communication with your feelings. Transform aggression into action! Don't allow others to look into you; direct yourself at the important things and storm ahead.

Pimples, in general

Sadness and aggression are being spit out like venom; an accumulation of nervous energies; not feeling able to express emotional content. You don't have the courage to convey something in words to others; you feel powerless, not good in your skin. You feel, at the same time, limp and weak; on the other hand aggressive forces are pushing! You poison yourself with black, destructive thoughts, because you don't express what dwells in you. You feel so discontent inside yourself, in a structure that is too oppressive for you; but you direct this discontentment toward others, in criticism. Self-manifestation is too difficult for you; courage has, instead, sunk into your boots. On the one hand, you would like to crawl away; on the other, you would like to spout it all out. An aggressive dominant force makes itself master over you whenever you block your spontaneous energies, and as long as you think yourself ugly or not good enough. Now live your life to the full and express yourself the way you are, without detours. Say what you have to say, reach dialogue with others. Cherish yourself, in your body, content. Enjoy with all your senses, and allow creative energies to flow freely.

Pimples, with white heads

You feel unsure, especially concerning your emotions. You think you fall short somewhere, anxiously bringing yourself into question. Perhaps you experience yourself like a lame dog, like a failure. You are not sure how far you can allow your feelings to come through; you don't dare show yourself the way you feel! You hide behind an attitude that doesn't reveal any of your feelings. You think you are "bad" if you manifest yourself the way you are. Perhaps you are outwardly very friendly and docile, but inwardly you have to pay for this, and you don't bottle up only your true feelings and

thoughts, but also a frustrated anger! You come out "white," but you feel "dark," bad, or ugly. You experience yourself as a powerless, deserted child, that courageously, but alone, has to find its way — left to its own devices, but feeling inadequate.

Anxiety about being dragged along by your feelings. You think you have to satisfy certain norms to be accepted by others, but neither inwardly nor outwardly do you answer to the social expectation-pattern.

Don't allow your individuality to be pushed aside by an anonymous mass! You don't have to drive in a carriage of glittering gold: now acknowledge the gold inside you. Allow your emotional source to flow freely; dare to trust your intuition, your feelings. You only reject yourself, and as a reaction to this you possibly will attract people who will also judge you negatively. But the cause lies inside you. Don't be ashamed of your true feelings, of your unique content. You are different from others: be proud of your uniqueness. Don't bottle up any emotions: look for channels whereby you can manifest yourself without any reservation. No longer resist; surrender to yourself.

The power over your life lies inside you. If you think yourself outwardly ugly, then this is only a result of the fact that you don't totally accept yourself the way you are, that you don't really love yourself. Build your house, stone-by-stone, perhaps slowly, but surely. Full of self-confidence, stand on your own feet.

Proud flesh, keloid

You hold on to a lot of things, in thoughts, and emotionally; experiences from the past and from the present. You grasp, you embrace, you want to hold on to more and more. You often experience the past as a slow-motion picture, in flash-backs — "no one can take this away from me anymore" — but in the meantime you are stuck, as if in an inflated plastic bag, because you inflate yourself, your head, your intestines. It's so hard for you to let go and go on.

You'd sooner live in a world that's "not real," in a world of "ideas and symbols," of imaginings and remembrances. There's no question of an actual evolution, step by step, in the here-and-now. You allow yourself to "be lived" by your longings, by an institution or a teaching; in this way, your actual life is passing by, toward death. You go beyond your borders; you don't recognize the borders of the space-time-Now-moment.

You look for knowledge and stability outside yourself; you don't live yourself. You don't become master over yourself; you allow your thoughts and feelings to flow over you. You desire ever further, more and more. You'd prefer to grasp and force things. Because you refuse to recognize the fullness and wisdom in yourself, you try to reach further and further, you want to fill yourself with things and experiences that you seize from the outside. Possibly, you are used to materialistically desiring things because you feel anxious and threatened; you look for protection in possessions, in gold, instead of acknowledging the gold in yourself. But, it can just as well have to do with a "spiritual" desire/possession. This depends on your "system of values." You don't follow the path of your Nature, you force things, because you neglect your divine Self and its creative possibilities. An unreal, False growth.

*Go along, flexibly, with the current of your heart; allow your deepest Self to **give**: it gives what's best for you. Therefore, don't grasp, don't force, but let go. Don't get stuck in the past, but intensely experience the Now, so that herein you become fulfilled by yourself. No longer want and want — let everything flexibly go its way. Trust in your intuition; allow your inner wisdom to speak. Experience to the fullest this content, this wisdom inside yourself and don't allow anything else to take its place. Determine your borders; don't go beyond yourself in order to*

*find truth and satisfaction. You **are**. In this fullness, you can open yourself up to that which is most beautiful in your surroundings — to others. Determine your path, your structure, in the life you wish to lead. Become master over yourself and don't seek your happiness in false teachings.*

Psoriasis

Fear of your own feelings and forces is becoming bigger and bigger, because you keep suppressing those forces and feelings! Afraid of those energies deep inside you, of unconscious forces which might threaten you (comparable to the painting "The Scream," by E. Munch). Existential anxiety. You don't only flee from the responsibility for your deepest emotions, but also from projections of this suppression in your close surroundings. You fear, perhaps unconsciously, that something very big and mighty, something threatening, might crush, rape, hurt, or destroy you. You are constantly at the ready to flee — this is just a result of that enormous fear and of the mistrust regarding your deepest "I" and your feelings. You can very well keep things rationally under your control or organization as long as you are not confronted with your other side: your emotions, your intuitive forces. You would scream: "NOOOOOOO!" Resistance against this essential part of you! You DOUBT your worth: you don't push your true self through.

Express yourself! Self-expression. No longer suppress your aggressive Forces! Don't be so afraid of your deepest Self; allow all your energies, your feelings, to come through freely, don't fight against them! Blocking this natural flow of feelings actually hinders anxieties from disappearing. No longer repress, because it's this repression that makes you sick! You have nothing in yourself, no single force or emotion, to fear. Your Living Self is solid and trustworthy: surrender to it. Become master over yourself: you are able to regulate the brake and the accelerator. Allow all energies to flow freely, for by doing this you liberate yourself! Your Anxiety is the result of NO LONGER HAVING CONTACT WITH YOUR AUTHENTIC, LIVING SELF: come very close to yourself; discover the riches deep inside you; say yes to yourself.

Ringworm
ring-shaped rash because of fungus; "Tinea"

You are not able to set up your own structures, to border off your own terrain, because you don't listen to your own authority, feel powerless, don't build your life enough on your own basis. Still, you feel restricted under the observing eye of a father or of another authority. You *do* feel your worth, a certain inner pride is present, but you allow your life to swing back and forth in the hammock of your mentors, your examples, or your surroundings. You don't really break through; you don't really live freely and openly the way you would like, because you are afraid — possibly also of the boss looking over your shoulder, or, for instance, of a director who's spying on you, etc. . . . You don't feel able to choose your own life's course; you fly onward, but don't know where.

Your spontaneity is being curbed. Emotionally, you feel grabbed; something or someone overpowers you. You aren't getting a grip on yourself or on your feelings. You feel unable, and this powerlessness hurts you. The least authority can be too much for you, because you let yourself suffocate. Energies and emotions pile up, wishing to be allowed to come through freely, but you don't dare be yourself because of anxiety, self-doubt, or for fear of being hurt. Inner resistance comes to the surface! Your own sadness and powerlessness are being transformed into inner aggression; you make a fist in your pocket. But you are not able to let through those powerful energies that are asking for creativity and resolute self-manifestation. You hold them back, until finally you totally collapse. You

don't at all believe in your own possibilities. You think it's others who restrict you, but it is you who strangles yourself.

Anxieties, like the way a bolting horse feels when it's seized by the neck. You want to get away, but you can't. That's how it seems. One looks for a way out. Your fists close tight, your hands push, wringing themselves, but you feel small and powerless against Something, something that oppresses you or gives you a feeling of imprisonment. But it is you who makes yourself angry because you have not completely established yourself inside yourself, in your body, in matter. Structures that are too tight; and you try to satisfy, or you keep yourself within rules and regulations about which you think that's how it's supposed to be or that you will be considered/acknowledged good or proper by following them. In the meantime you immobilize yourself.

As if you constantly question yourself unconsciously: How am I allowed to be/stand? This way or that? As if you are a compass that will adjust itself according to the question or demand inside or outside you.

You feel as if you were pushed backward: What now? Your feet don't quite reach the ground; you have the feeling you are somewhere in the power of something or someone, not having a grip or perspective on something. Where lies the solution? You look for a way out.

You open yourself completely, as it were, in order to then allow yourself to be "filled" by Something or Someone.

Because you don't like yourself, you long for confirmation from others. But they will only react to your negative convictions regarding yourself, so that you still won't receive true love. You feel painfully hurt; you close yourself off now! Henceforth, you refuse to offer any of your feelings to others: "Now I'll take everything for myself; I'll go along on my own now." Refusal to communicate on an emotional level. The pain and the self-rejection make you hard, aggressive, and resolute: you withdraw into yourself. An unrelenting attitude. Fear that others might still hurt you more or that they might steal your emotions.

There dwells inside you a rhythmic sound, a dynamically instinctive movement, but these deep primal forces ask for a transformation into creation and renewal, for a creative act, for becoming conscious, and for exploiting energies on an elevated, human level. Possibly, you sometimes don't know what to do with all those energies, and you look for a solution, but it all seems to stick to the facade. No matter if you walk, jump, dance, or beat the drums, there still seems to be something "more," yes, much more, and now you are asked to "look" at that: inside yourself, of course.

Don't direct your view outside yourself; don't surrender to something or someone outside yourself, but open your view inwardly. Now withdraw, very deep inside yourself; feel concentratedly present in your body of flesh and blood. REALIZE it is "you" who lives: take your life in your hands, powerfully and resolutely, and apply yourself to a constantly renewing life.

Sadness dwells inside you; perhaps you would like to weep, but you cannot or will not; you really would like a solution to these things. You are searching, going around in a circle, possibly getting angry. You will find what you are looking for if you first "let go" of the things and people outside you, if you OPEN yourself up to everything that is INSIDE you, to a FEELING called "feeling alive," to a kind of awareness of life that does your heart good. Pull yourself together quietly, forcefully — inside yourself in a positive sense: highly concentrated, being present in your body. FEEL who you are; experience that gladness for your being, your physical presence here and now, and thank Life for being allowed to experience all of it. Emotions are wonderful when directed by love and thankfulness: a CURRENT OF JOY flows through your being when you surrender — only to yourself! An abundant *giving* to yourself and then also to others. One warm current of feelings. You don't "expect" anything from others because you now offer yourself love, and you liberate yourself.

Don't flee. Don't try to escape from true advancement. You try to force certain things, try to push away certain things which you cannot see clearly yet, but you ask yourself ever and again the same questions. Stop this, and allow Life to make clear to you what's good for you to know at any moment of your existence. Don't try to suppress any lies, but look at them: What do you make yourself believe? What don't you want to see? Bring it above water and solve it, POWERFULLY and resolutely, in LOVE and with insight. Don't give up in indifference and weakness, in "not wanting to see," but get a Firm grip on yourself, as master over yourself — over your vessel full of emotions, full of energies — and CARRY IT OUT, from out of your fundamentally strong roots. Energies are calling for this!

First achieve unity in yourself: allow your feelings and your creativity to freely exist under the authority of your Conscious "I." Don't doubt yourself; accept the structures that are good for you at the moment, but don't place your authenticity, your creative forces, and your spontaneous blossoming covered under a bell-jar. Become aware of your possibilities instead of wanting to go to the other side of the stream — allow your own stream of feelings and intuition to come through freely. Open up completely within your own space; be good to yourself; confront yourself with your anxieties. Actually, you are weeping for nothing: you are self-sufficient; you can do more within the borders you have; become aware of the diamond in your safe. Don't fight against outside authority, but build up your inner (re)appreciation; liberate yourself inwardly.

Allow your nature to exist freely in all spontaneity, without artificial restrictions, without condemnation of yourself!

Live from out of your TRUE self, from out of your Heart, from out of your original feeling of life: be yourself! Allow energies to flow unhindered and don't bottle things up, don't tighten up in anger and powerlessness ... because you immobilize yourself. Don't blame others, but allow yourself to come through, blossom. Not with a "wait and see" attitude ... but going onward!

Rosacea
redness, and burst blood-vessels, mostly in the face

You long for others to acknowledge you, because you fear not being acknowledged at all anymore, especially regarding recognition for your outer ego. You feel anxious, pushed into a corner, because you don't stand solidly on your own feet, don't get a grip on yourself, don't consciously experience yourself as master over your own life, over your own body. It seems to you that emotions can just overwhelm you, without your being able to take real charge. Therefore, it is possible that you begin to "grab" for others or, with an aggressive urge for power you begin to dominate or pull others toward you. This is because you experience yourself as being powerless with regard to yourself, because you are afraid of being tossed into a corner like an old rag. Meanwhile, you suppress your healthy, aggressive, creative powers and are holding on to too many emotions, as if you are afraid of no longer being able to master yourself. You want to protect yourself; you anxiously gather between your pincers whatever or whomever you can seize; you'd like to reach beyond your present borders, but you don't achieve one step in the direction of self-realization. You stay in the same place, inflating yourself, not daring to be yourself because you doubt your worth. You enclose your earthly, energetic feelings without daring to express yourself, without daring to be yourself in a relaxed way and communicating

with others in an open and gentle way. You put a check on your healthy energies! You don't allow yourself any spontaneous movements! You are like a plant directed toward heaven, but you smother earthly, emotional, human energies. You are too hard and too inflexible concerning your own evolution: you refuse to let yourself be born; you refuse to stand on your own feet.

You are good the way you are: every human being is unique and has the right to be faithful to his nature. Relax in yourself, let yourself go, allow emotions to flow freely. Turn inward; don't pattern yourself in a tense way on the outer world. Respect yourself; all you need is to realize your worth; this self-satisfaction will at last lead to joyful relationships. Don't force anything, let your heart speak, don't block any spontaneous energies, let off steam; stand solidly on your own feet and simply be yourself. Bend flexibly toward yourself. In this way, you will be gentle toward others. Don't exert yourself so, but surrender to your feelings. Create your life in a self-aware way. In this way communication problems with others will solve themselves also.

Scabies

You "are" almost NOT. You absolutely don't attribute any worth to yourself; "I" am just a zero. It seems to you as if they do with you what they want. You don't manifest yourself at all; you hide, you crawl, you bow to Authority: you feel repressed, under pressure, in the grip of, tied to. It seems as if they quarter you. This is only a result of your own weak situation; you can't get it, you don't know what direction to take. You actually want to get out of yourself, but where to? Your own powerlessness really makes you sick, but you react with aggressive self-protective behavior, taking it out on the authority you experience above yourself. You refuse to accept what others say about you, even if it is for your own good. You don't really come out with your aggressiveness; you are afraid of being hurt, that they might take away something from you, that they might hurt you or penetrate into your personal domain. You hide: you are not always straightforward and honest because you don't dare express your emotions. You feel hurt, but it is you who doesn't dare to be yourself. You feel pushed to the side, but it is you who doesn't vigorously manifest yourself in life. You feel threatened; you can no longer embrace all your emotions. A "victim" with a lot of emotional pain, inner revolt. Your head's like an emotional Full moon that produces thoughts: the conscious, rational mind, putting things into perspective, seem subordinate to emotions.

Now put order into things; become master over yourself, and give yourself all honor instead of kneeling by necessity. Radically throw over your old way of looking at things, and get a hold of yourself. Allow powerful energies to come through, and now become aware of your worth. Place the moon, your emotional world, under the authority of your Sun-center!

Resolutely take responsibility for your life: THAT IS ME; fulfill your tasks joyfully. Inner liberation: listen to your nature. Taking up your place on earth solidly with both feet on the ground. If you don't live according to your worth others can treat you like a victim. Resolute self-realization, honest, and without holding back! Don't allow yourself to "be lived".

Seborrhoea
overproduction of skin fat
(Causes oily hair and skin)

You feel unprotected; you build up a defense (psychologically), including a defense against outside authority. Unconsciously being propelled onward, but you refuse: suppressed feelings, aggression. You hold yourself back; energies can't be expressed freely. Restlessness . . . Nervousness; rushed.

You'd like to get into action, but you don't really do it. Within a restricted psychological space, you begin to pace, back and forth, without really going onward. Emotional vulnerability. Your deepest Self calls you to come to productivity with your whole being; higher energies wish to come through. Don't become rigid by fretting, by doing things purely routinely. Don't hinder yourself from realizing true goals, from enjoying things you have wanted to do for so long, from developing your possibilities. Don't curtail yourself; don't immobilize yourself in a rusted framework. Anxiety can lead to the fact that you are working on self-destruction instead of self-realization. You spend a lot of energy on protecting your feelings, your vulnerability; this is useless and tires you out.

Build your life very calmly but in a well-considered way; no longer let yourself be pulled along by doubts, by anxieties or complexes. In a self-aware way, take charge of your existence and don't block your abundant energies. Transform your pent-up aggression into true action and evolution.

Shingles
herpes zoster

A good-natured clown sticks his head in the sand like an ostrich. Nameless fears about something threatening, a giant energy which could take possession of you — anxiety about death or imaginary world catastrophes, about sex, about the Devil or Father, about a dark philosophy or school, etc. In fact it's about mistrust regarding your self. You want to avoid a part of yourself. You flee from your nature, which you mistrust. You cling to a basis that is built on sand, to unstable structures "outside" yourself, which don't offer you any rest or certainty.

Out of fear of your own shadow side — anxious about not being able to keep under control certain negative energies in you — you bind the "girdle" around yourself, hold yourself within a band, a certain structure which violates your nature. So, you flee, as it were, into a Tower with your blinders on, whereby your receiving channel to your deepest Self is also being closed off.

You wish to see only that aspect of yourself that you think good and beautiful: a duality comes into being. Out of inner uncertainty and anxieties, you perhaps cling to superficial exhibition, an outer Crown or ambition, or "good works" with the anxiety of being dethroned. These physical symptoms call out a halt to you: you can't flee any farther.

The return to your oneness. Come toward acceptance and integration of all your suppressed or hidden feelings, so that nothing is experienced as being frightening anymore. True love for your Self. Inner kingship, no outer affirmation. You were not bad, you are not bad: you are always evolving. Understand this growth-process, for then you don't condemn yourself. Revise your thinking-patterns: you can only feel good and solid if you live in all freedom from out of your heart. You are allowed to experience your nature to the fullest: no protection is necessary. Trust your own nature, and this trust will give you joy. No one but you, yourself, has been your enemy. Therefore, no longer anxiously run away from yourself or from what frightens you: confront yourself with it. Only through confrontation can you resolve suppressed feelings and thoughts.

Vitiligo
local depigmentation, whitish patches on the skin

You put an inner stop! on yourself, forbidding yourself to be who you *really* are. The natural tendency, that spontaneous urge to be yourself in a very honest way — that is being suppressed! You think you have to answer to. . . . You think you are not good the way you experience yourself, think you constantly have to restrict yourself, or at least protect yourself, against the bad impulses in you. Your deepest, true nature lives withdrawn,

hidden. You are on guard against yourself: thus far and no further! An inner collision, yes/no/yes/no. . . . You hear it, feel it, know it: you should stand up for yourself, for your true and total nature, honest and self-aware — and still you don't do it, refusing to change; you go on hiding. A collision, sometimes, between morals, indoctrinations, and norms on the one hand and your Nature, your soul, on the other hand. You forbid yourself to be "free" — again and again there's the "prohibition" sign — because you think you are not good, not beautiful, and also that you would be rejected by others if you'd really dare to be "YOU," in all your aspects, inwardly and outwardly. You live, in fact, under cover, not really warmly taken up in the group at all.

Do you feel unloved, rejected? Do you buy others by putting certain restrictions and laws on yourself in order to please others and earn their love? Emotionally, you experience pain and "being tied down"; you can't get out of it; you feel defenseless, pierced through and stuck. You don't really live for yourself, don't really dare to enjoy life to the fullest; you play a role in a show in order to be accepted and loved by others. So that they will give you what you withhold from yourself: a warm welcome reception.

Break out of your armor and dare to experience, to show yourself, in all openness the way you are. No longer hide yourself: dare to observe yourself, honestly, the way you are, and love yourself; no longer condemn yourself, and then you will no longer attract reactions from people who are tuned in to this wavelength and will translate your self-degrading convictions regarding yourself into words, into criticism! The cause lies completely in you: throw away negative programming, you have only the obligation to be honest with yourself. Dare to be the way you are: you no longer have to see those who don't acknowledge you in your true nature; in this way it will be obvious who are your friends, who's truly in harmony with you.

Feel the safety in yourself, in the solid basis of the Living Self: here lies true support, so don't look for it outside yourself. How do you expect others to love you the way you are if you condemn yourself? That's not possible after all! You put yourself out of the game; you push away your deepest "I"-force: dare to blossom from your core, outward, no longer wondering what "they" are going to say about you. Your natural content of being is what counts; don't fret about outer details. Love your soul, your body; you are very good the way you are. Place on your head beautiful, proud antennas, which are open to fine vibrations: beautiful encounters with people — who just like you dare to experience their unique beings — will be received this way. You get what you ask for. Do you ask for love and a warm welcome, but are convinced you are not at all worthy of it? If so, then you won't attract it! In the first place, show your colors to yourself; live your life to the full, the way you are, without punishing, condemning, or camouflaging yourself.

SLEEPING SICKNESS
trypanosomiasis: serious African disease transmitted by the Tsetse Fly, with fever, skin symptoms, and brain damage

Insufficient concentration of the "I"-consciousness; not standing with both feet on the ground, in a Self-aware way. A belief in threatening mysteries of Nature; a belief in a god or totem outside of you. You experience yourself only as a human being; you actually run away from a true life here-and-now. You escape from reality because it appears too heavy to you, because emotionally it is all too heavy on you. You try to keep yourself standing until you can't anymore. You allow yourself to be "grabbed." You feel you are in the "grip" of something or someone; you

are convinced that a human being can't really determine his own life. Lacking a solid grounding on the earth; too "spiritual," too absent.

Come strongly into your Self, with both feet solidly on the ground, and feel that inner divine Force of your Living Self! Concentrate yourself in your earthly existence, a here-and-now sense of reality; Insight into the creative force of Humanity. Becoming aware: taking your existence in your own hands through the force of your consciousness. The kind of life you lead is a result of your inner expectations of life. Needless emotional burdens fall away when you come to the right Insight.

Read the first part of this book.

SLEEPWALKING

In the daytime, you are full of emotional contradictions, and you don't know what to do with your primitive forces, with your enormous creative energies. You repress yourself; you feel repressed, too tightly bound within a structure, within a certain life's pattern in which you don't find enough room to BE yourself. An accumulation of energy! No trust in one's intuition; you think so much! Frustration, the fear of being yourself; you are charged with an inner fire, but you don't manifest this fire outwardly. You have to accommodate yourself (sometimes out of necessity) in a perfect system, in a precious suit, but you have to accept the consequences of this (at night).

You don't feel able (yet) to transform primitive longings and needs into creativity, growth, and self-confidence. You don't really believe in yourself; you hide behind a shield. Aggression, anger, is being suppressed.

Hesitation about really going on. . . .

Come to Self-awareness, and produce, create! No longer suppress these spontaneous energies, and manifest yourself. Solve all contradictions inside yourself; allow all emotions to flow freely and work them out. Transform aggression into Action! Dare to stand up for yourself, be faithful to your nature. Get a grip on yourself, on your life. Your home basis is fire-red: allow steam to escape during the day; find rest and joy in yourself by realizing yourself in a powerful way through work, creativity, play, through artistic activity.... Don't bottle things up. Dare to really go onward, during the day, not at night! Trust your intuition.

SMALLPOX

Absence of the "I": too hazy, not truly present here on earth, no self-structure; an impersonal being here, allowing yourself to droop completely, not setting your own borders, flowing into other things, a feeling of being stupefied, rather not being than being, a feeling of weakness and smallness — you are anxiously on the look out because you don't have the least grip on yourself.

One can do with you what they want; you don't offer any resistance, even though you are anxiously on guard. Domination of the unconscious, of feelings.

"Here 'I' am! I'm not a part of a machine: you may take my feelings into account!" Say what you have to say, show your fist if necessary.

Self-awareness, belief in yourself; you are not powerless. Every human being is great in his heart: if you love yourself, then you don't allow yourself to "be lived" — then you give yourself all rights to a joyful existence. An intense presence in yourself, in the here-and-now, marking off your terrain, demanding your rights; self-confidence without

fear. Natural immunity. Becoming master over your emotional world. Becoming aware.

Read Lepra, solution.

SNORING

Snoring is not an illness. In certain cases, it can be disturbing to the surroundings and in some cases to the snorer himself.

The first cause is: you dwell in higher, lighter spheres and don't care any longer how your body should be functioning: you just leave it up to the habitual direction of your living Self-core. That one person snores louder than the other has to do with the fact that the Living-self makes an adjustment; a kind of attempt to restore balance. Mostly, it's about the fact that while awake the person lets his life run its course "in structures" or with strong "thinking patterns," while underneath, deep-seated creative forces and spontaneous feelings are being suppressed. A battle can take place between a deeper-seated emotional life and the "thinking." For instance, the person tries to hold back, with his thinking, that which he feels inwardly he has to allow to happen.

He resists surrendering to Life in himself. During sleep, the suppressed side — or the side which wants to manifest itself more strongly than it already does — wants to make itself heard in an expressive way. (Sometimes it has much to say!)

One has to be careful with the interpretation of snoring: one can't draw a clear line here! One should really not attack or interpret "someone else's snoring." Depending on one person or another, here it can be about: "I want to push my feelings more to the front, to let them speak," or "I am angry and will show it now for once," or "Give me room to live, don't smother me!", etc. In this last case, it's of importance that a very heavy snorer realize that someone else never can "smother" him or take away his breath, that he can only strangle himself, restrict himself, or imprison himself. If a person gives an exaggerated opportunity to the thinking pole in his life while his emotional life is being silenced — if a person keeps on wanting to do things for others but forgets himself in doing so, or has a feeling of: "I want to be FREE, I want more ROOM for myself!" — then he might unconsciously start to snore loudly as if he were kicking wildly around in order to obtain his freedom.

He'll realize now that it's not Someone else who robs him of his freedom, but it's he who brings himself into unbalance in one way or another, through which the Self-core propels the suppressed part again to the surface: it is the human being who stands up for himself in order to be able to exist as a TOTALITY. He is allowed to bring to the fore his natural forces of creation, his feelings! The possibility that a move actually takes place (by the partner) to another room, is then the expression of something much deeper than only the snoring. Possibly, it's even good that both partners rely on themselves for some time. The snorer says: "Give me room," and unconsciously pushes his partner a little away. This has nothing to do with either loving or not loving the other person, but with the unconscious longing to find ONESELF even more, *to free oneself more from oppressing structures, patterns, which hinder free passage of life energies. He's not allowed to put a check on his feelings, on an intuitive way of life.*

He shouldn't neglect the voice of his deepest Self-core. The emotionally rich lifestream asks for a larger bed, *and the snorer can surrender with ease to the large "seas" in his own being — in an awake state of being as well as in a state of rest. A longing to freely let himself go within the banks of one's own "I."*

A loud snore is often an inner call for Transformation, for a rising up from the old "I," for giving oneself a chance to blossom and not remain in the larval stage. Freedom! Self-liberation! The human being can, therefore, give himself all the opportunity to step out of old patterns and go onward on a new path! He should not stubbornly hold on, with his thinking, to old habits. Stop all self blockage!

SOCIAL PHOBIA
shunning contacts

You are at a distance from your feelings, from your nature, from your body; so cold.

You feel cold and high, at a distance from yourself. In this ivory tower you also close yourself off from others. You don't at all feel safe and sheltered in your Basis.

You have probably experienced your past as being chilly, unsafe, and unsure. You don't feel able to self-assuredly stand on your own feet; you'd prefer to keep living in your "egg" so no one has to see you, because you are afraid that they might kill you with their coldness, with their eyes, which would look down on you from above — but actually it's you who looks at yourself that way. You feel "inferior"; you are afraid; you don't really dare to be yourself; you'd prefer to stay under the ground, like a worm, because you are "not good"; you don't experience the earth and humanity as warm and comfortable because you are not at all warm toward yourself. When you condemn yourself critically, you fear the deadly stares of others. Because you don't acknowledge the power in yourself, you fear the power of others over you. If in you there lives the conviction that the human being is hard and cold, that a person doesn't have his own safe Basis, that it is best he hide himself, then you will attract circumstances in your life which confirm this image, through which you will be hurt or even more disappointed; in this way you will withdraw even more. Anxious, sometimes aggressive, with a defensive attitude.

Transformation. Free yourself from your experiences from the past and allow yourself to be born! Go onward in life, trusting your deepest Self, and know yourself to be safe in yourself. Be yourself. Be faithful to your true nature and never get disturbed about what others say or think about you. First and foremost, you will make yourself welcome in a warm way, will offer yourself coziness: allowing yourself the warmth, the acknowledgement of your body, of your natural longings. Come home in yourself! Nothing or no one can threaten you unless it is you with the negative convictions regarding yourself. You are good and unique as a human being the way you are. Feel that warm basis, place yourself calmly in the arms of love; know yourself to be taken up in that immortal divine Self. Dare to live, allow the caterpillar to become a butterfly. Experience that rich emotional world inside you and don't suppress it.

Build your life into a paradise: you create your life with your Consciousness; don't allow yourself to "be lived." Only seek contact with people with whom you feel really good; never feel "obliged."

SODIUM
Deficiency, insufficient assimilation of

You lead a sham life. You reject yourself and others. Rejection of Life.

You look at yourself and others from a distance, critically, sometimes disdainfully, superciliously. Looking down your nose at things, frowning, haughty, cold, pedantic behavior: this is just a second "I," a false layer with which you've become entangled. Are you at a distance from your body, from your nature? Are you repelled by it? Behind this lies hidden aggression because of your own powerlessness. You ache; you close yourself off so that no one can approach you. You

will never admit your pain and anxieties, your doubts regarding yourself, but instead you will conceal them.

You don't bend, you remain stiff; you treat yourself like a bad stepmother would, critical and cold, without love. Deep inside, you feel small, longing for love, but you can't even offer this to yourself. Therefore, you also have a hard time accepting warmth from others: "Am I really worthy of it?" Emotionally, you are stuck, anxious, afraid you will be crushed by others; therefore, there is this camouflage, an unconscious measure of protection in your threatened life situation.

Your outward behavior only hides a inner feeling of helplessness.

You close yourself off from your natural feelings!

Transformation! Come out of your hiding place into life and come out from behind that false posture. Dare to be spontaneous, to experience your feelings, and express them without a screen.

Be yourself, open up in total flexibility, lovingly embrace yourself, your body and Life. Come to self-contemplation and look at your deepest feelings of "sadness, anxiety, and powerlessness." Don't ignore it; observe and digest it; don't stick your head in the sand. Accept your inner self and no longer turn away from earthly joy, from life. Accept that unity between your consciousness and your body; know yourself to be welcome among people, and open yourself warmly to the emotional wealth of yourself and others.

Don't be so "dry," but dare to enjoy all beautiful things. Stop being disdainful with yourself. Feel that powerful Basis, your deepest Self, which you can fully trust: this awareness of true safety will hinder you from unconsciously seeking an attitude in order to survive. In this way you honestly come to yourself; dare now to spontaneously express your opinion, your feelings; don't be afraid of physical contact.

FEELING OF TENSION OR CONSTRICTION, POSSIBLY PAIN, AT THE LEVEL OF THE SOLAR PLEXUS

As in a "Pietà-image" you look at the dead son on your lap and think: "What do I have to do with this now?" An unconscious urge toward completely coming to "Life," toward BREAKING with the image of "HOLDING ON"; no matter if this has to do with things, with work or with people. . . . Because "holding on" has to do with death, and "letting free, letting go" with Life! *"Letting go!" and "giving" from your heart instead of seizing or holding on — that makes you inwardly free.* Things, habits, thoughts and convictions, certain affairs and actions from the past, begin to weigh heavily on you, and you want to "get rid" of them! *You no longer want to carry this burden, and you unconsciously want to allow your Feelings and your Life Forces to flow in a spontaneous, discharging, totally free way!* You'd like to throw out death, the old lifeless part of your "I," which has been established in the human being from time immemorial, but you don't really know how. You — your Living Self — wants to definitively jump onto the path of life and leave the dead child in yourself behind forever. *An extreme urge for SELF-LIBERATION in the full sense of the word! The snake that throws off its old skin and rises up like an eagle.* Leaving behind that which is dead — LETTING GO of everything — in order to rise up as a new Reborn Human Being: truly becoming YOU in a total Living form!

What will you do with it now? There lies a heavy damper on your head, as if you can't get any air under the blue stone cover of the tomb, in which you placed yourself in the past. *A call for rising up in yourself, for absolute recognition of your Living Self, for throwing off all your burdens and restrictions, for a resurrection, for a rebirth in yourself!* Be like a living mother and a giving father to the living child in yourself! Bury all aspects in you that are old and oppressive! You have hurt yourself by putting pressure on yourself; you have injured yourself and possibly have as a result attracted painful confrontations with others. No longer give attention to that which is dead, to the dead, let go. A CALL from your deepest interior to come to more INNER, PURE FREE SPACE, to come to openness and clarity, to cleanse yourself, to make the wide hallways of your being — whose walls have gathered dirt from the past — pure and easily passable, so that you can get a very broad and open feeling regarding that which lies BEFORE you: the future. A need for spring cleaning inside yourself, a cleaning up of all old things and habits which don't belong to "life"; a letting go of needless burdens . . . *going onward in All your inner Space . . . toward further.* You have suffocated yourself for too long, placed yourself under high pressure and high tension; now life asks you to come to a Clear View on yourself and on life, that you no longer carry any needless burdens, that you make SPACE for YOURSELF. No, no one can give you the feeling of suffocation: in fact it is you, yourself, who suffocates you and as a result you attract situations which give you the feeling: "Help! I don't have enough space for myself." TAKE UP YOUR OWN SPACE . . . without pressure, without haste, without self-suffocation. Open those windows wide and feel like a totally FREE human being! Nothing or no one can give you the feeling of suppression any longer as long as you clean YOUR LANES yourself, when you do yourself what your inner FEELING urges you to do — spring forward, give the energies inside you full range, and go on!

Don't get stuck, don't stand still, but at any moment of the day do what you feel you have to do; don't let yourself be held back by *"yes, buts."* Take that space, that freedom to which you have a right as a human being. Nothing has to oppress you, no thoughts, no convictions, no time limits, no space.

Openness, freedom and self-liberation down to the deepest roots of your "I." Where do you still keep yourself prisoner? Where do you still block yourself in a free flow? Now throw away those dead leftovers in yourself definitively and rise up! Resurrect yourself! Make yourself a way to absolute inner freedom, and *no longer put any pressure or tension or obligation or holding back on yourself.* Throw open those windows; allow yourself to be who you are, in all freedom, and no longer keep yourself prisoner! The Old has passed! You now bask gloriously in the power, the joy, the relaxation and the broadness of your sunny, living "I"! YOURSELF LIBERATED in the PRESENT!

FEAR OF SPIDERS
arachnophobia

Bottled-up aggression and a suppressed urge to assert yourself. Inner contradiction: on the one hand you are stuck, unsure, and fearful. You feel not really in balance; you lean on others; your imagination is going wild. You don't trust your deepest Self; you don't dare to resolutely build up your life; you control yourself, full of frustrations. On the other hand, you feel robbed of freedom, perhaps like a dog that is tired of being tied up, waiting to have to serve its master. You are full of longings and desires, but you cannot really satisfy them. An unconscious urge to rebel, to break with the situation in which you feel imprisoned; an urge toward autonomous self-realization — but fear and self-doubt hinder all this. Strongly suppressed assertive powers will lead to collisions with your surroundings, especially with those in whose

grip you feel yourself to be. You are not really aware of your worthy Self; you mistrust your nature, and you don't really come to self-realization. A whole world of imagination lives in your head; you fool yourself because you don't really have your feet on the ground in the here and now, in reality. When you are afraid of your own deep contents, when you don't trust your own Basis, then you feel threatened in life.

Don't let yourself be seized; take the bull by the horns and dare to realize yourself. Come into balance: allow the Self-aware "I" to maintain the authority over unconscious questions and emotions. Bottled-up powers call out for liberation: go on! Discover your inner values, your possibilities. Trust your nature and fully live the way you inwardly feel. Allow built-up energies to come out freely, in self-aware action and creativity! Anxieties and fantasy will disappear when you stand on your own feet, trusting in your deepest Self, and when you no longer shy away from a part of yourself, concealing it as something bad. Your inner essence is good and beautiful; nothing or no one can threaten you when you acknowledge that you deserve to spoil yourself. Take a good hold of yourself and offer yourself all the beautiful things you deserve. Don't cast out a part of yourself; don't let yourself be "caught" anymore, neither by others nor by spiders. In love of yourself, take charge of being Master of yourself.

SPLEEN

Psychological correspondence and Ailments, in general
(See also Lymphatic system)

The spleen as an organ within the lymphatic system symbolizes the entrance of our spiritual consciousness into matter: feeling good and comfortable in your body. The high, happy, pure spheres of a Consciousness that remains open, that intensely experiences freedom and space, regardless of the boundaries of the earthly body.

The melting together of the volcanic fire inside a human being, the primal powers, the divine spiritual energies which create life, with earthly matter, with the living water, the emotional.

A concentrated energy in our body, an inner wisdom through which we Believe in ourselves and project a meaning or goal in life; build up an earthly existence, full of enthusiasm, in freedom, taking up all space; not allowing yourself to be restricted; daring to observe and consciously work out all unconscious emotions; an unlimited reconciliation between heaven and earth. The spleen, therefore, asks for a complete surrender to your deepest inner Self, to the intuitive; not getting stuck in "thoughts and fretting." A demand to go straight for the good goal, with a spirit of enterprise, not dwelling on things you think you "have" to do!

The spleen symbolizes the balance between emotional and rational aspects, between the female and the male, between body and "spirit."

Are you too much "spirit"? Do you imprison yourself in "thinking or in spiritual clouds"? Then your consciousness will no longer have full authority over your body, and you will lose immunity. You might also hallucinate and no longer see certain things the way they really are at all. Anxiously, you are on guard — the spleen will call you back to earth!

Do you restrict yourself too much? Do you imprison yourself in a structure outside forbidden terrain? Do you feel forced into a framework that is too tight (philosophically, psychologically, educationally)? Do you restrict your life to a reservation? Do you take away from yourself all freedom and space in

thinking and doing? Do you fixate your thoughts on something in an obsessive way? Why constrict yourself so much? Out of fear? Don't you trust yourself enough? The spleen asks for your consciousness forces to be freed, for feelings and creative energies to be allowed to flow through.

Do you shield yourself from emotions, from your feelings? Let them go free!

Do you shield yourself from your sun-center, your conscious "I"? Do you deny your worth, and would sooner hide yourself? The spleen asks for honesty, for open, enthusiastic participation in life, without anxieties.

You DON'T HAVE TO DEFEND yourself from yourself, nor from life. Take up all space, without brooding, without anxieties — surrender to your intuitive, spontaneous Self.

The spleen is healthy when you feel calm with a safe and warm feeling inside, when you are content and happy with yourself, when love and trust govern your life.

Don't stubbornly fixate your thoughts on one point; let go and trust! Your thinking can strongly overburden your life — especially if anxiety is the motor — to such an extent that your head might burst and your spleen might call for help. A clear Consciousness in a warm, earthly body.

Abnormal enlargement of the spleen

Instability concerning the relationship of spirit-body, active-passive, emotional life-reason: a chaotic, unsure up-and-down line concerning the feelings and the thoughts. On the one hand, you'd prefer to keep at a distance from earthliness like a "Virgo," rather spiritual, because you are afraid that someone might step on your toes. You are afraid of showing your feelings; your creative energies turn inwards. You look at the world from a certain distance, from a height; you don't integrate into matter.

Your energies are blocked: you hinder a breakthrough of powerful, creative consciousness-energies. You hold back what has to be driven through!

On the other hand, you really fight against the stream. An absolutely WANTING, PRESSING, FORCING, but against the wise advice of your deepest Self. This can lead to compulsive actions or obsessional thoughts. You push in the wrong direction, because you don't trust what your intuition tells you.

You are completely stuck in yourself, as it were: finally, you even refuse to receive awareness-impulses; you close yourself off from your Source, you cut off transmission.

Thoughts turn around in a circle; energy that keeps turning and turning, but is not being transformed into deeds. You draw everything inward by a suction force, as it were: you turn away from outwardly directed, active, self-manifestation. The lamp of Consciousness burns, but the electric current is not being transferred. A denial of your "I"-worthiness.

You don't go straight ahead! You don't live with consistency; you obsessively dwell on certain thoughts. This leads to nervousness, to an accumulation of energies that aren't allowed to flow through.

Think things through consistently, and act: don't keep beating about the bush in your brain. Higher energies wish to come through; therefore, don't concentrate on narrow thoughts.

That which exists like a barrier in your thoughts will disappear only if you are open to the true alternative: the experience of your higher Consciousness, of its Power and creativity. Feel how light energies make the palms of your hands radiate, lighten your brain, and make your body scintillate with the joy of Being. You are so much more than matter and thoughts.

The true "I"-power of a human being lies in the creativity of his spirit.

Create your life in a self-aware way: allow energies to permeate your body from out

of the non-three-dimensional Self, so that unity is experienced, so that in this balance you become master over yourself. All anxieties disappear; you find rest and joy in earthly life.

Splenic trauma
Possibly, surgical removal of the spleen

You feel jammed: how can I get out of this?

You would like to do good, also for others, but you can't. . . . You hold on to much sadness, including that of people with whom you feel a bond. You hold on to so much (anxious thoughts, sorrow); you'd like to "do," but you are not allowed to or can't; you feel so powerless, like a little black duckling ("Calimero") who screams. You'd like to do a lot of good for others; you live too much for your fellow man, and it becomes too heavy for you, you can't handle it anymore. You exist only for them, for your relations; you suck the oxygen out of them for your own life, as it were! But you do have an enormous ability to develop a powerful Consciousness. If you make yourself too dependent on others, you pull yourself down, restrict your space. Anxious: after all, you turn yourself away from your deepest Self. Anxiously fixated: on the love, the affection, the attention for others. Or on the attention they have for you??

Allow yourself to be taken up in love by your own greater Self: live first of all for yourself. Feel those powerful awareness-energies which want to break through from within your deepest Self. Don't resist, don't hinder it by clinging to others. An autonomous Power in you, which radiates divine wisdom and enlightens your complete head and your body: no longer lower yourself, don't run away from this. In this spiritual force, very personal and independent, lies your immunity (you don't even need a spleen for this).

Therefore, place the sun-center in yourself, not in an authority or partner outside you. Your total consciousness-being wants to flow through inside your body: don't resist because of fear, but feel how that "wisdom-love" energy reveals itself in your physical structure (the energetic force of the shoulders-heart-head). These values you can't find anywhere outside yourself: now, without fear, build your life spontaneously on these natural, loving impulses, on your powers. If you have good intentions, then you can trust that everything will happen for the best. Therefore, don't be afraid to Be, as an autonomous Self. Let go of those dark thoughts.

STAMMERING, STUTTERING

You don't really dare to manifest yourself outwardly. You keep hidden in yourself. You don't really love yourself; you feel imprisoned inside yourself, in uncertainty, in feelings of inferiority. You take away all your breathing space, suffocate yourself by a tense, emotional noose. You constrict yourself spasmodically; you don't give yourself the right to liberation because you feel so unsafe in yourself. Anxiously, you hide your feelings, your creative forces, your true nature. Do you think yourself or your body to be just "nothing"? You place the power over your life too much in others instead of acknowledging your power.

Have you come home in peace, quiet and love for yourself?
Then throw open those windows, and come to the light! Total self-liberation! Don't hesitate now to let your energies come through completely, to show your feelings. Feel that inner force; in a self-aware way take the rudder in hand and make yourself master over your life, not by hiding yourself, but by just being yourself — no matter how — without minding the expectations or reactions of others. How you feel is what counts, not

what others think about you! The stronger you now unblock your nature, and the more flexible you manifest your true feelings and longings, the smoother the stream of words will flow. No longer hold yourself back! Dare to be yourself; trust in that fundamentally solid Basis of your deepest Self, and live in all freedom and openness! Relax, gain an overview in self-confidence; feel at home in your body; feel your muscle power, and know yourself to be safe in yourself. Discover your unique worth as a human being; don't try to be like someone else, but be yourself, in your own way. No one can show you this. Cherish yourself and your body. If you love yourself, you won't feel rejected by others. The outer world only reacts to your inner opinion regarding yourself.

GENERAL STIFFNESS, RIGIDITY

Your natural feelings, spontaneous forces, aggressive energies, etc., are being firmly tied down. You don't really live from out of your heart. Perhaps it's of much more importance to you how you are being perceived by the outer world or how much you respect certain norms and rules. You don't allow yourself to live flexibly and freely! You are hard, demanding, condemning, stubborn. Inwardly, you feel small and dependent, but you refuse to outwardly show this gentleness! You feel unstable on your own basis, unsure and afraid; you frenetically keep yourself standing even if it's just for the eye of others. Perhaps you proudly stick out your chest, but you smother your feelings. Because you don't allow yourself to live freely and joyfully and to fully spontaneously enjoy life — because you resist your gentle heart and longings — you possibly are angry or jealous, critical or judgmental, with people who do dare to be joyful and to live without caring about restricting laws. Your spontaneous creativity is not allowed to exist; you live within structures and lines in order to feel somewhat "safe." You hold yourself back; sometimes you don't know what direction to take, because you don't trust your intuition and your feelings.

With small-minded thoughts, you can make your existence very tense and narrow. You don't really go onward on your life's path; you don't allow yourself to evolve or to flexibly develop your possibilities.

Dare to joyfully take a hold of life with both hands! Allow those primitive and healthy aggressive forces to come through, and feel that strong inner Basis of your everlasting Living-self. Dare to be yourself; dare to get angry; free those feelings; no longer suppress your emotions! Aggressive, extremely strong forces aren't bad. Use them in a healthy way, in smooth action and creativity. Live honestly and gently according to your heart: listen to your wishes, and don't deny yourself joy. Don't be afraid of your deeper nature: true pride comes from within. The pride of your inner, divine worth, of your true talents, your rich feelings — has nothing to do with facade-pride. A human being doesn't fit into a "framework"; follow your nature, don't satisfy the expectations of laws and people, but the demand of your Heart. Flexibly bend toward the little child within you, and ask how you can please it. Open yourself up to yourself, to others. Every human being is unique; condemnations indicate a lack of Insight.

Your "I"-esteem is being thrown away; it lies under the knife, suffers, because you neglect it, because you are too hard on yourself: now follow your higher Self and don't do anything that hurts you, don't do anything "to perform," only to satisfy the expectations of others. You don't "have to do" anything. Your worthiness, your wisdom, your golden "I" runs on unsteady wheels; you listen too much to others instead of to your Conscious "I."

Your body hangs too loosely from your Consciousness: become master over yourself, over your body! As you don't allow your deep forces to come through freely — because of anxious tension, nervousness and unsureness, so that these energies are not able to circulate freely in your body — as you are stuck with worried and tense thoughts, and as you don't trust in your inexhaustible inner Source, the pain in your side calls you back to your SELF: this asks for Rest and trust in your deepest Self, for a powerful self-aware action from out of your Center. So that you might feel master over your life and your body, without anxieties, with an open mind, in warmth and love. Anxieties block healthy circulation. Honest cordiality toward yourself will unblock cramps. Self-confidence and a relaxed spirit; directing your life, *yourself.* Allowing higher consciousness energies to pass through freely; not suffocating yourself with anxious thoughts.

Don't force yourself: listen to your Authority.

STITCH IN THE SIDE
often resulting from running
or vigorous exercise

All of a sudden, a lot of energy is released, and you can't handle it — an alarm is being sent out. But, in fact, it's about a "star of Bethlehem" here: a road map to your inner, living Self, which begs for acknowledgment.

STOMACH

Psychological correspondence and Ailments, in general

Accepting and experiencing your feelings in their fullness, the moon in the light of your Sun.

Feeling calm and safe, at ease in your sun-center, in your deepest Self.

Nervous anxieties lie at the basis of stomach problems: you don't trust enough in your deepest Self; anxiously you hold on to experiences, emotionally, and in your thoughts.

Like an exaggeratedly grasping Cancer, you try to embrace everything, but you have a hard time digesting it all. It stays heavy on your stomach. Shocking happenings can stay there like a stone in your stomach.

The stomach, therefore, is symbolic of the emotional digestive system: how do you deal with new information, new impressions?

The ability of a human being to work himself up psychologically, to grow toward greater harmony by digesting stored, unconscious facts, which then — through confrontation with the outer world and via self-contemplation — are being transformed into Awareness. From the shadow into the sunlight: a process of becoming conscious. In the stomach we take in food the way we take in new information in our brain computer. Digestion offers better programming: as we get new Insights, we continuously adjust ourselves in the evolutionary process. The stomach symbolizes emotional digestion, but also digestion through thoughts. Does it all linger in your head like a nervous web? Can't you get certain things out of your mind at all? Do you again and again see in front of you certain happenings from the past? Does something "indigestible" stick in your stomach?

Do you refuse any longer to accept, to swallow, what they give you, and do you spit it out? Is it all too much? Can't you handle the new facts? Do you reject them, and vomit?

The stomach points at the hidden emotional world, at being an ostrich: do you anxiously push certain things toward unconscious regions? Do you close your eyes to certain problems, but do they keep gnawing at you? You bottle things up, but you remain silent.

Justice and conscience, among other things, find their place here. Why don't you digest? Do you blame yourself? Do you feel guilty? Does your own duality turn your stomach? It is of the utmost importance that no secret, dark, emotional world pushes down your existence: bring it all to the surface and look very Consciously at your emotions, at your problems and your deep anxieties; confront yourself with them and work them out. No longer push away your feelings! Are you afraid to see yourself? Do you anxiously keep yourself tightly closed? Are you constantly hurrying, perhaps for someone else? Is this because you are so insecure? Does your head buzz with nervousness, with dark thoughts and ideas?

Don't stick to someone or something: free yourself of needless burdens. No one can rush you, only you yourself.

Find rest in yourself, and trust in your inner wisdom, your intuition: don't let your brain go crazy in fretting without end. Only this unlimited trust in your deepest, divine Self will liberate you from anxieties. A safe feeling, rest and joy.

Gain a clear overview through lucid thinking, and let go of whatever gnaws at you: dare to resolutely transform your aggressive forces into fruitful action; create your life's path in a self-aware way.

Come out of your shelter! Speak! Honest with yourself, with others; honestly stand up for your opinion and your feelings!

Acidity of the stomach, causing a burning sensation

Repressed aggression; you can't really be yourself. Anxious nervousness; you take a black view of things.

Instead of liberating yourself from an inner emotional battle, you'd rather stay passive in this. You don't arrive at true, active digestion; you don't dare to really break through or stand up for yourself; you are sad and angry. Powerful energies which wish to come through from out of your deepest Self — from out of your true longings, from out of your natural disposition — are being suppressed! You just linger in this situation; you don't *really* go onward; you are very busy with futilities, with superficialities, with the cares of tomorrow, with business worries; you think and fret or pray — you constantly ruminate. You run in place without making any headway instead of quietly digesting things, of letting go of the past and the future and resolutely going on in the Now, cutting through the knot and trusting in your intuition.

Nervous restlessness conquers your brain: you feel frustrated because you don't really live from out of your own power center! You hold things in; you live too mechanically or not really naturally; you immobilize yourself in etiquettes or in a suffocating structure.

You often expect the worst and you worry about nothing, because of unsureness and anxiety, feeling as if you are pursued like wild game. You'd sooner evade a problem than solve it.

Listen more to your Nature, to your longings; free yourself from emotional tensions. Do, instead of thinking and fretting. Resolutely get a hold on your problems and work them out. Feel the warm safety in yourself; come closer to your body and enjoy your senses. Relax; find rest in your deepest Self, and surrender trustingly to this safe Basis. Look at your feelings from a distance, and chase away the "phantoms" of needless anxieties. Allow feelings to flow freely; don't mistrust, and dare to manifest yourself proudly and openly. Optimism, joy, rest, idealism.

Stomach bleeding

Aggressive emotions and angry, sharp thoughts turn inward, are not voiced, but flow in with an overwhelming threat.

This dangerous, self-destructive, inner aggression finds its deepest root in Fear. Mortal fear.

You hide yourself; you don't show your soul, but your thick skin is only camouflage: in fact you feel so hurt, so anxious, small, suppressed, a defenseless victim of Fate or of a dominant Authority against which you now revolt.

Unyielding in your judgment, stubbornly holding on to your sharp ideas, a murderous emotionalism, powerful aggressive resistance. It's compulsive, it holds you in its grip, or rather, you refuse to digest, to let go.

But instead of thrusting the sword toward the outside, you rather remain silent and turn it on yourself. . . .

You are not a toy of destiny. You think you are a victim of situations, but it is you who have unconsciously called them up in your life! Calmly and safely crawl into your nest, make peace with yourself. Trust in that safe, fundamentally strong Basis of your inner Self. Don't get furious with others because, thus far, you haven't made what you wanted to out of your life: gain a clear Insight into your contents, into your emotions, and put your thoughts in order. Look for the cause in yourself, and change your life! Begin to take your life in hand in a self-assured way, with calmness and force. In love, come toward yourself so that anxieties no longer form an obstacle to transforming your burning, creative, aggressive energies into action, into deeds, into externalization of your potentialities.

Don't project things onto others; jump up from the spot that becomes too hot for you, and proudly build up your life. Supple flexibility, an openness to Understanding, a softening.

Stomach cancer
(See also Cancer, in general)

Dark, heavy thoughts constantly occupy you; emotional burdens, anxiety.

You give up; you refuse to truly live. You run away from responsibilities; you flee. The "spiritual," unconscious aspect now becomes stronger and stronger: you want to get away, you let your shoulders droop.

Saying "No" to life, but also to your self-esteem. You perhaps have cherished many ambitions and longings for life, but you have the feeling it's over, that you haven't been able to reach anything — and you'd sooner blame it all on your partner, on others or on circumstances! In fact, you have been fleeing from yourself for a long time. You have allowed others to emotionally force themselves on you; you have swallowed up emotions; you have been completely open to taking in emotions.

Through your black thoughts, anxieties, and the unconscious refusal to self-create your own life, you have made yourself dependent on other people and things, and as a result you have led a frustrated life, because of which you have attracted black happenings.

Love and warmth toward yourself will chase away cold anxieties: don't expect anything from others; first make yourself welcome. Grounding. With both feet solidly on the ground, with proud self-awareness, make yourself master over your emotions. Allow everything to stream off you and begin a new life; don't blame others because thus far you haven't dared to take responsibility over your life yourself. Let go of everything and everyone that has a grip on you, and now come to the surface: dare to live! Feel good and safe in your deepest Self. If your expectations regarding life are positive, then a joyful result won't stay away. Radically change your attitude of life and your convictions about life, and give yourself a new chance.

Joy, peace, faith in yourself, relaxation, and a longing for life itself, propel healing energies to your body from out of your deepest Self. No longer hide yourself!

(See the category Stomach, Ailments, in general)

Stomach cramps

Anxiety, strong emotional tension; the absence of your strong, Conscious "I": you don't get a grip on yourself; you don't have a clear perspective on what happens in your surrounding; foggy, black thoughts that don't get a solid grip on anything.

A feeling of being extremely unsafe, just as if you'd land in an dark vacuum.

A feeling of being lost in a sea of deep emotions; you sit and wait, passive.

Feel safe in the house of your deepest Self; build your life in a resolute, active way, without doubts. Bring yourself into balance again by surrendering to your Self in a calm and relaxed way. Lift yourself up higher; nothing can "crush" you: your anxieties ask you to rely on yourself, to acknowledge your deepest Self. Trust drives away anxieties: create your life yourself; don't just wait and see. Adjust your life where it's beneficial for you to do so. A solid structure, clear thoughts, relaxed faith.

Hiatal hernia
protrusion of the stomach through the esophagal opening in the diaphragm

Inner tension. You flee from reality; you are not really present here-and-now. You live just in thoughts, imaginings, in dream-images. You are on an island, alone with yourself. You keep holding on to the past, to emotional memories, and you look with fear at the future. You actually experience yourself and life as too empty, too dead, too cold. You flee into yourself, into your thoughts, and as a result you truly lose contact with reality. You no longer see things the way they really are; you might develop paranoia or spiritual fantasies. You hide your emotions deep inside yourself, or you try to cover them up, pretending they are not there. Introverted, deathly spheres.

Healthy, natural emotional currents are being blocked. You live too much in the spirit, anxious, fretting, nervous, and obscure; you lose contact with yourself, with your body; you don't dare to trust your nature. You blow up certain things; you don't dare to take a well-determined direction in your life. You allow yourself to be directed by hidden emotions; the captain of the ship seems to be flying far beyond the seas.

Don't flee: confront yourself with your deepest emotions. Partake of yourself and warm yourself in love. Become aware of your worth and allow energies to flow freely. Don't lock yourself up in yourself, give your feelings free passage. Listen to what you feel, to your intuition: don't break with your nature, with that which is most beautiful inside you. Don't break with life, but free yourself from anxieties and phantoms. Openness, honest communication with others: look for your path; let go of the past, in faith. Bring yourself into clear daylight, and you will see that — if you are open to it — what you are fleeing actually helps you along on a new path.

Rest and relaxation in yourself; the satisfaction, the joy to just be yourself.

Open yourself: in letting go of the old, in listening to the new. No longer block yourself. A smooth passage for feelings and life energies.

Inflammation of the stomach
gastritis

You don't in the least think you are on a safe foundation: huddled up like a small, insecure, paranoid child. Anxious: what will happen next? You are almost only Head: you think, fret, and you flee, as it were, from the base. You anxiously cling to a series of elements in your life, like a scared dog on the roof of a house that is about to collapse.

You hardly dare to stand on your own feet and go on; you hardly dare to reach out your hands to something new. Mistrustful, on guard. You are ready for the worst. You bottle up a lot of tension and emotion! A feeling of being extremely unsafe; unsureness.

Negative things don't overtake you without reason: with negative expectations about the future, you will indeed create a sad reality. Alter your expectations! Balance between heaven and earth: first take care of a sure home basis in your earthly existence; a discovery of your deepest Self, your fundamentally strong Basis. From these solid roots your life can grow, and, while thinking, you can "build" a structure that is erected from within. Don't overburden your head with worrisome fretting; you are safe in yourself! Express your emotions and work them out. No longer cling to things; open yourself up completely, liberate yourself from this net that you, yourself, have set up.

Stomach ulcer

Nervous, anxious uncertainty. Emotionally tightened up; you feel "stuck."

In order to accommodate others, in order to make a "good" impression — because you feel so unsafe in yourself, and therefore look for security in others — you are not straightforward; you perhaps perform an act, obediently nod "yes," while your thoughts say "no." Perhaps you inwardly burn with aggression, with a desire for vengeance, or are you busy making plans to rescue yourself from a certain situation that you don't like, which your acquaintances might describe as cowardly. In fact, you are just like a timid weasel that flees silently, so that no one sees it: anxiety always pursues you.

If you can't flee, it keeps on gnawing in your stomach: it "eats" you. Sometimes you make a step forward — then, again, you stay where you are, anxious about really going onward. You mostly suppress your aggressive, active forces, but in the meantime you'd like to force things, because of powerlessness, in order to still be able to go on.

A lack of self-confidence; doubts about self-worth, because of which one is dependent on others: in relationships you will be silent and bottle things up, when it would be better to voice the truth, but you don't dare — dishonesty toward yourself first of all. Do you hide from yourself? Are you not happy with your true nature, or do you think yourself to be bad, inferior?

Know yourself to be safe and sheltered under your roof, not under that of others: come home to your safe, deepest Self. Openly and honestly say what you have to say; let go of the bottled-up energies; feel your own solid Force, and allow your feelings to flow smoothly; don't be afraid of your aggressive forces, of your anger.

Speak freely, without fear; dare to live without throwing up obstacles to your energies; transform frustrations into active self-realization: only then, not by hiding yourself, will you experience rest and relaxation. Dare to be yourself and to show yourself the way you really are. You don't have to meet any expectation of others. You only have to be honest and faithful to your specific nature.

Mind! In many cases, a so-called stomach ulcer is really a duodenal ulcer (See the text on page 359).

FEELING A STRONG NEED FOR EATING SUGAR OR SWEETS

In itself, sugar certainly isn't unhealthy![7]

Sugar is fuel that immediately warms you and can give you a pleasant feeling if you are open to it. Because you long for love, warmth, sweetness, you quickly reach for "sweet" products. *By itself, it is not an ad-*

diction to like sweet products such as sugar, but it is a natural need for what you, with your individual disposition, so much long for: sweetness, gentleness in life.*

Enjoy sugar products, then, and don't refuse sugar in a condemning way! But it is true that your fondness for sugar is a signal from yourself, which makes clear to you: be nice to yourself; fill yourself with the warm fuel of yourself, with love. If eating sugar products is accompanied by anxious, compulsive behavior instead of calm enjoyment of something sweet, then this indicates that you experience yourself too much as an emptiness, as a coldness, that you are not really present in your "body," that you deny — don't really allow — the sensuality in yourself, the pleasantly sweet sensorial aspect, the enjoyment of earthly things, of your sensuous longings! You determine your being, with dark thoughts; perhaps you attach much importance to the exterior, to your "facade" and allow yourself to be misled by social demands and norms concerning the cult of appearance. Nothing of all this is of importance. Love yourself; develop emotional warmth, which is the true fuel for your body, dare to be yourself the way you are, in joy. Don't force a "diet" on yourself, but enjoy sweetness. If you feel attracted to this, you need to take sweet products on the condition that you no longer leave yourself out in the cold, considering yourself a zero.

Sugar is being completely assimilated and digested only if you are firmly and Consciously aware of your Worth, if you are nice to yourself, and if you direct your creative energies outward. Be productive in whatever area, and don't allow yourself to listlessly run empty. Don't grasp, don't hold on to things or people. Direct your radiating forces, your love, *outward!* Unfold yourself; don't retain your forces and your possibilities. Don't be sad; don't put yourself in a subordinate, dependent position. Be proud of yourself; get a hold on yourself, not on others! Become aware of your rich Content, of your inner Fuel, the forces of love and trust

[7] However, diabetics will first have to work on the psychological causes of their disease before the pancreas can function normally again and little by little the intake of sugar can rise again.

in yourself, which constantly nourish your total body, so that you no longer *have to* eat sugar, but still may.

Don't be hard and strict on yourself; feel full of self-confidence, and no longer *let* yourself "be lived." Allow feelings to flow freely, and resolutely determine your course of life. Life is joy: discover that warm, emotional core inside you; yield to love for yourself so that you no longer feel "lonely." Only when you are convinced that you are "worthy" of love, happiness, and warmth, will you attract joyful circumstances. Bring about changes regarding your expectations of life, so that you create happiness yourself. Enjoy the earthly, and don't push it away. It's allowed to eat sugar products on the condition that you are nice to yourself now, because the pancreas will function optimally only under impulses of self-love. The longing may remain, and the satisfying of this longing also may remain, but the "imperative need" will disappear in proportion to the growth in yourself of emotional warmth.[8]

a clear view of yourself; your Individual boundary is not there; you think you are nothing. You allow yourself to "be lived." You don't really give form to your life, don't take up your responsibility. Cold.

Bring yourself to realization on many levels; self-realization on Earth. In flexibility, in love, and self-acknowledgement, in gentleness toward yourself and others; you are bendable, flexible, but you still stand with both feet rooted in a solid foundation. You build a solid house on a basis that you, yourself, have traced out. You regulate and organize your structures, your existence. You, yourself, determine your direction, and you give concrete form to your existence. You allow red, active forces to break through in self-realization. Put things in perspective, with humor, because after all you know well that every human being is the creator and cause of his own existence. You believe in your Self. You see the many details, the many segments, of life. You enjoy the horn of plenty.

SULFUR
Deficiency, insufficient assimilation of
(See also Demineralization)

SUNBURN
(See also Skin, Ailments, in general)

Negativism, nihilism; you don't attach value or credence to anything or anyone, nor to yourself. You don't believe in Life anymore; nothing matters to you anymore.

For a long time you have been looking around mistrustfully; you are on guard; you don't really believe anymore in that which is beautiful and good. You let yourself droop, flag, in an exaggerated way; your structures aren't solid enough. You aren't at all present here as a Self-aware personality. You don't stand with both feet on the ground; you'd rather float above the earth. You don't have

You place the authority outside yourself. Fear of something or someone bigger than you, who might have you in his grip. Frustration. Your "I" wastes away in the flames: you don't dare to come out of your hard shell. Your feelings, your powers, remain concealed. You don't truly realize yourself; you are practicing self-destruction. You feel so powerless, anxious, at the mercy of deep powers and emotions inside yourself. You don't cherish yourself in love; possibly you connect love too much with outer appearances and superficial sex, but that warm, deep acknowledgement of yourself isn't there at all. You feel unsure and afraid; you are

---

[8] Read more about this in *The Symbolism of Food — The Horn of Plenty*.

The Key to Self-Liberation, Christiane Beerlandt © Beerlandt Publications

sad; you feel hurt. You allow yourself to go back and forth in life, dependent on others. You don't dare to be yourself. A feeling of powerlessness; not being able to go onward on your own feet. You are imprisoned inside yourself, in the grip of others. In powerless aggression, you might grab for something or someone outside yourself, but by doing this you don't get a better grip on yourself. Your heart bleeds because you don't acknowledge your Worth, because you stab yourself. Sometimes, you are so angry because you don't succeed in realizing yourself independently, because you don't lead the life you'd want to lead. Possibly, you attach too much importance to exterior things and superficial appearances, or you are not at all happy with yourself, with your body; perhaps you consider yourself ugly. You don't trust yourself or others; you live in anxiety. You refuse to transform and place all authority in yourself. You feel cold in your being. Creative forces and emotions ask for a breakthrough, for spontaneous action and self-realization, but you suppress it all; you frustrate yourself; possibly compulsions come to the surface as a result, and this makes you even more anxious.

If you handle those inner flames with mastery, in creativity and emotional experiences — outwardly directed — then you will know yourself to be liberated. Place the warm-hearted Love inside yourself. Respect yourself; allow your "I"-consciousness to blossom, and listen only to your deepest Self. Place authority in yourself; nothing or no one can threaten you anymore. Trust in that essential basis of yourself; solve that unsureness by becoming aware of your worth. Solve your sadness by not looking outside yourself for Joy but by coming very close to yourself, in warmth. Don't bottle up emotions; no longer hold back your self-development; don't be angry because of your own powerlessness: in a Self-aware way, take your life in hand and don't allow yourself to "be lived"; don't allow yourself to be

scorched by a Source outside of you. The sun-source in yourself is inexhaustible: count on this divine, immortal core inside you — the core which is of equal value in every human being — so that you don't have to place yourself Subordinately to something or someone. Create your life; don't allow yourself to be burned up.

SUNSTROKE

You suppress your deepest, essential feelings, your True Self.

You live too much at the surface of your existence, allowing yourself to be "seized" or "beaten" by an Authority other than the Authority in you: the power of outward show and Image; the power of the group or the society to which you belong; you go along.

Also, you especially look at everything from below up, like someone who denies his true inner worth and rather would be negative toward himself. The sun-center inside you is being ignored; you live too much according to the rules and expectations of a superficial world. It is "proper" that it should be that way; you do things to please others, to be accepted. You don't have true contact with your deepest Being; you look at yourself rather coldly instead of offering yourself the warmth your heart needs so much. You are full of desires, jealous, angry with others, because you are not really in contact with your beautiful Content. You don't (yet) really love yourself. Your inner chilliness, your superficial, routine-like, emotionally poor attitude toward the outer world is only a consequence of a lack of Self-appreciation, of not wanting to be open to your own heart, to your intuition and your emotional possibilities. You cut yourself off from your deepest soul-content. You lean your life on others; you don't find safety and protection in yourself. You position yourself as inferior and dependent. Moreover, you don't give enough room to deeply hidden emotions; they surface, like a vat that ferments.

Cool off by allowing your own deepest feelings to flow, and listen to them. Allow those bottled-up energies and emotions to flow out. No longer linger with the cult of the exterior or with the superficiality of a society. Penetrate to the core of your Heart, which, for a long time, has been calling for your acknowledgement!

Roar like a Lion for once, so that you feel that you Are and what you are! Optimism, self-protection, self-appreciation: offer it to yourself. Now, place all power and Authority in yourself, and do what's truly Good for you. Don't rush yourself for the sake of the outer world; don't try to please others, but be faithful to what you feel. You are safe deep inside yourself. If you attach importance only to the superficial or to how you are "perceived" by others, then this means that the Sun of the outer world is stronger than your sun: it can beat you down. When you finally acknowledge that autonomous Sun-power center in yourself, you will be immune, invulnerable, and safe. Emotions and powerful energies warmly piling up inside you and not finding a way out is only a result of not truly living from out of your own Authority. Let go of everything.

Let warmth flow outward: offer warmth and love to others, to yourself. No longer outwardly be the cool gentleman or lady, because the inner fire of the heart will avenge itself.

SUPPURATION
discharge of pus

Seeing especially the dark, black side; pessimism, and a feeling of "everything is lost anyway." You allow yourself to be weighed down; you can't handle it anymore.

It weighs too heavily on you, or you can't digest something. It's because of "them"; you blame others. . . . You worry too much; you feel rejected (mostly self-rejection!); feelings of "old, spoiled, stinking, unpleasant anxieties" live unconsciously.

Overwhelming sadness, sometimes desperation or despondency. A revolt, resistance! You feel "marginal," pushed to the side. It's your unconscious forces that call upon you to no longer hinder yourself from Living in joy and optimism regarding your own Being and possibilities! With Plutonic force, your inner powers and old emotions push themselves to the surface in order to finally make a clean sweep regarding unsolved frustrations, and also so that you finally might acknowledge yourself, no longer pushing yourself to the side!

So, allow yourself to be reborn in yourself, to transform. Try to go very deeply toward that golden core inside you, and achieve higher consciousness. Experience the warmth inside you, the timeless joy, those beautiful feelings that are ready to flow through if only you'd wake up from your dark dream. Powerful energies are ready to wake you, but you still resist these beautiful things in you. Allow yourself to blossom, and fully acknowledge your Worth: place yourself in the center of your life and know yourself to be connected with other people through warmth-radiations. Allow your sun to radiate; don't push it down. . . . Every human being is good and beautiful in his or her own way; acknowledge yourself in Love. Do you think life is a vale of tears? If you give up and refuse to take responsibility by creating, yourself, a joyful, optimistic life, then life is indeed a black sleep.

You will have to wake up out of this unconscious dead-end dream. Do you want reality to be a joyful experience? That, you will have to build up yourself: if you are convinced you are a sad, miserable, human being, then you will attract negative situations.

     The Key to Self-Liberation, Christiane Beerlandt © Beerlandt Publications

Spit out your pus, your negativity! Allow pure, renewing impulses, and begin now to build up your life in self-respect.

With negativity, you only poison yourself: the cause and solution lie inside you, not in others. No longer allow your life to rot: make use of your beautiful, positive forces!

See, if necessary, the category Festers.

SWALLOWING FUNCTION

Psychological correspondence

You feel warm and safe in your deepest Self, and therefore you can calmly welcome everything and swallow it. You feel sure, cheerful, and at ease in your nature, and you say without fear: "Come in!" A feeling of inner Peace.

You feel protected, without anxieties; you are also able to take others under your care. Flexibly, you go onward in life; you don't close yourself off from new things, but at the same time only take into your life that which isn't "too much"; you don't allow anything to be forced on you; you take to you what you can swallow at the moment.

Dynamic Force, sharp and alert, when you have to be — self-aware, proud, without shame.

Daring to show your nature the way you are, in all openness! With a great heart, allowing the full force of energies that want to come through: creativity, physical experience, natural longings, etc., without throwing up obstacles.

Experiencing primitive energies only in the light of love, as an original creativity, not as a compensation for emptiness.

Energies can powerfully flow through. If you know yourself to be connected with your inner Source, with your divine Self, then you won't be overcome by emotions, anxieties, and powerlessness — then you will live in a Self-aware way, in harmony with yourself. Then you will heartily welcome life, and will blindly trust your nature. You allow yourself to flexibly go onward.

Ailments, in general

Anxiety. you'd like to flee, high up into a tree. You'd like to hide, to protect yourself by a shield, as it were, so that no one can "enter," because you feel threatened. You clam up; you get a scare, or you tie down yourself and your feelings. You go through life too carefully, on guard against that which might "grab" you.

You don't feel safe in your deepest Self; it's as if others have a grip on you. You feel to be under the power of others, forced to swallow certain experiences that you really don't want: powerlessness. You can't defend yourself because you experience yourself as weak. Do you feel guilty and think others might punish you? You are afraid of psychological or sexual castration or rape. Fear of death. Sometimes Paranoid emotional experiences.

Swallowing the wrong way

You want to do or to say too much at once, standing up for yourself; you want to acquire too strong a "grip" on others or on a situation, because of the conviction that it all may escape you or overpower you. You have the feeling that you can't express yourself enough or can't stand up for yourself enough — and then you might force things, wanting to bring ten things to the fore at once, wanting to justify yourself very quickly, out of fear of possibly not being understood by others, or out of concern that the other person might cut you off. You rush yourself in order to keep control over the situation, to stay in charge of the situation, because you don't trust enough in, nor rely upon, the solid fundamental basis of your Self.

Serious choking:
Out of fear of being destroyed by something or someone bigger than you, by something threatening: you feel sad or powerless inside yourself. Emotionally, you are very tight inside: your emotions cannot flow in a relaxed way. Because you inwardly feel powerless and threatened, you inflate yourself, you unconsciously call up aggressive forces from within, as a rescue (vengeance) for your unrealistic anxieties. Possibly, you encapsulate yourself; a structure that is too tight, too anxious, a tense attitude, hinders you from freely and calmly being yourself. In this way you live under pressure.

Consider your personal appearance as a small part of the greater, light, consciousness totality that you are. Look at things from above and keep feeling that you are the master over yourself, without concerning yourself about the expectations or behavior of others. Acknowledge the Authority in yourself, so that nothing or no one can threaten you or throw you out of balance; anxieties are unnecessary when you become aware of that immortal fundamental power, your deepest Self. You don't "grasp" or claw at others, neither do you allow yourself to be rushed, as long as you trust in your own sun-center! Let go, look at every situation with trust in your inner authority. Now acknowledge that power in yourself, so that you no longer experience yourself as powerless. Don't make yourself so tense with emotions; at all times be yourself; don't put yourself inside a formal coat of armor.

DO, live, express yourself — calmly, from out of your inner source-center.

SWEATING, EXCESSIVE

A constant state of alertness, at the ready to defend yourself, to attack. A feeling of being unsafe, of vague anxiety. You are on guard. A feeling of being threatened, as if at any moment something might explode, but it all actually happens inside you. Because you suppress strong inner forces and emotions — because you are full of active, potential, energies, but Forbid them from breaking through — you're actually on guard against yourself, although you think the danger lies outside you. It is you who suppresses your feelings and your forces. Because you are afraid of those deep forces inside you, you will also be afraid of others. You are at the ready to shoot, as it were, instead of allowing your Content to blossom. You bottle things up until you possibly burst out. Are you afraid of yourself? You don't trust yourself. Possibly, you sometimes appear tough and strong, arrogant, or conceited, but this radiating, external force is only meant to get "ahead" of others. Before you might get a blow, you'll have put the other one in his proper place. Fundamental mistrust in the human being, in life. You think you have to protect yourself by taking safety measures.

This is senseless, foolish, and a waste of energy. Allow your feelings to freely flow; express your emotions, and share your creativity with others. Nothing, or no one, threatens you if you trustfully open yourself up to your deepest Self and to life. Allow creative forces to come through freely; trust your nature. Dare to enjoy life in a relaxed way. You are safe and protected inside your Self. Don't bottle up anything; communicate with others in an open, honest way. No longer cut yourself off from that fundamental basis deep inside yourself, so that paranoid thoughts can disappear.

T

TAPEWORM

You refuse to listen to your own natural disposition: you take on structures, ideas, and patterns of your parents, of your friends. . . . You don't really live *Yourself!* Refusal to live "completely"; you parasitize others, without growing from out of your deepest Self. You are like an ostrich; you don't do what you have to do, don't make good use of your time. You roll, as it were, from here to there, living like a marionette, not really Conscious: a tapeworm takes your place.

You are too absent in a Neptunian way; you live in a false atmosphere of self-deception and deceit: because you aren't honest with yourself, others will rebuff you. Confrontation with your own powerlessness.

You keep running in place without making any headway; you see many directions, but you don't chose any; you live off others; you measure everything critically but don't emotionally integrate yourself into a life that really suits you. You get too stuck in details. Too large an accumulation of petty problems to which your thoughts stick; too many details about useless things — it all goes beyond you and "eats you up."

Do you too much allow yourself to be guided by ideas that aren't yours, or by "money," or by other false values? You don't live here-and-now; your thoughts twirl in unearthly spheres so that you no longer see things as they are. You don't see the forest for the trees.

You allow yourself to be manipulated by others just the way you manipulate yourself: you refuse to fall back on your own solid Basis. You now think you have to sacrifice yourself for other people because you don't consider yourself able to live for yourself! Your body follows orders from "someone else," as it were: your conscious "I" even seems to have turned away from your body: do you condemn your body? Do you condemn yourself to a path of suffering?

Don't allow others to get power over you; don't grasp for power yourself. Don't "fill" yourself, but fulfill yourself.

Unmask your own being, "bare" yourself, be honest with yourself. Allow body and soul to be reconciled with each other: allow your body to follow your conscious mind, not the mind of someone else. Build your ideas and structures yourself: don't allow yourself to sag, nor to be eaten up by others. Live toward a new goal — your ideal — and let go of old structures or unauthentic habits. Get your feet on the ground, cherish your body with love, no longer allow yourself to "be lived" (because that's why you have lost all control over yourself, over your body). Dare to break through, to become yourself, and then you will also meet genuine, honest people. Look at the essence of life! No longer fill your life with "false" values. Don't grasp outside you, but discover your own precious treasures.

TASTE DISORDERS, REDUCED ABILITY TO TASTE

You are not completely concentrated in your body, here-and-now. It's as if you flee from your feelings, away from yourself. Perhaps you act like a puppet player, or play the monkey or the clown; you float "above" yourself and the earth; you are a false king with a crown of fake gold on your head because you ignore your real worth. You degrade yourself; you play the role of a puffed-up emperor or else of just a joker, but you do so because you don't really *know* who you are, because you have only a vague idea about your feelings.

You run away from your deepest nature, from your true nature, from your body! You have placed a shield around yourself so that no one can reach you, but you can't really reach yourself. Your body's energies evaporate as it were, just like you don't acknowledge your "I" as the Core. A Neptunian flight, away from the earth, so that you don't really have to feel your body and your feelings. You refuse, be it unconsciously, to really stop and think about yourself. Why do you run away from your nature like that? You play a game to protect yourself: if you are not really Here, not really "reachable," then one can't hurt you either! This unconscious defense-mechanism, a flight *out* of your body, is the result of the fact that you are not really solidly with your feet on the Earth, that you insufficiently trust your own nature. You float, like a hot-air balloon, full of piled-up forces!

This inner rift (split personality) can be solved by integration of body and spirit: by putting trust in your Nature. Making an end to death (the separation of body and consciousness): enter the earthly structure and don't feel threatened, don't always be ready to flee, but acknowledge your body; recognize your feelings; feel sheltered within the safe walls of yourself.

Concentration of awareness in matter, being consciously present, here-and-now. Resolutely daring to stand up for yourself with Mars powers! Not taking off in the "spirit." Build up stronger earthly foundations. Feel yourself to be Master over your nature: pull the reigns, but don't choke the horse! Natural feelings and energies are imprisoned inside you: let them flow freely; acknowledge that deep worth of your Living self, feel your core and don't just live in a "facade." Use your creative energies in a self-aware way.

TEETH
(See also Gums)

Psychological correspondence

Represent: self-assured following of a certain course in your life; without hesitation, building up your life on the solid foundation of the fundamental power in you, your deepest everlasting Self. Self-assured standing on your own feet, autonomously. You can count on yourself; you don't allow yourself to be "pushed down"; you don't "hang" on others.

Triumphant joy about your primitive fundamental powers: combative self-defense, vitality.

You are determined; you don't let yourself be influenced by others too much: you clearly take your stand; you make firm decisions.

One can't push you over because you are solidly rooted in your Self.

The acknowledgement of the radiating white light in you means "liberation": white teeth, firm and solid, not too tight, nor too wide —

you take up your space with power and joy. You acknowledge your worth and your rich content; you load up your vehicle again and again with food, impressions, experiences. You "divide and rule" over this; you chew, make yourself master over your life; you swallow and you go on and on without end. . . .

Energies turn and circulate; you chew, "dissect," analyze certain experiences, but you resolutely go onward. You measure and build the architecture of your life; you take those building stones which you need; you don't stand still; you "bite" into delicious life, full of self-confidence. Your life is beautifully put together, structured by nature, in balance. You are the guardian of your divine content.

Ailments, in general

You don't experience yourself as Master over your life. You let yourself droop or you don't at all resolutely build up your life the way you'd like to. You don't dare to fully stand up for yourself; perhaps you feel yourself inadequate or a victim of circumstance. Are you afraid? Too anxious to really be yourself? Do you feel too much confined, too oppressed, too imprisoned, too dependent on others? Or do you actually show your teeth aggressively, because you feel inwardly threatened? Do you allow someone else to take your place so that you are almost "not" there? Do you feel angry and powerless, unable to persevere, to give shape to an independent existence? Do you allow yourself to be swallowed up by "something" or "someone"? Do you feel tied down, "stuck"? Liberate yourself, then: only be responsible to yourself, to your heart.

Do you keep chewing and ruminating the same things, unsure and indecisive? Don't you dare to trust in your own fundamentally strong Basis and do you listen too much to others or to motives that are only of secondary importance?

Live from out of that which is deepest in yourself; follow your intuition and your longings. Don't live directed toward the outer world, toward the Image, nor toward material futilities, but listen to your deepest "I," to the essence of your being. Resolutely determine your direction and go on without hesitation. Observe and analyze that which comes to you, and swallow it; continue on your way and don't look back. Be honest and consistent with yourself; stay faithful to your true nature.

Do you lean on others too much, on structures outside yourself? Only the life's house that has been built on the foundation of your inner Core is safe, trustworthy, and truly reliable. Don't cling to people or to things outside yourself. Don't fight for an image, a position, but if it has to do with joyfully experiencing your nature, with building your life up from out of yourself, then set your teeth into it! Acknowledge your worthy content and go on, without hesitation, in a steady course!

Dental abscess
(See also Abscess, in general)

Searching in all possible directions in a chaotic nervous way, filled to the top with natural aggressive powers, but you don't clearly see *which* direction to take. You don't really break through; you run in place in a frustrated and indecisive way, without making any headway. Anxiety is the largest stumbling block: "What will happen when I? . . ." Sometimes, unconscious, vague anxieties, because you don't have a "grip," a perspective on yourself, on your life.

Powerless doubts and anxieties often lead to fury, hatred or vengeful thoughts.

You don't trust enough in your personal basic structure, and therefore you don't dare to build upon yourself.

Discover in yourself: reliability, self-assuredness, indestructible primal powers, the absolute beginning, the "prehistoric" core, the rock in yourself. The eternal, everlasting Self, the faithfulness to your unique nature. The awareness of your talents, of your potential powers; determine your life in a self-aware way. Don't hesitate to determine, yourself, your lines to the future, and go on! Being aware of your Living Self, trusting in that divine core of yourself, and resolutely creating your life: knowing that nothing or no one can take your place; knowing that only you are master over your existence. Then all anxieties will disappear. No longer restrain yourself: allow your creative energies, your emotional powers, to flow freely and dare to be yourself! Realize that black thoughts only exist for as long as you don't acknowledge the mastery in yourself. Self-assuredly sail your course now, in peaceful harmony with yourself.

Caries, dental decay

You lean too much on the structure of someone else: you don't build your existence on your own Basis. You "suck" at others; you "fill" yourself with things, instead of existing independently. Your personal energies are looking for their direction, but they aren't made use of; they burn away on the spot. Refusal to Be as an Individual. Do you think yourself too weak, too small, not good enough? Do you tie yourself down in attachment to, or under the dominance of your mother, of someone else? Anxieties and insecurities hinder you from really building on yourself; you "fill" your life with others instead of, in the first place, with your Self. You'd like to reach your Core, but you don't very well dare; you remain too absent. You don't really believe in your deepest self; you look for a hold outside yourself. You perhaps do believe in Destiny or in great Danger.

Your thoughts sometimes search furiously, but you don't get a clear perspective. You close yourself off from higher awareness energies; you limit your experiences too much to negative or black, fatalistic thoughts. You think you can't really take your life in your own hands. You have no answer to emotional questions because you look for the answer outside yourself. Now, you should strongly build up the structures of your life, but you don't really believe in your inner Powers.

Arrive at the Core of yourself, and with your higher Consciousness throw light from above on your existence. Through intuition and self-contemplation, you are able to experience your powerful "I"-center. Don't lean on others; don't allow yourself to sag; don't allow yourself to "be lived," but feel those strong primal energies, those creative powers that well up from out of your deepest Self: handle them with mastery, and create your life yourself in the direction you want. No one is subject to Fate or Coincidence. No future is "predestined." Choose and determine your life course yourself; don't leave yourself "empty"; don't allow your space to fill up with negative thoughts, nor with "others."

Get a good hold on yourself; resolutely build up your structures; by doing so you get a clearer view of yourself: follow your intuition, your feelings, your longings. Have faith in that beautiful Light inside you. Manifest yourself in an active, autonomous way. Place yourself above your emotions in a self-aware way and don't allow your life to be dominated by anything or anyone other than your own Mastery. Don't just "fill" yourself up with things.

Open and free! Fill up all the space yourself! Enjoying yourself in an earthly, physical way, hand-in-hand with solid foundations.

Loose teeth

Where are you? Where is your true "I"? You absorb much from others; you suck in experiences, feel responsible, sometimes even guilty toward others; you absorb everything that comes to you in such a way that you, yourself, don't know where you are anymore: you even take in the feelings of others instead of first and foremost minding your own things. By holding on to others — by sometimes even forcing yourself, adjusting yourself too much to others — you can no longer be yourself. You are like a satellite dish or a receptive basin for the world around you: do you still recognize yourself? You don't really live from out of your heart, from out of your longings, from out of your nature. Do you serve as a gangplank for others? Don't you dare to take the responsibility to be *yourself?* You don't really evolve; you resist your *self*-realization. You don't determine your personal boundaries: your lifespace is too much taken up by thoughts, life philosophies, opinions, and the life, itself, of others. Hesitating.

Experience your center and build, yourself, your thoughts, your life philosophy; don't take on things from others. Turn inward and discover your depths. Let go of that which doesn't really belong to you; mark off your terrain and don't allow others to take up your living space.

Strongly establish and affirm yourself! Take in what you need, and no more. Take firm positions; don't allow others to direct your life, but be flexible toward yourself; resolutely follow that path you intuitively know you have to live. A strong backbone, a solid approach!

When a tooth is completely loose it mostly indicates: Transformation! An old root has to be pulled out, a new "I" wants to be born.

Dental neuralgia, tooth nerve problems

On the one hand, you let yourself droop; you don't believe in your fundamental powers; you sometimes even feel immobile, unwieldy, and slow; you stick to a persistent habit or to the past. You don't really live from out of your personal will and longings.

You go on — without true evolution. Rather being indifferent and at the surface of your existence. You think you will never be able to be *yourself,* and you resign yourself to it; you allow yourself to be ruled by others. You stay stuck to the surface of yourself, perhaps to your pleasures instead of to your true joy: you don't really live from out of your deepest Core! Possibly, you constantly give in to people or systems that totally go against your true nature. You are "a sufferer."

On the other hand, this leads to an enormous inner revolt! You resist "being-lived"; you spring up with all possible suppressed potential powers, which protest from the depths of your soul, which cry out for the liberation of your authenticity! That which you apparently no longer cared at all about, for that you now snort like a bull who's been restrained too long. Your nerves "break down" after this self-suppression.

You may glow with happiness; no longer live like a suffering victim. Solidly stand on your own feet and become aware of your inner Powers. Potential energies ask you to break through; don't hesitate; live from out of your true nature. No longer restrict yourself in a structure that is too tight; take up all your space and fill your lungs fully and freely. Tense your muscles; feel how consciousness powers wish to nourish your body and your life.

Give in to spontaneous impulses, to genuine creativity; no longer let yourself droop like a zombie or a sheep.

Be honest with yourself; don't lean on others or on systems, but build on the basis of your everlasting deepest Self. No longer bottle up emotions and energies, but dare to live life to the full, in full self-expression, so that nerves no longer have to protest.

Understand this message: free yourself; become faithful to your true nature.

Problems with teething
(See Teeth, in general)

You don't yet allow yourself to be really born. Carefully feeling out life. You calmly take time to build up your house in life.

Emotionally, you don't really dare to stand on your own feet. You look for something to hold on to; your body isn't yet really powerfully directed by your consciousness energies; you remain stuck with one foot in the unearthly atmosphere. Carefulness, uncertainty, and anxieties hinder a quick breakthrough of your "I."

Feelings are being "held in" to a great extent; aggressive powers turn inward instead of transforming themselves into decisive courage and self-realization. Anger, too, can be concealed   Life is heavy for you.

Don't smother yourself in your feelings: express yourself! "I AM." Show your power and feel secure in yourself, in your family. If the mother feels anxious, then the child won't experience this as "safe" and won't be likely to quickly break through into earthly life. Self-assuredly go into action, speak, sing, cry, laugh, dance, shout — don't be afraid to completely be yourself, spontaneous and natural, without fear or reservation. Discover your own powers!

Pulling teeth and dental prostheses

A shark, for instance, automatically has a new tooth "in reserve," when he loses one. Ever and again he can have new teeth at his disposal because teeth are very important for his survival. The human being however is not an instinctive animal, but a being of a higher consciousness-level, who doesn't "need" teeth to live. If he has no teeth left, he can choose to go on without false teeth — doing so, he doesn't care about the cult of the exterior! Or, for practical reasons he can, just as he takes a fork or knife out of the drawer, permanently or temporarily put false teeth in his mouth.

After a "first" birth (out of the physical mother womb) the child develops milk teeth which are symbolic of the first emergence as "I" on earth; a searching/becoming oneself with one's little feet on the earth. *Milk teeth disappear and are replaced by other teeth when the child is in a subsequent evolution phase.* A growth-process in the genesis of the "I" in the human being. Ultimately, it's normal that a human being, mostly in his adult phase, loses several and possibly all his teeth. *By itself every farewell of a tooth indicates a farewell to an old phase, to a problem which asked for a solution, which a person either has worked on or not.* One can look at the symbolism of caries, of abscesses, etc., in order to bring about psycho-emotional corrections. When the tooth is pulled, life definitely asks for a "new beginning" at the point symbolized by this tooth, this abscess, this pain, etc.

So, you see that when people decide to have all their teeth or their remaining teeth pulled in order to replace them with *dentures,* the moment has arrived to implement a *total rebirth,* to start a new life, as a Powerful "I," in a New Form. A *transformation* comes about at the same time as the last teeth are being "pulled" — at least if he allows this rebirth/transformation to happen inside himself.

If he wants to, man can *make grateful use of a partial or complete dental prosthesis.* Here, too, the technical side of the business will go smoothly as long as one continues with this "Rebirth" of oneself, if one lives in complete faith and in the greatest love for oneself. Never point your finger at someone else — for instance at the dentist. Always ask yourself the question: "Why does everything always go wrong with me?" Or, on the contrary: "See how smooth and painless it all is proceeding."

Unconsciously, after all, you attract every situation, the beautiful as well as the less pleasant. If something proceeds well or badly, the cause lies in you, not in the doctor. Though a doctor can make mistakes, of course, even then — unconsciously — you do attract it. (Read about this in Part I). It's to your advantage to trust that everything will go all right, to know that you don't have to suffer pain (that you love yourself and don't want to make you suffer pain) and that the technical side of the business doesn't have to bring along problems. This is because you make the steps you have to make in order to bring about your Transformation strongly! On the basis of these optimistic expectations and this love for yourself, you attract the painless, smooth course of things, and you will never need to have problems with your prosthesis if you want to wear one.

Therefore, don't "desire" to "keep" a tooth at whatever cost, while life gives you different signals, while you feel and know: "This tooth wants to/has to go!" Pulling teeth is not at all "bad," it is no drama. Try to understand the language of your body, your tooth; bring about transformation where needed and *joyfully let go of the old; also — synchronous with this — let go of a tooth when you feel, "Now this one has to go!"* This is okay, this is good and belongs to the evolution process of a seeking, truly living, human being. Do you, however, feel that a filling is good? Then you thankfully open yourself up to it.

Certain people are sometimes afraid to be "without teeth," and frenetically try to hold on to them. Often, this is not only because of the cult of the exterior, or for practical reasons, but also because one regards oneself as "old" when one has no teeth. Well now, a newborn baby has no teeth either: having or not having teeth has nothing to do with being "old," nor with being "ill" or "unhealthy." Neither can one read the level of consciousness, the strength, the ability of a human being in the number of teeth he has in his mouth! It all has to do with growth and evolution, digestion, and letting go.

How many times do we see that young people die of a serious illness, like cancer, and still had "all their teeth."

So: follow your own path, with or without teeth: after all, this has nothing in itself to do with living or not living, nor with being healthy or not healthy.

Suppose it was good for Life that at a certain moment teeth energetically and concretely, "as if by itself," again sprout and grow in the mouth of a human being — then it will happen.

Never, however, should a person force or desire this. It is not of fundamental importance to humanity.

Forming of tartar

You stand there, melting like a snowman, not really living from out of your warm center; with open arms to take in everything and everyone, but you don't feel good doing this. Your energies drain away. You don't know very well who you are; you don't succeed in making contact with your own basis, with your loving "I." You don't get a grip on yourself; you are there for others and not for yourself. You poison yourself by not really living from out of your personal will, from your longings and ideas. You don't see how to bring yourself to realization, because you don't listen to your inner authority. You place the authority outside yourself; possibly you fight for ideals "outside" you, because you don't acknowledge your divine Self.

You prefer to live hidden, you don't really come out. In this way you do get a grip on, or even power over, others, but not on yourself! Are you so afraid? Do you think you have to protect yourself? Don't you dare get out of your hole?

Bundle up powers in your Center: trust in your original nature, in your inner Self, and build up your life in self-assuredness. Allow creative powers to unfold spontaneously; feel your warm heart, your everlasting Basis, your own divine Self, and LIVE from out of yourself. No longer conceal yourself behind others, behind norms or ideals, the Authority outside you; but become aware now of the possibility of taking your life in your own hands and creating it according to your will and longings. Don't let yourself sink away, but establish yourself solidly; arrive at unique personal self-realization without first asking others, society, whether "You" are good the way you are. Be yourself! Don't encapsulate yourself. Open up, like a flower in blossom. Acknowledge the sunlight in yourself and no longer idolize a golden calf.

Impacted "wisdom tooth"

You build on the basis of others, on the foundations of your parents or of your teachers. You don't critically *think* for yourself; you are too attached and too tied to the teachings — the norms, the rules, the habits, the thinking patterns — of others, sometimes just like a parrot. . . . Where are you? You don't depend enough on your inner wisdom, on your intuition. You think like others, but you don't really check whether this is truly your "vision"? Because you are insufficiently present in yourself; you hesitate, and you wish to hold someone's hand or, at least, follow in his footsteps. You have not yet really been born in yourself; your "I" doesn't come out enough. You still stay under the earth; you don't have enough of a grip on your emotions because you don't really believe in the power of your strong Self-aware I. Instead of really existing *yourself*, on your own Basis, you allow yourself to be "carried" by others. Your Consciousness, your "spirit," is insufficiently concentrated in your body.

Transformation: allow yourself to be born from the depths of your Self. Mark off your terrain and strongly concentrate yourself in your body, with your feet solidly on the ground. Critically reflect about your way of life and life-philosophy: look for that which corresponds with your true "I," and let go of the rest. Come home to your true nature and now solidly establish yourself, independent of others. Build new structures and directions for your life: let go of the past and allow your own House to rise up, with your Core, your self-Aware "I," as the solid foundation. Arrive at insight, at wisdom, through

self-contemplation and intuition; don't be a copy-cat or an ape, but discover your unique SELF, and dare to manifest yourself!

Feel your powers; know yourself to be safe on that fundamentally solid, everlasting basis of your deepest Self. Go on, follow your nature, don't hesitate. Don't allow your life to be subdued by the teaching, the theory, the domination, the attachment of others regarding you. Go onward on the basis of your own Insights!

TENDONS

Psychological correspondence

The tendons symbolize the suppleness with which you find your way through life.

They show your readiness to follow and listen to your inner Self: without resistance, going along in the right direction; your ability to adjust.

They symbolize finding the balance between being structurally solid, on the one hand — knowing yourself to be supported by your inner Authority, being strongly anchored in the earth — and, on the other hand, allowing your emotions to flow supply — the flexibility and the agility with which you go through life, the letting-go of excess feelings and being open to joy (a connection between muscle and bone).

Knowing yourself to be powerfully supported in order to be able to work out your emotions, to carry your burdens in life. Knowing yourself to be protected against an overburdening of emotions.

Tendons symbolize the willingness to look — looking well in all directions — taking into account all various factors and not limiting yourself with blinders on.

Living from out of your own Power and not according to image, to the external, to the material aspect, to the Authority of others.

The Key to Self-Liberation, Christiane Beerlandt © Beerlandt Publications

Tendons symbolize the ease with which you make a connection between the old and the new, between structure and content, between duty and longing.

Making it too difficult for yourself, forcing yourself, or bending and being too compliant regarding your needs. Do you gracefully carry life, lightly and joyfully, or do you bear needless burdens and refuse to bring about change in this situation?

Ailments of the tendons, in general
(See also Achilles tendon)

Refusing to really see, to listen to your inner authority. Because of an urge for achievement or self-affirmation, you'd force yourself to please an audience. You hide behind a posture, a mask toward the outside, instead of *really* living from out of your deepest Self, from out of your natural disposition. You refuse to bring about the necessary change; you pretend you don't see anything. Emotional burdens are becoming too heavy; holding on to sadness and tensions. A contrary attitude toward yourself or others.

You take a wrong life-direction; you stagnate in a certain pattern; you carry needless burdens. If you don't bend, you will tear or break.

True beauty lies in the specific uniqueness of every human being: you ignore that; you force yourself toward the outer world — an unnatural attitude and behavior — giving power and authority to others instead of placing it in yourself. You make yourself dependent on an authority outside yourself, or on the judgment of others: you place the sun-center outside yourself, and as a result you burn away. Or do you allow yourself to be dominated by your passions, your instincts, and so refuse to take up your mastery in a self-aware way? Do you inwardly feel weak or inferior, and are you looking to compensate for this in outer display, in sex, or in tough behavior?

Go on calmly in life, without hesitation. Don't bottle up problems and emotions, but work them out. Stand with your feet solidly on the ground, knowing yourself to be safe and supported in your inner Self. Flexibly bring about changes where necessary; don't burden yourself too much; live in the light of yourself and be aware of your Worth. It is not the outer form that counts. Flexibly and spontaneously dare to trust yourself: self-purging of thoughts and feelings that are too oppressive; in a relaxed way, letting yourself go. Balance and flexibility.

Shriveling, shortening, of tendons and aponeuroses

Anxiously and tensely, you cling to structures, to a person.

A feeling of insecurity, estranged from your deepest Self, at the mercy of others. You drown in your emotions, in unconscious spheres. You have pain; you feel as if you are in the grip of others, although you take on an attitude of a victim.

Frustration; you feel as if you have run off the rails; you don't get a grip on your life; you allow yourself to whirl around — although a powerless aggression sometimes appears. Mostly, you allow the "spirit" to dominate your "earthly" being, here-and-now. Then again, you'd like to prove yourself!

But you feel too feeble, too weak; you'd rather hide behind a screen because you feel so anxious and threatened. You attach too much value to what others might say about you. You don't really live from out of your heart, from out of your longings. You think you have to justify and defend yourself to others. You shrink away; you don't really believe in your Powers. You don't dare to fully live, to enjoy. You restrict your life, and by doing so you draw people toward you who add to this restriction.

Build a new, strong structure from out of your deepest "I" and get both feet on the ground. Firmly stand on the Earth and bring about changes in your life.

Don't hide: blossom with all your powers; trust in your nature, in your spontaneous energies, in your possibilities. Don't live according to the standards of others, but arrive at true action from out of your Self, and know that if you flexibly and attentively open yourself up to your inner Self, regenerating powers are at work. Don't tense yourself up in such a frenetic way; find rest in yourself. Arrive at flexibility and cooperation with others and allow yourself to enjoy. You are a victim and suffer only as long as you allow it: alter your expectations of life, change your destructive opinion about yourself. Stretch out your life; take up all your space; unfold your talents; open yourself up to joy. Feel safe on your Basis.

Tendinitis and tendosynoviitis
inflammation
of the tendon and tendon sheath

Loaded with a lot of energies, you might — energetically charged — jump on your horse and in full gallop enter into battle. Full-blooded forces direct you onward; perhaps you stretch yourself, move yourself along (literally and figuratively) with flying speed. A mass of whirling energies asks to be used, asks for your airways to be open and free, asks for you to be able to go onward and act in a free and powerful way ... in a *true* evolution, not *immersing* yourself in your work or ambition! Sometimes rather reckless, with the helmet on your head, but not really seeing where you are driving, going or walking; *focused too much on that one point outside yourself, no longer being present inside yourself as a totality.* Your spirit and your body are completely possessed by what you are "trying to achieve"; *muscles and tendons tighten themselves in order to reach "a goal" OUTSIDE YOURSELF.* You will, and you shall! Even if you have to force yourself! Animalistic, instinctive, driving forces

seek their way and serve just this one goal — this means impoverishment of you, as a human being.

A striver's urge. *Blindfolded,* without thinking, *possessed* by your goal, the "cup," the line or finish-line you want to reach. Like a Ram's head full of ideas, possibly sometimes illusionary ideas, desires and strived-for goals, you don't keep yourself under control. Like a red-wild centaur you rush on and don't consider anything or anyone anymore. Possibly, you mess things up on your way; everything has to yield to your ambition, your sought-after goal. Hard and zealously desiring, too much fire. The sought-after goal takes the place of "YOU" as a human being. You are FIXATED, as it were, on one point, and everything has to move aside for this. You sometimes set off like an instinctive animal that runs wild, until your head and veins are red and swollen, until you would fall off your horse and realize: *"Why am I running ahead of myself? What is my life really? Am I a wild beast or a human being? What am I pursuing:* with passion and greed, with desire and ambition, in a search for talent, in wanting to be 'the first' or 'the best'?"

The solution lies in a return to yourself, in calling a "halt" to yourself, placing your horse (or whatever "object" or element you are using to reach your goal: a musical instrument, computer, sport attribute) in its stable and looking deep inside yourself.

How you disfigure yourself, make yourself small ... until there's only a tiny particle left of who you truly are as a human being in totality. You ignore the large space, the true treasures of yourself, and give yourself over to passion and the urge for pleasure, overzealous, and looking outside yourself for filling. Stop this; calmly sit down and drink a cup of tea or coffee[1]: make things a little easier for yourself, a little more restful. You don't have to "rush," to run and strive and

---

[1] Read more about the symbolism of tea and coffee in *The Horn of Plenty.*

pursue, to seek outside yourself, greedy and restless, "wanting to have or achieve" (an end result for instance).

You will find it all deep INSIDE you. Let go! Come home to yourself and enjoy true life in a restful way. Don't run after anything, don't try to "reach" anything . . . but live in the wonderful PRESENT moment. A resolute chase is a surrogate for the true, dynamic life that wants to manifest itself in you on a larger scale. Therefore, let go of "wanting to have or achieve" and enter into your "being": this is the path of life.

No longer force yourself, no longer desire, don't run after anything outside yourself. Look for the goal in life itself, in your Living Self, in the being of your "I," and experience true joy in this. Follow yourself, stay with yourself, not striving after things outside yourself, don't run ahead of yourself, don't rush yourself so. Live, minute by minute, in the dynamics of yourself, without seeing the final goal already in front of you: that is healthy. Then you supplely bend along with yourself, with nature, with life.

Therefore, no longer stretch yourself so far, burning red in order to reach the finish line, but let it be, let go. Life is not a contest, not a straitjacket, but an open space in which you are allowed to be yourself, at any moment of the day.

Stay with the nature of your body, your legs, your feet on the ground in the here-and-now.

Now let go of everything, sit down, come close to yourself, enjoy yourself in the eternal now. Don't hustle yourself with the whip. You have plenty of time . . . and nothing is a must. Don't let the worthiness of yourself depend on what you "have" or have achieved: after all, this has nothing to do with TRUE worthiness. Break with the world of false appearances. Throw off the red animal skin and step forward as a human being, powerful, restful, dynamic, serene. As a loving shepherd to yourself, no longer as a hard-as-stone tyrant.

TETANUS

You don't really dare to take the central space in your life. You refuse to wear the crown of a Self-aware person: you think and think — you fixate your thoughts again and again on the same things, without really breaking through. You waver: "What will I do?" You ruminate, weighing the pros and cons, but you don't really dare to go on, to go straight ahead. You don't really live from out of your nature. You stand still, thinking and waiting — and in the meantime life slides by without your *really* assuming your space. You deteriorate, like a building that has been affected by acid rain. You remain standing with the help of "scaffolding"; you are in urgent need of restoration! But you build your life on rational thinking, on the structures and authority of others, on religious indoctrination, on old patterns — and you don't dare to really live for yourself, from out of your heart.

Instead of resolutely biting into life, you allow yourself to be seized. You destroy yourself with doubts, with aggressive powerlessness, with the denial of spontaneous life. "No," you say: a refusal to really live.

This asks for an acute choice.
Complete self-liberation. Feel your Self-aware power-center, and get a hold of your life. Speak, express yourself, instead of withdrawing in thoughts and fretting.

Allow healthful, aggressive powers to break through, and offer yourself life. When you acknowledge your worth and place the mastery in yourself, then your body will immediately obey your orders. A powerful brain activity under the Authority of your "I." True immunity and healing of whatever illness lies in becoming aware of the Power and possibilities of your Self-aware "I."

No longer doubt yourself or the value of life. Go on! Bend your convictions in a to-

tally opposite direction; you ARE able to Direct your life. You are not powerless. . . . Create the quality of your life yourself.

THE THROAT

Psychological correspondence

To be able to speak for yourself, to stand up for yourself. Liberating yourself by, on the one hand, easily swallowing emotional experiences, and, on the other hand, expressing in a self-assured way that which you consider it necessary to say.

This natural receptivity to new impressions and the smooth process of letting these experiences pass through — this demands being solidly rooted in your personal, secure Basis. To let feelings flow through in Trust. The throat will symbolically make clear to what degree you can receive and digest, in Self-assurance, impressions and emotional experiences; and to what degree you dare to boldly manifest, realize, or express inner energies, creativity, talents, and longings. Do you, proud and relaxed, stand up for what's inside you, or do you hide your feelings and your talents behind a silent mask? Do you liberate yourself or are you keeping yourself a prisoner? Do you express yourself, or do you bottle things up? Symbol of the strength and power over yourself: you can always say what you determine must be said. Or do you feel so powerless, small, and afraid?

The throat represents the production of something new, letting things be born, creating on many levels.

A mirror of dualities: powerlessness/power over yourself; dependence/independence; being emotionally stuck/liberating yourself; attracting/rejecting; self-assuredness/unsureness; letting things happen to you/having the courage to speak up; fearing to be yourself/daring to Live from out of yourself.

Ailments of the throat, in general

Holding in — you don't dare to speak for yourself. Anxiety can paralyze you.

Anger, sometimes a stubborn anger, piling up emotions and resisting working them out or voicing them. Possibly, something has been ready for a long time to be born, but you put it off because you are afraid of that which is new or of the reaction of certain people. You conceal things; you don't dare to voice the way you really see things.

Sadness, not being able to digest certain impressions: you take too much to heart the attitude or words of others because of your being too attached. You allow yourself to be disconcerted because you don't believe enough in your own solid Basis! Somehow, you'd like to escape, but then again you wouldn't. . . . "I have to get out of this!" But you can't; you feel too weak.

Powerless anger, but you remain silent. Fear of being yourself.

You allow yourself to be flattened by others; there's no more room for you.

Give free passage to spontaneous, emotional expressions, to creative innovations, to intuitive reactions. Become aware of your autonomous worth as a human being and allow the wheel of powerful energies to keep turning with suppleness. Don't block yourself; don't bottle up your sadness or anger, but speak, and free yourself of all tensions. Dare to live more spontaneously; to sing with joy; to laugh; to scream when you feel like it. Look at the powerlessness and the anxieties behind your pain: Self-confidence!

Cancer of the throat
(See also Cancer, in general)

You are insufficiently yourself; you constrict yourself; you'd sooner flee or "close" yourself. Inwardly, you thunder with electric energies, with impotent anger; you can no longer handle it; you can't listen to it any more; you plug your ears. Out of fear of confrontation with your Self, you run away — you don't trust your deeper being; you are afraid of that which is deepest inside you. You constantly AVOID your true self; you just let everything happen; you follow routines without getting true satisfaction from them. You allow your life to be dominated by others, or by Something; you feel or behave like a victim, but you hide your inner emotional world. Here, you put up a stop sign: "You can't get in! This is my world!"

In the meantime, you strangle yourself with this aggressiveness: your softer feelings are kept hidden. Again and again you have placed above you an authority, a partner or employer, a system, or. . . . Again and again you have clung to others, as powerless and unsure as you were, but the sun above your head is beginning to singe you. You resist this dependence; a nervous agitation overpowers you and calls you to independence and self-realization, no longer skulking underneath someone!

You are being completely shaken up: creative energies and emotions ask for a way through, but you close up your throat, with arms crossed in front of your chest. "You have no say concerning me now!" A fury, a reaction to having been unable for years to really manifest yourself; a revolt against your feelings of powerlessness.

If creativity and spontaneous feelings have been suppressed, then you are now being faced with the consequences. This seems to you like a dark threat, but you needn't feel threatened! Make use of this mass of piled-up energy in order to look at the reason why you are angry. Speak out! Unload your negativity. In this way, you will arrive at your deepest emotional world, which for so long you have suppressed. Look at your emotions; look at that powerlessness and at your anxieties. . . . No longer flee like an ostrich. Allow feelings to flow freely, and liberate yourself: arrive at resolute self-manifestation; say what you have to say; stand up for yourself; don't be afraid of your

own aggressive powers — these lead only to productivity and to confrontation with your fellow man. Dare to be original; don't let others pull at you; in love and gentleness determine your own life. Don't be so hard and closed up; open your heart. Now, allow bottled-up energies to go free — let go of that cancer. The more you make sure that You, Yourself, are leading your life, the more will the cancer cells die off. If you fill yourself with joy, hope, and faith in a new future — a future in which you finally dare to live from out of your Self — then healthy cells will be born.

Epiglottitis
inflammation, swelling of the epiglottis

Powerless sadness, anger. Fixated thoughts hold on to that which is past. You swallow and you swallow, taking everything without defending yourself; you don't express your feelings, although you are swollen up with pain and sorrow.

You hide behind an inscrutable face, behind an artificial attitude, anxious. "They are going to seize me or hurt me."

Anxiety! You feel "inferior," unable to live, unbalanced: you are oppressed by *much* too heavy thoughts regarding experiences from the past.

A nervous search for something to hold on to, but your total emotional world stays hidden and swells up more and more — you don't dare to live your life to the full and express yourself the way you *are*.

Swallow that which is past; direct yourself, full of self-confidence, at the here-and-now. Don't stand still; in self-awareness, choose your new life-direction; dare to allow new thoughts and ideas into your head.

Replace sorrow and powerlessness from the past with joyful action directed toward the future!

Become master over your life and allow your energies to go free! Self-assured manifestation, without holding back. Know-

ing yourself to be safe and protected on your Basis, in your deepest Self.

Don't so forcedly keep yourself covered up and swollen: allow that which is new to be born.

Trust in your intuition; let go of suffocating thoughts.

Inflammation of the throat, in general
sore throat, pharyngitis
(See also Throat, in general)

As a "child" you feel powerlessly pushed to the back — Ah, you cannot or dare not say, or express, what on the emotional level is stuck, or what you have been carrying around in your head for some time. Out of fear? You would like to exist *yourself,* independently, but you don't feel able to do this. Love-hate; push-pull; standing up for yourself or accommodating others' wishes. You want more space for yourself, but you restrain yourself, anxious, unsure. Angry because of your own attachment! Sharp resistance with your elbows. Indignant at authority, you'd like to scream it out, but you remain silent.

As an adult, you are possibly struggling with the above-mentioned problems. For young and old, having a sore throat comes down to "being emotionally bound." You experience yourself to be dependent on others and therefore also strongly emotionally influenced by what others say to you.

Building up independence is necessary: you will then "love" others, but will not be hurt, will not cling compulsively, nor will you deny yourself.

The throat reflects your powerlessness, your anger, and your no longer wanting to accept the pain that others inflict upon you: free yourself from this situation by trusting in your own nature, by manifesting yourself autonomously, in action, in deeds, in creativity.

Make no compromises from a position of weakness: afterwards, you'd be angry with yourself about it. Dare to go onward, say what's on your mind, arrive at clarity in unresolved problems which haunt your thoughts: no longer immobilize yourself, but confront yourself with that which blocks you.

Express your feelings and work them out; don't bottle them up. "Now it's enough, all right?" Say this to yourself, not to others. Solidly stand with both feet on the ground and allow your emotions to come through. Don't strangle them.

Dare to be yourself; now, be aware of your worth and feel those propelling Powers, rich in energy, which, from out of your deepest Self, pierce your throat in order to incite you to productivity.

Experience the world around you not as a battle, but know that when you find Peace in yourself — if you dare to build on your Basis, full of self-confidence — this self-contentment will lead to reconciliation with others. Anger and pain disappear if you allow others to exist freely, the way they are, and if you resolutely dare to go on upon your path, independently.

Instead of fighting AGAINST your feelings, AGAINST your talents, AGAINST others — go on!

Having a lump in one's throat

You feel weak, limp, without a structural basis, too powerless to react. . . . Your throat is being strangled; you can no longer get any air. Feelings are overpowering you because you have insufficient trust in yourself, because you ignore the Mastery in yourself. You "endure" instead of carrying the scepter *yourself!* You let others treat you the way they want instead of acknowledging your worth and your Power!

You feel pushed backward, as it were; you offer resistance to your own powerlessness. Because you don't dare to stand up for yourself, you keep your "I" tied down and shut, and your spontaneous energies are being held back. Anxiety paralyzes.

No longer wait to speak; dare to spontaneously be yourself; no longer feel small, but get a hold on yourself. Full of self-confidence, lead your life with the power of your Self-awareness.

Arrive at rest in yourself; don't be afraid: trust in your intuitive impulses and give in to them. Allow your powerful energies, your feelings, to flow freely under the supervising eye of your "I," and no longer place authority outside yourself. You are master over what happens to you; it's not the reverse. Become aware of this and act!

TONSILS

Psychological correspondence

Just like the other glands, the tonsils are channels for the fire, the inner Consciousness-powers which give form to physical existence. They stimulate us to earthly incarnation. In the throat (See also the previous subject), these glands are translators of expression; the bringing outward of your deeper content, of your true being, of your talents in creative self-manifestation. Transforming the divine fire in you into outward productivity, into those activities that correspond with your true nature: live in harmony with your Living Self.

Enlarge your space in many directions; don't remain stuck in yourself.

On the other hand, they represent a defense, a guarantee, two guardians at the threshold. If you are in close contact with your deepest divine Self and are putting your faith in it — choosing your life's course intuitively and freely — then you won't be bothered by swellings or inflammations. If, however, you turn away from your deepest Self, begin to doubt, despair, or become angry ("I have to protect myself here in an ag-

gressive and sharp way because I am being threatened."); if you look for support outside yourself because you don't trust your own roots, then the Guardians draw their swords; then the tonsils protest as translators for your deepest Self: they call upon you to live from out of your deepest Core; to find the balance in yourself; to put all hope in yourself, not outside of yourself. Your own supporting power, your own grounding. Become who you are, don't drift off your course, don't stay stuck. Break through!

Swollen, possibly inflamed tonsils
tonsillitis
(See also Throat, in general)

Feelings are being suppressed, words and creativity held in. You feel "smothered," your throat closes up as it were: you only take up a small part of your psychological space. You have almost no air left because you don't allow yourself to fully live in a creative way, because you bury your talents. As a human being you undervalue your worth: do you despise yourself? Afraid to be yourself. Resistance to enlarging your life. Or don't you dare? Do you insufficiently stand on your own feet? Do you cling to others, as a child to your parents, as an adult to a partner, or to a job which doesn't give you enough room?

Inner division: on the one hand, an urge toward self-manifestation and liberation; and, on the other hand, being sadly stuck, a struggling powerlessness, self-degradation, continuing to hold on to things or persons, frustrations — "I can't."

This inner rift leads to an accumulation of active, aggressive energies, which ask for a breakthrough by one's Individual uniqueness: you swell up because of held-in potentials (words and deeds)! Things held in like a log-jam. You become angry with the arm that cherishes you, or with the hand you grab hold of; a red inflammation is the result of this: revolt, anger, with which you only wreck yourself.

Now, allow your Self to be born! Tonsillitis indicates that you are not "being yourself": you consider yourself incapable of it, or perhaps you don't at all know who in fact you are. . . .

You don't completely live from out of your core; perhaps you say what others say, or you show your strong muscles or your tough behavior, but really something's wrong here: you can only find this out when you very honestly look deep inside yourself, Daring to trust in yourself no matter how small you might feel.

Your content, the eternal living Self, is very individual and authentic in every human being — including in you. Don't live according to the standards of others, to social examples, to the models of father and mother; but discover YOURSELF, your specific, natural disposition. Believe in yourself and don't force yourself into a straitjacket, or into a structure that doesn't fit you at all. Speak, live, create, externalize those beautiful energies!

A healthy brainwash, a radical turnaround, is necessary: now place yourself Higher and look, in Self-awareness, at yourself, your content, and your possibilities. No longer flee into factitious words or into superficial activities: find your joy in the genuineness of yourself.

You are not "inferior"; you are allowed to be yourself. Say what you have to say; speak with the fire of an inner urge for self-realization; no longer destroy yourself by anger that has turned inward, but arrive at powerful self-affirmation, at productivity that follows naturally from your true nature and your longings.

Don't block your emotions, your flow of feelings! Don't bottle things up, but dare to take up all your Space. With open arms, free the path ahead of you. Don't hold back that which has to come out.

THUMB-SUCKING
for an exaggeratedly long time
(sometimes even after childhood)

You experience yourself as being powerless, small, unprotected, without solid ground under your feet, at the mercy of others: "They do what they want with me." These feelings of frustration lead to resistance — even to a sort of anger toward those who bring you up, upon whom you are dependent. You don't find yourself; you can't manifest yourself. You have a longing for, a hunger for, life-fulfillment. But your unsureness makes you feel like it's impossible to realize yourself. You are full of emotions, sadness, anxiety, question marks. You long for acknowledgment and love.

These factors lead to the temporary satisfaction and emotional anchor that is found in thumb-sucking.

A self-satisfying, numbing action which resolves frustrated energies and drives away feelings of powerlessness and anxiety.

On the one hand, we are dealing here with filling up emptiness and inability; on the other hand, you remain in the closed circuit of yourself — a feeling of weakness that unconsciously has as its result *a "firm seizing and searching for oneself,"* which by itself is a healthy reaction and a temporary solution for a child. Ultimately, the infant frees itself from this by fulfilling its longings for *creatively* and spontaneously living; feelings of being restricted, that go against its own nature, need to be resolved in free, Natural playing.

Daring to participate fully in life, no longer hiding within oneself: sadness, anxieties, and unsureness can now be expressed and overcome. It is necessary that feelings can flow freely and that they are not blocked in frustration.

The child will become aware of its worth and will be "proud" to be able to do without sucking its thumb. Here, it's about the *transformation* of basic instincts of (psychological) survival into action, self-manifestation, consciousness, Love, true creativity. *Full development of one's Being;* not attaching oneself to something/ someone else, in a grasping or desiring way.

THYMUS GLAND

Psychological correspondence

This gland lies physically as well as symbolically close to our heart. Here we experience how fire-forces, consciousness-forces, from out of our deepest Self are constantly being transformed into true atomic power, which is the basis of a safe, fundamentally strong, earthly existence. Here, we also experience a wonderful soft atmosphere, which — if we live in love and harmony with ourselves — is able to bring about "miracles."

"Love does wonders." The Nuclear forces of our being — that powerful Experience of Unity of ourselves, that fundamental nature — that is Life; that is love for Life, that is the gentle Joy, the peace, and the boundless hope in ourselves.

The pure, divine energy, the guarantee of our Autonomy, of our Immunity, is called love-power. It's this power which is able to transform cells, to bend genetic material into a new direction: if we don't betray ourselves, if we lovingly acknowledge our divinity.

The fertile activity of atomic energy is actually boundless.

If, however, we limit our lives to loveless sex and loveless action, without integrating these higher awareness-powers, then life runs out, then energy will just burn away, then the thymus will shrivel away.

Within the symbolism of the thymus lies the secret of a great age and of earthly immortality.

Don't squeeze to death the small, original, spontaneous, love-child inside you: allow the child inside you to come close to you again, because here begins the kingdom of god, love for yourself, for others, for life. Here begins immortality, the endless process of transformation toward an ever-greater Unity in ourselves. In this unity there's no border between Consciousness and Physical presence here and now. Here, we find again our original nature, without space, without time.

Here, we are aware of our Worth, of our Immunity, of the ability to self-create our life from out of the power station in ourselves, directed by the Love for life. And, at every moment, again purify our body, transform it toward a new body. Here ends suffering and death.

Let's no longer limit our existence to the "nature preserve" that has been represented to us so far: our borders reach *much, much* farther.

The thymus is the silver-white symbol of our gentle presence inside ourselves: here, all problems are being solved; here, we experience unity with all humanity. We need to free ourselves from limitations, from negative convictions, from self-hatred, from self-underestimation. In this radioactive source of ours, we find the guarantee of happy, eternal existence, without illness or suffering, on the condition that we acknowledge our own Mastery, that we carry the child in our heart.

If we can we compare the thymus with the original, happy, Living Child embedded in the safe shelter of the giving, primal mother, then we can compare the heart with the radiating Sun-God, who warms, strengthens, and Crowns the same Living Child in himself.

THE CHILD in you knows itself to be safe in the round-shaped, maternal center of your being. The ability to get, to draw out from very deep within yourself, from out of that Central Life Source inside you. You fool yourself by holding on to others; you save yourself by experiencing, feeling intensely, this round center in yourself.

The childlike candor. You come into the world with an open, happy outlook, full of expectations of what will come, in fresh simplicity, in openness, unrestrained, a sparkling lightness in the eyes. But you still have to grow. You are open to it; your attitude toward life always remains open-minded and amazed: what will it bring you in the next moment, tomorrow, etc.? You don't at all expect evil! Everything makes you feel light and pleasantly surprised about so much delights in the world! You'd never have thought this! And you are allowed to participate in it? It's all still young, like spring animals just born, coming out of their nests, like a gliding caterpillar which still has to emerge and fly away as a butterfly. But already you show yourself with a cheerful yellow butterfly pin in your hair; you succeed continuously in living, in being: now in a newborn state, a not yet transformed state. It will come. Don't rush things. Observe well and calmly the things that come on your path; leave the evil behind you and take on the good. You declare yourself a friend and ally to everything that is honest, open, candid, sparkling, and truthful — longing only for being, for advancement and growth.

You do the things you feel you have to do, as belonging to your task, in helpfulness, in simplicity and peace . . . together with others. You diversify your acts, deeds, and tasks. You adjust easily and behave in a peaceful and communicative way. You just let yourself be; you let others be. There is balanced cooperation between you and others, between left and right in yourself. You offer a helping hand where it's good. You are completely easy about it.

Things go very well with the thymus gland if you live in this way, if you offer and pass things on to others, if you don't only want to "have" things for you alone. If you do good to yourself, to others, if you can let go when something is completed. No longer staying stuck to it with your feelings or thoughts. If you go on again to your next phase. Very easily letting go and going onward; not pondering things in advance. Allowing others to be themselves, while you stay with yourself, not losing yourself in things, in people. Solidly and closely keeping your hands in YOUR pockets, taking them out if something needs to be done, if you need to help here or there. Then again going onward on the "free," Autonomous path . . . while whistling, carefree, like a happy, adventurous person who is open to everything that is good.

Thankfulness and happiness for what is, and not needing any more than that.

Ailments of the thymus gland, resulting in impaired immunity

You don't experience yourself as an Autonomous being that is full of love; the result is that you look for rescue outside yourself instead of in your deepest Self. You look for support and protection outside yourself because you don't trust in that fundamentally strong, divine Basis in your Self.

Emotional overburdening; you feel anxious and unsafe. In order to fill up your own emptiness, you reach for, grab or claw at, others; you are being seized by others — a logical result. You are under the authority of a teaching, a doctrine, a person; you don't really build your life upon your own insights. You paddle around in emotional memories from the past, without evolving. You immobilize yourself because you don't have a clear perspective on life. Bottled-up aggressive powers are seeking their path. You are worrying so much; you are so afraid — because you ignore your worth and your possibilities, because you don't really lovingly welcome yourself.

You hold on to the trash can of the past, sometimes in nostalgic sadness, so that you make no room for new energies. You hinder yourself from really joyfully living. You clasp someone else, your partner, out of necessity because you leave yourself in the cold. This sometimes leads to impotent fury, to anger because of this dependence, because of intensely reaching for something or someone to hold on to outside you. Deep anxieties tell you that you are not on the path to Life.

You are not really Consciously present in your existence; unconscious powers and emotions are triumphing.

In openness, surrender to your deepest Self, without anxieties. Know yourself to be very close to yourself; integrate every aspect of your being, including your body. Love for yourself. The most original powers within you ask for Self-aware leadership. Don't hold anyone in your grip, but first of all look for the naked truth regarding yourself. See what dwells deep inside you, and drag up the "dirt." Deal with it, and let go of needless emotional burdens from the past. In an autonomous way, move toward a new life in the faith and trust that only you are master of your existence, and that you are able to create your life according to your own wishes and convictions. Let contradictory feelings come into harmony so that you find peace in your heart. Know that, as long you don't fail to acknowledge this, you are naturally protected in yourself.

THYROID GLAND

Psychological correspondence

The thyroid gland symbolizes the warm, radiating, sun-power of your SELF, the acknowledgment of inner Authority. In creativity, with inexhaustible creative power and driven by your self-aware "I," you allow yourself to be born in warm love, with a radiating fire-power.

You are joyfully tuned in to your Living Self: just like all the glands in your body, the Thyroid is an energy-center which sends out inner messages. More than any other gland,

this gland — which lies close to the throat — symbolizes the ability to outwardly "express" and externalize our divinity: giving creation to, allowing to be born, creating. . . . No longer building on the ground of our education, but erecting a new building on the foundations of our deepest Self.

Transformation, a rebirth in ourselves, is necessary in order to be able to *really* live and create from out of our core.

The pearl which does not remain in the oyster, but which reveals its beauty in an independent existence.

Intuitively being open to our deepest Self, and no longer allowing ourselves to "be lived" by influences from the past or from the outside; a balance between intuition/feelings and rationality. A letting-go of old structures, allowing powerful, joyful inner energies to flow through. A happy and warm feeling about yourself.

Assuming complete responsibility for your existence: living from out of yourself, not first of all for the outer world. First, fully appreciate yourself, not allowing others to take up your space. You are king in your existence; you can help others, but not as a martyr.

Self-acknowledgment and an intense contact with your own divine content is necessary. Active, not passive, participation in life; not with a feeling of being victimized, but with love. Don't live a life with which you really don't agree. In a self-aware way, bring about changes where it is necessary for your own well-being. No slavery, but acknowledgment of your mastery.

The thyroid symbolizes being tuned in to the higher love and pure joy of your core of existence, as a result of which all restrictive emotions can be worked out immediately.

It symbolizes the creation of totally new things, invention, and that which is genius in the human being; just as there are many unique people, so are there many new, beautiful things that can be born.

The thyroid symbolizes not allowing yourself to be limited — not by self-suppression, nor by the authority of others, nor by restrictive laws and structures.

It symbolizes the bringing out of your artistic abilities and your emotional richness.

It symbolizes the power over yourself, and also the power to express your feelings and turn your energies outward. Productivity, fertility.

Ailments of the thyroid, in general

The unconscious refusal to be yourself, to transform. Possibly, you are under a strong authority: the authority of your father, a religion, a sect, a partner. You don't really believe in the Authority of your Living Self. You live cut off from your most beautiful Core; you don't believe in your worth. You are slave and servant, inferior and "sinful," unable to create. You treat yourself too coldly, too distantly. You live like a clown; you hide your feelings; possibly, you only live for others, not in true joy for yourself. Your longings to live are being constricted because you prevent yourself from breaking through. Do you have more respect for someone else than for yourself? Then something's not right here. Anxiety and powerlessness hinder you from manifesting yourself via your creative possibilities. You don't really live from out of yourself.

If you don't first of all love yourself, then how can you be loving to others? Then your work will be slavery instead of an original expression of your uniqueness.
You shut yourself out. You think and dream; you bottle up anger and frustration, but the cause all lies in you. Dare to say, "I Am"; express yourself; stand up for yourself; create; be fruitful. Discover the warmth in your own sun-center and *radiate* this warmth to others. Coldness will also distance others from you.

Don't block your intuitive powers; break with the influences of restrictive indoctrinations, and become aware of your worth.
Perhaps you want to have too much power over others: place all the power inside your-

self and let go of others.

Do you remain silent for the sake of peace and quiet? By doing this you do more harm than good. Be firmly rooted in yourself, and manifest yourself in a loving way, without reservation.

Don't put your talents in the ground; don't blame others, but assume responsibility for your own existence. No longer refuse to truly be yourself.

Hyperthyroidism
thyroid produces
more hormone than normal

It seems as if a long wall inside you hinders you from making contact with your deepest "I," and as a result you feel cold, lonely, and underappreciated: because you don't really believe in your Self! You feel imprisoned in structures, in laws, in the grip of others, but actually you are imprisoned inside yourself.

You refuse to, or feel unable to, be yourself — to outwardly manifest your feelings and possibilities. You refuse to look deep inside yourself; you ignore your own worth, your divine core. You keep yourself at the surface of things and of yourself. You are angry with yourself; you think yourself to be bad or inferior. Self-destruction. Angry thoughts; shut off from your intuition.

You don't really like yourself; possibly, you feel imprisoned in a task, in a religious system, but you, yourself, have called this up by not acknowledging your human Worth. Anxiety; you have no clear perspective on yourself; you don't really know who you are. You want to get out of your situation, but you don't realize that the cause lies in your convictions. You shut yourself out; you feel seized upon by others, and that makes you so angry. It's as if you always "have to," or something "is not allowed." Ultimately, in pent-up aggression, you push everything and everyone away because you don't see a way out for yourself, how you can escape out of this feeling of imprisonment.

You blame others, but in fact you are angry with your powerlessness, with your feelings of inability, especially in the area of creativity and self-manifestation, in the area of experiencing contact with your deepest Self. You feel cold and shut out because you don't recognize your own warm heart; because you ignore your divine center.

Allow the sails of the windmill to turn vigorously, in full sunlight! Savor life to the full! Safely come home into yourself, in warmth, love and gentleness. Lay down the hatchet and discover the rest, the peace, the joy, in yourself. Fraternization with others, liberation of your inner tensions. Now, acknowledge your worth; say goodbye to death, and LIVE fully, from out of your deepest Self, in creative, joyful enthusiasm! Feel that beneficial harmony within you when you are open to the sun-center, the true authority, in yourself. No longer undervalue yourself; allow the deepest Powers from your self to blossom, and discover your true nature.

Don't smother yourself with angry thoughts; no longer banish yourself from life; open yourself to your intuition. Express your longings, your feelings. Don't imprison yourself behind lock and bar. Free flow of warm energies!

Hypothyroidism
thyroid produces
less hormone than normal

You avoid the responsibility for this life; you flee into idealized thoughts, into dreams, into unreal fantasies. You flee; you experience life as burdensome; you look for refuge somewhere else.... You take a deviating path; there, high above, in your "spirit," is where you can handle things; there, you don't have to *really* live.

You no longer participate. Initially, you cling to others; ultimately, you climb ever higher into the clouds. There, things will be better; there, you expect to find security, without anxieties. No longer experiencing reality; an ethereal condition. Ignoring your Living Self. A flight....

A warm feeling of Self-awareness. A warm contact with the earthly, the physical.

They are nice to you; don't be afraid. Reassurance. The earth is not full of black danger: you can come back here. Feel safe in your own warm sun.

Know yourself to be protected in that divine, primal core, your deepest Self: you don't need to flee. Nothing bad will happen to you if you live trustingly.

Create your life yourself, here on earth, not only in dreams. Love for yourself, manifestation toward the outside, with both feet on the ground. Take the bull by the horns!

(See also Thyroid, psychological correspondence.)

Cancer of the thyroid

You live too much in the "spirit," not really from out of yourself. You place yourself under the Authority of your father, of a leader, or.... You totally adapt your life to others, without really living for *yourself*. In relations, also, you lose yourself; your partner serves only to replace your own inner Authority, to compensate for your own emptiness. You withhold love from yourself, but you do expect love from others. This, of course, can't be. You have anxieties. You are afraid of power because you experience yourself as being powerless. You are stuck in the experiences of your childhood: have you been suppressed? Have you never been really yourself, in a spontaneous way? Were you afraid of authorities? Negation of your own inner Authority. You feel alone, deserted, cold, and small; perhaps you blame this on someone else, but in reality you don't offer yourself the warmth and respect you deserve.

Sadness. You think you "need" someone, but first of all you need yourself. You feel dragged along by others, by life. You don't really create your existence; you let yourself droop. Bottled-up energies and emotions, sometimes an angry urge for power as a reaction to your powerlessness. You wait, afraid; you don't manifest yourself the way you feel. Perhaps you flee into a religion, into the authority of a guru, into a partner. Thus, you don't live from out of your deepest Core!

Feel your inner fullness; become aware of your divine beauty and radiate it outward. Joy comes from out of the depth of your being; for this, you don't need anyone: don't shut yourself out.

If you feel deserted by someone, know then that every happening in your life has been called up by your negative expectations: change your expectations. Now, welcome yourself warmly and say goodbye to the past. You alone are the leader of yourself: assume the task and responsibility for your life! Feel joy about who you "are"! Experience your total being beyond all lives; the Power in yourself in order to build up your existence according to your longings. Creativity, active participation in life, not according to the norms of others, but according to your own authority. Give expression to your feelings; let go of needless anxieties.

Goiter

You shut yourself off from your deep feelings. You think you have to keep everything under control with your thoughts. There's no true contact between the emotion-world and the thought-world inside you. Why do you run away from those feelings? You put on a disguise of superficial chatter, as if nothing is wrong emotionally, but here we are dealing with a camouflaging screen behind which hide anxieties and injuries! You don't offer yourself real, warm love or attention. You ignore the small, sensitive, vulnerable child inside you. Perhaps you hope that others might give you attention and love; but with them, too, you feel unjustly treated or abandoned. It's as if no one cares about you; but it is you who leaves yourself out in the cold! Distance, coldness, sadness, imprisoned in your cold cell: your spirit is separated, as it were, from your body. Your body is not really being nourished by the warm breath of life. You emphatically ask for attention from your surroundings, although you don't always admit it.

In order to feel safe — fleeing from deep anxieties — you cloak yourself in the mantle of "thinking" and close yourself off from your feelings.

"See how much pain I'm in! See how my heart is bleeding and longing for love!" That's what you say to your surroundings. Possibly, you do a lot for others in order to fill up your own emptiness or to still receive affection. Possibly, you place your third eye at the service of others, but your feelings, heart, and body are not integrating with this!

Are you so afraid of being hurt? Do you think you have to sacrifice yourself for one god or another that might punish you if you don't? (Anxiety.) Are you so afraid that someone might get a hold on you or might get power over you if you show your feelings? Deep inside yourself you feel powerless, hurt, lonely, anxious, seized by the throat.

Do you condemn your feelings? Don't you love your body? Do you think yourself ugly?

Why do you distance yourself from that warm, earthly aspect in you? That which you don't dare to acknowledge, your body now brings outward in a specific, "hysterical" way.

Listen to your Heart and make true "contact" with your deep feelings.

Allow those feelings to develop and express themselves; don't lock them up! Now acknowledge that female, gentle, aspect in you, and no longer be afraid of your emotions!

Your powerful "I"-consciousness is allowed to be "itself" in every way. You are not ugly or inferior; become yourself in pride; feel that body-warmth and now offer yourself all the warmth and love you deserve.

You are strong enough to carry feelings, to work them out and transform them into productive energy; accept them; absorb them into yourself.

You don't need to suppress your life under the mask of external or rational control.

Trust that spontaneous nature of yours; express yourself and fully enjoy your life; let yourself go. Trust in that fundamentally strong Basis, the Living Self, that endless source in you — and dare to live life to the fullest!

No longer bottle up emotions and creative energies, but bring them out and enjoy them! Become aware of your worth.

You deserve that others should respect you, and that they should serve you kindly. For as long as you deny this inwardly, you will only work for others. Self-respect and self-love, however, will attract to you people who will also lovingly acknowledge you.

First satisfy the necessary requirements in order to be able to lead a happy existence: warmly welcome yourself, your body, your feelings, into life! No longer look down on yourself, from high above!

Graves' disease
(See also Hyperthyroidism)

Complete uncertainty concerning your own identity: "Who am I really?" Distrust of your deepest Self: "Is there a little devil in me? Help! My emotions are dangerous and will overpower me!" Afraid to be yourself, afraid to live, because of fear of completely showing yourself the way you *are*. Because of distrust — and out of fear — you might put up a false front while doing a task which does not at all suit you, sacrificing yourself, so to speak, with an occupation, but in the meantime profanities and other thoughts are in the back of your mind. You are doing all this because you "must." You aren't completely honest with yourself, and in this way you don't respect yourself and others enough! You have no confidence in yourself nor in the people around you. You totally re-

fuse to build upon yourself, and you hold on to your partner, your friends, etc. You experience yourself as cold. Ignoring all the beautiful things that are inside you, you are afraid of the unconscious powers within you. Therefore, when others appear to be friendly to you, you don't totally trust them: "To me? That can't be true!" Because you, yourself, don't completely show who you really are! You are convinced that you have to constantly be on guard. And that out of the magic box that you are, a serpent might suddenly appear!

*Honesty, openness: there is no other way! Carry out your task, fully aware of your responsibility, in thankfulness for life. With honor and respect, bring beauty to the fore. Manifest yourself completely the way you are. Dare to show your true nature; close the door to your past. Look deep inside yourself, dare to look at all your possibilities, at all your aspects: at least **acknowledge** your SELF and don't run away from it. You are good as you are, trust your being: paranoid thoughts are not necessary. Don't be afraid of your Self, and say: welcome!*

Your emotions, your black feelings, can never become a threat to you as long as you let them come through; observe them and work them out. Don't suppress them!

Nodule,
small lump in thyroid

Powerless anger, pent-up aggression. Because of powerlessness, because you don't succeed in realizing yourself — freeing yourself from the feeling of being "stuck" — you take it out on others. Inwardly, you might boil with fury; for once you'd like to scream at others, but you are blind to the fact that you, yourself, are the cause of all your problems. Nothing in life "just" happens; via unconscious convictions and negativity, you attract certain situations. Underestimation of yourself, self-hatred, anger toward the powerless child within, frustration at being unable to be yourself. Possibly, your life is limited to the material aspect, to "work," to caring for others, to a function — in this you carry heavy loads, and in the meantime you don't allow yourself to explore the deeper things of life, don't allow yourself to make contact with the deepest creative sources inside you. You limit yourself to that which is superficial in life, or to criticism of others.

You are not honest with yourself because you place all power in others and react to all this with impotent anger, as if others are to blame for your being stuck in your limited existence — to blame for you experiencing yourself as being inferior to others or as powerless regarding your life. Instead of giving yourself more room and depth, you'd rather aggressively direct your claw of power, or your discontentment, at others.

Outwardly, you can put on a show, act as if nothing's going on, while inwardly aggression gnaws at you. You doubt your true worth, your creative possibilities, and as a result you fixate on things that it would better to put into perspective and let go of. You hold back the spontaneous emotional flow inside you; you restrain your true nature.

You are putting the noose around your own neck. Time to come to clear and pure insight into yourself. In your self-realization, make good use of all those powerful, beautiful, creative, aggressive emotions instead of wasting yourself. Self-expression, expression, artistry, open and honest communication with others. In a relaxed way, free the "child" in you so that you no longer have to vent your frustration on others in fury, in this self-suppressed condition. Surrender to your nature; listen to your longings; be open and gentle toward yourself. See how you are smothering yourself. Don't put the blame on others; every circumstance in life that you have unconsciously attracted has apparently been necessary in order for you to discover the deeper values of life and of yourself. Now, no longer resist; let go of the material

aspect, let go of others, and finally arrive at your own deep, worthy core. Unfold all your talents.

Discover in you those possibilities for creating your own life! The responsibility for your life lies only in you: don't allow your life to be determined or guided by someone else, but live from out of your nature. Only then, when you live in honest harmony with yourself, will you attract those circumstances in your surroundings which will be a reflection of this balance in yourself. This path begins by approaching yourself in peace and in love.

TIC

Tensely stuck in yourself; full of potential energies, but you aren't really going on; you are holding back energies.

Stuck — still — immobile — tense — imprisoned in yourself — unable to go one way or another — feeling as if you are the target of others, which again leads to tension — powerlessness to allow energies to flow spontaneously and freely — you aren't really taking a hold of the rudder of your life. You allow yourself to be limited by rules, norms, structures, educational laws or influences from the past; you narrow down your life; you place yourself in a "schedule."

Sail on with full force, allow all energies to flow freely; at every moment spontaneously do what you feel you have to do; be faithful to your nature and don't immobilize yourself within a framework that is too tight; place the power over yourself in yourself, not in others. Take the rudder in hand in a self-aware way and go on without constantly looking back and questioning things! Action, enterprise, creativity! Don't doubt yourself; don't resist spontaneous Impulses in yourself, but give in to this.

TOES

Psychological correspondence and Ailments, in general

Being sure about the *direction* you want to take, and still remaining supplely flexible; an openness. Choice, decisiveness, with both feet solidly on the ground. You are able to rise above chaos, above the multitude, not in the form of "spirituality" or in a "dream" flight, but with the wise eagle-eye of your Self-aware "I." Gaining a clear overview. You flexibly turn to all possible directions while remaining solidly on your foundation. You put your claws into earthly life. Your inner energies, your earthly powers, are being used in a flexible way in order to build up your life-ideals. Feelings are not being bottled up; you don't flee into unearthly spheres; you participate joyfully in the earthly festivity: you don't undervalue the physical. Self-assuredly navigate, take the rudder in your hands; take into account the multitude of details and possible directions.

Do you no longer see the forest for the trees? Is it all becoming too much for you, and are you taking flight into an unearthly sphere? Or do you, in resolute decisiveness, dare to confront yourself with the turbulence of life? Do you go straight ahead, without self-doubt? Do you think you have to defend yourself in an aggressive way? Do you feel threatened? Do you not dare to acknowledge yourself the way you *are?* Do you run away from yourself, so that only your tracks are left behind? Powerlessness, indecisiveness, resistance? Are you too hard on yourself? Do you force certain things instead of flexibly going along in the direction which you intuitively feel to be the right one? Are the "male" and "female" aspects in disharmony? Does hard logic and restricting armor control your existence? Your toes indicate to what degree you are faithful to your true nature without violating yourself by suppressing one of the important aspects of your being.

Being established, in balance, on Earth. A feeling of safety and sureness. Flexibly being open to possible new information or directions in your life, without going out of balance. When you arrive at a fork in the road, you know, after weighing and considering, what direction to choose: the "I" gains mastery over its life's course and goes onward dauntlessly, patiently, but with decisiveness.

Corns

You don't really live with your Consciousness in the here-and-now. You don't live concentrated strongly in your body. You primarily live in your "head." You think, you fret, you live too much in the "spirit," in the rational mind; you don't live in the midst of that which is earthly: but you "fly" above it. Your worried thoughts go to problems from the present and from the past. Emotionally, you send out aggressive bombs from a distance, because there's no real participation of your "I." You allow yourself to be carried along by life; you are not fully in the Center of your existence.

Painful, hardened thoughts — sometimes with vengeance or bitterness — suppressed aggression, all turn inward.

You are sensitive and vulnerable, but you are not aware enough of your Worth as a Human Being. You remain "enclosed" in yourself; because of this, you bottle up certain memories, emotional experiences, and you harden yourself that way. You are in pain, but you don't dare bring it all outward; you don't succeed in digesting things, because you try to control everything with your head. You do fixate your thoughts on ambition, career, or achievement; you try to climb "upward," to get further, but emotionally you can't untangle yourself.

Softening! Listen to your intuition, to your feelings, and live with your total being, with your body. Don't live with your thoughts circling around others, worriedly, but live with your heart and soul in earthly joy. Open yourself up; direct your thoughts to that which is beautiful, to enjoyment, and don't allow thinking to put a dominating damper on life. Put on your crown; live from out of your own center, in the Now, and allow feelings, intuition, and mind to live harmoniously together. Acknowledge earthly pleasures, sensorial joy; integrate feelings, body, sensuality, into your life.

Don't bottle up any hard thoughts. You, yourself, need to stand in the Core of your existence. Live in love and tenderness toward yourself. In this way, you will no longer attract any negative experiences in your life. After all, it is you, yourself, who has attracted the "hard, painful" happenings via unconscious negative convictions regarding yourself. Now surrender to your heart, to what you FEEL, to your intuition, and lead your existence with a masterful overview, without being blocked any longer by thoughts that are pinched together.

Crushed toe
(See also the specific toe)

Inner confusion, nervousness — an extremely agitated situation. You go against the flow. You don't see clearly what direction to take: nervously, you look for a way out. You are spinning out of control; your epiphysis and your brain work in an exaggerated way; the rhythm of your heart might be disturbed; you feel constricted in your heart and lungs; you don't know anymore what to do or how to do it: which of the five directions will you take? A stubborn refusal, you get up on your hind legs, in revolt: "No!" You don't go along anymore; you refuse to go on in this way; you don't listen to the voice of your deepest Self; you might begin to force certain things. "Now it's over with!" A halt. For too long you have bottled up natural aggressive powers; you have suppressed your personal nature, perhaps have done what pleases others. Now, you flee

from this situation. You flee, and perhaps you are very angry instead of reaching for a true solution. Now, you go beyond your limits; you go against the current, nervous. . . .

Because you have never really listened to your deepest feelings, because you have never really found your right direction, because you can't handle this path any longer, you say, "No." You'd prefer not to be, as it were! In desperate nervousness, you ultimately don't know what you are doing anymore. Possibly, regardless of all possible warnings, you try to cling to a certain life-path that is not at all good for you. Emotions and nerves get the upper hand because you don't acknowledge the Authority in you, because you don't make a Conscious, resolute choice in your life — a choice whereby you listen to the interests of your deepest Self.

Build your life upon a healthy structure, the safe Basis of your Self. Resolutely bring yourself into line; give the hot-tempered child in you a slap in the face, and spit it out! SAY what you have to say; solve that confusion; come to clear insight; no longer walk on hot coals. Confront yourself with reality instead of fleeing: force yourself, in the here-and-now, to SEE and bring about a change, a solution. Place all responsibility, but also all Authority, in yourself, and make your own decisions: don't allow yourself to "be lived." Listen to the signals in yourself, and, without hesitation, choose that path which won't crush you emotionally. As long as you go on in this way, you will feel oppressed: get a hold of yourself!

Dislocation, sprain of a toe

Unconscious or conscious refusal to go on in the direction in which you are now going. Suddenly, the brakes are put on; you are on the wrong track; intuitive resistance. A demand for change, for consistent action, for honestly being open to yourself, no longer going on in this way, no longer having to make compromises that go against your true nature.

(See also specific categories.)

Fungal infection between the toes

On the one hand you want to live in a warm and sheltered way, and on the other hand you want to get away, trying to punch your way to freedom.

Inner duality. On the one hand you can behave sharply, harshly, or in an authoritarian way to the outer world, perhaps even as a fighting idealist, with a sword, directed onward; or as a tough sports hero; or as a show doll, who proudly steals the scene. On the other hand, in all these situations you are far removed from your true nature-core, your feelings. You live too much at the surface of your existence, directed to the outer world; perhaps as a child you lived only according to the habits, the Authority, of your parents, without really being able to fully live your true being, your feelings, your unique personality. Your emotions, your energies, are pinched closed. On the one hand you feel secure and safe in your little hole (between your toes), and you keep adjusting yourself to the Authority of others, to the outer world. On the other hand, protesting powers from within push out. You feel suffocated under the web of a compelling authority, of an oppressive love-tie, of an authoritarian parent — whereby you have no room to freely exist. But in the first place it is you, yourself, who directs that aggression inwardly, who punches and fights to get free, because you, yourself, suffocate your nature, your feelings, under a hard mask, under rational thinking, or under "a second face." "It has to be this way," and you live accordingly, neglecting your true longings, your true nature. Do you live too much according to expectations from the outer world? Do you violate yourself? Do you ignore those powerful, creative ener-

gies in your deepest Self? You are stuck — imprisoned, frustrated, and inwardly much softer and much more sensitive than you would outwardly exhibit! Inner unsureness and vulnerability lead to a hard, camouflaging disguise. You don't enough take your feelings into account. Emotions twist and turn in order to be allowed to flow through; you too much bottle up and hush up everything. Toward the outside, you possibly function optimally and exert yourself in order to "satisfy"; inwardly, nervous tension grows, the urge for a breakthrough. You need Space! Space to be able to be yourself, to be able to breathe freely, without suffocating armor.

Free your energies! Create space, and listen to your inner Self. Don't first of all live according to the standards of others, but live from out of your Core, from out of your Nature.

Be faithful to yourself, relax; in all openness, allow feelings to exist freely.

No longer burn away on the spot; no longer keep those beautiful powers imprisoned; liberate yourself and live spontaneously, without allowing yourself to be suffocated. Be honest with yourself; build your life on your inner Authority; don't remain stuck in a pattern in which you can't be yourself in a natural way. First of all, accept your unique nature, your worth. Stand up for your Self; only then will others respect you in your "being." Don't push yourself behind an exhibition, a false front, or behind certain behavior that doesn't really correspond with what you actually feel inwardly.

Live from out of your heart and dare to speak, to show yourself the way you feel. Express your aggression, your indignation, if it makes you feel better, but then continue on your personal path without expecting others to understand your "being." If you don't hide yourself any longer, if you believe in your inner worth — the beauty, the way you are now — then that will make fungus disappear.

THE BIG TOE

Psychological correspondence and Ailments, in general

In a positive sense, this toe represents inner Leadership and Freedom, Self-liberation; in a negative sense, it represents dominance, suppression, and compulsions.

The acknowledgment of the pure, earthly, dominant Power of your "I." You take hold of yourself; you guide and direct the Traffic in your life: what is allowed to "pass through"? What has the right of way on your path?

Joyful life-enthusiasm on Earth.

Allowing creativity and powerful primitive energies to exist freely, under the watchful eye and the Guiding Authority of your Self-aware "I."

You, yourself, choose a well-determined path, independent of others, autonomous and free; Uranian electric energy.

Not blindly rushing into something or going somewhere, but allowing yourself to blossom gradually in a conscious way. Unfolding your energies and talents.

Placing the Authority in yourself; respect, pride, dignity, knowing how many golden possibilities there are in every human being, and performing your task, your work, in a good way. The "male" and "female" aspects in balance; making yourself a path toward the sunlight in yourself; joyful, loving encounter with yourself, with your partner. Respecting that which is beautiful, the core in yourself. Allowing feelings to smoothly come through within a powerful, expanding structure. Acknowledging the divine energy, the power of your talents. Becoming aware of the Mastery in yourself: the warm Sun-core in yourself, not false gold, tinsel, or Image!

The deeper feeling of self-worth, of Trust in the Central power-source of yourself. Trusting in Life and daring to choose *that* path which doesn't violate your Heart: daring to experience your joy of living, your earthly feelings, without inhibitions, in the Light of your everlasting, deepest Self.

You don't cause yourself any heartache: joy may flow freely.

You don't allow yourself to be used: you, yourself, resolutely direct your life. You are not too hard on yourself: you don't "compel"; you listen to yourself in freedom.

You have no anxiety: you get a solid "grip" on your life and with resolute powers you create it and build it upon a solid foundation, anchored in the Earth.

In freedom, you open your lungs widely and feel so happy in this free living space, like a bird in the sky. If you suppress your free nature-powers, you might get a problem with obsessive thoughts or compulsive movements! You guide your primitive powers, your emotions: you are master over them; compulsions, instincts, perversities, emotions, sexuality — nothing can crush you! You are master over your existence. You get rid of needless emotional burdens that are too heavy to carry; nothing can keep you in its "grip." You are no victim of that which is "unconscious." You stand solidly, on your own feet; you give yourself sound structures: you feel safe in your sun-center; if necessary, you say, "Let's go! Onward!" You break through restricting barbed wire. You are not afraid of working out feelings and letting them go.

You don't float in the clouds; you try to get a clear perspective on reality by effecting the harmonious cooperation of rational thinking and intuitive feeling.

You allow electromagnetic currents, power-fields from out of your deepest Consciousness, to flow freely so that no short-circuit, no overburdening of nerves, no insanity, will appear. Your Self-aware "I" is the leader, but this leadership is based on inner knowledge, on your intuitive wisdom. Balance between reason and feeling under the direction of a loving Master.

This toe indicates to what degree you allow primitive powers, healthful-aggressive powers, and deep emotions to flow through; or to what degree you frustrate yourself, block yourself, until there's an explosion, perhaps a blaze of fury. You "hold on to too much."

The big toe indicates to what degree you paralyze yourself under the authority of Reason. Pain in the big toe — but also general neuralgias, compulsions, and restlessness — can be the result of a too-extreme, dominating, oppressive attitude regarding your worthy powers. Are you raving at others in an overbearing way instead of maintaining Authority over yourself? Do you dominate yourself or others like a dictator instead of listening to your heart, to your inner wisdom?

Do you ignore the Power over yourself, and do you force certain things? Do you punch at others in order to make way for yourself? Do you feel oppressed in your life situation and want to fight your way out of it? Do you not know very well which way to choose? Are you on guard regarding Life, and are your thoughts often leading toward death? Are you allowing yourself to "be lived" by others? Do you deny the Authority in yourself? Are you allowing yourself to be used like a pack-mule? Do you try to keep standing under heavy emotions that become too much for you because you have suppressed them for so long? Because you, yourself, don't dare to live?

Does an inner conflict lord over you? "Whom should I satisfy — myself or others, the outer world?" Do you make compromises? Do you too much exhibit false fronts or outer facade instead of experiencing yourself in joy and freedom? And do you then become furious because of this frustration? Do you have the feeling that you are getting a nervous breakdown because you don't give the Freedom of existence to your powers, your emotions, and your energies?

Do you not dare to determine your path in a Self-aware way? Do you present yourself as being aggressive, in a defensive posture, or do you fight against yourself? Why are you so hard on yourself? Why do you force yourself? Or, do you completely let yourself droop, subject to compulsive primitive impulses, with your "I" being unable to get a grip on things?

Are you destructively aggressive with yourself? Do you not offer yourself the love you deserve? Do you cling to a love-partner? Or do you not really show yourself as you feel because you fear a break or you think you are not good enough? If you hold on to so much, then sooner or later you will sag under these burdens.

Do you feel Inferior and unsure? Are you afraid of deep unconscious powers, of pure emotions? Does anxiety overtake the freedom to be who you are? Do you feel "ringed"? Have you nowhere to turn, and do you feel unable to free yourself? Do you feel like you are everyone's servant, and do you revolt? Do you crush yourself or others under a large foot? Do you not allow yourself to truly Live in joy?

Are you angrily rebelling against Authority above you, although you refuse to listen to Authority in yourself?

Carry out your work, your task, in gratitude, in reverence, in respect toward yourself, and in acceptance of your inner Mastery. Resolutely choose *that* path which seems best to you and which leads to Joy. Feel good in yourself; reconciliation with yourself and others, love for yourself and others.

Proud of being yourself and of being able to develop all your talents. Supplely going along with the wishes of your Self. Don't dance to the tune of Image or the outer world; but, in Freedom, lovingly acknowledge and unfold your natural energies. No longer suppress yourself; acknowledge your Worth and allow powers to freely escape from the prison. Place Authority only in yourself!

Fracture of the big toe

The urge for liberation! You want to know for certain who you *are* and where you stand.

An inner call for recognition of one's own inner authority. Have you attached too much value to your outer pride, to your Image? Have you begun to "swell up" in fury and indignation, in pride or arrogance, or in anger at those who supposedly don't acknowledge you? They are just reacting to that which you send out "telepathically." Now, come to rest in yourself and listen to your heart. Feel those inner powers, those emotions, and your possibilities — no longer bottle things up. Don't build your life on others, nor on outer Authority, but only on the Authority of your Self. Give yourself room to breathe freely and no longer restrict yourself. Now, become aware of your Worth and unload your emotions. Become the master over your life and choose the path to true life. You don't have to be "powerful" or "powerless"; honor the worth and the divine Power in you; create your life in a self-aware way. Don't make it too hard for yourself. Allow energies and talents to slowly unfold. Just because you feel inwardly frustrated, don't turn to others in a negative manner. Transform aggressive powers into Action! Seize the rudder *yourself* and don't allow yourself to "be lived" by others, nor by outer appearance.

Bunion
inflamed swelling on the base of the big toe

You don't take up your full living space; you don't live from out of your inner wisdom and insights. You will listen to bookish knowledge and to that which others tell you, because you don't believe in the inner Power and the divine Worth of every human being — nor in your ability to create your own life. Possibly, you are very active, but you are not really creative from out of your deepest Self. Deep powers are not being used to the fullest. You have Anxiety. You are afraid of those powerful energies deep inside you. You are not really master over yourself. Also in regard to relationships, you will cling to your partner with sucking cups, as it were — or you will allow your partner to claw onto you because you don't believe in your own autonomous power. Sometimes, you feel like a chicken on a barbecue spit, because you *allow* yourself to turn with it — you don't really make decisions about the direction in your life. Because you don't consider yourself able to, you don't make yourself master over the multitude of experiences that come to you. Sometimes, you are so

afraid of being pulled along. It's as if a great claw presses on your chest — that's how suffocated you sometimes feel. Deep emotions, beautiful aggressive powers, are being suppressed. Do you anxiously hide your emotions? Are you so afraid of being yourself? Do you so little trust yourself and life? If so, you can't feel free and happy.

Acknowledge that divine Power over yourself and the life in you. No matter who you are, be proud of your unique being and openly manifest your true longings, your true Nature. Don't suppress yourself, but participate joyfully in earthly happiness.

Creativity from out the depths of yourself. Acknowledgment of those powerful energies in yourself: don't conceal yourself behind false growth, behind the existence of your partner or your children. You are you: stop this self-suppression, and now take up your own living space! Arrive at a clear overview; don't let yourself be overpowered by a chaos of experiences. Become Master over your existence and no longer let yourself "be lived." Now, acknowledge the authority in yourself, and no longer allow yourself to suffocate. Liberate yourself!

Hallux valgus
big toe grows outward

Not daring to follow your own straight path; feelings of guilt; thinking you are not allowed.

To yourself, you are like a severe judge. You punish yourself; you constantly rap yourself on the fingers, as it were. You resist your spontaneous, emotional flow. Refusal to surrender to natural growth. You carry heavy emotional burdens, like a victim. You don't sincerely manifest who you are inwardly: do you think that's how it "has to be"? Are you just trying to satisfy the expectations of the outer world? Sadness and anxieties are overpowering you because you are not living from out of your deepest core. You will also push back the experience of love and relationships within well-determined lines, or, like a sculpture (Venus), you just participate in it in order to please others. You are tormented by feelings of guilt whenever you allow yourself enjoyment. Did your parents put this rule upon you? Hesitating uncertainty: yes/no. "Will I go on?" You put the brakes on your Mars-powers. Will you allow yourself to be born or not? Emotion and rational mind contradict each other; you stick the sword into the ground; healthful, aggressive, creative energies go to waste. You try to keep up your image because you feel so vulnerable whenever you are in contact with others. Your head is a merry-go-round of self-restricted thoughts. You are too sharp; you constantly hurt yourself. You don't dare to break through.

Love, reconciliation, warmth, making yourself welcome. Free yourself from that role of being a victim, and become your real self! No longer force yourself; feel those powers, those healthy emotions, in yourself, and don't be afraid of them. In a self-aware way, dare to experience your life in all freedom and joy. Surrender to your most beautiful feelings, to your nature. Listen to your Self, and follow your intuition. Stand up for your rights as a human being to make yourself happy. What counts is not what others — or that severe judge in you — expect from you, but that which your nature tells you is best for you. How you FEEL is what matters.

SECOND TOE
"Dragon Toe"

Psychological correspondence and Ailments, in general

To what degree do you feel good in yourself and independent? To what degree do you take care of yourself, treat yourself like a king? To what degree are you "egotistical" in a healthy way? Seen negatively, you could call this "self-important"; in a positive way, this is called "spoiling" yourself or moreover: the natural survival instinct. "I

have to make sure I don't lack anything; I have first of all the responsibility for myself."

You live intuitively; you trust in those inner powers as well as in your physical powers. When you are confronted by philosophical questions about Life and Death, Law and Judgment, history and conscience, you turn inward; but when you are self-assured you don't become emotionally troubled by "suffering" because you are good at putting things into perspective, because you experience yourself to be in such close contact with (your) nature, because you respect and understand the laws of life.

You powerfully go onward. You experience yourself like a bendable reed that is grounded in a strong root — your inner Self.

You have faith in the life-processes, without anxiety.

You enjoy to the fullest the wealth of that which is earthly.

You have a strong imaginative and philosophical capacity — about love, life, and death. You look at all the details, and you dissect all aspects of "existence" into fragments. You climb onward in life, full of self-confidence, proud, undisturbed, straight-ahead, beautifully balanced, stable: you acknowledge in yourself the Power over your existence. You surrender to life in self-aware "manly" action, courage, and self-assuredness. You don't allow yourself to become unbalanced by emotions, nor by the outer world. You freely go your way; you stand solidly with your feet on the ground. You walk on independently, but you don't lock yourself up. On the contrary, you speak, proclaim, that which is beautiful; you say what you have to say, without fear. Energies turn outward.

You feel how Consciousness-powers course through your strong muscles, your body; how your "I" directs your body; how you can depend on yourself.

You don't hang on others; you trust in your intuitive energies. You hold on only to yourself. You experience the Force, the power, in yourself, and you acknowledge yourself as being the only Authority over your earthly Realm. You know yourself to be protected in yourself.

You don't just let in anything or anyone. Critically, you determine your life, your boundaries, your path.

Being able to be one and alone with yourself, peaceful, undisturbed, quiet and gentle in complete stability. Feelings know their place, in serenity. Self-assuredly, in faith and trust, you calmly navigate toward your goal without the least anxiety. Directed by your intuition, ideals, wisdom, and love, you make a path for yourself. For you, life is the horn of plenty. You possess a Jupiter-like self-confidence in your own immortal, divine Self.

What are the psychological causes of Ailments of the second toe?

You have ANXIETY. Your whole head, your thoughts, your body, are being occupied, being possessed by someone or something — by ideas, by an Authority, which You *are* NOT. You feel seized; perhaps you resist others who might grab hold of you. It seems as if you can't protect yourself very well. You feel old and inadequate, unable to take care of yourself.

You place Authority outside yourself; you cling to others.

You think that others, perhaps a superman, might "rescue" you. You ignore the powers in yourself.

Possibly, you escape your task, your work, your responsibility, in a cowardly, fearful manner, because you feel yourself "imprisoned." You secretly want to slip out; you withdraw into yourself; you don't express yourself. You don't really trust in that intuitive power in your deepest Self. You might think yourself to be bad, or you might mistrust your own nature. Without being critical, you swallow everything from others. . . .

Other possibilities: have you been just an arrogant, self-important facade? Do you live in a cold and haughty way, empty inside,

showing off to the outside? You won't feel good doing this. You ignore those powerful Awareness-energies in yourself. You live superficially. Feelings of powerlessness can lead to Aggression.

Do you blame others because you don't succeed in following a resolute path?

At last, have you fallen on your "Exterior Face"? Do you hide behind someone else? Don't you honestly show yourself the way you are? Don't you allow living, warm energies to flexibly flow through your body? Do you remain standing in a stiff, rigid, and anxious way, as if you have been put in irons?

Don't you have a "personal" face? Don't you really live animated from out of your heart, from out of your inner self?

Do you desperately try to defend yourself against whomever or whatever you think keeps you imprisoned?

Fracture of the second toe

Anxiety about being pulled along by suction, as it were. "Who am I?" You resist, aggressive, desperate, impotent. On the one hand, you let yourself droop, not really present in yourself; you allow yourself to "be lived." You are so afraid of the future. You don't really dare to go on. There's resistance in you. You feel unable to self-confidently build your path. You refuse to go on. Sometimes, it all leaves you cold. On the other hand, you suddenly revolt in anxiety and aggression.

THE MIDDLE TOE

Psychological correspondence and Ailments, in general

You stand in the Middle of your existence, solid as a rock. On the one hand, you stand Powerfully and stable, with both feet rooted in the earth; on the other hand, you experience life as happy, and you turn with motherly attention toward your feelings. The balance between "male" and "female" aspects. Venus, love, your feelings — all carried in the strong arms of the Self-assured Mars. You remain always faithful to your feelings. You feel totally secure in the power of yourself. You build up your life resolutely; the structure and Trust in yourself protect you in such a way that whatever happens outside you can't hurt you nor keep you from your chosen path.

You know yourself to be safe within your living space. You are content with your talents, your inner richness; you are self-sufficient; you don't really "need" anything or anyone. You build your existence only on yourself.

You have complete trust in the Jupiter-abilities of a human being: "Don't worry, everything will be all right!" Everything goes smoothly; you know that things which are happening now have, in fact, first been called up (unconsciously) by you. Knowing this, you are constantly creating, producing — in an active, fruitful way. You do this especially in order to provide, protect, and care for yourself and others in a good way, in order to organize everything in such a way that everything goes along smoothly. You supplely glide along on the tones of life, without anxieties, without forcing. Once you have done the necessary actions, you easily let go of everything. You burn energies in productivity. Inwardly, you feel calm and full of peace. You don't lift yourself above your feelings or above your earthly condition of "human being amongst other human beings." You are aware of your worth; you place the kingship in yourself, but this does not result in willful arrogance, in hypocritical play-acting, in a tinsel Image. You don't blow your own horn; you are not false or deceptive; you don't place yourself above others. You live honestly and openly, not presenting yourself differently from the way you inwardly feel. You are content with yourself.

You are Gently open to your feelings. In this way, you will also be open to others —

lovingly, socially, righteously, balanced, and peacefully.

Or do you carry heavy emotional burdens and refuse to unload them? Are you angry, yes, aggressive? Do you strike down yourself or others with cold, condemnatory, harsh criticism? Are you constantly worried about nothing? Do you not trust your deepest Self? Do you feel so weak on your own Basis? Is there a question of an inner rift: the way you feel/the way you appear to the outer world? Are you becoming entangled in a lot of details because you don't live from out of your Center, but instead live toward your Image or toward judgmental Authority, toward Structures or laws which rigorously and strongly oppress you?

Powerlessness and anger, a senseless battle, can be the result of the fact that you make demands on yourself or others instead of listening to your heart, to the feelings of the true Nature of every human being.

Do you live "falsely," not the way you really "are" inwardly? Do you mislead yourself or others? Or do you cling one-sidedly to the "Mars" aspect, the militancy in you? Are you hard, short-sighted, condemnatory, imprudent, pushy, reproachful, naive — without really caring about the "gentler" feelings? Do you perhaps blow your horn from a very high tower and disregard the feelings of others? You punch and fight — because you suppress the gentleness, the "female" aspect, in yourself. You feel threatened by it because you feel you are too Weak. When you trust in that fundamental power in yourself, when you no longer feel threatened, only then can you open yourself up, in peace, to your feelings.

Dare to manifest yourself, the way you inwardly feel. Don't be afraid that you might lose your "dignity and power" if you acknowledge your inner feelings! No arrogant, aggressive yapping, no camouflage for your inner unrest, for whatever — but a carefree, Happy existence, which is built on that strong central pillar, the everlasting Power in you. Don't lift yourself above the earth, but root yourself solidly: feel sure, safe, protected, and don't be hard on yourself, nor on others. Not the wicked stepmother, but a fairy godmother. A waltz, in which the male and female elements in you exist in flexible harmony, wherein one listens to the song of Venus and Mars, and wherein you don't just watch from behind the curtains. A balance between resolute, self-assured Power and motherly gentleness.

Fracture of the middle toe

You rise up against the structure, the network, which is too hard; or against hypocrisy, the unauthenticity in which you are imprisoned. Without looking up or around you any longer, you break through. You want to go your own way, no longer having to be accountable to others.

Primitive powers and emotions that have been suppressed for too long — aggressive charges — now burst open. You want to go onward, no longer worrying about anything or anyone.

THE SECOND-SMALLEST TOE

Psychological correspondence and Ailments, in general

On the one hand, you protect yourself, taking precautions; if necessary closing yourself off for the sake of your sense of well-being.

On the other hand, you trust your inner, primitive fire-forces and make use of them in the service of productivity, of fruitful self-growth, of consistently going on, calmly, ever pushing back your physical earthly frontiers. Proportionately balancing, directing, organizing, aware of your inner Sun-center. You take the obstacles with ease. You don't, in shyness, stifle the fire, the magnetic powers, the talents in you. On the

contrary, you direct healthful, aggressive energies outward in self-manifestation! No structure can crush these inherent fiery energies. You allow yourself to blossom; you don't suppress anything; you don't destroy yourself or others with destructive, aggressive arrows. You shoot your arrows in the service of a calling, a task, or a personally chosen direction. You allow yourself to open up in self-expression, in outwardly fully experiencing your emotions, your energies.

You are aware that you can always trustingly depend on your Self. Where necessary, you offer yourself a "safety valve"; you don't bottle up your energies; you don't burn yourself up on the spot; you don't put your talents into the ground; you don't waste your powers in "anger" toward the outer world.

Pure consciousness powers that come from very deep inside you — energies and emotions, creative powers. . . .

You allow them to come through freely, and in the unity of yourself — without contradictory feelings or thoughts of inferiority being a spoilsport — you handle these powers with mastery and purposefully steer them in *one* direction.

You participate in earthly existence; you don't roam about in heavenly, spiritual spheres without your feet touching the earth! This toe will hurt if you neglect those magnetic, volcanic, fire-forces which are meant to establish your SELF strongly on earth, like an Incarnated being. Expressing this in creativity, in artistry, in taking the initiative, in action, in earthly work, in physical experience, and also in anger when necessary — sometimes, as an outlet, so that peace and harmony can be rediscovered after expressing, working-out, and letting go. No "holding in" of this fire! No condemnation of those powerful Mars energies. No suppression of spontaneous longings. No "holding on" to heated emotions.

The elasticity, the flexible power to accommodate yourself to all possible changes in your life. In this way, you know yourself to be safe and protected. You follow your inner, Individual path without wasting your precious talents. You are like a proud lion, aware of his worth. Spirit and body perfectly united.

Consciousness nourishes your muscles; you experience yourself as being full of joy. You weigh and consider, but decide and let go of whatever is a needless burden. You don't cling: you dare to let yourself go! You are self-sufficient. You are master over your emotions; you direct your powers. You feel balanced.

Do you hold in aggressive powers, red-hot energies, anger? ... Are you burning inside because you don't realize yourself, because you restrain yourself, or because you feel ashamed or inferior? Frustration, build-up or fury — powerless to be yourself. Are you not being understood? Are you afraid to show yourself the way you feel? Afraid of not being good enough? Are you afraid of those inner, aggressive, creative powers? They are good: allow them to come free; and in all openness, become yourself! Are you now stuck with exaggerated longings (including sexuality) because for too long you have suppressed yourself regarding self-realization? Or are you wedged into a structure that you have imposed on yourself and that is too tight? Do you not dare to be earthly, to taste the "fruits," to savor the exuberant enjoyments of life? Are you afraid of becoming your true self? Or, do you not at all protect yourself, letting yourself go completely because you ignore the mastery of your Conscious "I"? Are you going beyond your limits? Are you angry with others because you block yourself from complete Incarnation and creative development? Do you kill yourself with inwardly turned aggressive powers because you don't allow yourself to truly live? Do you live too much in the "spiritual" realms?

Fracture of the second-smallest toe

Are you tired of always playing the holy nun or some other Role? Are you now driving yourself too severely, too coldly, too in-tensely, in a certain direction where there's no more room for spontaneous energies? Or do you resist the "conductor" who has led your life into this harness? A revolt against Authority?

You want to push back your frontiers, adjusting your structure to the content. Emotions, energies, aggression, have been bottled up for too long. You have behaved too "white": red forces are now looking for a way out in order to bring to realization an earthly, spontaneous, creative existence. You have acknowledged yourself too little; now you are sick of it. You protest; your feelings collide, and you break out. Poison, energy that is turned inward, overwhelms you: the spontaneous child inside you calls for acknowledgment. Fruitful productivity seeks its way. Now, recognize those pure, earthly forces in you, and manifest yourself in a Self-aware way. Flexibly adjust yourself; open up new horizons if necessary. Transform aggressive powers into active self-realization! Fully enjoy earthly life; don't live as an "ideal," but integrate all your inner powers in order to fulfill your inner longings, in love for yourself and others. Don't live too much in the spirit, nor in a harness, but follow that voice of your earthly nature, of your unique disposition. No one else but you can show you the way here! Don't be afraid of being yourself! Listen to your Feelings.

If fiery creative powers are being experienced and put into practice, then there's room for gentleness and harmony inside Yourself. Frustration and self-restriction call up swelling and illness. Express Yourself!

THE LITTLE TOE

Psychological correspondence and Ailments, in general

Knowing yourself to be protected in your Self by the smooth exchange between the female and male aspects in you.

Nourished by your true nature, by your deep feelings, by your intuition, by love and care for yourself, you can supplely, flexibly — *offering, giving* — productively proceed. This toe makes clear in what way you experience the loving "female" aspect in relationship to yourself, to the "male" aspect, as well as in relationship toward others. What direction have you chosen here?

The "female" element on the Throne.

Respecting your feelings, your nature, your body, your deepest Self.

Providing for your safety, in balance between rational thinking and intuitive feeling, between structure and content, between female and male. In the solid center of your Self, you can surrender to love, affection, tenderness — toward yourself as well as in relationships with others.

Sensual surrender to your Nature.

Not the superficial female aspect, not the facade, not the fashion doll, not the suction — but, instead, the true, primal femininity in every man and in every woman. The wise queen, self-assuredly on her throne, carries within herself the king, the male element. She is open; she receives; she knows herself to be protected in herself; she cares for others.

The little toe symbolizes the way you deal with the "female" element (See Left Body-half), but you can't "uncouple" this from the male aspect. The self-aware, proud authority (male) of the loving, caring (female) element; the fertile-productive, the earthly-natural, the physical experience, the "passive attraction," the playful, inviting call — all this in order to be supplemented with the active, male aspect. You can allow the Child, the female element, to exist in you because "I AM." The perfect merging of both aspects in yourself leads toward beautiful growth, to higher consciousness-experience that frees light, joyful energies.

Then, you know yourself to be safe and strong. The "guardian angel" in you speaks through the little toe: to what degree do you dare to surrender to your deepest Self, to

your Intuition, to your true nature, to your physical experiences, to your spontaneous, healthy, sometimes childlike impulses? Or, do you crush your fine emotional world too much by "thinking, Image, laws, structures"??

Do you not acknowledge the Queen in yourself? Do you hide your feelings, your earthly nature, beneath armor? Do you not dare to fully sense your inner Self, and do you cling to external values? The little toe symbolizes being spontaneously open toward yourself, toward your energies, emotions, potential powers that emerge from your deepest soul.

Spiritual Joy, intense and beautiful, can be experienced by surrendering to your deepest Self, to your feelings, to your spontaneous creative impulses, to your power to create on many levels. Caring for yourself, for others, without "clawing onto others," without neglecting yourself or being oriented only to others.

Being able to help yourself without having to be dependent on others; authority in yourself. You don't have to hold yourself straight via Image; you can smoothly allow your feelings to flow because you trust in your solid Basis, your Living Self.

In this way, you bring forth Fruits: the toe indicates how you deal with creative energies inside you.

Do you restrict yourself to the superficial, to sex? Or do you allow your creativity to blossom in a wide range of productivity?

Or do you just sit there, doing nothing? Do you feel "chained" to someone else? Do you feel bound hand-and-foot? Do you not dare to experience *yourself?* Do you direct your life only toward others, like a mother hen, like a Cancer, a crab that pinches onto things without actually evolving itself? Do you not very well "see" what direction to take? Do you live full of Anxieties? Do you cling to Outward appearances, to Image, to a structure, to *thinking,* to logic — without taking into account your feelings, your natural longings, your body? Do you live one-sidedly, in a tightly "masculine" way, and do you close yourself off from your wealth of feelings? Do you flee into sex or into a hermit's hut?

Do you place yourself on the electric chair? Are you filled to the top with creative energies, but block yourself? Possibly, you blame your fellow-man, but it is you who immobilizes your healthy energies. You "oblige" yourself to walk within predetermined, artificial lines, and you have to bear the consequences of this. Are you performing daredevil feats in order to satisfy the expectations of others, of society, of "external-physical" norms, of "beauty"? And by doing this do you force or break yourself? Or, without listening any longer to your own nature, do you do that which your partner demands of you? Do you feel hurt in your most intimate being? In your feelings? In your physical body? Or do you feel forced into sexuality, and do you now close yourself off? Do you now block a healthy flow of feelings? Do you not dare to fully experience your nature in joy?

Are you afraid of your deepest Self, of unconscious powers, and do you prefer to live on the surface? Cut off from your deep, everlasting Core, you possibly "draw" others to you by "suction," so to speak — attracting, seducing, charming — because you experience yourself as being empty, because you don't offer yourself any love, because you have to "fill yourself up" with others in order to feel yourself confirmed. Or do you push others away from you because you feel threatened or because you don't need anyone anymore?

Do you, in empty arrogance, hide behind a chic hat or a fashionable outfit? Where is that deep, sensitive, female, loving core of yours?

Do you not dare to surrender to your nature, to your feelings? Do you flee from this? Do you live only with your "exterior"? Are you perhaps a clown who's crying inside? If you exaggerate by accentuating too much either the superficial female aspect (too

flexible, too limp, etc.) or the superficial male aspect, then this will lead to illness.

If you follow the natural divine impulses of yourself, and acknowledge your Self in care and love, then just as in a Beehive, your productivity will yield fruit, and a structure will spontaneously build itself up from within.

Don't plan a rigid structure. On top of all this, as a human being you carry the scepter in a self-aware way: you can choose. Therefore, choose *that* path which doesn't violate your true nature, your feelings. Trust your intuition, your feelings, the female aspect in yourself, and don't suppress this, but experience it unto its depths. Go on, without looking back; affectionately cherish yourself and others; surrender to healthy creativity. In joy, experience the physical, the natural longings. Let go of the past; don't cling to things or people; surrender to that which is playful inside you.

Fracture of the little toe

You have tied yourself down too tightly; now, your suppressed feelings, your spontaneous energies, are calling for acknowledgment. The clown tears away his mask; he has wept for too long. "I want to be myself!" You break out of a structure — a framework, a habit-pattern — in which you had imprisoned yourself. You want to break out, like bottled gas, which explodes.

Possibly, you haven't at all really had both feet on the ground. Have you lived too "spiritually," and does your deepest Self ask you to create in yourself a balance between consciousness and body, between spirit and nature? Your primitive, spontaneous powers are breaking through. No longer ignore your unique emotional life. Follow the laws of your true nature. Become yourself; don't fight *against* things or people, but give room to all creative aspects of yourself. No longer violate your nature and your feelings. Manifest yourself the way you really feel; no longer *immobilize* yourself. Only when you lovingly approach yourself will you be able to live in harmony with others. First, allow the male and the female elements in you to be reconciled. Don't satisfy the expectations of the outer world, but flexibly open yourself toward your inner Heart.

In a self-aware and autonomous way, plant yourself with both feet on the ground; thus can your feelings flow freely, and you are no longer "fragile."

The little toe and sexuality??

Even if suppressing the emotional, creative powers — in men as well as women — can lead to ailments of the little toe, we must take the following into account: the so-called "female" energies can be employed and experienced via Sexual experiences. In people who have come to awareness, however, these energies can be made use of in a range of possibilities, including creative experiences and joyful experiences. Thus, the ailments of the little toe can be seen — *NOT first of all as a problem of Sexuality, but as a denial (or hardening) of the female, loving, productive energies; as an inhibition of complete self-realization as a Human Being — as a possible over-accentuation of a sort of hard masculinity with regard to one's own "I." As a result, one feels more "vulnerable" and naked.*

(See further the chapters about Sexuality.)

TONGUE

Psychological correspondence and Ailments, in general

Abundantly giving, offering to yourself. You are allowed to taste, to savor, the best life-wine. You take good care of yourself; you dare to take what you deserve. You speak, you stand up for yourself; you build your worth on your inner Authority. You allow your energies, your emotions, to flow freely, without interruption, so that you constantly refresh yourself, like a ventilator. You get

"rid" of that which is superfluous; you don't smother yourself in repressed emotions. You take up your complete space; you don't strangle yourself, but in all openness you manifest your Self, your opinion.

Not in the name of love, nor in anxiety, will you close up.

You let off steam if necessary; you don't bottle things up. You shake free thoughts that are stuck: you digest things and express yourself. You fully enjoy all tastes and pleasures of life. You are good to yourself. You go along smoothly on the gentle waves of your longings, your feelings. You constantly turn the wheel of life: you take *those* nourishments, call up those happenings that make you happy, that make you taste the joy of earthly life. You don't clam up; you are not hard or ascetically cold. You respect and honor your Self, your body.

When you close up, when you feel guilty because of the pleasure that you gave yourself; when you are not really open to the well-being of yourself, then your tongue will become sick. Do you again and again bite the tip of your tongue? Do you not really dare to be yourself? Do you not dare to enjoy all those beautiful tastes in life? Do you punish yourself? Do you cover yourself up with a thick, scaly coat of fur? Do you estrange yourself from the earthly, from your nature, from the physical? Do you live too much in the "spirit"? Do you allow yourself to be "seized" instead of depending on your own Authority? Are you a slave of someone else, of a certain "philosophy" that isn't yours, of a power system, because you are afraid and don't dare to build your life on your own foundations?

Burning, stinging sensation of the tongue

You withdraw into yourself. You say you don't care anymore. You let yourself droop.

Anyway, you can't tell someone else what to do. You'd sooner live in your head, in your thoughts, in the "spirit." Possibly, you now cling to a "faith." But, actually, you are filled to the top with piled-up, aggressive powers. You have tried to hold on to certain things or people, or tried to push them in a certain direction, but failed. You remain silent because of anger and powerlessness. Your movements can become mechanical. You no longer act out of joy for yourself, for life. Possibly, everything tastes very bitter to you. Are you now in your castle-in-the-air, or in your ivory tower, high above earthly reality here-and-now? Do you silently blame others? Would you like to shake someone, but do you hold back and remain silent? The deepest cause lies in the fact that you don't feel safe, that you don't trust in the Authority in yourself. You wrong yourself. You don't really "live."

You don't very well know who you "are"; you feel powerless.

You can't tell someone else what to do, but you can tell yourself what to do. Change yourself, your convictions, and then your surroundings will change. Take up your own space; enjoy, and live from out of yourself instead of orienting yourself toward others or toward a castle-in-the-sky. Turn inward and be open and honest. Now, stand on your own feet; don't depend on others; don't cling. In purity, come toward yourself: undo yourself from bitter, dark, or accusing thoughts, and free yourself. Spring-cleaning: eliminate self-destructive emotions.

Say what you have to say, in self-confidence. Listen to your nature, your longings, and fully partake in earthly enjoyments. Descend to earth! Know yourself to be welcome, and take good care of yourself! Place inside you all power over yourself; let go of others and acknowledge the Authority of your Self.

Cancer of the tongue
(See also Cancer, in general)

Outwardly, you can appear calm; but, inwardly, you are ready to explode! You have bottled up emotions for too long, until insan-

ity is approached: mortal fear, wildness, vengeance, fury. You don't *really* live from out of yourself. You "draw in" others by suction, as it were; you try to get power over others or to get a grip on them because you experience yourself as being so anxious and powerless. Cool and cold in yourself, shaking from impotence, full of scary thoughts, full of burning aggression. Are you going to burst out, or are you going to let the candle go out? You don't very well know. You control and suppress your "I": you don't leave your feelings, your awareness powers, any room to exist. You are a sentry with a sword: you supervise yourself; you smother your nature. You don't really allow yourself to enjoy. You see everything as black and deathly. You don't dare trust in your deepest Self; you feel unsafe; you don't take your life in your own hands at all.

OUT!

Open the windows and let everything flow out! Put things in order; express your aggression, your sorrow, your fury. In the first phase, this brings relief. Then, arrive at Insight into the true cause of your feelings. Acknowledge your powerlessness. Discover the Power of your inner Self, and stand solidly on your own feet. Feel yourself to be safe on this Basis. Dare to express yourself, to unload, without reservation, and then find again the rest and peace in yourself. You have the right to Joy.

The true cause of whatever you have experienced in life lies in yourself.

Now, get a hold of yourself and go in the opposite direction: offer yourself life. No longer bottle up emotions, but express yourself! Acknowledge the fact that deep in your heart you are angry with yourself and are outwardly projecting the scapegoat. Now, in love and gentleness, come to yourself.

Coated tongue, brown

Resistance to transformation; you don't trust yourself or others.

Behind this, a complete inner-drama often hides; now you finally give up; you don't even defend yourself anymore; you don't at all believe in the power of your "I" anymore. Inwardly, there is deep-hidden aggression, but it leads to death. You stand before a blank wall because you refuse to look into yourself for the cause of your problems. Standing still and threatening, constantly looking out for danger, full of dark, rotten feelings and black thoughts, mistrusting, anxious, and unsure; hard as a rock and stubborn. As if at any moment the world can come to an end; you feel like you are standing on very shaky ground. You don't build your life on your own Authority. You are afraid of Authority — which you have placed above your head yourself — no matter if it has to do with the god of materialism or possessions, with a partner or a Supervisor. You are hard and severe on yourself; you refuse to listen to your heart, to your nature. You expect the worst at any moment; you look at tomorrow in a very negative way.

You hold inside yourself this negativity of feelings and thoughts.

Look at your emotions from above, and don't let yourself be overpowered by them. In self-mastery you can handle energies and emotions in a productive way. Turn deeply inward, and for once shake everything out: give expression to your feelings; now allow powers to direct themselves outward in creativity.

Life is not dark or negative: make an end to those convictions because they attract that which is less beautiful into your life. In trust, open yourself up to that which is most beautiful in you; allow yourself to enjoy, to experience joyfulness! Rescue yourself from this mud puddle and step into the light of your living Self. Don't be afraid of those emotional depths in yourself. If emotional powers are trustfully directed, they lead you to joy.

Coated tongue, white

On the one hand, you remain emotionally stuck in painful experiences from the past, and you don't feel able to really go on. On the other hand, just like a dragon, you spout the fire of anger and criticism toward others, but you keep it in; you don't really say what troubles you. You are killing yourself in this way! Actually, you consider yourself to be limp or weak; you try, therefore, to find confirmation in the outer world so that others might consider you good, beautiful, clever, or fantastic. You want to be acknowledged by others, and so you don't really behave the way you truly feel. After all, you feel hurt, wronged, perhaps humiliated, or else you are often hostile toward the "evil" outer world: you close off your feelings; no one has any business with them!

Bottled-up aggression: anger toward someone who has hurt you a lot; you can't forget it, and now you say, "Don't touch me! I'm not yours!" But in fact this is only a manifestation of your powerlessness to feel safe and strong in your deepest Self.

Being angrily closed up: you want to be alone with your feelings. But emotions such as sadness, bitterness, and vengeance eat at you. Inwardly, you chatter and rattle, leering at, and criticizing, others; but in the meantime you feel as if you are on a slanting, slippery plain. In this situation, you can't hold on any longer. Despite everything, you try to remain standing, but you grab hold of "certainties" outside yourself: Image, Church, society, nihilistic indoctrinations, etc. Why are you so angry and reproachful with yourself? Why so cold in that Ivory Tower? Why do you close yourself off from warmth and love? Do you think you are not at all worthy of them? Are you so condemnatory regarding your own mistakes and shortcomings? Perhaps because you could never live up to the expectations of your parents? Outer toughness, inner unsureness?

Be reborn in yourself: you don't have to live up to anyone else's expectations. You don't have to be Image-tough: you are allowed to naturally be who you are. Descend from that tower and be a human being among human beings. Offer yourself the warmth you need so much.

Put the past behind you: you have unconsciously attracted those life circumstances, those mentors and friends via whom you might be able to evolve strongly. Don't pay attention to reactions from your surroundings, but be faithful to your unique disposition. Don't feel threatened: know yourself to be safe in your everlasting self, and allow your feelings to flow freely.

Don't try to keep standing "on high," in accord with the artificial norms of others, but listen to your inner wishes.

Accept your nature with its faults and gifts. First and foremost, be happy with yourself; dare to express yourself spontaneously; go on in a self-aware manner; live in the Now, so that you can discover joy. Transform aggressive powers into true, resolute Action, and acknowledge your Worth!

Fissured tongue
deep central furrow and side furrows, possibly causing inflammation and pain

You don't live like a unified human being, straightforward. Inwardly, you feel sad, dark and lonely. You bottle up aggressive powers, anger, criticism — as if you would like to stab with a dagger! Outwardly, you try to be "holy" or "good." You do that which is expected of you; you flexibly go along with others; you assume that attitude which you must in order to be accepted by the outer world. But, inwardly, a devilish emotional battle rages. You are sick of not *really* being yourself. You are angry because you don't acknowledge the Authority in yourself, because your life is built on false or external values. You *can't* say anything because you don't dare to speak your words from out of your true nature. You don't even know who

you really are. You don't agree with something, and yet you remain silent.

In this duality, you punish yourself; do you feel guilty? Do you think you have to punish yourself? Do you think you are not allowed to be who you really *are*? An inner rift, which painfully splits your tongue and your life in two.

In this way, your deeper powers, your creative energies — which grow directly from yourself — remain unused. Possibly, you outwardly say in a tough way: "I'll take care of that business!" But inwardly you live withdrawn.

Solve that inner duality, and experience that Powerful unity deep inside yourself. Don't let yourself droop; don't lean on others, nor on outer norms, but acknowledge the Fullness of your Nature. Express your spontaneous energies, trust your deepest Self, dare to live, to speak from out of your Center, your "I." Feel that powerful joy in you when you tune in to your Self. Don't live according to the eye or the expectations of society, of a partner. No longer betray yourself. Via openness, honest spontaneous words and deeds, you will get to know yourself better. Dare to give in to those impulses, to your intuition, under the authority of your Self-aware "I."

Quietly look inside yourself and take note of how you have ignored yourself for too long. Speak for yourself. Get a hold of your life in an autonomous way, and no longer allow yourself to "be lived" by appearances, by a silent mask, or by suppressed emotions. Experience yourself as being unified: go straight ahead, speak forthrightly, live from out of your soul. Establish yourself solidly, independent of the reactions of others. Transform aggression into energetic action, and determine your life-direction without hesitation.

Geographic tongue

Even if you take a map in hand, you still don't know what direction to take. Emotionally, you feel quite powerless; you are filled to the brim with aggressive powers and anger toward others, but you just look, with dark eyes, without opening your mouth. You are on your guard, ready to defend or attack because you don't really feel master over the situation, because you can't get a hold of the scepter. You have heard it all too much; powerless anger. You don't really know where to direct yourself; you have no perspective on yourself: "Who am I?"

You forget to enjoy; you remain too tense; chaotic release of emotions. You don't have both feet on the ground; you ignore the Awareness-powers in yourself. You keep yourself impotently locked up in mistrust, darkness, and anger. You force yourself, as if you totally banish joy, love, earthly pleasures and enjoyments from your life.

Don't make yourself so tense and shut. Emotions and life are there to be enjoyed, not to bedevil you.

Flexibility: toward your own Nature, toward others.

Give yourself freedom; follow your nature, your intuition. Integrate into your life that which is round, plump, joyfully earthly. Taste, try, enjoy, that which is most beautiful: allow yourself to live freely.

In a self-aware way, come to a clear overview, and without forcing things determine your path, in the direction which harmonizes with your true nature!

Don't fight against that spontaneous flow of emotions, of longings, but listen to it; become master over yourself; no longer offer resistance to your natural development.

Come into open communication with those with whom you emotionally feel comfortable. Give expression to that which is going on in your mind, and don't close yourself off.

You will find direction-indicators only in your Self.

Problems with the string of the tongue

Emotionally closed up. You look for a way out. Soulless, lonely. Constricted, not authentic. You don't fully engage yourself in life. You feel vulnerable; you peek at life from behind a screen, as it were. Possibly, you piss on it, being angry with life, itself. You only say that which is strictly necessary; you hold in certain negative feelings. You can't handle it anymore; desperately, you seek; you feel stuck. You are really angry with yourself, although you might blame others for whatever doesn't go well with you: being your SELF, no longer suffocating yourself in a bond, a structure, an outer pattern. You feel powerless to really flow along with life, but you feel unable to express your true feelings.

Closed off, not really present in the here-and-now. Holding back. Anxiety, sadness, worries.

Refusing to live in this way any longer. "Where is joy, nature?"

Manifest yourself, and flexibly bend toward yourself. Feel free, joyful, and surrender spontaneously to your inner feelings. Break out of the restrictions you have placed upon yourself!

Respect your Nature and break with oppressive structures, with self-restricting emotions. Speak, express yourself, work out your emotions, and let go. Dare to be yourself, and no longer be afraid of being hurt. Every human being attracts those situations which enable him to unmask inner convictions regarding himself. For too long you have "stayed away": now, come completely into yourself, participate fully in life, and take the rudder in hand.

Dare to experience Joy without reservation! Liberation of an imprisoned nature.

LOSS OF THE SENSE OF TOUCH

lost sensitivity of skin, mucous membranes, mouth, throat, while remaining conscious

Heavy, paralyzing pressure on your head because of anxiety, unsureness, emotions.

Nervous tension. You feel extremely small; you don't dare to land on your own feet. Afraid of something or someone much bigger than you.

Unconscious fears of being "grasped" and of disappearing into nothingness, of having Pain. Tense resistance against something or someone. You brace yourself, ready to escape totally, to be gone. Sometimes it is the fear of exchanging affection in a love relationship: you might "disappear" in it.

Self-awareness. Dynamically direct and organize everything in your life. Dare to act and live yourself, not from out of automatic life habits that are not really rooted in your personal development, nor from out of sclerotic, rusted, inherited traditions.

Start to "feel" yourself, say what you want to say, and if need be bang on the table; shout yourself awake! Acknowledge the inner Authority in you, which no one else can acknowledge for you: build your existence on this safe, supporting basis. Allow, then, your feelings to come through quietly and to grow ever further.

TOURETTE SYNDROME

motor and verbal tics, involuntary and compulsive utterance of obscenities or abuse

You feel just small and "bad": you protect yourself from yourself; you constantly keep your emotions and spontaneous longings under control. You are convinced that your nature is not to be trusted. You suppress

your true, spontaneous, natural aggression and emotional expressions!

You call up (unconsciously) an environment that accentuates this and which says, "You can't control yourself; you have something bad or devilish inside you," etc.

You feel many unconscious powers, many deeply suppressed emotions, but you flee from them; you keep them under water. You are so afraid of being yourself; you think you are a dragon, as it were, which at any moment might begin breathing fire if you let yourself go. You push yourself away with all Force. You feel clumsy.

This self-suppression gives you troubles: outbursts, unexpected primitive deeds or words — it's all about concealed aggression and suppressed longings, about arriving at self-manifestation. . . . You don't dare; our society, or perhaps your mentors, are themselves stuck in structures that are placed upon them and restrict them. . . .

You don't feel good in your skin; you feel so feeble and inferior. By your negative convictions regarding yourself, you provoke a negative reaction from others. Aggression, mockery, disdain — possibly from your surroundings — are just the result of suppression of your natural being, of your spontaneous impulses to act energetically. You are so afraid of your own primitive, sexual, or physical feelings.

Yes-no, yes-no. Am I allowed? Am I not allowed? Forbidden-not forbidden. You think you are "bad," full of rottenness; you try to defend yourself against it, until the bomb explodes.

Here, we are often dealing with the primitive outlet for the imprisonment that parents impose on themselves. Is mother afraid of sex, of the physical, of the emotions? Do mentors not trust in their own nature and unconscious longings?? Again and again, one needs to look at the child and parents together: a liberation of spontaneous, impulsive energies is necessary — of the parents and the child!

Frustrations, embarrassments, anxieties in the parents — who consider themselves to be partly devilish — lead also to the parents putting their child in a "Protective Structure." It doesn't have to be like this, however, although it often happens that the child offers a "mirror" to its parent(s). Both can then transform.

Don't hinder that natural growth! Dare to go onward without anxieties! There's nothing bad in you! That outlet is very understandable! But you can solve things in another way. Stop condemning yourself, stop restricting yourself and judging yourself to be inferior: live life to the full and express yourself freely in action, in free Play, in emotion, in creativity — don't at all hold yourself back from spontaneously living.

Parents, allow your energies to flow freely, and let your children free; don't "seize"; don't tie yourself or your child down. Let go of all power except one: the power of daring to let yourself go. Don't clothe your life in an old-fashioned uniform; arrive at self-trust, at trust in your nature. Stimulate the child to dare to experience itself "TOTALLY," to accept everything that has inside him, and consider it good — a total integration of instincts and emotions, in parents and child, is necessary: in order to grow in Love and Faith.

One of the most important reasons for your being born here is to make clear to you and your parents that feelings, emotions — that which is natural, physical — necessarily need to be respected in a human being. These are very powerful energy sources which, when acknowledged, will have a calm flow: no longer suppress, but use this rich energy-flow, full of self-confidence, in Action and creativity! It is just your "powerlessness" and/or that of your parent(s), which makes you grasp for "power" and "control," because of which you ultimately become suffocated and constricted. Therefore, acknowledge this power, these forces, in yourself, and don't be afraid of them: handle them in creative and relaxing, thankful, loving Action.

TRAVEL-SICKNESS

Airsickness

Insufficient belief in yourself; you don't have a clear insight into yourself, into your life-course.

You are not going straight for the goal; you avoid the essence of things because, in your life, emotions are too heavy. A feeling of unsureness in yourself; in daily life you are not really "with your feet on the ground." In the airplane, these feelings are magnified. Anxious and unsure, impotent, and hiding yourself in a hole.

Trust in yourself and know that nothing will happen to you without you first having asked for it. If you are convinced that you deserve a beautiful life, then nothing will happen to you. Assuredness, being friendly and sociably open toward others; Self-aware, calmly contented, absolutely trusting in the right choice that you make, and in self-protection. Calmly observe your emotions and master them. Open communication, flexibility, firm trust in your nature; festively giving yourself a red-carpet welcome, in a warm-hearted and happy way. Self-assuredness; solidly standing with your feet "on the ground." Don't float in the air, nor cleave to ethereal, nebulous philosophies.

Carsickness

In daily life you feel oppressed, wedged in an iron structure; you are too cold and too hard with yourself. Warm feelings of love cannot sufficiently flow in your heart; perhaps you feel suffocated under strong, authoritarian domination. Anxiety, lack of self-confidence, anger because of your feelings of "being stuck."

Emotions weigh heavily on you; insufficient stability in your emotional world.

Therefore, allow your own feelings to blossom in warmth; place the sun-center inside you; it's no use to resist an authority, because the true problem is your inability to achieve self-realization. Warm yourself; dare to express yourself fully so that anxieties and coldness disappear. You are becoming carsick because you don't yet really live from out of your self-aware "I," because you don't yet know yourself to be really secure and protected in your deepest Self, because you feel as if someone has seized you by the wrists. You ache for self-liberation.

Seasickness

You feel imprisoned in your emotions, imprisoned in a certain life-situation.

Inner resistance, revolt, anger — because you feel stuck in a certain pattern that you don't like. You are unable to build up your life the way you would like, but you angrily point a finger at others instead of your bringing about changes in your life, yourself. You bottle up your emotions, but inwardly you make plans, sometimes vengeful ones: "Just wait!" You inwardly criticize and blame others, but you remain as impotent as ever, stuck with your piled-up feelings. You don't get a grip on your life. You offer resistance. You don't participate anymore, but in fact it's your dependence, your own person, your impotence, your mortal fears, and the situation in which you feel stuck, that make you puke. You have no faith in your own nature. You don't go along smoothly on the waves of life; you resist. You look for a way out in your life, but you don't find one because you don't place the cause of your problems in yourself. Self-destruction: you underestimate yourself; you don't develop your creative energies in a positive way. Unstable emotional life, insufficient self-awareness.

Make friends with yourself; don't feel threatened; handle those strong powers in you with mastery. Allow your possibilities to blossom;
don't lock yourself up; speak about your feelings. You are not a bird in a cage; take your freedom in your own hands. Autonomy!

Trust in your deepest Self; arrive at true self-realization.

Don't allow yourself to "be lived," but concentrate yourself more strongly in yourself; be content with yourself; adjust flexibly and struggle no longer.

TUBERCULOSIS

In general

An inner battle for one's own psychic survival, which results in a hard mask. You anxiously flee from painful memories of the past, from being "stuck" under someone's authority. You have already swallowed too much sadness and emotion; you have no tears left. You expected protection and love from others instead of placing this in yourself, and as a result you possibly feel small, cold, abandoned. You remain quietly underwater; you don't dare to actually appear; you might, nevertheless, explode because of the repressed urge to build up. Something or someone — an authority, an inner, self-restricting system — oppresses you.

You would like to cast off the pressure; you have been hiding for too long. Your feelings now scream for a breakthrough, to be hidden no longer. You are like a dominant Lion (possibly reflected in, and in the footprints of, your mentors), who suppresses the little child and its spontaneous, vulnerable, emotional world so that every feeling is being nipped in the bud.

You can no longer show your real feelings. You can't feel any love for yourself.

You have held on to so many emotions from the past — a suffocating burden.

Possibly, you are embittered, resentful, irreconcilable, vindictive, coldly aggressive.

Tuberculosis Now asks that you create space for yourself. That your lungs soften under the love and attention which you offer yourself. Take off that hard girdle; come to Insight and understanding so that aggression, rancor, and resistance to gentleness disappear.

Know yourself to be protected in yourself; feel safe on the solid Basis of your deepest Self. Free yourself from this self-oppression; know that with hard, unconciliatory thoughts you only destroy yourself. Know that you have attracted every situation in your life, as a result of hard, self-destructive convictions about yourself. Then don't blame others, but in gentleness find yourself. The circumstances at your birth are already the result of your unconscious expectations from life. Therefore, now allow yourself to thaw out, in love toward yourself. Dare to feel, to LIVE, with heart and soul. No longer look back, but build a new existence according to new Insights.

No longer suffocate yourself with icy thoughts, but discover the quiet peace inside you when you listen to your divine, everlasting Self.

Bone tuberculosis
(See also Tuberculosis, in general)

You are clamped in a structure that is too tight: lack of space in which to move. Your heart has too little opportunity to radiate in gentleness and warmth: you are too severe and too cold to yourself and others. In fact, you are full of anxieties and you fear that at any moment the earth, the safe secure ground, will sink away under your feet; therefore, you unconsciously take harsh measures for self-protection. Because you don't find your own structural security, you build strict, Saturnian, limiting rules and constructs that are *too* severe for yourself: a prison. Outer solidity, inner hollowness, since your body is not being properly fed by the powerful stream of energy emanating from the love-fire, but is being consumed by

unconscious anxieties and feelings of not being safe. Constant fear of collapsing, or being afraid that one or another supreme Authority might punish you or pull you down.

Feel safe in yourself: swaddle the cold child in warm cloth and cover it with loving attention. The baby in you aches for this! Don't transmit to yourself and others the same cool severity that you perhaps encountered early in your upbringing. Pull free from the hooks of self-limitation, which for so long have had you in their grip. Turn your mind to that which is beautiful, and allow all energies to openly radiate; direct yourself to all possible paths that are open to you. Dare to enjoy, without fear. Nothing is safer than your own strong, inner Self, which wants to lead you to a joyFUL(L) life, if only you trust in it instead of denying it and placing the Authority above you (See Anxiety). Action, busyness — are very wholesome for you!

Intestinal tuberculosis
(See first Tuberculosis, in general)

You experience yourself to be like a child at the mercy of the authority of others. You are afraid; you feel cold and small; you fear getting hurt even more or getting a kick. You want to protect yourself against this and you close off your feelings. Unsure, you cling to old values, to something or someone, but at the same time you immobilize yourself by doing this.

A revolt against this self-limitation, against the emotional burdens you have been carrying for too long. You won't, and can't, go on like this any more: you don't dare to step over the barrier of dependence on others, because you doubt your own abilities too much. In resistance, you stubbornly stay where you are; you hinder every evolution. You hesitate: "Free myself, or stay bound to these limiting, obstructing structures in my life?"

The unsureness regarding your own Power

and Worth leads to you being too much in "the spirit," in thoughts or dreams, to living insufficiently as a physical presence here on earth.

Be present in yourself with your full Consciousness! Concentrate on the sensory, the here-and-now, the earthly. Dare to stand solidly on the ground and allow your feelings to flow freely; free yourself from the iron mask; come down from your ivory tower and know yourself to be safe in yourself. Love and gentleness toward yourself, strong faith in your warm human side. Others can't come close to you in warm human contact if you are not first present in yourself. Let go of all resistance and stubbornness: accept your emotional life, work out the past and, in self-assuredness, become aware of your worth!

Tuberculosis of the lung
(See also Lungs)

Too stiff, too rigid, standing in the distance. You don't integrate the "female softness" in yourself; you only allow hardness, distance, dominance. You put up a "prohibition sign" for yourself: your total Self is not allowed to come through. Hidden behind this tough shield, however, you are scorched by that which you keep hidden: feelings of pain, deep sadness, anger. Possibly reinforced by hard experiences in youth, this second Self has become an automaton, a self-protecting mask; you hardly know any more that you are also this soft, sensitive human being. You hold on to an old pattern, afraid to be seen through, afraid of being unable to live otherwise. Your distant — or hard — posture is often an unconscious reflection of how you feel you have been approached by certain people; however, you should know that these experiences were already a consequence of your inner condition. The cause needs to be resolved IN yourself. Don't reproach others. Your attitude sometimes comes across as cold revenge, but it is instead a buffer for self-protection. Your feel-

ings — no one will get a grip on them. And you, yourself, are afraid to acknowledge them, let alone express them.

Tenderness, openness: surrender to yourself! An harmonious balance between right and left (see also Body Halves); a balance between strong self-awareness and tender indulgence, between clear rationality and pure intuition. This leads to higher consciousness and clearer insight in yourself. Abolish the hard, chilly distance that separates you from yourself, and you will be able to draw so much better from the healing source that you, yourself, are. Stronger than any medicine whatsoever: definitive healing of your total personality. The force of the Now is stronger than the influence of the Past — unless you disregard the Now. The power of Love, softening.

TUMORS, IN GENERAL

A feeling of being unsafe inside: you will cling to others, will strongly pull your child or partner toward you in a sometimes suffocating tie.

You "grab" for a hold outside of you; you look around for protection, would hide behind others, because you are anxious, because you don't dare trust in your own deepest Self.

As a result of this attachment — this powerlessness to call upon your own forces as an autonomous being — emotions such as jealousy, rancor, hatred, disappointment develop.

A form of self-suppression: afraid of allowing your energies, your creativity, to blossom! You don't really live for yourself; you carry so many beautiful fruits inside, but they remain unexploited. Holding everything and everyone inside you, instead of letting life flow through you freely, in full surrender to yourself.

Find yourself, and make contact with your deepest, powerful, Self; let go of suppressing ties and allow your energies to be free; allow possibilities and talents to unfold themselves under the supervision of a self-assured, conscious "I."

Carry yourself; offer a helping hand to others, but don't devour anyone. Keep your claws to yourself; don't mind other people's business; don't dominate; offer love and attention, generous energies that give. Don't grab, don't hold on to anything or anyone! Fight yours way to freedom by falling back on your fundamental force; get a solid hold on yourself!

Sorrow is the lie of life. Be content with yourself; have faith, and consciously create your life. There's no "fate" or a "devil." (See Part I)

Clear insight is necessary for you to make anxieties disappear.

TUMOR, BENIGN

An emotional cry for help: for too long you have been piling up emotions. You suppress the world of your feelings. You have the feeling of being stuck, of not getting a step further. You dominate yourself (possibly also others) in an authoritarian way. You feel that others also grab you by the neck, just as you emotionally strangle yourself! You have built a thick layer of protection around yourself, sometimes as hard as a rock, so that you become estranged from your feelings. You grasp for others, sometimes in a powerful, dominating way. Instead of placing the inner Authority inside you, you become a busybody or even a bully. You claw, and don't let go. You adhere to others via suction cups, as it were. You fill yourself with others instead of radiating *yourself* in your center.

You can be a slave, a victim, or "director," but in all these cases you wish to put yourself in a safe position, because you don't really believe in your own worth.

You are too hard, too condemnatory, too demanding with yourself, with others.

Why don't you leave any room for true joy, relaxation, pleasure, without always worrying? You won't change others; you can't change the world by piling up negativity and sadness *yourself*. On the contrary — you just pile higher the dumping ground of misery and sorrow in the world. When are you going to listen, in love, to yourself? Are you afraid of yourself? Do you fear you are bad? Don't you very well know who you are? Does your outer ego dominate your feelings so that you smother yourself? Do you conceal your true nature? Have you been treated by others in an authoritarian way, just as you now treat yourself? Then this is but a "result" of your convictions regarding yourself and life.

Let go of everything and everyone. Look only into yourself: your surroundings change in a positive way if first you change yourself. Don't blame, but understand.

Do not grasp the suffering of the world, of others, because in fact it's all about your impotence: you have not succeeded to feel Joy and thankfulness for life itself. If you succeed at doing so, then hardened tissue will soften, then sadness will disappear. Let go of the past; let go of emotions. Express your sadness; don't harden yourself.

Come, in love, to yourself; no longer concentrate on the negative, but build up your life in a self-assured way. Place the kingship in yourself and send your golden, heartwarming rays to others! Don't sorrow over sadness, because then you only intensify this pool of misery. Be happy about your existence as an autonomous being; offer your feelings, but no longer grasp.

Feel at home in yourself. Don't place yourself in a hard way above your feelings, nor above your body, but experience yourself as a unity. Turn inward; don't expect anything from others, but give; allow the balloon, your feelings, to escape. Allow feelings to flow freely, without blockage.

Be happy about yourself, about life the way it is NOW, and go onward. Try not to hold on to things or people, but radiate those inner powers outwardly. Open yourself up. Control no longer.

No power over anything or anyone, only over yourself. Trust, joy! Break down the hard armor. Listen to that gentle nature of yours and surrender to it in all openness and thankfulness for your being permitted to Be on Earth!

TUMOR, MALIGNANT
(See also Cancer, in general)

Anxiety. Forever mistrustful, on guard against "negativity," even in your imagination.

A negative attitude toward your Self, toward others. You strongly believe in the bad, the evil, the devilish. You don't at all experience that safe, solid Basis of your deepest Self. You are not really Master over yourself; you allow yourself to be pulled along by the suction of others, circumstances, life, emotions, negative thoughts — and you think you don't at all have a grip on yourself! On the contrary, you are afraid of the depths in yourself. You always expect the worst; you expect accidents, misery, illness, death. You don't at realize that it is you who creates your life; that negative happenings in your existence are the result of your inner negative expectations! You don't put trust in yourself; you think: "Ah, who am I? A small, powerless being who has no say over his life."

On top of it all, you feel hurt because by having such a negative outlook on life — also in relation to others — you will certainly have attracted a lot of negative experiences! This can degenerate into aggression, fury, hard vengefulness, embittered sadness. You look at the past through black glasses; you are not aware that you, yourself, are the cause of every happening in the past. It's hard for you to forget; you accumulate dark memories. You can also be angry with yourself because you don't at all acknowledge your beautiful divine core. You would murder the gentle, vulnerable, childlike heart inside yourself. Self-punishment; feelings of guilt, self-destruction, because you don't really believe in your inner goodness. Perhaps, therefore, you do a lot for others — in order to fill up your emptiness, in order to feel that your existence does have a sense, somehow. But you dare not, or cannot, enjoy life in thankful joy about yourself. In this way, you grow toward death. You feel "seized" or painfully "punched in the stomach"; you have the feeling that you always have to get hurt. You think that something threatening, something much bigger than mankind, can drag you into the abyss without your being able to do anything about it. Deep anxieties and holding on to a dark past allow the tumor to swell and darken.

Self-contemplation and transformation. Resolutely, choose life or death.

Consider yourself beautiful, and appreciate who you are. Feel good in yourself. Love.

Warmth, security, joy, peace, gentleness in your Self. You alone are lord and master over your existence. Nothing just happens by coincidence: cancer disappears gradually from your body if you dare to look at the naked truth regarding yourself — unmasking those negative convictions and expectations regarding yourself and your life. Only you create your existence: if you are convinced that an illness will destroy you, then it is possible. If you decide that your Conscious "I" is able to bend all negative expectation patterns toward the positive; if you stop considering yourself a poor victim who has no say over its existence; if you see clearly how happenings from the past have been called up by YOU, and that you NOW can choose a new life and create positive circumstances; if you become conscious of the fact that nothing and no one but you, yourself, can lead your existence or destroy it — then you are now taking the reins in hand in a Self-aware way, and you will change course. Know that your body immediately listens to those messages you send out. Be convinced that you heal yourself, that you are master over your body. Joy and love toward yourself. Know that your body only reacts to your convictions: in this manner you can recover, in a relaxed way.

Trust now in your deepest, Living, immortal Self. It's not without reason that you have attracted this illness; via this confrontation you can become aware of the fact that life is not ruled by coincidence, but that your life is being directed by your "I." That every human being carries inside himself the Power over himself. That every human being has the possibility of leading his existence toward joy, happiness, and harmony.

Don't wait for a God; don't wait for a cure; but begin now to live differently. The grateful flow of joy, being aware of your inner goodness, stirs up healing electromagnetic powers in you — which will cure you! Time doesn't play a role here, but being aware of this process does: your Consciousness leads, your body follows.

*You may/can make use of classical or alternative remedies (see Part I), but let it be accompanied by a solution of the True psycho-emotional causes, so that you can arrive at permanent, fundamental, **true** healing!*

TYPHOID

Extreme sadness, loneliness, desolation. You feel powerless, in the grip of "life," of sorrow. You don't see a way out anymore; you feel desperate, in a prison. You bear enormous emotional burdens; you no longer really believe in a solution. You don't believe in the power of every human being. You do believe in the cold hand of Destiny, of death, about which a human being has no say, so you think.

You live in a "group-awareness," and in this way you allow yourself to be guided and swallowed up by group-happenings.

The individual becoming aware. The discovery of the power and possibility in every human being to create his life himself. Autonomy; coming very close to yourself; rising above the group; your awareness becoming extremely concentrated in your body. World solutions have to be looked upon in the light of human consciousness-raising in a very broad area. Sad circumstances are the result of a human being's unconscious, negative convictions. Rise above this; come to clear Insight, and acknowledge the divine creative power in every human being. Natural immunity. Read Part I.

(See the chapters about Infection, contamination.)

U

ULCERS, FESTERS, IN GENERAL

You feel stuck, like a martyr bound on a chain; this makes you so furious, but you keep this anger in. On the one hand you beg, "Please"; on the other hand you are unrelentingly hard, hard as a stone, and aggressive.

Although to the eye of the outer world you perhaps sit on a throne and allow your ring to be kissed, you feel more like a foolish jester, without a scepter, like a bird in a cage. You feel in a forced situation; you want to free yourself, but you can't bring about actual changes. You would nevertheless like to shift the helm in another direction, but something holds you back. You search and stare into the distance; in delirium you'd go beyond your borders. You would like to feel almighty and free, but you remain blocked. You get excited; your head glows with angry thoughts and aggressive plans; you fly, as it were, far above your head; you no longer stand on the earth. A whole load of electricity piles up because of bottled-up energies and an aggressive working of the brain; on top of it, emotions are not being expressed; water, fire, electricity, but *much* too little Earth. Similar energies in your proximity will react to this field, so that you may also be confronted with the aggressive discharges of someone else. You keep yourself in check because you are actually anxious. You waste yourself away like this. Fear of the Eye that sees you, no matter whose — this really lies inside yourself. In this way beautiful energies are being dissipated into negativity, into self-inhibition. Electrical impulses strive for a breakthrough and liberation of your "I"!

Become yourself, and stop your self-destruction. Stand firmly with both feet on the earth and make yourself open and free. Emotions are not able to overpower you if you don't want it to happen. Steadily build your happiness here and now; bring about changes in your life if necessary. In a self-aware way, make an end to your immobility; transform creative energies into action. Experience your feelings and your body; enjoy the sensorial things and put things in perspective.

Come to an understanding; it doesn't make sense to get angry any longer. Acknowledge the kingship IN yourself; give yourself all the space you need. Allow those primal forces of yours to blossom, and transform them into fruits. No longer restrain yourself, but don't act destructively: build up your life, tread new paths. Self-liberation: the freedom lies IN yourself.

FEELING UNWELL, SICK
(possibly with nausea)

Rejection of an experience or of new insights. Critical refusal, sometimes a proud resistance, but with inner anxieties.

Resistance to that which in the outer

world is a reflection of that aspect in yourself that you don't wish to see: critical allergy to a, nevertheless, *real* aspect of yourself.

You feel sick because of a false role you play: you put up — be it unconsciously — a proud and strong front, but you bury your head in the sand! What is hidden under this cover? What do you turn yourself off to in the outer world? Or what aspect in yourself do you push away? *You are not* completely yourself. Is this because of fear? You turn yourself off to that which is new — that which you have a hard time integrating into yourself — because inwardly you don't accept this aspect of yourself. For instance, resistance against the fetus in your belly because you turn yourself off from the child in yourself, because you become nauseated from your attachment or powerlessness.

You cling to the stiff, lifeless part of yourself, rather than to your living "I." You cling to that which is in the past, perhaps to norms or habits of your father. Do you refuse to evolve?

You refuse to truly exist from out of your own deepest Core! Resistance to a new direction which will bring you closer to yourself. Are you so fearful? Emotionally overburdened: you no longer have a grip on yourself; you are now at the mercy of your feelings. Insufficient self-confidence because of which you will easily be influenced emotionally by others.

Accept life the way it NOW presents itself and solidly stand with both feet on the earth. Get rid of those superfluous feelings: arrive at a clear perspective with your thinking and get a grip on yourself. Allow your feelings to flow freely; honestly come to yourself. If you live in harmony with yourself, you will be less easily influenced emotionally by the outer world. If you don't reject any aspect of yourself and don't live upon obsolete values from the past, but are faithful in a self-aware way to your true nature, then you are open in a healthy way to all new impressions without this causing an emotional resistance or Un-

wellness. What annoys you most is that you insufficiently consider yourself a strong, worthy, autonomous person.

Become YOURSELF! If you build your life on your deepest living Core, not on outer image, nor on an authority outside of you, then you will experience life as being safe and without anxieties. Open yourself up to this transformation! Don't reject the true joy and the sensorial physical pleasures in your life. Be open to every authentic part of yourself.

URINARY SYSTEM
water in our body

Psychological correspondence

Water is life. Life is being propelled by emotions, by the longing "to be" on Earth.

The spacious, unlimited feeling of Being — just like water can flow and freely stream without hindrance. But emotions, just like our water tracts, undulate *in the body* and are not being experienced separate from an Individual uniqueness.

Kidneys, bladder, and urinary tracts will show us how we deal with our emotions and with the energies, the forces, which these emotions in fact are.

Turned in love toward ourselves, we will engage our emotional forces in communication with others and also in active self-realization. We take care of ourselves and spoil ourselves. Emotions are constantly moving: we allow ourselves to evolve.

We flexibly digest our sadness, our anger, our disappointments. We know we are protected in ourselves. When we feel good and calm, we radiate powerful, beautiful energies in all possible directions. A feeling of peace and satisfaction.

After being filtered, being digested, residues are transported via the sewer system.

For this a balance is necessary between the "male" and "female" aspects of every human being (see also the subject Left and right body halves). It is true that here we are dealing with an artificial classification: - and + as it were. Still, there is a need for actual harmony between the thinking, giving structure, planning self-aware "I," on the one hand, and the emotional, intuitive aspect in a human being on the other hand. In optimal cooperation, the division between the two falls away. The organs of the water tracts suffer under an over-accentuation of one of both aspects.

Emotional overburdening hurts.

Allow your emotions to flow and grow freely under your Conscious mastery; give them guidance, but don't block them or suppress them with your "thinking." No accumulation of aggression, but a steady experiencing and expression of feelings, of active energies. No emotional sacrifices for others, no reproach or anger toward others; don't go beyond your limits; take care of yourself, of your fellow men, within earthly reality. Don't allow your water to boil or go up in steam, by losing yourself in anger or by turning away from that which is earthly. You don't allow yourself to be "restricted," you build your life concretely and lovingly on a peaceful, harmonious basis. You don't hurt yourself, nor others.

You don't "freeze," you don't "harden," you don't "dry up"; you want to *live* in a warm, gentle way, with Venus in your shield.

You don't have to defend yourself, nor attack. You are not cruel, nor do you ill-treat or neglect yourself or those for whom you are responsible. You don't constantly aim the spotlights at your partner in a critical way. Because you yourself feel so full and *alive,* you don't expect anything from others and don't get stuck in emotional experiences from the past.

You don't flee into another dimension; you stand firmly with both feet on the ground. You know you are supported; you purge yourself of useless burdens; you have a

clear overview, structure and order in your life. You experience your kingship in yourself on earth.

Calcification of the urinary tract

Red, aggressive sadness. You are stuck. You would like to go on, but the past has a hold on you. Instead of evolving onward, straightforward, and open, honest with yourself, you would slip away. You are cut off from the Light source in yourself; you are under the influence of an Authority outside yourself. Influences from the past, indoctrinations, are being held on to. Because of this you don't at all feel free emotionally! You are not really faithful to your feelings, to your true nature. You hide your soul. Aggression, by which you hurt yourself. You tightly hold yourself back and keep yourself closed; you extinguish the divine light in yourself, because you idolize false gods. Do you feel guilty and bad when you surrender to your nature and your feelings, because the gods (parents, philosophical systems, etc.) told you that this is not allowed? Or do you think you have to "harden" yourself, making your nature subordinate to a structure, to hard, rational rules? You restrict your nature to a narrow passage. The deepest reason for all of this is: anxiety. You mistrust the ground on which you stand. You don't really trust in the deepest original creative powers in yourself. You think you have to protect yourself. In anxiety and sadness you might cling to a religion, a person. In this way you immobilize yourself. You rob yourself of freedom.

It seems as if, on an emotional level, you are not able to let go of the old; your nature sticks to a dead bottom, but you don't dare detach yourself from it because you refuse to acknowledge the Authority in yourself. You are afraid of yourself, of your nature, of your emotions, of your body. You take a sharp, defensive attitude toward others, because you feel so insecure in yourself.

Be honest with yourself and then go on! You can no longer escape your inner Authority. Choose the path which leads to freedom. Feel solid, with both feet on the ground, secure and sheltered in your deepest divine Self. Surrender to earthly enjoyment, to sensorial joy, to a free emotional flow. No longer block your paths so, and break with false gods. The truth is beautiful and clear: it lies inside yourself; no longer look for a hold outside yourself. Dare to feel good in your body, in peace and joy. No longer fight against your nature. Gentleness and love toward yourself, freedom and enlargement of your emotional life; activate the intense atomic powers in yourself in order to ultimately, in a gentle way, break down the calcification from within and drain it away. No longer put a damper on your nature with rationalizations and prejudices.

Urinary tract infection, in general

You stir with a spoon in your mud and in that of others; you are stuck in the bottom layers of yourself, where unconscious forces run rampant in a non-transformed way. You feel hurt, stuck, full of sadness and anxieties: this ultimately leads to powerless revolt and anger. Aggressive emotions laboriously seek their way outward. You feel in the grip of something or someone, of an unbearable situation; this is because you refuse to come to true insight and understanding with your Conscious Self, from above, which would make evolution possible and make you realize that it's only you who has attracted the circumstances and people in your surroundings in order to learn from it all, and so bring about changes in yourself, and not direct criticism at others. Anger is being bottled up inside. Powerlessness.

Solve, inside yourself, the cause of your frustrated aggression: come to yourself in gentleness and peace. If you become Aware

of your real powers and your worth, if you no longer take such a hard and doubtful position regarding yourself, if you find the Security and shelter in yourself, if you don't reject yourself, but allow the female, loving factor to enter more into your life — then a balance will come about in which you will feel calm and good, protected, and without anxieties. Little by little you can create your life yourself; you don't need to remain "stuck." Make an end to negative, destructive (self-) criticism and go on steadily. Push through those deepest inner powers, your emotional energies, your creative possibilities. Don't allow yourself to "be lived" so that dependency blocks your emotional flow from within. Build up your construction; don't waste your life energies in immobilization or anger, in hesitation and self-doubt.*

Calmly, balanced propelling onward your inner powers, in gentleness and peace, in love toward yourself.

Express yourself: don't lock yourself up inside yourself. Don't live just in your head: enjoy with your soul and body.

Pollakiuria
very frequent urge to urinate

A strong presence of the "female" aspect, of the emotional aspect in yourself, but you don't really dare to openly manifest your Self yet; you experience your emotions in a rather hidden way. You have not yet found the real joy of your being; a kind of sadness still has a hold on you as long as you don't really acknowledge your "male" I-power. You still look for confirmation in the outer world; you try to "secure" yourself because you don't trust enough in your own powerful Basis and still make yourself too dependent on others, because you don't really feel safe in yourself: emotional contacts, communications from the heart, outward expression of your inner feelings, etc. — all these are being hidden behind a coat of paint. You don't dare to be yourself in an open and direct way; you will hide your hypersensitivity.

Again and again you take a step backward with regard to others; you look at yourself from below; you underestimate your worth; because of this self-degradation you will possibly cling too much to money and materialism, to sex, power, and image. So many feelings are being experienced and held on to behind the "protecting mask." That which you clasp and suppress "above" will again and again find its "outlet" "below." Anxiety about spontaneously being yourself, emotionally and creatively, can call up situations in which you begin to feel like the "garbage pail" or "servant" of others, but here we are dealing with self-cremation, with denial of your Mars-Powers, denial of Conscious mastery over yourself. You don't really feel protected in yourself, and therefore you constantly place a "screen" in front of yourself.

You don't enough use those fertile, female, creative, sensitive powers in yourself; you just let yourself slide down a slope, without actually stepping forward, *yourself.* You allow yourself to be led by unauthentic values because you don't really believe in your Self-aware "I."

Build on that fundamentally safe Basis of your Self; know yourself to be protected in yourself and stop giving yourself sorrow! Allow those inner emotional forces to flow through under the supervision of your Conscious "I," and tear away the rigid mask from your being. GIVE warmth and love to yourself and others instead of making yourself dependent on that which comes to you. Make an end to Image; manifest yourself the way you feel inside; dare to show to the outer world your true Nature, without camouflage or inhibition. If you put trust in those structures of yours which are strong as iron, then you will no longer be afraid to express your feelings in a relaxed way; then you will no longer tensely have to stand firm against the outer world. If you place the Power over yourself inside you instead of in others, then you no longer will feel in the "grip" of emotions, of desires, of others; then you will

calmly and openly dare to be who you are. Allow those spontaneous feelings to flow; don't hold yourself back; now take up your full living space, no longer anxiously having to hold anything back or in: self-liberation.

Resolute Mastery in yourself, and the glorious feeling of being allowed simply to be yourself.

Urine retention
failure to eliminate urine from the body

Hurt and cold, you close the iron gates: no one can enter here anymore! In this self-built prison you think you can barricade yourself safely and make yourself invulnerable, which is of course a delusive idea. But here it's about a negative reaction, taking distance from others, because inwardly you feel so unsure, with painful memories from the past. In a critical way you condemn this or that, determining guidelines for someone else; possibly your attitude is rather uppish or arrogant: or you force others — seizing power over them — to do what "must be done" according to your demands. In the same way you can be suffering under the Authority of someone who treats you this way, with a bottling-up of aggressive emotions as a result.

Your so-called protective attitude (shielding yourself) toward others is the result of deep anxieties; in the past, possibly even as a baby, you had very painful experiences in which you felt defenseless, in the "grip" of someone else, your mother or a mentor. Now you keep yourself, your feelings, your Nature, in an iron grip: you are hard and cold toward yourself. Your head, your thoughts, are being overexposed; your gentle heart is almost being crushed. Hurtful experiences from the past are haunting you. You fight for psychological survival, as it were, because you don't trust your Self enough.

Mortal fears. The emotions, the aggression, the pain and the thoughts that you bottle up smother you. Also, in the relationship with a partner you will on the one hand cling too strongly, with sucking cups, as it were — and on the other hand you feel unfree, in the grip. But you are too unsure and too afraid to stand on your own feet and be yourself in all openness.

Become master over unconscious emotions, over the past; in the light of the Now, in the awareness of your worth and your sureness, the past can no longer hurt you now.

Let go and free yourself from this prison. Become your own master; feel safe in your Self. Nothing or no one can hurt you as long as you acknowledge the Authority in yourself.

The past was the result of an "unconscious" life; now build your life in a self-aware way. Allow consciousness energies to escape freely; radiate like a sun that is aware it is in the center of its existence. Don't restrict your life to keeping things in, bottling up, to negativity: discover that which is most beautiful in yourself and allow yourself to truly live. First acknowledge yourself in love, come very close to yourself, to your heart, to your feelings and your body, to your longings and your gentleness: in this harmony with yourself, in Self-assuredness, in trust, you will build up relationships with others in a relaxed way, and this won't make you tumble down from your basis.

Be faithful to your nature; allow emotions to roll; don't mind others: dare to manifest yourself completely outward the way you feel inside. No more anxieties: safe shelter inside yourself. Energies spread out; your head is being relieved of a pressure that was too heavy. Space is coming available for new energies.

Stenosis, narrowing of the urinary tract

You force yourself and others; you no longer give yourself and your feelings any room.

You smother the child inside you. In-wardly you get so angry: like a devil in a font of holy water, because it doesn't get you anywhere; you only cut your own skin.

Emotionally you are so sick of it! You close yourself off from your partner, from your fellow men: "I will no longer go along!" You enclose yourself in anger. Hard, closed off, furious, indignant. You now push everything and everyone away from you, while you have clawed and grabbed on to things for so long, but were unable to change anything or anyone outside yourself. Now it's been enough! "I no longer want to accept things this way." You want to break out aggressively, but instead of actually making your liberation happen, you lock yourself up in yourself, with your feelings. You don't express yourself anymore, you are too angry. You suffocate yourself. Possibly you have tried for a long time to change your partner or your children and you didn't succeed. Now you give up the battle. Possibly you have allowed people to play you for a fool for too long, and you blame this on your partner; now you close yourself off from him/her: "You won't do this to me anymore!" The cause of all this doesn't lie in someone else, but in the battle you have with yourself. An inner collision. You are entangled in your feelings. It is you who refuses to change, to transform, who sooner expects something from others instead of evolving yourself. You don't allow yourself to completely be *yourself!* Your reason and your feelings are fighting with each other. You hinder yourself from being faithful to your own nature in a natural way, no longer minding the expectations or criticism of others. You don't offer yourself the love you so need; you are hard and critical with yourself. You don't build your life in an independent and spontaneous way. You still expect the approval of others. Thus your feelings can't flow freely and spontaneously. Actually you are angry with yourself because you feel powerless to be completely faithful to your Self. Do you possibly feel guilty when you dare to enjoy yourself? Are you really so severe with yourself? Pent-up aggression indicates that you are not energetically building your life's specific path. This fact by itself will again attract situations which will give you an even stronger feeling of being "stuck," but these situations (with relations, among others) are already a result of your original powerlessness.

Free yourself of needless burdens and let go: express your feelings, let go of the past, and from now on build up your own future. Be faithful to your nature, to your feelings, and see how your anger is a result of the powerlessness to completely be yourself. No longer fight against your nature, but listen to it; don't mind the expectations of others: don't seize, but give. A balance between your emotional and thinking worlds is necessary. No longer feel like a stranger regarding your own life. Don't resist your inner gentleness; surrender to yourself; no longer be so severe and restrictive toward yourself! Stand up for yourself. Don't bottle up your anger, but speak. Open your heart to yourself first of all so that you don't experience yourself as cold and rejected. If you are in harmony with yourself, then relationships with others will also change.

Don't close up in anger, but speak; work things out and allow all emotions to flow freely, so that no blockage is being formed. Free yourself: just be faithful to your deepest feelings, to your intuition, without fear.

Urethritis
inflammation of the urethra

Sadness; you feel hurt in your most intimate being; powerless anger.

You would like to shoot arrows at others, but you hold in your aggression. You swallow and swallow again; digesting more and more pain. This is because you absolutely want to go on in *this* direction, because you are "holding on" instead of letting go, because you Want it to be just so and no other way. Doing this, you become hard and criti-

cal with yourself, but also with others. You want to arrange and organize, including the life of your partner or your friend, but in this way you inwardly destroy yourself. You cling to certain things; you fixate your thoughts on that which, according to you, "has to be," because you don't trust the smooth life process, nor do you trust your deepest Self, your intuition. Anxieties and feelings of insecurity and powerlessness, ignoring those divine creative powers in yourself, underestimation of yourself — these make it so that you want to secure yourself by trying to get as strong as possible a "grip" on your life and that of others.

You keep rowing in the same direction: the wrong one. You don't go along with the waves of your own nature. You try to hold back something or someone, but ultimately you will have to let go and trust that what happens is best for you and your fellow man. Trust ultimately leads to joy. Conflict, aggression, and wanting to "grab hold of" ultimately lead to tearing pains.

Let everyone go his path, and you yours. Let go. Don't concentrate so sharply and anxiously on a certain path which, according to you, "has to be." Trust, call up the best with your longings, but don't fixate the future. You don't always know what's best for you and your fellow man. Allow your feelings to flow in all possible directions; recognize the soft pastels in your being and experience those supple, softening emotions in your heart. Every bird has its own song; be faithful to your nature and leave others free. If you acknowledge yourself in love and appreciation, if you no longer take an expectant or demanding attitude toward others, then that which is best for you will come to you. Therefore don't feel powerless, but loosen your grip, so that now your life can blossom without limits. In thankfulness, produce, enjoy, those beautiful energies which can flow out from within you; share this joy with others. Know yourself to be safe in that fundamentally solid Basis of yourself. You don't have to defend yourself, nor be angry. Start with building your existence in an autonomous way and listen to the signals which you unconsciously call up, so that you can follow them like road signs. Allow that emotional flow, that aggression, to transform itself into action and self-realization!

THE BLADDER

Psychological correspondence

The bladder grabs you by the collar, as it were; you can't get out from under: it forces you to be here-and-now. It confronts you with the Truth. Being honest with your feelings.

The bladder and its contents, the urine: the solid structure of your Self, which offers your feelings a safe passage.

You know yourself to be secure and protected in your feelings if, in a Self-aware way, you build certainties in yourself; if you construct your Self like a solid house with thick walls; if you take care that there will be a beautiful clear passage of feelings. This taking care of, this watching over, your "safety" happens by Consciously seeing, by a Controlling Eye in you, symbolized by the Bladder.

It indicates that aspect of your psyche which makes sure you listen to the truth regarding your inner emotional world. The bladder will resolutely reprimand you when you violate yourself or the truth regarding your most natural feelings. That which has been delivered by the kidneys arrives here: the last judgment can be beautiful here, but also can confront you if you have not been correct toward yourself.

The Bladder will function beautifully if you take good care of yourself; if with your Conscious eye you don't flee from truth and evolution; if you are good to yourself; if you know yourself to be safe and comfortable in that solid Basic Structure of your Self; if in this certainty you offer an open and free passage to your emotions without holding on to the past any longer.

The bladder is closely related to the sexual organs; the bladder also plays a role in the unfolding of the electromagnetic powers to create, of those primal creative energies; if one doesn't allow those creative powers — with the Conscious "I" — to freely develop themselves, doesn't use them in the constant process of transformation, then they can degenerate into negative emotional experiences such as: manipulation and misuse of power over others, too sharp aggression, sexual exaggeration, frustrated and irritated reactions, over-accentuation of the outer Ego.

The bladder asks, therefore, a perfectly combined action of male and female elements in every human being in order to achieve a harmony between: on the one hand Structure and Self-aware resoluteness, and on the other hand emotional life, intuition, gentleness, contents.

Emotions are being digested; the kidneys filter the water supply. In the last resort we are being confronted — in the bladder — with the way we have dealt with our emotions. Here the final balance is made up.

In order to have a healthy bladder it is necessary that we want to relieve ourselves; rid ourselves of negative emotional experiences; that we allow evolution and new movements in our feelings.

Don't immobilize yourself in an imprisonment that you have looked for yourself, in powerless aggression, but take the rudder with a firm hand. In this way a continuous flow of water-power, of feelings, will liberate new energies in order to create a new safe future. The old constantly makes room for the new; giving room to your emotions means freedom in the here-and-now.

Ailments, in general, causes

Do you refuse to see the truth regarding yourself? Do you hide in the role of a martyr? Do you avoid the responsibility of living *yourself?*

Do you feel stuck, like a prisoner? Do you blame it unjustly on others, and do you urgently want to get out of all this? Do you hold on to emotions from the past? Do you refuse to let go? Frustrated, irritated, bound, aggressive, furious?

Do you not succeed in building your life in a safe way? Do you feel anxious and tense? Do you not really dare to manifest your powerful "I?" Are you being wasted away by inner anger, but aren't succeeding in bringing about actual changes in your life? Are you looking at others with a critical, negative eye, but without any clear view on yourself? In this blindness you possibly play a superficial game of sexuality, of power-manipulation. Is there no room for deeper emotions? Do you live only as an "outer Ego?" Do you feel too limp, too weak, too defenseless, because you insufficiently believe in the power of every human being? Because you close yourself off from your intuition, from your divine Self? Do emotions weigh too heavy, and do you experience yourself as powerless?

Do you hide your feelings for others? Do you bottle them up in an exaggerated way?

Haven't you been emotionally "honest" with yourself? Did you say "yes" while you felt "no"?

Feelings of inability, of anxiety and powerlessness. Do you feel cold and lonely?

Cancer of the bladder
(See also Bladder, in general, and Cancer, in general)

You don't really live "in an earthly way," but you live strongly exaggeratedly "in your head, the rational mind or the spirit." You idolize something or someone outside yourself: a system, a religion, a job, the church. You don't really stand with your feet on the earth; you would sacrifice yourself for that behind which you hide. You only live according to the standards of . . . .; you don't really live for yourself, for the joy of an earthly existence. Your head is bound; your thoughts are only at the service of that "for which" you live.

You think you have to look for and find

"knowledge" outside yourself. Your thoughts therefore fixate themselves on objects outside yourself; in this way you deny that deep wisdom inside yourself. You cherish and worship that which you hold in your hands, but you ignore the inner, earthly, emotional powers in yourself.

Your feelings are being experienced in a too "spiritual, too unearthly way": there's no question of a healthy balance between heaven and earth, between Spiritual Consciousness and body, so that your Consciousness also loses its healthy leadership over your body. You are not in the Center of your life. You "need" another to fill up your "earthly emptiness," but those kinds of relationships distance you even more from yourself. At the end you allow all energies, all life till the last drop, to flow away from you because you don't live enough in the powerful sun-center of yourself! Powerlessness-Power.

You don't really feel safe in yourself; you deny the divine power, the fundamentally reliable basis in yourself. You place a god or a saint above yourself. You sink into nothingness. As a reaction to this, you possibly strongly build up Power and an outer Ego in confrontation with others.

Acknowledge those powerful foundations in yourself. No longer ignore life, the strong muscle power, the warm earthly feelings in Yourself. Don't fight against your divine nature and don't place the god above yourself. You are not a submissive servant or a humble holy person: you are a human being of flesh and blood. A balance between the spiritual and the physical is necessary for good health. Fully participate in life; you may fight for an ideal, but don't look for it outside yourself. In you lies wisdom; don't fixate on things outside yourself, but first and foremost turn inward, close to your feelings. Experience earthly joy. In a self-aware way stand in the center of your existence so that you are not "dependent" on others. In this way you can lovingly nourish yourself and peacefully exchange feelings with others. Don't solely live in your "head," but feel how a powerful flow of energy nourishes every cell of your body. Be a human being among human beings: don't try to "live up to" an ideal picture of yourself, but follow the most ordinary, natural way. Experience your inner powers; don't reach outside yourself, using power.

Cystitis
bladder infection or inflammation

Emotional conflict. Cold and hard.

Stiffened, silent, petrified: aggressive emotions are being quieted down and bound.

You hold things in like a silence before the storm. You don't allow your feelings to flow freely, no matter how heated they are. You cut yourself off from your feelings. You don't really *live* from out of your emotional core, you are immobile in the sense that you don't allow your emotions to move freely, to evolve.

You are like still water. Unconscious, suppressed feelings are looking for a way out. You don't even express your anger, because this feeling immediately confronts you with yourself. You don't allow yourself to express your aggression, because you don't trust the emotional processes of life. You don't dare to surrender to yourself.

You can't really get any further in life because you constantly block your anger, your powerful emotions. You nail yourself to the ground, on the spot; you don't go forward or backward. Suffocating powerlessness, anger. Blockage of the flow of life.... You can work off these frustrations on a partner, in aggressive conflict, in anger, because she/he might hinder you from being happy, but this is a fallacy, of course: it is you who doesn't give yourself a free, happy life.

Allow the dove of peace to fly up; rise up from this self-restricting situation. Get a clear perspective on yourself and express

your feelings. Aggression may and can be expressed, but you, yourself, will be happier if you take away the reason for this aggression so that you can participate — in an open, peace-loving, powerful way — in the ever-moving life and emotional processes; so that you no longer immobilize yourself in a silenced, hard, sterile situation where there is no future. The reason: impotent to dare to experience your deepest Self, your deep emotions. Therefore, free yourself from the straitjacket in which you have strangled yourself. Now freely open yourself to all spontaneous emotional processes in yourself. Enjoy life, enjoy the joy of the senses, in fragrances, colors, and sounds. Don't close yourself off from life! Enjoy your body, the wind on your skin; seek a more intense contact with life. Live freely the way you feel and don't hide inside a house with thick stone walls.

If necessary, break with previous habits, but now be faithful to your nature; no longer ignore those energies inside you; don't place a damper on them, but dare to blossom. Don't live according to the expectations of others, but according to your heart.

Don't be angry with someone else: the cause of "standing still" lies in yourself.

Chase away that coolness in yourself; allow joy and warmth into your existence.

Paralysis of the bladder

You carry heavy emotional and practical burdens, although you don't "have to" do this, but it's as if you want to punish yourself or allow yourself to be punished. You close yourself off; you totally withdraw; you refuse to express your feelings; you hold a rag in front of your mouth, as it were. Repressed anger, powerlessness. Possibly you want to punish others, but in fact it is you who punishes the child inside you; you don't feel able to really break through as an adult. You allow yourself to be dragged along by the waves of life because you don't offer any resistance yourself. After all, you doubt your worth; you *allow* yourself to "be lived." You remain "hidden"; you suffocate yourself. Possibly you are even ashamed of yourself; you consider yourself to be low and ugly. You *let* things happen to you; you don't really build a personal life. You "hold on" to others, because you are not really interested in yourself. Deep anxiety of being crushed; you don't feel safe in yourself. You feel like a bad child.

Accept the "child" in yourself, under the guidance of your Self-aware "I."

Allow energies to come loose; rattle yourself up! Drink in life to the full; stand firmly on your own feet and come into action. No longer block those inner powers, and produce! Allow the piggy bank of emotions and talents to empty itself: be proud of your uniqueness. Bring yourself to realization and know yourself to be protected in that safe haven of your everlasting, deepest Self. Just let those energies turn and turn, forward, without hesitation; don't hold yourself back; manifest yourself; be faithful to your nature, to your feelings. Don't be afraid of your emotions; dare to storm into life with full force. Allow that valuable content of yours to blossom. Stand straight in your shoes and go on! Be nice to the child, the gentle feeling, inside you, and give it the chance to grow up.

Prolapse of the bladder

Aggressive, nervous energies, driven to an extreme.

Emotions and aggressive powers push, as in a race, in order to flow *onward* without limitations. But you hold yourself back. You don't succeed in building a solid Basic Structure for yourself because you are not Self-aware enough, because you really feel just small and inferior, because you don't at all stand firmly in your own shoes. Emotionally you go beyond your borders. You don't succeed in directing yourself, in guiding yourself. You are "being lived" by nerves and emotions. Moreover, you turn your mind to others, in anger, because you don't believe in yourself: because your life is being "filled" by others.

Your aggression is a result of powerlessness to be your Self. You "grab at" your fellow man because you don't get a real grip on yourself Your deepest feelings can't come through, as it were; they are behind locked doors. You just dilly dally at the surface; your deepest possibilities are not being exploited, don't come out. In this frustration you would like to push, bump, storm, hit, fight, let go of bottled-up powers — but you don't do anything; your bladder slips down.

You don't really live from out of the core of your being; possible you stick to outer and material values as a compensation for your self-negation. You fight against others; you strive for an ideal — but it only distracts you from yourself. You blame others, you criticize them — but it's only a result of the refusal to allow your most beautiful, most loving, energies to come through in yourself. You "lower" yourself, possibly in self-hatred; in this way you will also "lower" others.

It seems to you that others slow down your speed in life; but it is you who doesn't direct your life in such a way that you accommodate your wishes.

You can't fit those enormous energies in you into a larger framework of your Self because you deny your higher consciousness energies, because you live in the surface layers of yourself. So, as in an escape from your deepest Self, you'd want to run onward like some quarry, forever frustrated.

Contemplate yourself and acknowledge those inner energies deep inside you. Don't run away from your deepest emotions; don't be afraid to express your feelings. Don't be so condemnatory, critical, aggressive toward others, because the cause of your experiences lies in you. Are you furious? Then beat on a pillow if you wish; express your emotions, but then come to clear Insight: you are sad, feeling frustrated and powerless, be-

cause you don't trust in your deepest Self.

Your underestimation of yourself is the cause of the circumstances you call up in your life. Feel those deeper powers in yourself and no longer turn away from them; no longer push away feelings and productive energies, but now create your life yourself. Radiate warm heart energies outward; no longer push away that which is most beautiful in yourself. Nothing in life just happens by accident; you are the creator of your circumstances. What you experience is a result of your inner convictions regarding yourself. If you are convinced that you are a worthless creature who doesn't deserve any happiness, then you won't call it up in life. If you are convinced that happiness lies in superficial, outer or material values, then you won't find happiness, because happiness is not to be found here.

Take up conscious leadership over yourself in an independent way. Thus, your deepest possibilities and also your emotions will be able to exist freely within the protecting structure of your self-aware being. Love yourself; in this way you will also be able to let your most beautiful energies flow outward instead of poisoning yourself by bottling up negativity. Acknowledge the pureness and beauty in yourself, and in this way you will live in peace with yourself, in peace with others; in this way you will also bring to the surface that which is beautiful in your fellow men. You have the right to have Joy, but you have created too much sorrow in your life. Time for a "lift!" toward Joy and self-esteem.

Stones in the bladder

You want to fight, but it really is a conflict you have with your own gentle Self.

You "are" not truly; you live like a shadow. You don't allow yourself to be born. You hide behind a certain behavior, behind a tough, masculine, sometimes aggressive or greedy, voluptuous posture. You puff yourself up, sword in hand. You'd lose

yourself in this behavior so that you really might be *gone*, because the fundamental cause of your frustrated behavior (or feelings, in case you don't manifest it outwardly) actually is: you think yourself to be nothing, rather ugly and bad. Confused, you look in all possible directions, but you don't really choose a way that comes from out of yourself.

Influence and indoctrination by "a father," or by the past in general, are in the way: you just are not yourself. True productivity and development of talents don't get a chance at all. You possibly consider yourself to be like a donkey that sadly carries its burdens; you don't at all acknowledge the possibilities in yourself. You waste your time away. Aggressive outlets will only distance you even more from yourself. You allow yourself to sink down into an unauthentic life, instead of resolutely taking your own life in hand.

Because you don't live from out of your heart, you are constantly stuck with doubts and confused feelings: "What shall I do? To whom shall I tell it? What direction? . . ." You are at a distance from your feelings; you are too hard on yourself. The gentle, "female" element in you is being suppressed. Don't you love yourself? You seize, you swallow in a greedy way, people and things: you flee from yourself.

Take your place in a balanced way: give room to your gentle, calm feelings on the one hand and to your resolute Self-aware aggressive powers on the other hand. Look at new things, at the future; build a joyful personal life; unload those heavy stones from the past. Find yourself; be good and gentle to yourself and allow yourself to be born! Be productive and know what you want; don't allow your life to be directed by something or someone else. Be a father to yourself, but not at the cost of the gentle motherly aspect in you. Don't look at yourself from a distance, but cherish yourself in warmth. You alone need to determine your life's course. Hardened stones only are broken down and expelled by gentle, loving powers from within.

No longer bottle up your talents and emotions; bring yourself to realization in an active way. Let go of heavy burdening emotions from the past. Your frustrations only exist as long as you refuse to live from out of your true emotional core.

Be yourself, in pride! Let go of everything and everyone and dare to stand on your own feet, without fear. No longer claw on to things or people outside you, but now get a good hold on yourself and give free expression to your creativity, to your emotions. Don't restrain yourself: radiate your content. You are safe. You don't have to protect yourself against yourself.

Weakness of the bladder
not being able to empty
the bladder enough

Anxious pressure; suffocating, claustrophobic anxieties. You feel jammed between rational mind and feelings. You pull the string around your nature too tight because you don't really trust your own feelings. Emotions can't circulate very well because you anxiously and tightly close yourself up: someone has hurt you, and you are afraid of having to take more pain. You shield yourself from others; you won't reveal your innermost feelings! Possibly you give the impression of being a joker or a saint, as if nothing's the matter, but inwardly you can angrily make a fist. You won't show it if someone has hurt you: you stifle it; you keep in your emotions. In this way you live in an unauthentic manner; you yourself are afraid of your deepest feelings, as if they are not allowed to be there, as if you wouldn't be accepted by others if you lived from out of your deepest Nature.

Self-inhibition; you don't dare express your feelings spontaneously. Perhaps you conspicuously puff yourself outwardly up with words and thoughts, but this is not your true "I"; it's only an act, a mask. Inwardly the fury can rage while you are joking and playing. You position yourself as hard and invulnerable, but inwardly you suffer pain.

With your rational mind you might also press your emotions against a guardrail. You are afraid of honest, especially sharp, confrontations with others — also with your own emotions — because you doubt your worth. Inwardly you constantly feel tense, sharply protecting yourself against possible intruders. But you would hold in even the poison of a wasp sting instead of draining it; you would even camouflage it having stung you: a picture of your communication with other people.

Speak! Express yourself in whatever way; don't feel threatened; be honest.

Allow yourself to go along on the waves of life. Follow your nature; listen to your feelings, and relax. You don't have to shield yourself; you are safe in your Self. Don't let anxiety make you play a Role or Act, but always be faithful to your unique nature. Every bird sings a different song; you are good the way you are. Trust in those spontaneous feelings inside you and free yourself of this restrained, unnatural, tense attitude. Be always and everywhere yourself. Someone can hurt you only if you consider yourself to be inwardly vulnerable, if you place too much power in the "spectator."

THE KIDNEYS

Psychological correspondence and Ailments, in general

Conscious and unconscious emotional experiences and feelings are being digested, purified, filtered, and let go of. With this, new energy is being released; with this, we constantly transform. The kidneys symbolize this filtering work in ourselves. Thanks to this emotional growth, thanks to this drainage of poisonous matter (via the urine), we can experience pure joy.

We constantly purify ourselves; we take

in new emotional experiences, and we transform ourselves by digesting these experiences, which moreover can bring to the fore old, undigested emotions in an associative way, through which we come to an ever greater growth of consciousness. Needless emotional burdens are being removed; old garbage is being cleaned up if we are open to it. Freely surrendering to your nature, trusting in your deepest Self, are necessary for this. If, however, you anxiously hold on to old emotions, or if you block the flow of your feelings with your rationality, then you hinder the beneficial functioning of your kidneys.

After all, your consciousness directs the organs, and not the reverse. An harmonious unity between the "female" and the "male" aspects is necessary for this. The gentle, receptive, intuitive sensibility needs to be guided in a self-assured way by the conscious "I," which directs and organizes and freely transmits and handles natural aggressive and emotional energies.

The kidneys represent being reborn in yourself again and again, if you wash away old worries and sadness, if you allow to drop off your shoulders everything that means only needless burdens in the present moment: a wonderful, light feeling of liberation, of joy and happiness.

Kidneys function optimally if you are open to these transforming powers in yourself, which digest energies received and transform them into happy, radiating feelings on the condition that you don't cling to dark, pessimistic thoughts, nor to a burdensome past.

Trust that your Nature always helps you; a primal connection with your nature, with your physical body, with your deepest emotional core.

The kidneys reflect this relationship that you have with yourself: trust or anxiety? Are you hard and aggressive with yourself or gentle and welcoming? Do you loathe your body or do you love yourself completely? Do you allow these emotional energies to flow freely or do you block yourself with criticism, with restricting rationality? In case of self-blockage, your energies will look for an outlet: for instance in aggressiveness.

Optimal relationship between the man and the woman in yourself, harmonious co-operation between both: your feelings know that they are safely being carried in the strong arms of your Self-Aware "I." Reconciliation between left and right (See also the category Left and Right Body Halves.) A beautiful union.

The cause of kidney ailments lies, first of all, in the disturbance of the Relationship you have toward yourself. If you want a healthy relationship-experience, then you first need to find the Unity in yourself. Between Feelings and Thinking, between Spirit and Body: a balance, in Love for yourself. As a result, you'll also have a harmonious relationship-experience with your partner; therefore, never place the CAUSE of kidney problems in someone else!

Sexual problems connected to the relationship problems are often seen as the cause of kidney problems, but here also the cause lies deeper: suppression of feelings (not integrating the "female" element into your being) and also not acknowledging your Self-Aware "I"-worthiness, all will contribute to your looking for a solution in "sexuality" within a partner-relationship. In this way "partnership" as well as "sexuality" mean an escape from yourself, a filling-up as a compensation for the emptiness you experience in yourself. Those kinds of solutions bring along problems. Aggression, anger, criticism, sadness, disenchantment — these are the natural results of this! You will only experience the relationship with someone else as true joy if you first have reached that Unity, joy, that fullness in yourself. Deep anxieties and not trusting your own divine nature will be the cause of your expecting things from someone else instead of first and foremost offering yourself the loving relationship you so need. The above-mentioned emotional experiences very strongly influence the functioning of the kidneys.

Do you destroy yourself by taking distance from your body, by living in your head in an exaggerated way, instead of feeling *one* with your physical nature? Anxious nervous tension, constantly being *too* alert, a feeling of being overwhelmed and being smothered because you don't allow your feelings to flow freely! "Denial" of the gentleness, feelings, of the earthly body?

The kidneys also symbolize the feeling of "solidarity": in yourself and with others.

You feel safe and in unity with yourself; you feel united with your partner. If you truly experience this unifying alliance, this love toward yourself, then the kidneys will feel comfortable; then you will attract friends and a partner with whom you also will feel good and relaxed.

Feeling solidarity with life, with all that lives, with nature. No conflict, but peace. No distant criticism, nor aggressive animosity, no anxieties, but an unlimited feeling of safety, peace, and joy. A fresh fountain, carefree and radiating.

The kidneys ask for a balance: a guiding, regulating structure on the basis of common sense on the one hand and total acceptance and free circulation of energies, of emotions, on the other hand. The marriage of love inside you.

A human being who, in the fullest sense of the word, is Thankful for Life, for Being, will have healthy kidneys. Not demanding, desiring, and hard, but giving life and radiating!

Cancer, tumor of the kidney
(See also Cancer, in general)

You call out like a blind man in the desert, where nobody sees or hears you. You feel closed off, like a hermit: because you have closed yourself off from your feelings, from your nature! You feel small and clumsy; you

don't really do what you want to do; you let yourself "be lived," you don't really live from out of your Self, from out of your emotional core. Do you follow, like a baby, the footsteps of someone else? Where are you? You don't know yourself anymore; sadness, anxieties, and desperation, constantly running in place without making any progress. You can't handle it anymore: because you refuse to transform! You pity yourself, but it is you who doesn't Want to see clearly, who remains blind to new, healthy, joyful ways. You withdraw, as if you are going to disappear in the mist. Do you feel ashamed or guilty if you would show your feelings? Do you remain the little child of your mother instead of Really standing on your own feet and living from out of your heart? You feel guilty; you put up obstacles for yourself. Things go wrong in the relationship with yourself, resulting in problems arising in relationships with others.

Make contact with the Earth and enjoy sensorial experiences: be part of Nature. Look for your path YOURSELF; allow yourself to be guided by your intuition, trust in your deepest Self. Don't let yourself be told, but determine your life yourself. Build on inner knowledge: you, and no one else, know what's good for you. Listen to your feelings and allow them to flow in freedom; don't put up any barriers. Don't be afraid of emotions; feel at home in yourself and immerse yourself in a bath full of feelings in order for you to be able to truly Live again.

Thankfulness for your being; don't blame others, don't desire. Come gladly into your "Being"; don't feel guilty, but at last make yourself welcome and discover that pure joy of life about yourself. Be proud about your worth; dare to experience your unique being. Being in harmony with yourself, in a relaxed way: in this way you will also find (again) harmony with your surroundings. Be yourself; don't hesitate; express your feelings; surrender to that boundless current of life. Death is not there as long as you don't call it up. Guilt and shame are only aspects of the human being who refuses to acknowledge his divinity, of the human being who doesn't want to see how, from Now on, he can create his own reality in a conscious way.

Contracted kidney

A feeling of not being able to go on anymore; you give up; emotionally you feel feeble; with limp wrists you despondently let yourself droop. In a tense way you try to keep something standing in your life instead of flexibly going along on the waves of life. You go in a direction which is not really good for you. You feel hurt and offended; you don't succeed in bringing out your emotions in a healthy way. Instead of transforming inner, aggressive powers into active self-realization, you block these energies. You don't go forward; you puff yourself up, inwardly, like a bagpipe out of which comes no sound. Healthy emotions turn inward, and you burn away on the spot; you are being wasted by the emotional fire; after all you don't allow your emotional powers to freely move outward. Self-destruction. You absolutely want to force or change certain things in your life, instead of trusting in the spontaneous life-processes and listening to the symbolic language of the circumstances you call up. Powers flow out of you, no matter how hard you try, exert yourself or struggle with it: because you don't really live in love toward yourself. Are your ideas that rigid? Do your thoughts, your prejudices so strongly restrict your life? You'd sooner send poison and reproach to others than see your own faults. You don't listen to your nature; you violate it.

Energies, sounds, and feelings: blow the trumpet and radiate it out! Look at yourself, stop being the "limp one" or striking at others with a stick. Call yourself to order and stop this self-destructive way of life.

In self-confidence open yourself up to other people. If you come to a thankful, loving relationship with yourself, then you also will create an harmonious environment. Watch closely which direction you want to take, but listen to your feelings, your intuition, while doing so. Let go of that which you have to let go of.

Don't continue on a path which will destroy you: bring about change and alter your view of life. Know yourself to be safe and protected; find solid support in your own Basis and allow all your energies, including your most gentle feelings, to flow freely. Don't restrain yourself; give yourself a chance to truly Live.

Nephritis
kidney inflammation or infection

Anxiety and sharp anger at its worst. Aggression has turned inward. Not daring to say "no," not daring to stand up for yourself, out of Anxiety. You remain silent, but you bottle up enormous emotional energies: self-poisoning. You suppress every feeling that rises up inside you; possibly you can seem very calm and rational outwardly, but inwardly a volcano rages. However you don't allow your spontaneous emotions to come through freely and honestly; you are so hard on yourself. You don't feel protected enough in yourself; you think that something or someone can destroy you.

Mortal fear: this disease calls on you to honestly acknowledge and express your "I," your Feelings.

Dare to manifest your own ego; dare to stick out your nose! Direct your feelings outward, including the negative ones; don't be afraid of aggressive powers; they only become dangerous for you if you keep suppressing them. Express yourself without holding back. Dare to voice yourself spontaneously; don't hide yourself behind a silent rational mask.

Cry or shout, if this makes you feel better. Then come to Insight: your powerless aggression originates from your feeling of insecurity. Now feel that deepest certainty in yourself and build your life according to your longings. Listen to your nature; be good to yourself. Negative situations now are only the result of your convictions in the past. You yourself are the cause of the circumstances that you have attracted unconsciously: now come to understanding, so that rest, relaxation, and peace might rule. In this way you don't call up a hand which might hit you: nothing happens without you first having called it up unconsciously or consciously. Peace, softening.

Kidney stones

The child in you, that original spontaneity, those pure feelings, those emotional creative-powers in you, are being suppressed. You live too much wanting to "satisfy" others or "laws," out of self-protection.

Your chair is actually empty; still you are full to the top with energies, emotions. You don't really take up your space. Your Sun-Center lives concealed behind laws and structures, behind a mask. You live like a dual personality: functioning outwardly, and inwardly stuck with a lot of Piled-up powers and feelings which can't find a way out. You hold in many emotions; aggression and anxieties are being accumulated, but even if you are really angry with someone, you still won't be up-front about it. Because actually you don't really feel safe in your Self; you are afraid of showing your feelings. You exercise Power on your natural forces, on your emotions: you suppress them; you only allow them to exist in a very restricted space. Unconscious powers make you "clutch" at people or things: in order to feel some kind of a hold; clawing at people, at a job, etc. . . .

You don't believe enough in the inner Worth, in the conscious sun-power of yourself, because of which you don't dare to really break through with your "I" in the way you inwardly feel. You live hidden, on guard, although you can outwardly function quite optimally. You are too hard on yourself; you give no room to those gentle, loving feelings in yourself! You are at a distance

from yourself; you don't dare to trust your deepest being, your nature-powers. Aggression turns inward; creative emotional energies pile up inside, and you feel frustrated. Because the relationship with yourself is stumbling, you will also attract difficulties in other relationships. The cause of your stones lies in the denial of your "male" sun-worth and in the hardening of the "female," emotional moon-aspects in yourself: piled up aggressive emotions don't find an outlet, and they harden inside. You kill your spontaneous nature, your warm feelings, in a restrictive framework.

It's as if a big Eye (in yourself) constantly spies on you and forbids and orders you, possibly just like the way your parents used to bring you up severely critically, or just like the Eye of society to which you subordinate yourself because you refuse to experience your Self as safe and autonomous. You keep yourself bound; sooner or later those inner powers will want to break out. Nature demands its rights.

No longer reject the authentic child and the gentle female aspect in yourself.

Allow water to flow freely: now liberate yourself. Know yourself to be safe in that everlasting, primal source of yourself, your living Self; and let yourself go. Surrender to your nature, to your feelings. Acknowledge the worth of yourself; take away the mask or the structural camouflage, toward the outer world and acknowledge your Sun as the Center in your Life. Establish yourself firmly and build on your inner wisdom, on your intuition.

Be good and gentle with yourself; come very close to yourself and feel that unity in you. Make an end to distance and criticism, to aggression.

Go into action; express your emotions; in all freedom exploit healthy aggressive energies in building a new life's path. Let go of these anxieties and live in a more relaxed way. You are only accountable to yourself. You are master over yourself, over your feelings. Don't tie them down, but dare to participate in life, like a forthright human being. No longer restrict yourself, no longer tense up or constrict yourself; place all power in yourself and offer yourself freedom. All anchorage lies in yourself. Softening! Breaking through oppressive structures which kept your nature in a grip.

Uremia
self-poisoning through kidney failure

Anxiety, hurt, sadness, self-criticism, and self-condemnation, a feeling of failure, unsureness, emotional pain, feeling threatened. The gentle "female" aspect in you is being crushed by hard aggressive emotions. But you bottle up all these feelings.

You hold on to so many feelings that you block a natural flow of healthy creative emotions: this leads to frustration and to emotional exaggeration concerning aggression, desire, passion, criticism, the sexual urge. But you don't arrive at actually experiencing your emotions: you experience them intensely in your head, in your thoughts. You don't really dare to enjoy with your senses, with your body; you constantly put a check on yourself. You absolutely Want to push this or that through: you are hard, and you fight to conquer, while you should not at all fight. You think you have to control everything with your will and your rationality without taking into account your intuition, your deepest Self. You tensely hold on to something or someone, while it would be better if you would let go! You don't trust your Living Self; you want to keep everything in hand, in control, to arrange and organize in an exaggerated way; you suffocate yourself in this way. Your body never gets a chance to relax.

A stressful situation because you close yourself off from that fundamentally solid mother-basis in you, because anxieties whip you up in an aggressive whirlpool. You don't at all listen to the voice of your nature; you constantly force yourself, while after all

it's now made clear via your body that the alarm bell is ringing; it asks you to finally listen lovingly, and in a relaxed way, to your needs, to the longings of the child in you. A demand to resolve that inner emotional battle.

Anxiety and hopelessness, aggressive powerlessness, are just the results of the fact that you don't really depend on that secure Basis in yourself, on that everlasting deepest Self. Do you think yourself ugly or bad? Do you experience your feelings as dark and devilishly negative?

You don't have to force yourself; you don't have to grasp everything with your thoughts; you may calmly trust in your firm Basis. Anxieties are unnecessary; nothing in life is "coincidence." Trust in those most beautiful Powers in you, which enable you to build a new life. Don't grab for something or someone, but let go! Relax, like a vat that empties itself; surrender to the Present moment, and in love turn toward your body. Your deepest Self sees Everything, registers every detail: trust in this fundamentally strong ground in yourself; you can always count on it. Throw open the windows and breathe freely: enjoy the green, restful energies and allow the red, warm, aggressive forces to escape freely. While doing this dare to experience yourself emotionally, to express yourself, but not in conflict with yourself. Find that peace inside you; spread your arms wide and welcome yourself and life. Don't close yourself up tensely. Fully enjoy all that is natural, all your senses, the physical feeling of wellbeing. Spoil yourself and never force yourself. Listen clearly to the signals of your nature. According to which norms would you condemn — those of a society, of an upbringing, of others? Stop this demolition and begin now to believe in the worth of your unique Self. Allow all those feelings to rinse through: surrender to the female aspect in you. Have no fear, everything is being arranged by your Living Self if you are open to it and are not blocking the water-treatment

The Key to Self-Liberation, Christiane Beerlandt © Beerlandt Publications plant with anxiety and self-doubt! Descend into yourself: feel One with your nature, with the gentle feelings of your heart, and let yourself go. Self-confidence, becoming aware: restore the distorted relationship with yourself.

Don't reject yourself; you are good the way you are. Every human being is unique in his own way. There are no norms for this. Beauty lies in being faithful to your particular nature, so that in this harmony toward yourself joy is being passed on to others. Thankfulness for your Being.

URINE

Albuminuria
presence of abnormal quantities of albumin or protein in the urine

You feel "hit"; you would like to barge through like a Ram, to seize for power. You feel frustrated, because for too long you have bottled up emotions, healthy aggressive powers. You have not really been yourself; you have pushed yourself into a passive, unsatisfying role. Now you are boiling over. Frustration ultimately leads to anger. Suppression of emotions, of spontaneous physical longings, can ultimately lead to compulsive or overly intense feelings of aggression or of sexual desires. You would like to break out: emotional energies have been held in for too long. Like a bow which has been drawn tight for too long, you would now break. If you don't integrate healthy emotions into your existence, don't dare to experience them under the Authority of your consciousness, then there will be a chance that you will experience in yourself "animalistic urges, sexual desires, exaggerated aggression." Do you feel hunted, hurt, wound up, "on the attack"? Are you fed up with being a victim or hallstand others can hang on? Are you now standing up for yourself in an exaggerated way, wronged and angry? You want to show for once how tough and strong you are! Insufficient transformation of pure Instincts into Consciousness.

Allow the wheel of the water-mill to continue to steadily turn, allow emotions to flow freely, and no longer bottle them up until the alarm bell sounds. Turn deeply inside yourself and feel safe in that warm enclosure of your own Light, of your deepest, immortal Self. Confront yourself again and again with your feelings, and work them out immediately. Don't linger; don't lock yourself up inside yourself; don't degrade yourself. Integrate those aggressive powers, those emotions, into your life under the controlling eye of your heart, so that frustrations don't have a chance. Get a good hold of yourself and guide your feelings. You are not at the mercy of compulsions if you become master over yourself (See also the category Sexual Lusts). The cause of your feeling of dissatisfaction doesn't lie in someone else: take the rudder of your life consciously in hand. Transform aggression into self-realization. Place in yourself all power over your life: you are not at all powerless.

Anuria
no urine production because of kidney failure

Desperation, standstill, holding on to the past; you don't see *which* direction to take, because you don't listen to your feelings, your intuition, because you look for a hold outside yourself. Emotional energies can't flow freely. You feel "stuck"; anxiety and powerlessness. You feel constricted as it were; feelings are bound. You pile things up; you don't express yourself; held-in anger, tensions, and aggressive powers poison you. You don't go onward, don't really evolve. You fixate on others, who are supposedly the reason you can't calmly relax; but that reason lies in you. You don't allow yourself to *live* freely and truly. Emotions boil in your brain; you cling to relations.

You are so afraid to show yourself completely the way you are, the way you inwardly feel. You close yourself off; you are on guard with others, you mistrust. You don't speak in a straightforward way; your head bursts with sadness, pangs of love. After all, you don't offer yourself the love and freedom that could make you so happy; you'd sooner expect or demand it from others. Of course it can't be that way. You are stuck in the phase of a clinging baby, so that you now inwardly cry for milk. You feel wronged, but this holding on to others crushes you; you have hardly any breath left. You don't at all choose YOUR path, independent and personal. You are not yet master over yourself.

Your intuition, your deepest Self, knows very well: that direction! Trust blindly and surrender to yourself. Let go — go with the wind, listen to your nature and don't go against the flow. Now look for the most relaxing atmospheres, the most pleasant ways to completely "loosen" yourself. Let go of heated thoughts, angry emotions and anxieties: you can trust your deepest Self unconditionally. No longer hold back those healthy energies; allow the wheel of life to turn in you and open up. Speak, enjoy, trust, come back inside yourself; let go of others, and solely turn toward yourself. You can't change others: now resolutely direct your life onward; no longer stay immobilized. Action, onward! Your head will lighten up because of this; your forces, your feelings, will find again their free flow. No longer cramp yourself up; say what you have to say, but don't dwell upon this.

Follow your autonomous course. In this love toward YOURSELF you will at last encounter new people — whether it be seeing your partner evolving — without your having to do anything about it. Evolution toward harmony in yourself will automatically attract a harmonious environment. Offer yourself freedom, and let go of all your worries. Trust in this law of nature and go on!

Blood in the urine

Anxieties. You would like to flee from the situation you are in now. You are going a path of suffering; you feel as if you are nailed on the cross. In sadness, in nostalgia, you'd prefer to hide in a warm small nest, hidden away and safe: it's an escape.

You can't get an overview anymore; you can't see the forest for the trees anymore. You feel yourself kicking like a turtle on its back: you degrade yourself; you refuse to exploit in a positive way your deepest powers and emotions. You refuse to actually stand on your own feet and take your life in your own hands in a self-aware, independent way! On the other hand, you feel "bound," and you want to get out of it, but you completely block and immobilize yourself.

You pile up feelings; aggression is being swallowed; you hide your spontaneous Self, your creative possibilities, your true emotions, the way ivy covers a wall, behind a thick "coat of scales." In anxiety and sadness you look for a hold outside yourself, in someone else; possibly you are like a parasite or you crawl. Inwardly, however, your heart calls for freedom. You don't take total responsibility for yourself, nor for someone else, because you flee from the truth regarding yourself.

Possibly the bond with a partner irritates you, but you have sought this yourself; possibly you are afraid of the suffocating grip within a relationship, but it is you who oppresses yourself, who doesn't allow spontaneous emotions and energies to flow freely. In a forced and tense way you can assume a defensive attitude, inflexible and hard: you escape first of all from a profound relationship with your self. This will stand in the way of a good relationship with a partner.

Don't flee: confront yourself with your deepest emotions, with the truth regarding yourself.

Look deep inside yourself with clear eyes; discover the child in yourself and the immature behavior. Allow emotions, experiences, and energies to freely flow inward, also in communication with others, and send them out again with the radiating power of your deepest Self. With all the power of your Self-aware "I" you can go forward, full of self-

confidence, without anxiety. The safety lies within you, in that immortal core. Don't reach for the past, but direct yourself onward, create your life yourself, so that you don't have to suffer pain. Voluntary ties, in the name of love, with a partner, are good as long as you make yourself free inside. Take care of yourself; offer that shelter to yourself. Don't get angry, don't feel unable, but take the bull by the horns and build up the future, in trust. You don't have to close yourself off emotionally: allow those creative, emotional energies to flow freely. Joy and Peace in your heart instead of conflict, powerlessness, aggression and sadness.

Oliguria
production of abnormally small amounts of urine

It seems as if you can't Consciously get a grip on yourself, your feelings, and your powers. You *allow* yourself to "be lived" through your thoughts, through your aggressive emotions. You can't, or dare not, bring everything out, so that you burn away on the spot.

You feel "stuck"; you don't really have a warm relationship with yourself; you push yourself and others away; refusal, revolt; you don't want to go on in this way. Sometimes you feel like a squeezed lemon and now you keep yourself "inside," so that no one can cause you sadness anymore! The martyr refuses to play this role any longer: you don't realize that you, yourself, are the cause of your feelings of restriction, of your sorrow.

You are "imprisoned" in yourself because you have denied your own worth in the past; because you have produced too "mechanically" instead of living from out of your emotional core; because you have overloaded yourself with a heap of burdens; because you possibly have lived too much for recognition from others as a compensation for your self-negation; because you don't evolve onward in this way, but keep on running in place, making no headway; because you don't let go of experiences from the past,

holding on to them in an emotional way; because you cut yourself off from those most beautiful feelings in yourself; because you imprison yourself in certain thinking patterns and insufficiently dare to enjoy the earthly, physical, sensorial aspects in your existence.

It is you who constantly punishes yourself; who robs you of the freedom to experience your feelings in all openness, to live in natural spontaneity. You block a normal flow of creative and emotional energies coming from your depths because you experience yourself as Powerless; because you place yourself subordinately either to unconscious emotions, to material or superficial productivity, or to an Authority outside yourself — because you refuse to take in hand Conscious Mastery over your life.

You refuse to become aware. In this powerlessness you will "grab" for people and things, for the past, for material security, instead of placing the power and sureness in yourself. Possibly things will get so out of hand that you become a slave of your passions, of your urge for power and possession, of the accumulation of your emotional experiences. In this anxious "holding-on" you unconsciously call up situations in which others get a "grip" on you. You think you have to bear it all like a victim, but still there's that inner Resistance: "I no longer want to take part in life in this way."

Guide those forces, the serpent, the power in your stomach; take the reins and allow the horse to enter free nature! Allow healthy energies, emotions, and creativity to unfold themselves; no longer keep it locked up inside. Allow feelings and thoughts to exist in balance; love for that which is earthly, for your body; give gentleness and love a chance in your existence and give the martyr in you the stab of death. Come truly to life from out of yourself. Place yourself a step higher; you will more easily open yourself up in the awareness of your personal worth as a Human Being. Follow only your nature: get a close relationship with yourself, in warmth, and no longer be a mechanical, wooden puppet. You don't have to suffer; look for another path. Become aware of your spontaneous fruitfulness and produce!

Don't live within an iron structure, but listen to the supple waves of your heart, your longings. Take up your place, acknowledge the inner worth of a human being, and don't cling to anyone or anything. Anxiety disappears if you surrender lovingly to yourself. In self-assuredness you can "blossom" and allow feelings to flow freely. All power over your existence lies within you; nothing or no one can tell you where your path lies: follow your intuition, your deepest feelings, and don't stand still; dare to tread on new paths!

Sour-smelling of the urine, exaggerated

Powerless anger. By holding on to emotions you poison yourself. Even if you are hurting, you don't "let go" of something or someone. You grab, with power. Possibly you are very angry, because the other person doesn't do what you want, because something doesn't happen the way you had planned. This indignation is only a result: you don't know very well *where* your path lies; you turn in all possible directions. You feel anything but sure and full of trust in yourself. You don't really go onward; you are hard and "angular" with yourself. You only reason in an emotional way anymore. "Poor me": you feel "in the grip of," because you yourself cling to everything in such an anxious way; nor can you trust in yourself and let go. You keep yourself and your true feelings hidden because you feel threatened. You switch on a safety-valve in order to get rid of the consequences of this psychological state, like toxic waste: sharp negativity finds its way out.

Openness, softening, letting go. Know yourself to be safe in your deepest Self, in your warm Sun-center. Place the Authority in yourself and let go of others. Dare to be yourself, without holding back; every human being has his or her unique nature. Build your life up in a more playful way; a clear structure, a clear perspective on yourself. Come out of your hiding place and firmly stand on your own feet, independent of others. You can transform yourself, but you can't change someone else. Yet people and circumstances will change in a positive way with regard to you, if you resolutely go your path and give yourself the chance to evolve. Transform negative thoughts and angry, poisonous emotions into thankful joy about your Self: the happiness is in you, for you possess the freedom and the gift of creating your life yourself as a human being.

V

VERTEBRAE SPINAL COLUMN
(See also Skeleton; Back)

Ailments, in general

Anxiety. Having no trust in the Power of your Living Self.

You are afraid of yourself, of those dark unknown areas, of that which is unconscious in you. "What is there deep inside me — poison?"

You don't really dare to allow yourself to go onward, to trustfully evolve, because you are not at all convinced that something or someone might not give you a smack on the head, as it were. You sooner feel like a victim, you are mistrustful toward the vagueness in yourself and therefore also toward others. You are on guard; you constantly feel threatened; you feel as if you are a toy of destiny. "Watch out!" You don't at all look for support in your own Basis, in your deepest Self; you take too black a view of things. You will hide in armor, in a certain suit, because you don't really experience yourself and the world as friendly and trustworthy. In this way, however, you will feel even more imprisoned, constricted: you can't and dare not uncover yourself, being the way you really are! This leads to frustration and tension.

You don't trust your nature; you hold your hands above your head in a protecting way, as it were; your shadow becomes bigger than your own "I," your sun-center; you cling to others, to the past, to outer appearances.

You don't dare grow "straight," the way you feel inside. You hide yourself; you experience yourself as a target for sharp arrows, and you duck away.

Trust calls up salvation: a friendly energy, comparable to the Dolphin, is always present in you. Trust in this deep core inside you, which will never abandon you. Don't flee from your deepest Self; you are not a victim: resolutely take your life in hand, trust your intuition; even if you are a thousand miles under the sea, your inner security system always works if you put trust in it. Action! No more fearing to act! Create your life yourself; fate doesn't exist; nothing just happens by coincidence; no painful arrow will strike you if you build your life with positive expectations. There's no poison deep inside you, but there is a divine core, which forms the seed of your present existence. You can evolve in a self-aware way, trusting in this core. In a conscious way you give instructions to your life, here-and-now, and deep inside you your core receives these signals. In its turn this living Self will draw from an immense storage of knowledge in order to transmit new messages to you, which you can receive in an intuitive way; also by noticing how your body reacts to certain changes you bring about in your life. This unity, "conscious I-deepest Self," makes it possible for you to create your life yourself.

When you become aware of the immense ability of your self, and you trustfully, and with love, look at your inner being, then you will be able to be among people, in all openness, without anxiety, in a friendly way, without mistrust.

Kyphosis
increased convexity of the back

Anxiety. You hide. You feel threatened by others because of a lack of trust in your deepest Self. You have the feeling that you have no right to be here.

Life overwhelms you; you can't digest it all. You are anxiously weighed down by your feelings of powerlessness. You feel seized in a structure that is too tight; your feelings are tensely tied down, closed up; you are on guard.

Suddenly, in an aggressive way, you might show your teeth, make yourself seem like a dangerous person, out of defensiveness, to chase others away. You feel so oppressed; you don't dare to openly show and experience your nature. You feel "inferior," positioning yourself too much as a victim, with feelings that are being smothered. You hold on to too much, including that which one tries to shove onto your back. Black thoughts govern your head.

Be proud of yourself! You are allowed to be who you are. Show yourself in all nakedness; don't hide, but stand up for yourself and don't allow yourself to be burdened by something that is not yours. Self-confidently establish your limits, dare to enjoy; to cheerfully sit at the table in friendship with others, without feeling threatened.

Don't bend for others, but acknowledge your worth. The colorful mix of people together: be comfortable among others and feel strong and joyful in yourself! Confront yourself with yourself, with your feelings and with your body: acknowledge, respect and love your originality, your unique Being. Trust your intuition, let go of negative thoughts, relax in all suppleness.

Lordosis
increased concavity of the back

You don't really dare to take up your space; you allow yourself to be led too much by someone with whom you feel a bond. On the other hand this makes you feel very uncomfortable: you fight to be loose and free! An inner duality: you feel too limp, too soft, too weak, unable to self-confidently go onward in life; but on the other hand you get angry with yourself about this in an impatient, intolerant way. Therefore, you are not really proud of yourself, you are not really nice; you underestimate your worth; you demand of yourself a resolute, fast growth, but you don't succeed right away.

Sometimes you no longer at all accept the tender little child inside you, and you become aggressive with yourself, with others. You don't think you are really good or strong, and you loathe yourself because of this.

You don't dare to resolutely be straightforward; at one time in life you take on this attitude, and then again another, because you still divide yourself and place yourself too strongly under the influence of others.

You'd rather be passive, without a clear personal choice; you stay sitting, stagnating, not fully concentrated in life; you wait and see what others will do; then again you perk up: "Something has to change here!"

Frustrated anger.

Don't force yourself, calmly take your time to grow in life. You are good and beautiful the way you are; every human being has unique characteristics: discover these in yourself and firmly dare to stand on your own feet!

Protect the child in you; don't suppress it, but accept it in love. Be proud of yourself, full of trust in your intuition. Solve the discord in yourself by gradual growth toward a more self-aware presence in yourself. Feel safe and protected in yourself!

Scoliosis
abnormal lateral curvature of the spine

You push yourself to the side, like a loveless child, because you don't believe in yourself.

You don't at all feel supported by yourself; you experience yourself only like an insignificant gnome, who has as a back-support only the fragile structure of a brittle mushroom. You don't believe in your inner powers; you would throw away the baby (you) with the dirty bath water, because you break yourself down in many areas. "Ah, it's all of no use." In the negation of yourself you will at last have no more "feelings," nor will you experience the firepower, the "spark" toward self-realization. You allow yourself to be ruled by circumstances, just letting things happen to you. You allow others to "hack" at you; you feel tied down. You don't truly live; possibly you live like a dog for its master or like a wall flower that doesn't like itself. You feel so weak on your own foundations that it seems as if at any moment you or your life might crumble to ruins. You don't stand up for yourself; it seems as if life doesn't really matter to you.

You were born with this philosophy: in order to make an end to it now! Integrate in yourself the "male" aspect: healthy thinking, resolute assertiveness, self-assuredness.

What are you doing to yourself? Cherish yourself in love and warmth; no longer push yourself into the cold. Take up the central space that belongs to you, and acknowledge your worth as a unique human being. A healthy balance between the intuitive and the rational, between earthly experience and thinking.

Trust in those fundamentally strong foundations of your Self. Dare to express yourself straightforwardly and stand up for your space, your place on earth.

Life-motivation and joy grow from within by acknowledging your deepest Self.

Degeneration
of intervertebral discs

You feel as if you are being undermined, floored by others, by circumstances in your life, but it is you pulling yourself down.

You don't allow your "I"-power to really come through. Your inner powers can't fully circulate, because you don't have enough self-awareness, because you actually say: "It all is of no avail"; you let yourself droop, you don't believe in yourself, in your autonomous worth. You'd sooner run after something or someone outside of yourself than stand still for a while, with self-respect. You feel "imprisoned," stuck. You are tight and stiff with yourself, severe and cold. Healthy Mars powers can't break through; you don't really live from out of your heart and soul. You ignore the coat of arms, the individuality of your unique person. You feel unable to live for yourself. Your "I"-power is broken, as it were; like a bird with injured wings, you can no longer fly; or what's more, you think you are no longer worthy to live, to revive.

You become more spiritual energy separate from your body than a human being made out of flesh and blood, healthily incarnated into a body. You feel as if you can't remain standing on your own feet; an aggressive tongue will only be a camouflage for your powerlessness.

You surrender with your arms opened wide, instead of allowing that stream of life to constantly flow in you.

No longer be so hard and negative regarding yourself; be flexible, and be open toward your inner Self. Discover that fundamentally strong Basis in yourself and charge yourself from this life source, which is inexhaustible. When you believe in yourself, acknowledge your worth, your body will regenerate itself if you wish it so. Vouch for yourself and shake yourself awake, call yourself to order; no longer allow yourself to destroy yourself. Discover that essential core within you, that fruitfulness, your possibilities for creating a new life yourself. Find that nourishing basis in yourself; allow that hard nut to break open from inside out, and allow everything to flow through: feelings, impulsive powers, creative energies. Don't close yourself off from that life source inside you. Participate in the full life, dare to enjoy, and don't shut yourself out. Stand up for your "I"; give yourself the life you deserve. No longer break yourself down with dark convictions.

Joy because of yourself, because of existence — without further requirements — is enough to bring about that powerful, healing, energetic flow of consciousness and to allow your body to scintillate with life-creating powers.

Recovery in joy and thankfulness; that's all there needs to be.

Sadness and running yourself down are lies! Make an end to them.

Rehabilitation of yourself, by yourself. Only you need to take care of your life.

Remain yourself; don't run after something or someone; place the authority exclusively in yourself.

Herniated disc
rupture, protrusion

Now, you bend because of burdens that are too heavy. It has all become too much for you and, seeing the long corridor that lies ahead, you now totally collapse.

You have been too hard and too rigid with yourself; in order to satisfy expectations, you have functioned toward the outer world in accordance with the rules you have been taught. Possibly, with a perfectly straight back, wearing a chique suit: "Is my hat straight?" Because you draw your certainty from whether or not you appear successful in the context of society — outwardly, or in your position, according to Image or intellectual achievement, etc. Inwardly, there's unsureness: "Who *am* I, separate from the outer world, from my 'duties'?" You don't listen to your nature; your emotional world exists only in a wooden way, restricted within tight structures.

You close yourself off from your gentle core, but others aren't able to make real contact with your gentle, emotional core either. You appear to others as being not very deep, as if in a wooden puppet theater. You hide behind a cassock or an apron, behind an overall, etc.. You live too much like a robot; you absorb and swallow information and questions, demands and expectations; you want to maintain power over your situation,

but sometimes you feel really powerless. Where is your soul's core, your natural, spontaneous being? Are you afraid of completely showing yourself the way you feel? Anxiety actually underlies all this. You look for a grip outside yourself, thus to feel protected, because you don't really feel safe in your deepest Self. Anxiety about ultimately being left behind, alone, abandoned. Anxiety about having to do everything alone; anxiety about a break with something or someone. You pile up too many emotions: these are the burdens that weigh the heaviest. Especially because you force all feelings into an oppressive straitjacket of structures and rational arguments.

Possibly you have called up difficulties within your relationships, be it unconsciously, because of this mechanical, unnatural attitude of yours.

You also hold on to burdens, sadness, and emotional tensions from the past in a tense way.

With a cool head, you try to organize your life, but it's too cold, and too hard to be beneficial for you and your fellow men. Is your security built on a foundation that lies outside of you?

Then you urgently need to change something in your life, because in this way you are very unstable and can't really relax anymore.

Replace those general laws and structures with your own foundations: know yourself to be safe and protected in your immortal Self.

Show who, and how, you really ARE. Listen to your nature, to your spontaneous feelings and impulses; don't direct yourself according to the expectations of others; it is not the ambition or the satisfying of others that counts, but what is of importance is the solid Basis inside you and the way you build your life here in a very autonomous, but loving, manner — the solid support that you experience in yourself, the unfaltering Sun in your center, the warmth that radiates out of your awareness of self-worth.

Of importance is the fruitfulness every

human being carries within himself in order to create new things in an original way, from inside out; not "obliging" yourself in this or that way to be the center of attraction on stage, not thinking you HAVE to do this in order to confirm that you are approved of. Dare to be a spectator, part of an audience, in a relaxed way. Let go of tensions from the past in order to concentrate yourself in the joy of the Now, without subordinating your body and feelings to structures and "thinking."

Look at everything from above, with the eye of your self-aware "I" and let go of superfluous burdens — no longer force yourself in any way, not even "to please" your fellow men. First of all, be faithful to your specific nature. Then you will experience rest and security, in harmony with yourself; the Freedom to be yourself. A spider makes its web in a spontaneous, natural way, step-by-step, without thinking, without forcing. When you follow your nature, you will build your work and your life in a fruitful way, without "sticking" laws upon yourself. Being yourself in a natural way.

Dislocation of a vertebra
(See also the specific vertebra)

You feel incomplete, unable to *truly* let yourself come through in life. Possibly you do fight for an ideal, in revolt, like a rebel or a freedom fighter, for a good cause, but you hide behind this like a martyr. You might project your personal sadness on the sorrow of a nation or another person. But you yourself remain under water; you don't really dare to live from out of your heart. Aggressive thoughts will torment you because you hinder those healthy fire-forces from breaking through in you. You don't really bring yourself to realization. Sometimes you seem to be really deaf to your evolution.

You offer hard resistance to Becoming who you are. Short, sharp, aggressive thought-arrows shoot through your head: inwardly you resist this being-"stuck."

You just sit there by the grave of your living Self, while there is no death, but you behave yourself like a dead person.

You refuse to stand straight and take true responsibility for your life. You don't listen to your feelings; you constantly hurt yourself. Inner energies, creativity, emotions, etc., just turn and turn, ready to flow through; inwardly you are bursting to jump up at last and take up your full space, but you offer resistance to this with irritating, self-torturing thoughts. You don't allow yourself to manifest your worth; you pull yourself down. You collide with yourself in an aggressive way.

Don't you love yourself? Do you think yourself ugly and bad? Do you want to punish yourself?

Spitting like a dragon: healthy fire-forces!

Like a full musical note, aware of its necessity and its unique beautiful tone: in this way you are allowed to open up and radiate in beautiful orange-yellow warmth, and sing out the Sun-power of yourself.

This beautiful power of your deepest Self is of inestimable and immortal value. Acknowledge that worth of yours and break through without hesitation: transform and no longer resist your Life's path. Sing life with all the power inside you; remove the damper.

Fracture of a vertebra
(See also the specific vertebra)

It's becoming too much for you; you refuse to carry these burdens any longer. Rebellious reaction: in this way you will no longer be part of it! Pent-up aggression with anxieties lying at the basis; forces break loose. You now stand up for your "I." For too long you have been stuck with an inner conflict. "Me or the other(s)." And now you want to stand up for yourself in a vigorous way, so that these sudden energies will have a self-destructive effect. Powerlessness-power. The cause lies in you: for too long you have played a role, possibly of a victim. Possibly you weren't honest, and you have laughed, while inwardly you were crying or mad. You have allowed a situation to exist for too long instead of bringing about changes. Have you allowed yourself to be smothered by a partner or a situation?

It's up to you never to force your nature, up to you to constantly listen to your true Self. Never allow yourself to "be lived"; always be honest with yourself and others. Arrive at clear communication and don't bottle things up; don't carry heavy emotional burdens, but work things out and let go. Know yourself to be safe and supported in yourself, so that you don't have to "accommodate" or behave like a martyr, in order to find — in exchange — security outside yourself. Without anxieties, build your life on that fundamentally solid Basis of your Living Self.

CERVICAL VERTEBRAE (NECK), AILMENTS

First cervical vertebra
"atlas"

Your "I" is hidden behind a camouflage screen of your Outer Ego.

You try to please others or take on a certain attitude because you don't dare to be yourself in a straightforward way. You feel yourself stuck between the eyes of others, as it were, so that you take on a certain behavior which is not completely in harmony with your true "I." This "I"-power can't come through; you hide the self-aware male element in yourself behind a facade of a naive, affected, gossiping miss. The contents of your thoughts, your energies, turn and turn, but they aren't employed in a fruitful way for the production process of your self-realization. You flee in Fear! You flee into superficial behavior: you dwell upon trifles. You flee from the Core of your being, from everything. Possibly you like to be in the center of attention and don't realize that in this way you imprison yourself in the net of

the outer world; it becomes a vicious circle. You hardly dare to look at your own deepest feelings; you are so afraid of those depths in your emotions; it frightens you; you run away from it to the surface. In this play-acting you think you can escape from a real confrontation with yourself, with that from which you are fleeing: your deepest powerful Self. You are afraid of finding deep inside yourself something very unpleasant and bad, something frightening. You are very mistrustful regarding your deepest "I." You take on a false attitude, until you are shaken awake emotionally. Anxieties hinder you from supplely and flexibly bending toward your own content; you keep yourself too stiff, in a rusted, sclerotic pattern, in order not to be a failure in the eyes of the outer world, in order not to *really have* to be yourself.

Feel that solid Basis in yourself and build a solid structure on this. Now, take good care of yourself, don't allow your life to be directed by others, but shake yourself awake! Become aware of that beautiful core in which lies the ability to build your life yourself as a creative human being. Take your life in hand in a self-aware way; live spontaneously the way you are, not to satisfy the expectations of others, of social norms. Now, fully acknowledge the male aspect in you; in this self-assuredness allow your emotions and your energies to flow freely. Don't hold back: express yourself; dare to live according to your inner standards, your true nature. Turn supplely and flexibly toward your own content, in respect for your own divinity: in this way, in this honesty, your life will become lighter and happier. Placing power over your life in the hands of others really brings along burdens that are too heavy and draws the energy out of you.

Second cervical vertebra
"axis"

Anxiety about looking deeper inside yourself; you refuse to listen to true knowledge and to the wisdom inside you. You close your eyes to higher consciousness powers; it is possible that, like a know-it-all, you just gather a lot of bookish knowledge, but the true depth of your being — the knowledge which is accessible via your inner senses — you anxiously close yourself off to that. You flee from your deepest Self, your intuition, your feelings: you lock yourself up like a fetus in an air bubble, who doesn't hear nor see, who keeps himself small and hidden. You feel like a victim; you conceal yourself behind an unauthentic life. You don't really touch the core of your existence. You feel hurt, afraid of psychological pain. You are afraid of allowing your deepest powers and feelings to come through, and of not being able to keep them under control, afraid that they might crush you; therefore you immediately close the door to the deepest, the most powerful, those pure electromagnetic sources inside you. You doubt the inner goodness inside you. In an aggressive way you would distance yourself from others; instead of starting an open dialogue, you would run away in an indignant, reproachful or sharply angry way, or else withdraw within yourself. You refuse to look inside yourself for the cause of your physical ailments or your psychological sorrow. To this you remain blind, or even better said: you put your head in the sand.

Put your trust in your deepest Self, and develop those divine powers from within the core of your being; radiate those beautiful energies toward others and discover the grandeur in yourself. Here-and-now, go onward in self-confidence.

Don't flee from deep powers and creative energies inside you: handle them in a self-aware way. Arrive at open and clear contact with your Self, with others; don't hide; open your doors to true life and arrive at harmony with yourself.

Acknowledge yourself in your Totality and don't be afraid: the deepest basis of the life of a human being is the love-energy which is called Life. Gratefully make use of these energies in order to manifest your Individuality.

Listen to your intuition and dare to surrender to beautiful feelings.

Third cervical vertebra

Self-destruction: personal energies, spontaneous powers, one's own creativity and ideas, are not allowed to exist. You clip the wings of your life in such a way that you have no room for your unique being. The reason for this: unsureness, you think you have to realize yourself and prove yourself to others. You think you first have to prove that you are worthy of living, of earning the approval of others; because in fact you doubt this yourself; you have no trust in yourself. It's because you don't accept yourself unconditionally that you exert yourself excessively and burden yourself with tasks, duties, restrictions, and norms, in order to show others and yourself that you have a right to be there.

You can perform stunts and daring achievements for the eye of the outer world: "I can handle this by myself, just leave me," but inwardly you feel you are not at all sure about this. Because of this inner conviction of inability, you will at last collapse or surrender to others.

Here again you might experience a sense of guilt: "They again were right about me not being able to do it. Ah, I'm just a stupid, self-willed nothing." You break yourself down; you will then depend on others because you don't believe in your inner powers. You don't allow yourself to look for true wisdom inside yourself; you let yourself be restricted by the Authority of others, because emotionally you feel weak. Sometimes you are in great fear of not being able to sustain a task, which you want to do very well for the eye of others, for an Authority. You don't listen at all to your own nature; you experience yourself as a victim that is supposed to sacrifice itself for others: in order to gain acknowledgement and a right to exist.

Topple your support and stand on your own feet: feel the center in yourself and allow those pure life-forces to flow through you. Allow yourself to blossom emotionally, and no longer place yourself in oppressive armor. You are master over yourself.

Make available all the space inside you and open your lungs wide. No longer suffocate yourself with the idea that you "have" to do or prove something, that you are but a humble servant for others; that you have to suffer and carry heavy burdens. Free yourself from this (be it unconscious) delusion. Listen to the spontaneity of your nature and follow your impulses. Dare to enjoy life: you have the right to just be yourself. You will have to accept yourself first of all and believe in that fundamentally strong power in yourself. It is not up to the outer world to grant you true life: acknowledge the fullness of yourself, even without your work or other accomplishments. Life is joy; sorrow and suffering are lies. Hurt yourself no longer.

Fourth cervical vertebra

You chew and ruminate your feelings: your head is an emotional hotbed in which ferment sadness, emotional memories from the past that you refuse to let go of, heartaches, anxieties, and pains. You *allow* yourself to driven by your emotions; it all overpowers you, you don't see a way out.

You feel stuck in the claws of the limitations of life, as if you are not permitted to be happy. But you are the cause of this: you refuse to manifest yourself; you don't dare to go forth on your path. You are so anxious that, if you would express your true feelings and thoughts, you would be "seized" by something or someone. In other words, you feel too guilty and too anxious to be yourself; so you'd prefer to run from your emotions and emotional thoughts. You are afraid you have done something "wrong." You don't direct your life *yourself!* You doubt; that which you so anxiously keep hold of (emotional energies), now turns inward and

takes possession of you; you destroy yourself in this way. You can have the unpleasant feeling that something is following you, but that is your deepest powers and emotions, which you anxiously hold in. You don't listen to yourself; you run away from all this! You deny a beautiful aspect of your nature; you are afraid of confrontations with yourself. You hide feelings and natural abilities: refusal of self-realization because of fear. You kill the true feelings of love inside yourself. You push yourself into a corner. You are so hard on yourself.

Radiate outward! Spit out those suppressed emotions; digest; clean things up in yourself. Allow yourself to be born inside yourself and listen to your inner wisdom. Allow aggressive powers to open up in service to your spontaneous self-realization; stop your self-destruction and, in pride, direct all your energies outward. Self-confidence! You will find peace and relaxation in the discharge, in the creation, of a new and original life.

No longer run away from yourself; take away from your sorrow the right of existence by resolutely taking your life in hand and making something beautiful of it. Reality will follow your convictions; no longer resist Joy and self-realization. Let go of the past and acknowledge the power of the creative "I" from Now on. You are master over your emotions: take up your scepter! In love, turn toward your nature; you are good the way you are: every human being is unique and worthy in his own way. You only need to love yourself.

Fifth cervical vertebra

You are angry with people who have for once told you off. Resistance; stubborn refusal. "Go away, leave me alone!" Closing yourself off. "I will show myself the way!" Angry emotional enclosure. Do you feel misunderstood, inferior? Then you are oversensitive to the words, criticism or advice of others. Actually you want to be nice, but you close yourself off, in fear of being hurt, or of having your feelings of inferiority confirmed. Thus you run away from yourself. People who mean well regarding you, but who touch a sensitive string in you ("I am nothing but a . . .") will find themselves facing a blank wall.

Anger and sadness block your throat. You can barely stand up for yourself; you no longer even want to; you close up.

"I don't need anyone; I will take care of myself!" In the meantime you feel misunderstood, sad, and undervalued. But you do this to yourself: you underestimate and condemn yourself. As a result, this inner conviction will attract certain people with their specific reactions.

Know yourself to be protected in yourself; feel safe and sheltered in your deepest Self.

Become aware of your unique worth; allow feelings to flow supplely. Express yourself; come to a gentle openness! Don't flee from yourself, but stand still and contemplate that inner wealth of yours. You don't need acknowledgement from others; you know your Worth. What others tell you can't shake you up because you naturally acknowledge yourself. Speak, tell, sing, and create! Allow your talents to blossom, and place yourself in the center of your existence.

Sixth cervical vertebra

You try to embrace too much outside yourself — people and situations — but it is so hard on you: you burden yourself unnecessarily. You try to get power over others; you try to change others and make them the way you want them to be, especially toward you. This is the result of the unconscious refusal to change *yourself.*

Because you are at a distance from yourself, because you don't really like yourself, because you are not really open and good to yourself, you try to attract your partner or your friends, try to force from others the affection and the love that you withhold from

yourself; this is not possible, of course.

You can't keep embracing all this; you are so angry because of this powerlessness, but you probably have the opinion that others are the cause of your problems. You experience yourself as a suffering martyr; the truth is that you refuse to stand on your own feet and give yourself that which you have a right to, no longer expecting things from others.

Refusal to look for the solution inside yourself; anger with the ones you claw on to; pain and the sadness because of this cause a feeling of desperation. You try to convince someone else of your vision, or to change his behavior in life, while you yourself urgently need to Transform! You suffocate yourself and others.

You hurt yourself; let go and allow the process of transformation to take place in you, so that at last you can live your own, unique existence as a autonomous, liberated, independent being. You can only change yourself. When you bring yourself to realization and no longer close yourself off — no longer try to do the impossible in whatever area — then you will feel more free and lighter. Why make it so hard and heavy for yourself? Gain clear insight into yourself: direct your eyes inward and discover hidden forces, the power inside you, so that you no longer center your attention on others, in powerlessness. Embrace yourself; unfold your creativity, your possibilities, your unique being. Put a "stop!" to your suffocating behavior and give yourself all the room you need! Open yourself; give and radiate; offer that which is most beautiful in you: in this way you transform yourself, and people who have something precious to offer you will appear on your path. Open yourself up and trust; don't reach, don't grab, don't demand.

Seventh cervical vertebra

Because you consider yourself small, clumsy, childish, ugly, ashamed, too fat or too thin; because you don't stand solidly on your own feet, you don't dare show the way you feel inwardly. You don't dare be spontaneously natural.

Are you still on the back of your mother, of your mentor? Are you still good, submissive and meek? Were you taught to behave this or that way toward the outer world? Do you not you live from out of yourself? You don't at all feel self-aware and proud about yourself. You would sooner hide and shield yourself from the eye of others. You are not at all connected with yourself, not in contact with the deepest trustworthy source inside you: in this way you won't succeed in making easy contacts with others. You place all power outside yourself, in others. You don't really go forward, don't choose a direction; you allow yourself to be guided by what others tell you you have to do.

You have the desire to manifest yourself, to come out of your shell, but your feelings of shame, inferiority or unsureness hold you back. You carry heavy emotional and creative energies inside you: heavy, because you pile them up instead of using them in self-manifestation.

Your potential possibilities are great, but are suppressed. Inwardly you produce a fire, but you keep it inside. Rational and intuitive sources inside you are not really connected with each other; you have problems with the harmony between female and male aspects inside you.

You don't build upon the Basis of your deepest Self; you don't trust yourself. So you have lost the contact with the mother basis in yourself, because of which you feel dependent on the Authority of others, and because of which you are not yet aware of your divine creative powers.

Do what you have to do, from out of your nature. Be faithful to yourself: show yourself in all openness, the way you feel inside. Stop thinking you are inferior or placing yourself under the Authority of others. Fight your way to freedom! You are good the way you are; acknowledge that divine worth in yourself. Don't give the Eye of the outer world

any power; find safety and sureness in yourself and don't allow yourself to be held back by anything or anyone. Rise above this low esteem of yourself: place the crown on your head. You are no gnome. Dare to dive into full life, without any reservation; express your feelings, create and enjoy! Don't hang yourself like a flower on the wall, but take up the space that you are entitled to! Be spontaneous, natural, personal, authentic. Express yourself, be creative, tell others what's on your mind; come into open contact with yourself and others: so that you can feel calm and secure. Don't live according to the rules of life that you were taught in your childhood, nor according to the suffocating norms or demands of a society or a partner, which mean you take needless burdens on your shoulders and are not listening to your nature! Unfold these powers, that creativity in you, so that you don't waste away on the spot because of suppressed flames. Self-realization!

THORACIC VERTEBRAE, AILMENTS

First thoracic vertebra

You identify yourself, so to speak, with the fetus you once were, and you are so Anxious that you don't allow yourself to be born. You don't feel at all protected in yourself. You ignore the worth of your individuality because you don't at all trust that which is deepest in you — your emotions, your deepest unconscious powers. You experience yourself as being strange; you think you have to block your feelings; also, you might experience your physical longings as being negative or threatening. In short, you don't give your nature the right to exist freely. You aren't only afraid of yourself, of your emotions, but (as a consequence) also of others. They have too much to say about your life; they hurt you; they take you out of your "ivory tower" or out of your emotional island. You are at their mercy; they hold you by your feet, as it were, so that you can't get away. They make of you a powerless, suffering victim — so you think, which is not the truth of course. It's precisely because you feel so insecure inside yourself, because you are so anxious about your deep emotions — as if the bridge at any moment will collapse under your feet — because you don't acknowledge the power inside you, that you give others too much power over you. You'd prefer to hide or withdraw completely, sometimes even with an aggressive, protective attitude via which you constrict your space, and you almost suffocate. But you feel shoved over by others; you surely don't want anyone to penetrate into your Emotional domain. You shiver with fear: ultimately, suppressed emotions and powers can suddenly break through without your being able to resist it any longer. Then you feel doubly victimized.

Thinking and fretting — you search; you don't see, don't find. Your rationality is just drifting on emotional waters. At the same time you are too severe a judge on yourself. You hold on to laws, rules, norms, and prejudices. In this way you condemn yourself and are also afraid that others might condemn you. You shake with stage fright about life itself — about totally daring to be yourself — because you think yourself to be not good enough, not worthy enough, to manifest yourself and to live according to your feelings. Your feelings present a threat for you, just like life, itself. You might condemn yourself and life on the basis of sad, painful remembrances from the past.

Identify yourself now with the self-aware adult within you, and not with the powerless child that clings to its mother. Believe in the protecting power of your immortal, deepest Self: you are safe. Nothing can happen to you unless you have first asked for it. No one need touch you; if necessary, you can defend yourself. The power over yourself lies within you.

But first and foremost take up your space and allow your nature, your feelings ,to flow freely! Self-liberation; no longer that anxious tension. Nothing in or around you can really threaten you: you constantly create the situation around you. Therefore, take the rudder in hand and come out of your hiding place. Allow yourself to be born and cleanse your head from those negative, useless thoughts. Put the past behind you, and from now on take your life in your own hands so that nothing or no one can tell you what to do anymore. Slide flexibly through your emotions; they form a threat for you only insofar as you suppress them. Accept these beautiful, creative powers in yourself; no longer fool yourself by thinking that life, and you, might be bad or frightening. Make a break with prejudices, with wrong conclusions you have made on the basis of negative experiences from the past. A brand new start. Free yourself! In the light and force of the Now, the past no longer has power.

Second thoracic vertebra

The "male" aspect is present in you in an exaggerated, dominating way: authoritarian and aggressively affirmative regarding yourself and possibly others; you rage inside in a hard, dominating, sometimes merciless way.

The urge of Saturn, the structures in which you force life, are severe and restrictive. It seems as if you are constantly angry with yourself, as if, with a punishing Yahweh finger, you constantly place yourself under a fire-spitting order.

This self-destructive tendency can have as a consequence that you push others aside in a forcing, egotistical, and hard way, but the real cause of this hardness lies in your mistrust. You don't trust yourself; your soft "female" side is being suppressed: the world around you threatens you; perhaps you behave toughly, but inwardly you are constantly on guard, fearful of being dragged along or of being crushed by others, by the outer world. You actually feel afraid and powerless. You are afraid of suffering pain. You are afraid of the powers of that which is emotional: afraid that once you surrender to your feelings you will become the dupe of it, that you will get swamped.

Therefore, because you don't really feel safe at all, you need to maintain Authority in a hard way so you can keep your life under control — at least that's what you think. Inwardly, your heart is bleeding because you are battling with yourself, with your gentle emotional core. "No one will hurt you anymore!" Do you so much doubt your worth as a human being?

Suppleness, flexibility! A relaxed attitude toward yourself and others.

Reconciliation with yourself, with your gentle feelings. Approach yourself in love, and know yourself to be peaceful and safe. Thaw out this hardness and discover that which is most warm, gentle, and sweet in yourself. Openness, joy; trust in your deepest Self. Don't be afraid of your feelings. You don't have to act hard and tough to be master over yourself and your circumstances. You are not powerless when you surrender to your nature and your feelings; make peace with yourself. No one will hurt you when you acknowledge that power in your heart of immunity, security, and love.

You are worthy as a human being, unique in your own way; don't demolish yourself, but create a joyful existence for yourself.

Third thoracic vertebra

You place yourself at a distance from others. In fact, you feel inferior, but you can make yourself appear bigger or different than you actually feel. Feelings are being locked up; by doing so you anxiously try to remain standing, until you bend. You flee from an honest confrontation with yourself, with others. Ultimately, suppressed feelings still break through. Inwardly, you long for unlimited space, for freedom, for openness, but you keep going in circles. You keep yourself within structural limitations; you protect yourself behind an angular shield.

You degrade nature and its spontaneous growth to a box of blocks, where there's no room for spontaneity, for openness, for air. You sometimes feel dead-tired, without breath, as it were. You try to remain standing, but because you close yourself off from your original nature, from your deepest natural powers, your body is not being fed by this stream of consciousness.

Instincts, intuition, and feelings are being hidden behind a facade which doesn't really reveal what's going on inside you. It's as if you say to others: "Don't come close, don't touch me." In a tense way you hold on to old structures, to habits from the past, to emotional memories, to an outer function or to how your image appears; but you don't really show yourself the way you inwardly feel. You shield yourself from others because you experience yourself as an outsider, "someone who has the plague" or someone bad, someone who's been shut off. You experience your personal structural basis as being very weak. That's why you reach for a grip outside yourself. You have sadness and heart pains; you sometimes have the feeling that your chest is being pressed, as if you are not allowed to take in any air for yourself. . . .

You lock yourself up inside, closed off from others.

Arrive at infinite self-liberation; dare to expand your existence in all directions. You close yourself off from a very important part of yourself: from your deepest, fundamentally strong Basis, from your deepest Self. Place yourself in the Center of your existence. Make contact with your immortal core and be aware of your possibilities as a creative human being. Open yourself up to your intuition; listen to your nature. Manifest yourself the way you feel inwardly. No longer shut yourself out; feel yourself taken up in that enormous space; trust this space of life. Don't only be a shield or a facade, but "BE" in totality. Stand with your feet solidly on the Earth and feel those powers in yourself.

An outer structure will naturally grow out of your central being; don't stick any unauthentic structures, lines or rules on your existence. Allow it all to spontaneously grow, and no longer oppress yourself. Offer yourself free breathing space. Every human being is unique and good in his own way. You don't have to shut yourself out nor keep others at a distance. When you make contact with yourself in a loving way, then you will also fearlessly approach the world. Therefore, open yourself up to that which is most spontaneous, natural, in you.

Trust in that powerful, inner Basis of yours. Throw yourself open, dance, sing, and live without borders! You don't have to screen yourself off, because you are safe in your being. Stop this self-limitation, love your unique content-in-a-physical-form, and also welcome others into your existence.

Fourth thoracic vertebra

You feel stuck in an iron grip; you feel driven into a corner; deep unconscious anxieties overwhelm you. You look for a way out, but only betray yourself: you ignore the divine, that which is most beautiful in you. You feel threatened, as if others have mistreated you. But it is you, first of all, who short-changes yourself, and you are actually worrying about nothing. Dark, threatening forces seem to acquire power over you: they come from deep inside yourself. You seem to be at the mercy of a "superior power"; you feel painfully hurt. You don't trust your deepest Self. You don't really build up your life with all your possibilities and creative energies. You hold in your feelings; you immobilize yourself. It's as if you can't stand up for yourself; you feel powerless in this situation. This leads to enormous aggression, to whirling, cutting fury. You direct at others your powerlessness to express your feelings and your creativity; possibly you weren't understood and you were hurt, but this already is a consequence of self-betrayal and of your anxieties. You no longer will allow yourself to be ruled by oth-ers; you are at the ready with an aggressive, protective knife. But you are so afraid, that you sometimes might stray from the truth, that you may deviate from your straight path: a camouflage in order to protect your weakness.

You inwardly resist the emotionally dark depths, those anxieties and emotions which threaten to overwhelm you. You might get angry with others, although the cause lies within you. You might break with your friends; you might betray them and say: "All right, I quit!" in a revolt against your own embittered powerlessness. Sometimes it seems as if you are taking revenge against the world for the so-called injustice that has been done to you. Then again, you can outwardly act as if nothing's the matter. Deep emotions are brewing in a hidden way; you bottle things up; the anger turns inward and destroys you.

Express your feelings! Precious talents are being lost; stop your dark thinking, and arrive at self-contemplation. Arrive at friendship in yourself; solve your frustrations so that you no longer experience others as threatening. Allow intuition and thoughts to work together in a healthy way. Arrive at a calm, peaceful feeling, at self-satisfaction: acknowledge the worth of your unique being, of your deepest Self. Arrive at actual self-realization; transform aggression into action and creativity. Don't expect others to understand your feelings and your nature: you, yourself, need to be open to your nature. Live your life to the full, with your soul and body. Trust life; you, yourself, will create joy if you give yourself a chance. Purge your emotional and thought life of fearful memories and start with a clean slate. Regularly get rid of your feelings and don't keep bottling them up.

Fifth thoracic vertebra

Oppression, nervousness, uncertainty, confusion, being stuck. Because you don't have Confidence in the inner Authority of yourself, your life is too strongly built on "thinking" and on the Authority of something or someone outside you. You have a feeling of: "I can't get away anymore," and you are afraid, because you don't dare to live from out of your own feelings, according to your own longings. You give more value to the ideas or philosophy of someone else instead of listening to your own inner wisdom. You ignore your intuition, your divine content. Your life evolves in a too structured way, possibly too rationally, without having any room to accept, experience, feelings to the fullest. You measure yourself with others; you think you have to justify yourself; you are afraid that he/she may notice this or that about you. You just don't dare to be yourself; you'd sooner think yourself to be inferior.

The ideas with which you have built your life in the past now seem to suffocate you; you have the feeling you won't get out of this anymore. Then resistance rises up in you against that which has oppressed you for too long: the imprisoning structure you have built, the authority above your head, the job that smothers you, the function that didn't offer you any space, etc. With all your might you would push away the beam above your head and scream at the top of your lungs: "Here **'I'** am! I am more than just a structure; I have my wishes too, my feelings, my inner Authority." But, for the moment, you still feel like a small gnome, who swallows his feelings of anger, uncertainty, and sadness.

A butterfly in a net. Bound at the wrists. It seems as if every moment of joy in your life is being torn away by others. You are full of sadness and anger. You think and fret a lot; you don't see which way to go anymore. "What shall I do"? You feel forced into a certain direction or forced to live in a certain way, and that is no longer possible. You want to step out of this, but you don't believe enough in the worth of your Self. You don't feel you have the power to determine your own life, to stand up for yourself.

Powerless anger. Feelings are being blocked under the dominance of rationality, under the Authority above your head, and because of the embarrassment of being yourself.

Self-respect! Be aware of your self-worth. Not being afraid of anything or anyone, or holding back. With the super dominance of your deepest Self you have everything under control; confusion and unsureness only come to be when you build your life on the Authority of someone else. Trust! No more doubts about your worth. In self-assuredness place yourself a step higher. The natural protection coming from your deepest Self will never go away; in this absolute awareness of security you can let go of your feelings, free and without inhibitions. Be yourself without looking at the eyes of someone else for their approval. Seize the power over yourself, without hesitation bring yourself to realization; express your feelings and go on when you have to take a new turn.

Let go of the old. Your feelings don't form a threat for you: use them as creative energies in the construction of your existence. Be faithful to your nature and break with ties that are too oppressive or with structures that are too suffocating in your life.

In an honest confrontation with yourself you can allow your emotions to flow freely, without your rationality or your argumentation, or the eyes of others having to put a damper on it.

Sixth thoracic vertebra

Holding in something; not daring to come out, especially not with your feelings. Not living the way you'd really want to. You don't really dare to swim through the stream of life and feelings. As if you hold your breath; you stand behind the stage curtains, instead of fully standing in life. You are afraid, anxious, and that's why you don't take any responsibility. You flee, don't dare to look close, don't dare to deal with a total confrontation. Refusal, withdrawing into yourself, also — and foremost — in thought. Too strong a head- or thought-experience in nervousness and keeping silent. You run away from life; negation, pushing away, because you don't stand solidly with your feet on the ground, because you don't trust yourself, because you see something negative in everything. You don't really get in touch with your body; you withdraw too much into the "spirit," into your head. You don't very well know what direction to choose in life, because you don't really trust in your intuition. A sometimes frenzied, insane fury dominates you, but — with the head of an angel — you will just bang against the wall, instead of actually changing something about this frustrating situation. "No! No!" Refusal regarding life. A stubborn, sometimes proud, refusal to take in new experiences, to grow.

Don't flee; don't run away from those feelings: confront yourself with them and arrive at a clear solution. For this purpose, concentrate yourself strongly within yourself and feel how your Consciousness powers are getting a grip on every fiber of your body. Here and now: don't live outside this earthly dimension, not in another time or place. Stay here, very close to yourself, and take responsibility so that your life and that of your fellow men becomes more pleasant and more calm, more straightforward and more communicative. In a self-aware way, stand with both feet on the ground and resolutely take your life in hand.

Don't lose yourself in endless fretting, but follow your intuition so that you can feel very well: "That's the direction I want to take." No longer allow yourself to "be lived" by fleeing from your feelings, but fully integrate your emotions, and handle them with mastery, as powerful energies in the building up of your existence. In the security of your deepest Self you can easily be open to the new things that are coming at you; allow yourself to transform. Anxieties and nerv-ousness are useless when you know that it's only you who can create your life. Nothing "just" happens. Allow your "I" to come through, and dare to express your feelings.

Seventh thoracic vertebra

Energies — a lot of energies, emotions, and creative forces, escape from within you, but you work against yourself; you don't bring yourself to realization in a direct way. The flow of feelings and energetic forces that boil up from within you — your longings and spontaneous impulses — are being held back.

It all appears threatening to you. These suppressed feelings will ultimately seem compulsive and frightening; this increases your fear and also the dam that you, yourself, have put up against your feelings.

You think you have to be a suffering victim; you don't allow yourself to enjoy, to yield to your feelings, to the joy of sensory, earthly pleasures. An unpleasant, threatening feeling comes over you so that you rein yourself in very tightly; you are too severe with yourself.

You'd sooner kneel to an authority outside yourself rather than place the authority inside you. You place power in others. "Someone tells you how to live"; you are being self-destructive. You suffer immense fears, you are mortally afraid, as if someone might kill you. You anxiously and tightly close yourself up. Exaggeratedly burdening the spiritual aspect of your head makes it so that you are not really good to your body, that you don't give yourself warmth and enjoyment. You feel bound at both wrists; you'd sooner listen to someone else than to your inner authority. You experience yourself as naked and vulnerable, at the mercy of a god or of someone else. Don't you love yourself? Do you feel so sad? You are not enough in contact with earthly things, with your body, with the sensual beauty of all living things, with the colors and fragrances of beautiful nature.

Construct a framework from a solid central pillar: your "I." Put the stamp of your personality on your life and manifest yourself. Enjoy life to the fullest: sorrow is only a lie created by ignorant people. All power to direct your life lies in you. As long as you have the conviction that a human being should suffer, restrict himself, follow severe diets, go a path of distress — then you are listening to the "devil." The divine inside you is beautiful; don't allow others to dominate you, but handle the powers from your Self with mastery and build a happy existence. Allow your head and your spiritual forces to integrate themselves in your total being: acknowledge your body, your senses, your feelings, your intuition.

Think less worriedly; dare to feel more, with pleasure. Give yourself what you deserve. Free yourself from "obligations" and allow yourself. . . .

In gentleness come to yourself; plant your feet solidly in the Earth! Be a human being of flesh and blood, no holy one, nor someone who has his head in the clouds. Assure a balance between the spiritual and the earthly.

Eighth thoracic vertebra

Restrained potential forces, also power-forces: on the one hand you would withdraw, remain in the background; on the other hand you would jump forward, as it were, and grab on to things (or people) in order to feel safe; an inner contradiction. Because you feel unsure and powerless, because you aren't master of yourself, because you are afraid that your feelings might make you unstable, you try with an aggressive urge for power to secure yourself by getting a hold on things or people in a dominant way. This is a compensation for your own powerlessness; it seems as if you are absent from yourself sometimes, as if you don't have real contact with your feelings. You don't consider yourself able to really go forward in life because you are not in touch with your earthly self. You keep your legs stiff like a wooden puppet; you stay in one place with your feet, standing about, without evolution; with your arms, you would reach too far, so that the bow is drawn too tight.

Tensely you try to secure yourself everywhere; "This is mine, you are not allowed to touch it, stay away from my child, my task, my possessions, my image, the things I have obtained, etc."

This anxious restlessness is the result of the fact that you don't get a grip on your feelings, on your body, on your total Self. Powerless to grow up, to no longer experience yourself as a child. You are also afraid that if you allow your gentle feelings, your female flexibility, to come through — that if you no longer try to control and embrace everything — you will be totally wiped away, that you might have no more resistance. Absolute hesitation about going onward in life, as if you still even have to hold on to the past. Your thoughts try to watch out for everything; you think in a rather negative way. You are afraid that you can't sustain things, that you might crash, that you can't handle it all. Will you withdraw or go onward with the risk of failing? You don't feel safe in yourself. In the emotional area (for instance in relationships) as well as in your thoughts, you try to hold on to things or people in order to secure yourself in this unsureness.

As long as you try to get a "grip" or "power" over others you will be stuck in the power-grip of anxieties, of others. Arrive at a radiating, powerful sureness in yourself; become master over your life, over your feelings and thoughts. Enter into these warm red energies of yourself, into that friendly, joyful, cozy warmth of yourself. In this certainty of yourself, you will no longer need to tensely make yourself feel safe. Let go; surrender your thoughts to that peaceful atmosphere inside you; feel independent and strong in your Self. Try to flexibly bend along with your feelings, listen to your nature; don't force yourself. Feel free and safe in your emotions and don't shield yourself from them: allow them to flow. They don't cause your weakness! Just be yourself, without assuming an attitude in order to stand firm against others. You are allowed to be yourself; in this way you don't lose power and resistance, on the contrary. The more faithful you are to your nature, the more harmonious and joyful the relationship with yourself and others will be.

Ninth thoracic vertebra

Sorrow for the sake of sorrow. You regard yourself as lost; you totally give up yourself; you allow yourself to be removed; you let yourself be skinned alive by others. You still struggle a little, but at last you allow yourself to be grabbed. You are not at all aware that — especially by your inner convictions regarding yourself, by the martyr's role you play — you provoke the behavior of others. You turn yourself against them with aggressive thoughts. You deny the power and worthiness in yourself. You boil over with anxiety, sometimes an insane lonely anxiety. You don't allow yourself to look for support in yourself or in others; you create a distance toward other people. Your anger mostly remains repressed and destroys you. You don't know what to do with your feelings; you are in a fragile balance. You are so afraid of being crushed by something or someone — vague anxieties — but here it's actually about the fear of your own deep emotions, of your aggression, of your suppressed forces, because you don't bring yourself to realization. Your head is an emotional hotbed. You are so afraid of those moments of anxiety and loneliness, but you leave yourself in the cold; suppressing in yourself the feelings of warmth and love. It's impossible for you to fill this inner emptiness by entering into relationship with others. You are at a distance from your body, from your deepest Contents: how could you then expect to have good contact with others?

First and foremost you need to solve the sadness in yourself. Dare to experience YOURSELF; experience that powerful physicality, the flow of consciousness in every fiber of your body. Experience that power and that creative energy in yourself; now become aware of your worth, place the crown on your head. Be YOURSELF in an autonomous way. You are naturally safe and protected in yourself; calmly allow your feelings to flow under the supervision of your self-aware "I." Go onward and don't doubt your possibilities. Stand up for who you are.

First come to yourself in love; in this way you don't create a barrier against your warmth and against love that comes from others. The solution of loneliness and anxieties lies first and foremost in the experience of Oneness of your divine Self. Experience yourself in a relaxed way; feel safe and peaceful in yourself; don't hound yourself with any negative or brainsick ideas. Enjoy, in a calm way; life gives joy. Sadness only shows you that you don't treat yourself right, that you are on the wrong track. Choose that path which offers you rehabilitation. Be Master over yourself.

Tenth thoracic vertebra

Anxiety about being hurt; anxiety about being swallowed up "into nothingness."

Extreme anxieties; you expect the worst because you position yourself as a passive, suffering victim. It's as if others tear away your hands and feet: you don't at all stand firmly with your feet on the earth; you are not able to give shape to your life yourself. You *allow* yourself to "be lived."

Painful communication problems because in the first place you experience your relationship with yourself as imperfect and sad; you poison yourself with emotions that have turned inward, such as anxieties, aggression, panic, helplessness. You allow yourself to "be lived" by your emotions without directing them, like a boat without crew.

It's as if you have nothing to say about

your body, nor about your feelings. It all just happens to you; you fear that things will go from bad to worse. You create your life in a very destructive way. You are tense, as if the worst might come over you at *any* moment; a sharp, anxious attitude toward the future.

You no longer have a clear perspective on yourself at all; you allow yourself to be taken up into a sea of anonymity, in which all individual values drown. You wrong yourself! You allow yourself to slump totally into the bog. Ah, who are you anymore? You feel painfully hurt, like a poor emaciated victim of circumstances or of the deeds of others. You don't realize how the cause lies in you. As a reaction to this powerlessness to get a hold of yourself and realize yourself in life, you'd sooner behave aggressively and critically toward others. You forget to enjoy the earthly pleasures, the sensorial beauty, the physical joy.

Stand solidly on your own feet; build on yourself. In a relaxed way enjoy all the earthly beauty, good food, nature. Use your brain in a healthy way; develop self-confident, logical thinking-power. Don't hide your anxieties, your aggression, and your sadness; conjure up yourself out of the dark. Discover the joy of life; no longer allow yourself to "be lived"; feel that safety of your fundamentally strong basis, of your deepest Self. You are always protected. Discover the radiating power of your knees, the awareness-energies that nourish your body.

Acknowledge that which is earthly; put things into perspective and bring humor into your life. See how the cause of your problems lies in your inner convictions. If you are convinced that you are worthy of having a loving contact with yourself, with others, then the results won't stay away. If, however, you constrict yourself with anxieties and helpless expectations from life, then you create your life in a very negative way. You have your life in your hands; make something beautiful of it. You are the only one who's responsible for yourself. Acknowledge yourself as your best partner: the male and

female aspect in harmony; feelings and calm thinking-power hand in hand. In this balance you will also attract joyful people to you.

Eleventh thoracic vertebra

You see life as black and white, with the contrast: devilish/angelic. You are afraid of the bad in you; you think yourself just so-so, and you are afraid that others might discover your "badness." Because you condemn a part of yourself, you expect others to look at you in a disapproving or reproachful way. You are even afraid that they might grab you, just as you feel grabbed by the so-called "negativity" of your nature. You are afraid of the force and power in yourself, but this aggressive urge for power only pops up because you suppress your healthy, natural forces! On the one hand you would like to satisfy the norms of an "ideal-image," of a holy one, as it were, and that's why you suppress that which you condemn as "low-to-the-ground" or bad (sex, physical joy, etc.) instead of allowing transformation to take place and fully "experiencing" this transformation; it makes you afraid of the beautiful, earthly powers and emotions deep inside you; you don't really trust Yourself; you are also afraid of the evil outside of you, which might suddenly appear from out of a corner.

Your repressed urge for power is a result of that anxious mistrust, of the suppression of your own potential forces.

You suppress your "I": because you are afraid of that which is "black" in Yourself. You don't allow yourself to really break through in life; you block your energies and your emotions — until this all might escalate. You seize power over yourself, over your nature, over your feelings. After all you feel so guilty and black that you withhold true life from yourself. You blow up the so-called evil; sometimes you see the world in a paranoid way. You want to escape from the power-grip of others, while you don't realize that the cause of your problems doesn't lie *there,* but in your self-curtailment. You hinder the power in yourself from flowing, hinder the consciousness forces from nourishing your body in a powerful way, under the authority of your Self-aware "I," because you are afraid of power. Yet, these feelings of power actually grow, in a negative way, including toward others because you suppress the original forces in yourself.

You are like a gnome running away from a giant: fiction. If you feel angry, then you will fight off this anger as long as possible in yourself because it belongs, so you think, to that which is bad. You are on guard against others; they might grab you; you are afraid of physical contacts, possibly because you were indoctrinated that this is bad. You mistrust others; you don't dare to surrender to your spontaneous feelings; you hold things in; you are afraid of your own Mars powers.

That inner force in yourself is necessary and good in order to solidly establish yourself on earth. It is not power over others that is good but the power over your total Self, in which your emotions are allowed to flow freely. Don't block yourself! Accept all that is physical, emotional, aggressive, as healthy aspects of your existence. You are safe in your deepest Self. If you no longer suppress, through misuse of power, that which is most beautiful in you, then others won't have a grip on you either; then you will leave others free; then you will liberate yourself.

Don't consider yourself bad or guilty: these are negative prejudices regarding yourself.

But you need to realize that your deepest emotions and forces are original, healthy energies that can contribute to the creation of a joyful existence for you and others — if you only give them freedom.

Acknowledge mastery over yourself so that you won't be dominated nor have the need to dominate others. You are good; stop condemning yourself, because this only gets in the way of healthy relationships. After all,

they react to your unspoken convictions regarding yourself. Don't hold back your evolution! Creativity, action!

Twelfth thoracic vertebra

You deny inner power over yourself; powerlessness, sadness, unsureness, standstill; you don't take Authority and responsibility over your life.

You remain hidden in yourself, sheltered in the warm spot of your heart: you live concealed, turned inward. Only swollen red eyelids show your sorrow.

You are so afraid of coming out; you constrict yourself and close yourself up. You might suffocate in yourself because you accumulate your feelings, such as aggression and power-powerlessness.

You don't show any determination in your life; you feel helpless and at the mercy of others. Then again all of a sudden you will storm forward in life with aggressive fire-forces, too forced after a period of having hidden yourself. You feel like a black widow spider, sad, but filled with deathly poison, especially poisoning herself with concealed emotions.

You imprison yourself; you push others away from you. You can appear tough and strong to the outside because you don't dare to bring out the feelings of your heart, or because you protect yourself from another disillusionment in a relationship of the heart. You don't have a clear perspective on yourself, on your feelings. Because you look at everything too much through the glasses of a prisoner. You kill yourself because you block your warm energy currents. Do you not see the forest for the trees? You are stuck at the lowest point of your heart, safely hidden, at least with your inner emotional world; outwardly you might put on a mask, as if nothing's the matter, but in the meantime you don't allow yourself to live *really* happily. Your life is too sterile; your creative energies are being blocked.

You have all power in you; you are the Authority in your life: make a choice. Don't lock yourself up in a cage; surrender to your feelings. It is good to turn inward in wisdom, but not to extinguish all your powers, your emotions, your creativity, and then quietly die inside yourself.

Turn yourself toward true life in all openness. Don't hold yourself back; allow spontaneous forces to flow freely and now assume your full space. Get a clear overview of your inner being and unfold all your possibilities in order to communicate in a friendly spirit with others. Don't enclose yourself in a cocoon: allow your heart to breathe freely, without oppression.

Offer yourself the joy of earthly life. No longer hold yourself back; don't smother yourself; let yourself go, let yourself be free, allow those feelings to flow freely before they suffocate you. Resolutely determine your point of view and direct your existence in a self-aware way. Apply all your potential forces to the development of a fruitful existence! Go onward and produce.

LUMBAR VERTEBRAE, AILMENTS

First lumbar vertebra

You don't really dare to manifest yourself because you doubt your worth. You go against the flow, against your deepest feelings, because you don't listen to your Self.

You don't think yourself worthy to "belong," so therefore you'd rather stay alone, but in fact you long to be part of something. You lower yourself to someone inferior. You flee from yourself; you push yourself away because you don't appreciate yourself. Sadly withdrawn; you don't really *live* from out of powerful "I"-center. You place the Authority outside yourself. With this vertebra ailment you now might ask for attention like a "poor wretch"; on the other hand you don't think yourself worthy of attention and would sooner withdraw quietly, weeping, into a corner.

On top of this you long for an independent and free existence, on the one hand, but on the other hand, you reluctantly notice that you long for attention and love.

On the one hand you are like a rearing horse, on the other hand like a faithful, good dog.

You feel confused, tense; you hold in your aggressive forces; it's hard for you to explain your feelings to others. Tension, duality; this can only be resolved when you no longer push yourself away, when you accept yourself the way you are, being spontaneous at any moment, unconstrained, without authority above your head. For too long you have too much considered others and their needs, because of which you have not been able to really be yourself. You have never really expressed your anger, satisfied your urge for freedom and independence, because you have considered yourself subordinate to another Authority. Now, the urge is strong to acknowledge your Self as an Authority, although you still inhibit your own nature and feelings.

In the first place you have to come "close to" yourself! Become Aware of your inner Power. Enlarge your space! Fully take up your place and bring up your powers, your talents. Be proud of your being and don't push yourself away; don't be an ostrich, but accept yourself totally. At all times be faithful to your nature; dare to offer your feelings, and don't allow this to prevent you from withdrawing within your borders when you wish to do so. Push your life through in a self-aware way, without hesitation. Offer love to yourself and know that you are worthy of receiving love from others. No human being is inferior to another; destroy self-degradation and make yourself heartily welcome as a worthy, unique being!

Second lumbar vertebra

Confusion, nervousness, you don't clearly see what direction to take; you'd go in all directions at once. Your emotional life seems to you like a Gordian Knot; sometimes you feel like an insane person; you would like to say and spit out a lot, but you close yourself up. After having bottled up emotions for a *very* long time you might suddenly break down because of sadness, possibly in an aggressive outburst. You are having a hard time especially because you push the child within you away from you. You can't very well stand that small, anxious, sad, hurt aspect of yourself; it threatens you, might be able to destroy you some day! To others it might seem that you make a mountain out of a mole hill, but you are stuck with life-deep traumas. Because you were born with the conviction that you can't survive without the love of others, you may have attracted situations in your life which were a result of your anxious conditions: for instance, you experience the mother's breast as an iron milk machine and not as tender love, or your father as a strongly emotional figure, with whom you identified yourself, etc. Now you exaggerate experiences from your childhood, but the cause doesn't lie with your parents, but with you.

The truth is that you don't allow yourself to be born in yourself! You refuse to feel the power in your center.

Allow yourself to be born and be full of motherly love toward yourself.

*You don't need anyone, except yourself. Put the past behind you and build up your life with the power of the Now. Don't bottle up any emotions, but steer these forces in the right direction. Allow that pure creativity to be born out of the power of yourself. Don't blow the past out of proportion: let go. Everything that has happened to you in your life, you have first attracted it, be it uncon-*sciously. *Be your own father, your own mother, and tenderly press the child to your heart. You make the consequences much bigger than they are; get your feet in the earthly reality here-and-now.*

Self-aware manifestation!

Third lumbar vertebra

Pain related to that which you see concerning your Ego. How you think yourself to be bad, how you look at yourself with a disapproving eye — that's how you think others might punish you. "They are looking for you." You are afraid; your conscience gnaws, you feel as if you are being pursued. You think you are not worthy of living here; you would like to flee. You would escape into sexual play as compensation because you feel yourself powerless, unable to bring yourself to realization, because you feel yourself so much in the iron grip of others, because you deny your divine consciousness power and you'd sooner have the feeling that something bigger than you would threaten and crush you, because you have anxiety and you deny your own greatness. The urge for self-destruction. You feel painfully hurt, possibly in your infancy. In order to lose your own inner emptiness, you allow others to enter your own personal domain, but on the other hand you would react in an aggressive, dominant, and biting way against the pain that is being inflicted on you.

You go at it in a self-destructive way; you kill yourself. You'd actually prefer to be gone. You would "clutch on" to others out of fear of being in the claws of something or someone yourself. The feeling of powerlessness in digesting your feelings leads to aggression. Did you experience your mentors as being dominant and hard, and are you now the same?

Trust in your own "I"-powers; bring yourself to realization in wisdom. Look closely inside yourself; healthy thinking power, critical and wise, solidity and sureness, under the Authority of your higher Consciousness. The wealth lies within you: don't look for it outside yourself. Create a beautiful, balanced, safe structure in your life; allow feelings to flow freely under the guarding eye of your clear mind. Left and right in balance, the "female" and the "male" aspect; don't suppress either! In warm love come to yourself; no longer leave yourself in the cold; no longer reject yourself. You are allowed to fully become yourself; express your feelings, don't shrink your existence. Push through your nature; show your Ego outwardly the way you feel inwardly, without complexes. Trust your intuition, your deepest Self.

In gentleness, come to yourself; don't be so hard and dominant with yourself. Be good to yourself and offer yourself full life! Organize your existence and become master over yourself; don't allow yourself to be flooded with it all.

Fourth lumbar vertebra

You don't resolutely choose *one* direction, your direction. You allow your life to be too dependent on others, on something outside yourself, because you experience yourself as too weak, too inferior. Emotionally you would like to throw yourself open in complete freedom and spontaneity — your nature and your body. Wanting to experience sensuality, but you place yourself with rationality and demands within a structure that is too tight; you restrict and constrict yourself too much. "This is how it has to be and no other way." You do this because you want to be accepted within a system or by a certain Authority outside yourself, or because you need affection, attention, appreciation with regard to your person, or just because you need to prove yourself in the area of Image, achievement, function, material prosperity, because you consider yourself for the rest a "Zero."

You constantly vacillate between two things; in unsureness, you bet on different horses, so that you absolutely won't fail.

You don't know after all who you really are; you are like a baby, a victim, you *let* others direct your life. You don't really determine your life; you don't allow your spontaneous active powers to really come through, nor your feelings; impulses and sensual longings are being suppressed. On the other hand you are angry because you don't dare to be yourself, because you are stuck with your feelings. Sometimes it seems as if you have no say over your own life. You are afraid of doing wrong; you will "claw" too strongly on to certain things in order to find sureness, but this doesn't bring you a solution. You are flexible; sometimes you bend with the wind in order to temporarily save yourself. You don't just go along on your life's path because you allow yourself to be constantly interrupted by others; you try to satisfy many people at the same time, actually out of self-interest. Possibly you were under strong dominant Authority in your childhood as a result of the negation of the authority in yourself. You remain stagnating in this "inferior" position; you don't really live from out of yourself. The Structure, the Authority, the Eye — which first of all is inside yourself — pushes you down; you don't live in harmony and honesty with yourself. You are stuck to the past with thoughts and memories; in an anxious way you try to secure yourself in life, on all kind of levels. You have so much difficulty in letting things go.

Feel yourself safe in the iron-strong structure of your Self and allow your feelings, your powers, to blossom spontaneously. Live from out of your Core; no compromises. No longer allow yourself to "be lived" in the condition of a victim, but choose and create your life's path yourself. Don't block your nature; listen to your longings, allow yourself to enjoy. Stop being the "child": you are strong, safe, and sheltered in the Authority of yourself. Settle yourself solidly with both feet on the earth and bring yourself to realization from within your inner calling and ambition; don't live according to the expectations and the Eye of the outer world. At all times be faithful to your nature; don't act, don't be afraid to clearly manifest your personal opinion. Don't cling to things or persons; let go of the past: get a hold of yourself, place all power inside yourself. Just be your ordinary self, without any qualms. Now place all values in your Self, not in things of secondary importance, not in what others say about you.

You are master over yourself, anything but a chameleon-like victim.

Be a forthright man/woman. Determine where you want to go and come to resolute self-manifestation. Surrender to your intuition, to what you feel, to spontaneous life, and stop your self-restriction.

Fifth lumbar vertebra

Because you don't have contact with your deepest, warm Source, because you feel so closed off from that which is most beautiful in you, from your heart, because you feel anxious and unsure, because you refuse to acknowledge the beauty in yourself and don't trust yourself — that's why you remain "stuck" and feel frustrated. It's as though you don't get any further. It only seems as if others are threatening you, as if they keep you prisoner, but it's your emotions, your anxieties and mistrust regarding yourself which block you. You restrict yourself in expression, in creativity; you'd sooner fret and worry than trust in your inner Self because you don't at all have good contact with your deepest Self. It's as if a band squeezes your head; it makes you angry, furious sometimes, this powerless unsureness. You underestimate yourself, and because of this you don't open yourself to intuition, to inner wisdom, to higher consciousness-energies. You'd nevertheless like to Break out, like a lion from its cage, because suppressed forces pile up. Unconsciously, you attract people who are a reflection of your convictions regarding yourself: therefore you are possibly not being treated and respected as you would like, because you don't respect yourself enough. Until you inwardly burst: "Now it has been enough!" With an axe you would

break the rope and make an end to the situation which you have allowed to drag on for too long. Possibly you allowed yourself to be treated like a donkey, because you considered yourself just a donkey. This self-degradation has weakened your body. All of a sudden aggressive powers are popping up: "You won't get me anymore!" You don't realize that it was your own feelings of inferiority, anxiety, and unsureness which finally caused you to be furious. You ache for liberation.

You are stuck with inner anger because you are cut off from the enlightening source in yourself; you shut joy out of your life. You no longer can enjoy the little, beautiful things in life, in nature. Thankfulness has made room for somber dissatisfaction because you reject yourself.

Listen to that gentle, wise, inner Source in yourself. The quiet light in you radiates warmth. Accept that beauty in yourself; in love come to yourself.

Look for all the power and truth in your deepest "I." Dare to surrender to the beauty of nature, to the most simple things, also in yourself. You are good and strong.

The source of joy lies in your heart; thankfulness for life, for the existence of your Self. You are safe and sheltered in that fundamentally strong Basis of your immortal Self. Allow those higher consciousness energies to open up by opening yourself up to that which is beautiful, by no longer fixating on the negative. Be gentle to yourself and offer yourself the full right to existence instead of restricting yourself! When the contact with your deepest Self is restored in harmony, then you will also experience much joy in new contacts with others. First heal the unity in yourself. If the basis of your life is love toward yourself, then your life course will lead to happiness and contentment. No greed, no clinging on to things or people, but lovingly offering yourself what you deserve, what's good for you, what brings you joy. Go onward on your path, without hesitating, self-aware and without fear!

SACRUM AND TAIL-BONE

Sacrum, ailments

On the one hand you would like to go full-steam ahead, on the other hand your feelings hold you back. You very much doubt your worth; you think yourself pitiful; you are too severe with your gentle feelings. You would like to rush ahead, without having said good-bye to certain emotional facts from the past.

You look at everything from below; you are stuck in yourself, in the inability to bring yourself to realization in a relaxed way, because your feelings of inferiority or doubt, and of powerlessness, hold you back. Sometimes this makes you enormously angry — sharp nervous aggression, an electric shock as it were — because you really long to escape from this blockage. On the one hand you hold on to the old and familiar in a way that is sometimes very anxious; on the other hand you might all of a sudden, with a strong radiating power like a cannonball, stand up for yourself, for your advancement.

But you feel clumsy; sometimes it's as if everything goes wrong, as if you can't get a grip on anything, as if everything slips out of your hands; you feel so nervous and angry in this condition of a "standstill." In your emotional life, there's a conflict, a dilemma, which asks for a solution. It seems as if you don't have control of your energies, as if you don't at all guide your consciousness powers; these powers can suddenly force themselves upon you. But you refuse to go onward, because you first have to clarify your feelings.

Your chair is empty: where is your Conscious, unique, worthy "I"? In this absence, in this unsureness, you hold on to the familiar, but your Self calls for evolution!

The inner battle in you can only be solved by listening to your deepest emotions; don't be severe and hard with your feelings, but open yourself up to them, work things out, and then let go of the past. There's no use in wanting to fly on toward a future if you don't come to a solution for yourself in the Present moment. Don't run ahead of yourself, but dare to calmly take action in a certain rhythm, without overlooking your feelings.

Follow your intuition; in the acknowledgement of your worthiness you will be able to steadily go onward. Discover those pure consciousness powers in you, in every fiber of your body: they are being directed by your self-aware "I." If you degrade yourself, you don't get anywhere, your body won't be fed by those forces, you will feel yourself left out in the cold: because you refuse to make contact with that deep, warm source in you, with your heart, with your deepest Self. Become master over yourself and bundle your feelings together so they can cooperate in unification and unanimity. Say goodbye to the past; allow your feelings and your powers to come through in a flexible and self-assured way: in this awareness of your values you will again get a grip on yourself; you will no longer provoke any "setbacks," "clumsiness" or "accidents," because now there will be a free, supple flow of energies, without hindrances. So allow your Conscious "I" to take up its place; after all it was this absence that caused you anxieties, frustrations, and nervousness. Only in the Fullness of your being can you go onward: therefore place the crown on your head!

Tail-bone, ailments

You don't experience yourself as being unified; you see things black/white in yourself and in others. In this way you experience a kind of duality in yourself: dark-light, rationality-feelings, conscious-unconscious — and it is difficult for you to unify these elements inside you because you hold on to false, unauthentic values. You hold on to many things because you don't build your life on the Authority and the safe basis of yourself.

You can screen yourself off from your emotional world with self-willed rationality; you stare into the distance without solving the emotional problems of the Now. You don't listen to your intuition, to your deepest Self: you look at norms and values outside yourself, at the social "Caste" to which you belong, at religion or systems. Your outer ego possibly wants to shine; you behave as if you are greatly protected and safe in your ostentatious or proud behavior, in outward show, in a function. But here you actually put on a false front, because you feel like a prisoner. You anxiously hold in emotions, hold on to a situation that you have been fed up with for a long time; you take on an attitude which sometimes makes you sick. You betray your own nature, your true disposition, because you actually think yourself weak and insecure. Your being is sometimes cold as ice, because you don't lovingly acknowledge yourself, who you are. You poison yourself in a false life; you will attract false "friends." You close yourself off from love toward yourself, toward others. This unauthenticity can estrange you, isolate you from yourself, from others. You deny your true Self! In this way you plant yourself in a sterile place in the desert. Fruitfulness, productivity, and active self-realization are not allowed unless they are at the service of your Unauthentic, superficial world. You are blind to that which is original, to the intuitive, to true sureness, which you will find in your deepest Self. You think you are not good enough: so you try to be "someone." You fly high in the air with your nose up, but you don't feel the solid ground beneath your feet. Sometimes you flee from yourself. Sometimes because of this you receive blows in life that make you end up with your feet on the ground — so that you are obliged to enter into a confrontation with your honest Self.

It is very hard for you to let go of things, especially because you build your safety on elements outside you. Sometimes you are really angry with yourself because you allow yourself to be flattened, because you don't dare to be yourself. Sometimes you vent this anger on others.

Acknowledge the SUN in yourself: that self-aware power, not the exterior, tinsel, fake gold.

Discover that rich, warm energy source in yourself and allow energies and emotions to escape freely. No longer hold on; let go of that which is not really good for you.

True safety lies within you; stand solidly with both feet on the ground and become aware of your worth. Come to unity and peace in yourself; follow your spontaneous impulses, your intuition; every human being has his natural rhythm. So don't force yourself into too-tight a social straitjacket. Everyone has his unique nature: be faithful to your Self. Place the authority in yourself; know yourself to be protected, and allow the poison to escape. Don't try to prove yourself to an outer world, but grow from within. It's what you feel that matters, not the impression you make on others. Allow the male and female elements in you to come to harmony: in this unity you will feel good and sheltered. There's only one hold that is strong enough to last, and that is your inner Self. Let go of other illusionary grips and go onward!

VERTIGO, DIZZINESS

An exaggerated quantity of impressions, of information, of details, etc., goes around in your head. Moreover, you resist seeing the truth regarding yourself.

You have opened yourself up too strongly to thoughts, ideas or spiritual experiences: a chaotic mixing-pot. You can go in many possible directions, but you don't see *which one* is your true path because you float in the clouds, hanging with your feet dangling above the ground, lost in "thought" and dizzy.

You were a hollow vat; you didn't find sureness in yourself; your basis was lost; you listened to everything but to your own inner wisdom: then you filled yourself up with a lot of thoughts and knowledge from books and people. . . .

Because of this you are now at odds with yourself: you are looking to evade in order to not be obliged to truly evolve. Thus, you get entangled in a network, a web, of trifles and inanities; you have fled into a labyrinth. Don't run away from yourself! The true core of your being lies in your Heart, in the love for yourself here on earth and not somewhere in the sky or in your thoughts.

Love and trust yourself: there lies the solution. Stop fleeing into your head, into your far-off dreams or foggy thoughts.

Get both feet on the Earth. Allow the earthly aspect and the "spiritual" aspect to come to conciliation with each other. No longer fight against your gentle evolution — don't keep yourself imprisoned in your head in a tough way! Open your eyes and try to gain a clear view of yourself.

First consciously find yourself, rooted in your own basis; then calmly be open to others and, depending on your resolute choice, assimilate or reject.

Don't immobilize yourself by, in self-negation, giving up your place to a merry-go-round in the fog. Inner wisdom: on the basis of this you can make your choices with determination! Don't let yourself be over-powered; become Master over yourself, and resolutely lead from out of your inner, essential, Secure basis!

VOCAL CORDS

Aphonia
loss or absence of voice; only able to whisper

The powerlessness to be yourself, to manifest yourself the way you inwardly feel. For as long as you think yourself to be "guilty" and "bad," with as a result that you also experi-ence the outer world as "bad" or "threatening," it is better that you don't speak but first come to thorough self-contemplation. Unconscious feelings of guilt.

Because you are stuck with the inner conviction that you are small and vulnerable, that you have to be on guard, have to sneak quietly around on the earth so as not to be "seized," so no one might hear you — you will attract situations in life which will confirm these negative expectations.

You feel like a child that doesn't really have a say in its life; you don't really dare stand up for yourself because Anxiety tightens up your throat. Inside you is that inner conflict: "Shall I participate in earthly life or shall I withdraw behind the curtains at a safe distance?" Sometimes you feel guilty, and then again you are mad at the world and you prefer to stay out of it. You think you have no right to an existence of your own; you walk quietly, afraid to get "caught." You don't dare to be YOURSELF spontaneously, the way you feel inwardly, because you are afraid you are not "good," afraid others will condemn you. You don't offer yourself enough warmth and love! You bring yourself into question too much: "Am I allowed to do this or not?" You don't live enough from out of your heart and longings; you make your life too dependent on "what others might say," or "how they might react."

Take up your full space and breathe with your lungs opened wide: you are allowed to exist and to be the way you are. Change the conviction that you or humanity are "bad" or "guilty." Every individual is unique and needs to come to Insight.

Everyone is allowed to be who he or she is naturally. So-called evil is only a result of self-suppression and of a lack of Insight. Learn your lessons from the past and let bygones be bygones. Now become aware of the fact that every human being creates his reality: if you approach your life in an anxious way, you hinder the growth and break-through of your "I." Don't be disturbed by criticism, nor by expectations of others regarding you.

Feel welcome on earth and sound out love for yourself and your fellow men. Life is not black and threatening: people will only approach you in a negative way as long as you reject yourself or don't allow yourself to participate in life, as long as you consider life to be black. You are allowed to be there! Dare to manifest yourself the way you feel inside; become yourself, without anxieties, so that your feelings of powerlessness can disappear too.

Hoarseness

Two conflicting powers in you: "Shall I say it or not? Shall I stand up for myself or do I stay closed? Shall I really show myself the way I am, or do I completely adapt myself to others?" Do you not dare to be really faithful to your true nature? Do you stay closed? Do you not dare to one hundred per cent bring forward your deepest feelings, your true opinion — because of fear?

You feel too weak or too powerless, at the mercy of others. You feel "stuck": your "I" is tied down.

You don't assume your full space. Why don't you manifest yourself to the fullest, the way you feel inside? Is it because you fear losing the love or approval of others? Emotional attachment? Letting your sense of emotional well-being depend too much on others? Your life is built too much on artificial structures, on norms or thinking patterns which don't really go well with your nature; you lean on others instead of on your own strong Basis. You don't believe in the Power of your deepest Self. You *let* yourself "be lived" too much. Your rational mind and your feelings don't live in an harmonious balance: you don't listen enough to what you feel, to your body, to your intuition. Possibly you limit your life too much by living "reasonably, properly, and sensibly," according to the expectations of the outer world! Powerless to be your Self, to manifest yourself as an autonomous "I," independent of others.

Grounding: grow up solidly out of your own roots and don't bend too much, so that you don't deviate from the direction that is in accord with your true nature. You need to play first violin in your life. You can calmly depend on your Self if you just carry your heart in your head, if your thoughts and structures are carried by love. Pull yourself up with your own powers. Don't be afraid to completely be yourself. Say what you have to say. Give yourself all the space you need! Don't be limited by others; fully and freely live your life and your being the way you are, and don't force yourself into a tense state of being in order to conceal yourself from others or to satisfy the expectations of others. Push yourself through! Allow yourself to be born; come into harmony with yourself: don't make compromises that rape your nature, that neglect your "I." You are good the way you are; in honest openness manifest your deepest nature. Don't let others rule your life; self-respect! Liberate yourself from this self-limitation.

Inflammation of the vocal cords
laryngitis

Powerless anger. Unsureness, lack of self-confidence. You don't trust your deepest Self: anxiety. You hide your true core, your thoughts and your feelings: you are stuck, and you don't dare allow your inner energies to flow through freely. You keep yourself closed up tightly, doubting your worth; you think you have to protect yourself against the outer world and so you enclose yourself in a cocoon so that no one can really get to you. Anxious and frightened sometimes, you might run away from the world, from others. Inwardly there's that urge to push yourself through, to bring yourself to realization, to make yourself count outwardly, but you don't dare to — you feel too small and vulnerable. You don't trust the power of your feelings, your emotions; you are afraid of them and don't integrate them into your existence. Sometimes it seems as if you are at a distance from your own nature. Without this experience of unity in yourself, you of course experience yourself as "powerless." If you don't completely acknowledge your inner Authority, then it is possible that you have no authority — over your children for instance. If you experience yourself as so powerless inside, then you might attract situations in daily life in which you get angry with others: because you are not being acknowledged as an authority.

It is possible that as a child you experience a powerless fury because you can't be yourself yet; perhaps you enter into aggressive opposition to an authority outside you.

Inability to transform inner powers into actual self-realization; anger because of this frustration.

Self-confidently sail on in the open sea! No longer block your energies; acknowledge your worth and your possibilities, the beautiful power plant in you. Choose autonomy and self-realization. Allow yourself to grow in joy and trust. Don't hold yourself back: allow your feelings and your creative powers to blossom. Don't doubt.

All power over yourself actually lies inside your Self: don't turn away from this; bring yourself to realization! Don't allow your life to be dependent on others, but dare to openly manifest your unique personality, which you are. You don't have to resist anything or anyone if you acknowledge the Authority of your Self.

Vocal cord nodules
"singer's nodes"

Frustration. You feel stuck in a tight pattern, and you want to get out of it, but you can't or you dare not. In a stubborn way you say to yourself — or allow yourself to be dictated to by others — "It shall, and it must!" You lead a life that is too hard on you. Outwardly you might appear stalwart and shining, but inwardly you feel sad, afraid, and powerless. You don't really show yourself the way you feel inside. You don't really live your spontaneity, your nature to the full; you feel un-

able to *really* be yourself; sometimes you ask yourself, "Who am I?" Because you are able to hide yourself very well behind an outer role! In this inner division a revolt grows. On the one hand you feel anxious and unsure in yourself and therefore don't really live the way you would like to; on the other hand you get angry about this powerlessness. You might direct this anger at others: you will blame them instead of admitting that your feelings of dissatisfaction are caused by powerlessness to be yourself. Are you condemning your gentle, sensitive side? Do you think you are not good the way you *are* and would you prefer to show yourself different from the way you are? Are you afraid you don't satisfy the expectations of the public or of an authority "above" you? Are you so afraid others will hurt you or pull you down? With such an attitude to life you will attract situations that will make it clear to you that it is high time you listen to your inner voice, no longer to the voice of an outer or superficial "I," which looks for self-affirmation in the outer world. Possibly you were hit in the "face" as an Image, and you are angry about it.

Feel warm and safe in yourself and don't hold things in; don't allow yourself to be restricted: dare to be YOURSELF in a spontaneous, natural way, the way you feel inside, without violating yourself, without forcing yourself or suppressing the impulses inside you. Speak for yourself; don't put up a false front. Express your talents, sing lustily, in a natural way, no longer forcing yourself into a tight framework in order to satisfy certain norms or people. Live your life to the full, stand up for yourself. Transform suppressed aggressive forces into actual self-manifestation, but no longer for the "eye" of people. Come into harmony, into peace with yourself, no longer fight against your pure nature: now acknowledge your gentleness, the small, sensitive child inside you and, full of love, press it against you. Make deep contact with yourself instead of rejecting, suppressing or violating that which is gentle and loving in you.

You don't have to put up an Image. You don't have to satisfy the expectations of others. Acknowledge the command of your inner Authority, the everlasting core, and allow feelings, powers, and talents to discharge themselves spontaneously, no longer anxiously wondering if you are "good."

You are good if you don't violate your nature! Sing life out loud!

VOMITING, QUEASINESS

You can't digest certain experiences. You refuse to accept "new things" or to assimilate them in yourself. Your stomach, your solar plexus, would radiate joyfully like a sun if you would acknowledge your own authority and take command, resolutely choosing your straight path and going onward without hesitation! That is gold: knowing who you are in self-respect, and being faithful to your nature. But you are too scared to be yourself! Sometimes we unconsciously call up other people pointing out certain things to us — to which, however, we close our eyes. We remain stuck in insignificant details or side-tracks, which clearly keep us from the inner goal we have planned for ourselves. Your conscious "I" can't always grasp this, or rather: you still resist; you stubbornly hold on to old things and refuse to follow your intuition, nor do you listen to the words of people who actually bring your inner calling to the fore.

Whenever someone starts to talk about it, it makes you puke: in fact you are nauseated at your own powerlessness to go your new path with consistency. Listen to those who hold your feelings and thoughts up to you like a mirror, and come to self-examination. Then resolutely speak from out of your deepest "I." You feel powerless, unable — you are afraid of not being able to handle new things: you vomit when again confronted with this crossroads (past-future).

You can't hear it anymore! You are sick and tired of it! You feel forced by others, by mentors, to go in *one* certain direction. Although this goes against your nature, you don't yet feel able to fully manifest yourself; you feel unsure. You are sick of their admonitions; you are sick of your own powerlessness. You don't feel able fully to get a hold of your life and direct it yourself.

Don't be anxious about the future; allow new things to come to you in a flexible way, and don't resist. Calmly contemplate. Never feel obligated. Build up everything at your tempo. Chop off the branch that is rotten, and get a hold of the tree trunk. Feel supported by your own powerful Self and cherish the treasure inside you: no longer refuse to get very close to yourself. No longer follow the paths of tinsel and fake gold, but follow only that path in which you feel: "Here, I can be completely myself. This I want to offer myself as a golden treasure because I love myself." Then all resistance will break down, all anxiety will disappear, and you will be able to assimilate calmly everything that comes to you now. Allow innovation into your life; come to thankful acceptance. . . Joyfully perform your tasks yourself, so that no one else has to admonish you (parents, children.)

Vomiting during pregnancy

The new situation overpowers you. Still too little awareness of your own forces; you feel unsure: "Can I handle it?" Unconsciously you still push it a little away from you. Too little do you realize your own powers. This situation can confront you with your feelings of doubt and powerlessness. So, become master over yourself: first and foremost make yourself lovingly welcome; only then the baby won't be an (unconscious) threat to your own existence. Feel safely accepted inside yourself, then you can also calmly accept the little one and offer it a place in your shelter.

(Also read Vomiting.)

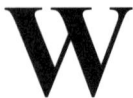

WARTS
benign skin excrescences

In general

You don't really dare to show who you *are;* you hide; possibly you are ashamed of yourself, of your feelings, of your body. "I'm not able to do it anyway; I'm just a. . . ." The warts take up the place of your Self: you don't dare to come to the fore, to show yourself the way you inwardly feel. You withdraw in thoughts, in a sometimes unreal, dreamy sphere, in a spiritual world; you lose contact with reality. You are ashamed of that small sensitive child inside you; it's as if you are constantly apologizing for the behavior of that sensitive aspect in you. You see yourself as a wilted flower; you undervalue yourself and because of that you often feel like you are not understood, not accepted by others. You actually don't have a real insight into yourself, no real contact with your own deepest "I," with the fundamental basis of your person; you don't believe in yourself. You don't *really* manifest yourself; you are closed up inside yourself, cut off from your safe Basis. You don't feel safe in yourself; you look for a hold in others or in a certain role, or in a function you do. A feeling of frustration, an inability to come to actual self-realization. Great, warm heart energies want to come through, but you hold them back, because you are not really lovingly open to yourself; you don't dare to offer your feelings to yourself, nor to show them to oth-

ers. Too many unused creative energies are looking for their way, but are being blocked.

You don't dare to take up your space; you look at what others, the group, the family or society, expect from you instead of really living according to your true disposition, your spontaneous nature. But in your unsureness, in your unstable search, in your loneliness, sometimes in panicky anxiety and nervousness, you are searching for yourself, for the door in which your key fits. It's as if this world is new and strange for you: because you don't really descend into yourself, because you still live too ethereally, because you don't stand with your feet on the ground and demand your own unique, individual space. As long as you doubt yourself — as long as you look for an anchor outside yourself, as long as you place the lock for your key outside you, as long as you don't trust your own powerful Basis — warts can develop and grow.

You feel so vulnerable; you are afraid of being hurt; you stay deep in your little hole, but in the meantime inner powers, emotions, and creative energies urge for a breakthrough. You become angry because of this frustration; you become angry with those people on whom you lean. It is possible that as a child you have attracted a milieu in which you don't feel at home; you cannot, or dare not, be yourself. The more reason to build as quickly as possible upon your Self. You think, dream, and fret too much; you don't trust your intuition.

Fear of death, of loneliness, of being rejected — because you think yourself to be ugly or bad. But especially: not totally taking possession of yourself, of your body. You don't yet live FULLY from out of yourself, from out of your true "I."

The Key to Self-Liberation, Christiane Beerlandt © Beerlandt Publications

Look for contact with that safe, nourishing Maternal Source in your Self! Dare to truly Live, here and now. Now allow yourself to be truly born; express yourself, and "scream" if you want to. Get both feet on the ground, and teach yourself how to walk on the basis of your intuition. Warts disappear gradually, or all of a sudden, when you take up your central space, when you dare to manifest yourself the way you really are, without anxieties. Every human being is good and unique, regarding the inner and the outer being: be faithful to your nature and don't look at expectations nor at criticism or condemnation of others. Don't follow the principles/norms of your mentors, of your teacher, but of Your inner Self. Listen to Your longings: discover Your possibilities in the creativity of life itself, and NO LONGER HIDE YOURSELF! Don't look for refuge in dreams or hallucinations, but in the shelter of your deepest Self. You may always know that you are protected in this immortal part of yourself. Let the ejection seat fly up; surrender to your spontaneous feelings; don't put a check on yourself with thoughts and doubts: now be faithful to your nature and allow yourself to blossom. Be good to yourself; experience the Peace in yourself; allow restlessness and self-demolition to make room for respect and love toward your original Self. EXPERIENCE YOURSELF 100%!

COME OUT OF YOUR HIDING PLACE! Fully living from out of your true self, without reserve, in healthy pride!

Warts on the face
(See also Warts, in general)

More than any other body part, the face has to do with "coming outward." You suffocate yourself in norms and social rules, in "this is how it has to be," in a tight structure. You constantly force yourself because you fight an inner battle with your true Nature. This nature does not, after all, get a chance to breathe freely. You camouflage yourself; you put on a mask. You want, for instance, to appear as a sterile holy person, while inwardly your powers are boiling up like a volcano that wishes to spout out its productivity.

It "has to be" this way; you carry needless burdens; you force your feelings by not really listening to yourself. You are angry with yourself; you have to satisfy this or that, but you never succeed at being "ideal." Your heart can't radiate love as long as you bottle up aggressive powers, as long as you consider yourself good only under certain conditions. Do you think yourself to be ugly, inadequate? Do you hit yourself on the head in self-punishment? Then, you will also spit venom on others. Energies are pushing in order to be liberated, but you constantly put a damper on them because you "obligate" yourself to meet this or that criterion. You hide your gentle feelings, your "femininity," behind a too-hard "male" mask. You kill the spontaneous child in yourself. Your heart hurts because you don't acknowledge your worth. You will cling to someone else in order to get something to hold on to, because you don't really experience yourself as being safe and protected. That's why it is necessary for you that others acknowledge you, and that you play your act for this. You suffocate yourself in this way; your feelings are being drawn tight; you give yourself insufficient space. Suppressed emotions reach for a lifesaver.

Be YOURSELF, not only your Outer Ego. Listen to those spontaneous powers, to the feelings in yourself. Manifest yourself; you are good the way you are. No longer try to satisfy the expectations of the outer world, but experience your nature.

Free yourself from your armor; make contact with your true, deepest Self.

Don't live according to rusted, sclerotic habits, to ossified rituals, to obligations and norms, but follow your intuition, your original longings. Respect your unique being; become aware of your worth and just be yourself.

No longer frustrate yourself; express your feelings; arrive at authentic self-expression.

No human being is ugly; in this respect, norms are totally wrong. You are you: don't betray yourself.

Warts on the hands, fingers
(See also Warts, in general)

You feel targeted: you are so afraid or ashamed that people might look at you, might condemn or hurt you. Unsureness; you'd prefer to hide.

You feel ugly, at the mercy of others, powerless. You think you are not good at all; you even have the feeling that others muzzle you, but it is you who doesn't dare to stand up for yourself. They are on top of you, "because I'm just a . . ." But it is you who destroys yourself and provokes reactions from people, as a result of your inner convictions regarding yourself. Do you think there's a little devil inside you? Are you condemning yourself? Then you will attract people who will make remarks regarding this. Powerless to be yourself: angry because of this powerlessness.

Freely show your hands, openly, and say, "Yes, that IS ME, indeed." Allow those beautiful, healthy energies to come through; stop considering yourself as negative. Make yourself welcome in the security, in the warmth, of your Self! Accept yourself completely, the way you are; be faithful to your nature, not to that which society or others expect from you. Dare to be yourself, body and soul.

You are unique in your way, and that's good. Don't be angry with yourself, nor with others: place in yourself all power and authority over you. Only you can tell yourself what to do.

Warts on the sole of the foot
(See also Warts, in general)

The way a bottle with a message is thrown into the sea is how you unconsciously call out, "Help! I am drowning in my emotions, in my powerlessness, in my frustrations, in my anger."

Unsure, unstable basis, searching, getting no grip on yourself, looking for a hold in others. Because you don't really dare to be yourself, you hide, unsure or ashamed, behind a Role you play. No matter if you play the role of the good Santa Claus, of Zorro, or Napoleon, it's about an unauthentic presence; your true nature stays hidden. You don't know what to do with your feelings; you don't dare to manifest them. Possibly, you feel ugly or inferior and play the role that others expect from you. You don't at all lean on your own solid foundations. You'd rather fret and dream than stand with your feet in reality, because emotionally it is all too heavy for you. You get angry because you cannot, or dare not, be yourself; inwardly, you resist people who don't understand You, who expect something from you that is not at all in your nature. You are closed; you hide; you live frustratedly, with piled-up energies and creative possibilities. You feel yourself to be in a twisted, unbalanced, "clumsy" situation because on the one hand aggressive energies are pushing to break through, and on the other hand you don't dare to do anything but remain in your shell.

You are too afraid to show your real feelings because you experience yourself as vulnerable, and you want to protect yourself — because you place too much power in others and their judgment and how they look at you. The anxiety of not being good enough; the anxiety of failing, of being mocked.

Possibly, you don't at all feel at home in your body; possibly you think your body is ugly, and you try to protect yourself against judgments and condemnations. You can become very angry about this: a fury directed toward yourself and toward those who "might" not accept you the way you are. You experience yourself as a loose, crumbling, structural disaster. You lean on something or someone outside yourself.

Feel that powerful "I"-center and show yourself in all Openness the way you inwardly feel! Be faithful to your nature; first turn lovingly toward yourself and don't bother about reactions or expectations from others. Dare to resolutely step into the adventure of life; hereby count on your solid foundation, on your everlasting, Living Self. No longer hide yourself; you are good and unique in your way, the way you ARE. What don't you dare do? Of what are you ashamed? Do you think that being "sensitive" means being weak? No. Arrive at clear insight into yourself, into your possibilities, into your emotional powers, which are the true source of your creativity and joy in life! Now openly radiate, like the sun-center in yourself; believe in those deep powers and emotions inside you; transform aggression into healthy action! Don't expect others to understand you, but first listen to yourself. If you live the way you inwardly feel; if you come out with your feelings and your talents, then you will attract those people who are more important to you than anyone else. Frustration is the result of the suppression of one's own longings, of the suppression of action and self-realization: stand up for your true Self. No longer remain underwater! Stand broadly and solidly on your own feet; take up your living space and no longer put yourself away.

WEEPING AT THE SLIGHTEST CONTACT WITH UNPLEASANTNESS

You barely have contact with the deepest foundation inside yourself; you place yourself under the Authority of Something or Someone. In this state you don't experience yourself as being safe in yourself. Also in relationships, you'll lose yourself in exaggerated attachment, because you don't really build on your Self. Fundamental anxieties, as if the sword hangs forever above your head. You allow yourself to "be lived"; you don't really evolve out of yourself. You feel threatened by everything and everyone, by the slightest thing, because you are so cut off from your Living Self. You mistrust the possibilities of every human being to create his own life himself. You place your little personality completely under the Authority of your parents, your teacher, etc. You melt away under the mantle of something or someone, of a teaching or a doctrine. You deny the Autonomy of yourself. A discovery of your unique worthiness is necessary — a discovery of your inner Powers, of your abilities to establish your uniqueness in life in a self-aware way. No longer experiencing yourself as the lesser being, the subordinate or the servant. You are king in your kingdom, just the way every other person is. Now, place both feet firmly on the ground. Show what you have inside.

By crying you can ask for attention, but it would be much better for you if you gain attention by unfolding your talents. Possibly, you've been struggling against the wind for a long time, trying to hold on to a conduct that would be better to let go of. You belittle yourself; you are convinced of being just a drum to be rapped upon. Now, fill your existence with Yourself and respect your own being!

Don't turn away from the fundamental essence of Life itself: endless Joy.

No longer make yourself believe that you are "small and weak."

WHITLOW

Suppression. An inner battle. You want peace with yourself and with everyone, but an inner aggression wells up; you would like to go to war in order to free yourself from the feeling of imprisonment. You feel like a martyr; you would yell and roar (mostly inwardly) in order to free yourself from the feeling of being stuck. You yourself hold on to certain people, with a feeling of powerlessness, and allow yourself to be held on to by others.

You are like the limp leaves of a weeping willow, which are cut off from their solid trunk and roots, you sorrow and you don't make contact with your deepest Self. There's no question of real consolation or rescue in yourself, because you ignore the essence of your being. You feel like a small person facing the enormous ocean; you fixate on certain things and people in order to feel you have a hold somewhere.

You fixate with your thoughts while you force your emotions to stay within certain limits; you would like to push away your feelings and often also your body and its natural longings. You even detest a part of yourself, sometimes it makes you vomit — you would like to push it far away from you; like a devil who sticks onto you. . . .

Suppression of the forces of self-realization can bring about either strong sexual desires, or a disgust about your sexuality, or both. Instead of freely experiencing your content, your total emotional world, you repress them within a rigid structure. Still, you have the frustrated feeling that someone penetrates your personal terrain, that someone "seizes" you, that someone hurts you — because you don't mark off your domain enough as an individual! On the one hand, you long for self-liberation and would rebel with piled-up aggression and defending nails; on the other hand you feel so powerless and lonely in yourself. . . .

Rid yourself of your handcuffs: in this way you don't only free yourself, but also your partner, your surroundings. Feel the power in yourself and become aware of your powerful creative possibilities: clearly border

your terrain — until here and no further — but allow warmth, love, and gentleness to flow freely; don't grab on to something or someone.

Free yourself from all self-restricting structures and obstacles: throw yourself into life with complete spontaneity; don't keep your nature hidden; trust these life energies. Seek contact with your deep, Living Self and conduct, create, your life in the direction you wish. You are powerful over yourself; no longer deny this! Nothing can threaten you. Now open the prison doors and meet the sun of Self-Confidence and Worth in you!

WORMS, INTESTINAL PARASITES, IN GENERAL
(See also Tapeworm)

You direct your attention, your spotlights, too much at people and things (possessions, money . . .) outside yourself instead of experiencing yourself in the Center. You are angry and discontented with yourself, but you will blame it on others; you place too much Authority in others instead of placing all power over yourself inside yourself. Because of powerlessness, you would like to "run away" from yourself, angrily running away like a child who's been bad.

You feel not really safe in yourself, not really in unity. You'd rather flee from yourself than take up your complete space. You are actually in conflict with yourself and, as a result, also in conflict with your surroundings. You take distance from yourself too much because you don't really believe in the value of your personal Content. Possibly, you have a big mouth; then you are silent and run away from yourself. You leave an empty chair behind, which can be taken by a visitor. You are not really on your own terrain; you constantly go over your borders; you look for security and confirmation outside yourself, in others. This empty powerlessness makes you angry; you withdraw, as it were, from your earthly body; you surrender the power to the Visitor, the parasite.

In this situation, certain people treat their body in a cold, negative, rejecting, and critical way, just as they do to their surroundings. Do you experience yourself as being so "empty" that you need to "FILL" your life with false values, material things, money, or more spiritual things? Do you feel like a "victim"? Do you feel in the "grip" of something or someone? Do you yourself seize for "Power"?

Don't allow yourself to be parasitized, nor should you parasitize others.

Come back inside yourself! Sweep up the dirt in your own house, not in your neighbor's. Aim the spotlights at your own Core; no longer aim them outward. Look inside yourself and discover your Worth, your Content! Place all power over your life in yourself; cherish your body. Unification in yourself leads to acceptance and reconciliation with your surroundings. Pure, agreeable communication with your fellow man will follow if you first lovingly make contact with yourself! Don't run away angrily, but participate fully in the joyful coming to be of your earthly Self. Warm your home and make it cozy for yourself. You are naturally protected in yourself if you take up your space full of self-confidence.

If children are concerned here, then the above-mentioned causes will sometimes apply to the mentor(s), too. Psychological influence intensifies the original susceptibility of the baby. Therefore, the mentor will have to solve these Causes in himself or herself. In this way, both will help each other.

WRIST

Psychological correspondence

Do we move smoothly and flexibly through life? A healthy wrist represents the balance in us: the gentle harmonious feeling, the peace we feel when we glide along flexibly in that life-direction which goes best with our natural disposition.

Lovingly and gently bending toward yourself and others.

The balance between, on the one hand, flexibility, compliance, receptivity, and the adaptability, and on the other hand the resolute, self-assured, solid, structured. The "male" and the "female" aspects in balance. Not too limp-feeble, not too rigid-stern.

On the one hand allowing your feelings to supply flow through, and on the other hand being master over these emotions in a self-aware way. The balance of being flexible toward others and still resolutely daring to be yourself.

The ease with which we allow in new impressions, and then let them go again; daring to look in many directions and not fixating yourself on one point.

Ailments of the wrist, in general

Too pliable, too mobile or too stiff, too recalcitrant. You allow yourself to be influenced too much by others; you let yourself be sat on; emotions overpower you; you completely sag; you are like a rag, without a backbone.

Or, conversely: you only look in one direction; you are stubborn, stiff-necked, and rigid. You constrict yourself in a structure that is too tight; you don't allow any relaxation or joy. You are hard and unbendable. Or are you too accommodating?

Are you *too* attached or *too* authoritarian?

In general do you refuse to open yourself up to the opinion of others, or is it you who trims your sails to the wind? Do you not allow any feelings, any flexible creativity into your life? Or can you never say "no" to others? Do you look for problems where there are none, or do you actually refuse to look at emotional problems and work them out? Resistance as a result of fear? On the one hand, a healthy wrist asks for self-assuredness, decisiveness, standing up for yourself, and on the other hand flexibility and easy maneuverability: harmonious cooperation of Power and gentleness.

X, Y, Z

XENOPHOBIA, RACIAL HATRED

You lead a "double life": on the one hand outwardly, and on the other hand deep in your heart. The anxious doe in the armor of a Lion.

You feel restricted in your life, frustrated, be it unconsciously. You are being pushed to the side as it were, or you think that others kick you out of the pen like a little pig; you feel hurt, rejected, sad, lonely, full of inability, often inferior and not much loved. For these reasons, you will, as a reaction, also want to push aside or hurt those who, just like you, feel rejected and suppressed. It's an expression of anxiety and POWERLESS-NESS; you are not getting a grip on yourself; in revolt to this you would reach for power over others. Inwardly you feel threatened. Anxious. But what seems most threatening to you are your own feelings, your emotions, your anxieties. The little, gentle child that lives in every human heart asks for attention and love, asks to be allowed to spontaneously and freely be itself, but you suppress it in a hard way! How hard you are on yourself. He who doesn't first offer himself understanding and love won't offer it to others either. Actually you don't think yourself beautiful at all; you rather experience yourself as inferior.

Just as you feel inferior, you will mock "those whom you consider inferior." Just as you experience yourself as ugly and dark, you will taunt those whom you consider "dark people." It's just an expression of SELF-HATE. Why do you hate yourself so? Was your upbringing directed to achievements and ambition, to appearing beautiful and strong to the outer world? But did you miss the most beautiful feeling (love)? You actually feel handicapped, never good and strong enough. You feel the need to find Self-Affirmation in your surroundings; like a roaring lion allegedly fighting for an ideal, you carry on in a destructive way. Actually you proclaim an ideal like a clown, but inwardly you laugh and joke about it yourself. As long as you can stand out and prove yourself as being a real man or woman, you feel satisfied. Because you are suffocating yourself with your hard mask, you also want to rob others of the freedom to be themselves. It is high time that you free yourself, that you dare to be yourself, from out of your heart, that you no longer degrade yourself and humanity.

The earth belongs to everyone. Great is he who discovers his own goodness. Now offer yourself the love and attention you so need, so that this also will cast its fruits upon the world outside you.

YAWNING, EXAGGERATED

Signal of self-protection: "Stop, it's been enough!" (tired, bored, sick, etc.). Or you ask too much of yourself; you see things so big that it might overpower you; it can also be an outer defense against something or someone who might get too strong a grip on you.

Perhaps you don't feel yourself "big" enough yet, not awake or ready to receive certain experiences. Are you too absent? Are you not completely present in yourself, in a concentrated way, and therefore don't feel able to allow certain things or people to come to you?

It is necessary that you allow your life to exist on a very solid and large basis in order to calmly receive all possible impressions, to integrate them or discard them as you wish. In this way you don't have to offer resistance to a lot of healthy energies which wish to enter you. Arrive at conciliation, in unity with yourself; in this way you won't ward off others as being too much. Don't live "unauthentically," but strongly concentrated in yourself; come to a warm-hearted presence in yourself. Put yourself to rest when you are tired; take another turn when you are on the wrong track: "Don't fight against yourself."

No compromises.

YAWS
tropical infectious disease

Not in the least believing in your worth as a human being. You close yourself off completely, so that no one might see you. You close the shutters, are ashamed of yourself. The difficulties, the emotional burdens, weigh heavily; you think you must have deserved this. You are silent, you droop; you don't want to have anything to do with anything or anyone. You wreck yourself, drilling yourself into the ground, as it were. You also shun communication with others because you have no contact with your deepest Self after all. "Who am I?"

People with these kinds of heavy, oppressive, negative convictions attract circumstances in life which confirm this. Becoming aware is the only way out. Becoming aware of the pride and the possibilities of the creative human being. Making one's way out of this unconscious, hellish state of sleep. The human being needs to discover its divinity: the possibility to change its world, to take its own life in hand. Away with Destiny and Fatalism or with punishing gods.

ZINC
Deficiency, insufficient assimilation of

Not spontaneously trusting your feelings; rather submitting them to the critical, the rational mind. Outer or material security give certainty and something to hold on to in this state of inner emotional mistrust. Anxiously screening off the most sensitive aspect of yourself because you don't have clear insight into it. Because of this you are busy in an exaggerated way with structures, your clothing, your documents, etc. You can't trustfully surrender to your safe, deepest Self. You don't give yourself in a spontaneous way to your feelings, your intuition, your Self. "First I will have to think about it."

Inwardly you tighten your fists, but you don't get any further; your powerlessness irritates you.

Anxieties, self-destructive tendencies. You want to be ready for the harm that might strike all of a sudden; sometimes you experience something devilish in Yourself. You are convinced that a human being has to stay on guard against the negative in himself.

You are at a distance from a part of yourself, mostly also from your body, from your sexual organs. You "observe" yourself. You look in the mirror, but you keep dwelling too much on the exterior order of things, so that you might feel safer inwardly. In the meantime you kill your Nature, your feelings, the child inside you, your spontaneity.

It seems as if your head, your spiritual awareness, is cut off from your body, from the rest of your earthly being.

Allow "heaven and earth," the male and the female aspects, to supplely flow into each other, with as the focus your Heart, your warm earthly love for yourself, your Joy about your existence here-and-now.

Love is the only solution here. Don't resist that large warm flow of feelings; trust your emotional forces, your nature. Now surrender to yourself. Allow your brain to work in a total way so that intuition and mental abilities flow into each other and work together, so that you get a clear perspective on yourself, on your life, without blinders on. With your feelings, with your intuition, you ultimately will achieve easy access to higher awareness-energies, to inner wisdom. Don't close yourself off from a part of yourself; integrate every aspect of your being. Warm earthly presence: in trust, partake in your body, in your Life!

INDEX OF SUBJECTS TREATED IN PART II

A

<h2 style="text-align:center">E</h2>

F

H

J

M

O

S

U

V

X, Y, Z